KU-111-006

HARRISON L. McLAUGHLIN, M.D.

PROFESSOR OF CLINICAL ORTHOPEDIC SURGERY, COLLEGE OF
PHYSICIANS AND SURGEONS, COLUMBIA UNIVERSITY

TRAUMA

W. B. SAUNDERS COMPANY

PHILADELPHIA 1959 LONDON

© 1959, by W. B. Saunders Company

Copyright Under the International Copyright Union

All Rights Reserved

This book is protected by Copyright.
No part of it may be duplicated or reproduced in any manner without written permission from the publisher.

Made in U.S.A.
Press of W. B. Saunders Company

Library of Congress Catalog Card Number: 59–5961

TO

WILLIAM DARRACH

1876.....1948

AND

CLAY RAY MURRAY

1890.....1947

whose tenets are reflected in these pages

CONTRIBUTORS

FRANZ ALTMANN, M.D.

Clinical Professor of Otolaryngology, College of Physicians and Surgeons, Columbia University; Attending Otolaryngologist, Presbyterian Hospital; Consultant in Otolaryngology, Bronx Veterans Administration Hospital, New York City

FREDERICK S. CRAIG, M.D., F.A.C.S.

Assistant Clinical Professor of Orthopedic Surgery, College of Physicians and Surgeons, Columbia University; Assistant Attending Surgeon, New York Orthopaedic-Presbyterian Hospitals, New York City

ROBERT H. E. ELLIOTT, Jr., M.D., Med.Sc.D., F.A.C.S.

Associate Professor of Clinical Surgery, College of Physicians and Surgeons, Columbia University; Attending Surgeon and Chief, East Surgical Service, Presbyterian Hospital, New York City; Civilian Consultant in Surgery, Station Hospital, U. S. Military Academy, West Point, New York; Consulting Surgeon, Southampton Hospital, Southampton, New York

J. VINCENT FLACK, M.D., Med.Sc.D., F.A.C.S.

Associate in Ophthalmology, College of Physicians and Surgeons, Columbia University; Assistant Attending Ophthalmologist, Presbyterian Hospital, New York City

SAWNIE R. GASTON, M.D., F.A.C.S.

Assistant Professor of Clinical Orthopedic Surgery, College of Physicians and Surgeons, Columbia University; Associate Attending Orthopedic Surgeon, New York Orthopaedic-Presbyterian Hospitals, New York City; Consulting Orthopedic Surgeon, Englewood Hospital, Englewood, New Jersey

DAVID V. HABIF, M.D., F.A.C.S.

Associate Professor of Clinical Surgery, College of Physicians and Surgeons, Columbia University; Associate Attending Surgeon, Presbyterian Hospital, New York City

MAURICE J. HICKEY, D.M.D., M.D.

Dean and Professor of Oral Surgery, University of Washington School of Dentistry. *Formerly:* Associate Dean and Professor of Oral Surgery, Columbia University School of Dental and Oral Surgery; Associate Attending Surgeon, Presbyterian Hospital, New York City

STANLEY L. LANE, M.D., D.D.S., F.A.C.S.

Associate Professor of Surgery (Head and Neck), Albert Einstein College of Medicine, Yeshiva University; Clinical Professor of Head and Neck Surgery, New York Polyclinic Medical School; Visiting Surgeon, Bronx Municipal Hospital Center; Attending Maxillo-facial Surgeon, Jersey City Medical Center, Jersey City, New Jersey; Consultant, St. Albans Naval, Bronx Veterans Administration, Fordham, Misericordia, Long Beach Memorial, St. Mary's (Passaic, New Jersey), Stamford (Conn.) Hospitals; Associate Surgeon, Sydenham, Jewish Memorial, Beth David, New York Polyclinic Hospitals, New York City. *Formerly:* Instructor in Oral Surgery, Columbia University School of Dental and Oral Surgery; Assistant Attending Surgeon, Presbyterian Hospital, New York City

JERE W. LORD, Jr., M.D., F.A.C.S.

Professor of Clinical Surgery, New York University Post-Graduate Medical School; Visiting Surgeon, Fourth Division, Bellevue Hospital; Attending Surgeon, University Hospital, New York City

HARRISON L. McLAUGHLIN, M.D., C.M., F.A.C.S.

Professor of Clinical Orthopedic Surgery, College of Physicians and Surgeons, Columbia University; Attending Orthopedic Surgeon, New York Orthopaedic-Presbyterian Hospitals, New York City

LESTER A. MOUNT, M.D.

Associate Professor of Clinical Neurological Surgery, College of Physicians and Surgeons, Columbia University; Associate Attending Neurological Surgeon, Neurological Institute, Columbia-Presbyterian Medical Center, New York City

CHARLES S. NEER, II, M.D., F.A.C.S.

Assistant Professor of Clinical Orthopedic Surgery, College of Physicians and Surgeons, Columbia University; Associate Attending Orthopedic Surgeon, New York Orthopaedic-Presbyterian Hospitals, New York City

EDWARD B. SCHLESINGER, M.D.

Assistant Professor of Clinical Neurological Surgery, College of Physicians and Surgeons, Columbia University; Attending Neurosurgeon, Neurological Institute, Columbia-Presbyterian Medical Center, New York City

LAWRENCE W. SLOAN, M.D.

Professor of Clinical Surgery, College of Physicians and Surgeons, Columbia University; Attending Surgeon and Executive Officer, Department of Surgery, Presbyterian Hospital, New York City

FREDERICK W. SMITH, M.D., Med.Sc.D., F.A.C.S.

Consultant in Orthopedic Surgery, Tobey Hospital, Wareham, Massachusetts, and Cape Cod Hospital, Hyannis, Massachusetts. *Formerly:* Associate Professor of Clinical Orthopedic Surgery, College of Physicians and Surgeons, Columbia University; Associate Attending Orthopedic Surgeon, New York Orthopaedic-Presbyterian Hospitals, New York City

THOMAS W. STEVENSON, Jr., M.D.†

Professor of Clinical Surgery, College of Physicians and Surgeons, Columbia University; Director, Plastic Surgery Service, and Attending Surgeon, Presbyterian Hospital, New York City; Consultant in Plastic Surgery, Northern Westchester Hospital, Mount Kisco, New York, and Phelps Memorial Hospital, Tarrytown, New York

BARBARA B. STIMSON, M.D., Med.Sc.D., F.A.C.S.

Director, Department of Bone and Joint Surgery, St. Francis Hospital; Consultant in Bone and Joint Surgery, Vassar Brothers Hospital, Poughkeepsie, New York. *Formerly:* Assistant Professor of Clinical Orthopedic Surgery, College of Physicians and Surgeons, Columbia University; Associate Attending Orthopedic Surgeon, New York Orthopaedic-Presbyterian Hospitals, New York City

JUAN M. TAVERAS, M.D.

Associate Professor of Radiology, College of Physicians and Surgeons, Columbia University; Associate Attending Radiologist, Presbyterian Hospital, New York City

NORMAN B. THOMSON, Jr., M.D.

University of Buffalo School of Medicine; Assistant Attending, Department of Surgery and Chief of Cardiovascular Surgery, Buffalo Children's Hospital, Buffalo, New York. *Formerly:* Instructor in Surgery, College of Physicians and Surgeons, Columbia University; Assistant Attending Surgeon, Presbyterian Hospital; Assistant Visiting Surgeon, Frances Delafield Hospital, New York City

ROBERT H. WYLIE, M.D.

Clinical Professor of Surgery, College of Physicians and Surgeons, Columbia University; Attending Surgeon, Presbyterian Hospital; Visiting Surgeon and Director of Chest Surgical Service, Bellevue Hospital, New York City

† Deceased

PREFACE

THE PREPARATION of a monograph on Trauma is not an easy task, for the surgery of trauma embraces the entire science of surgery. Consequently, much potentially pertinent material must be omitted, and for this there is no apology, only a hope that the material included will prove to be of value to those for whom it was intended. With one exception the authors are or have been members of the Attending Staff of the Columbia-Presbyterian Medical Center in New York City, and of the Faculty of the College of Physicians and Surgeons of Columbia University. These busy surgeons have pre-empted time from their full schedules to write the following pages, not so much for the edification of other surgeons as for the innumerable medical students, residents, and practitioners who will not receive a complete training in surgery but who, nevertheless, will be called upon to cope with the great majority of all civilian accidents.

The first section of the book is devoted to a consideration of the local, regional, and systemic responses to injury, an enunciation of established principles in the treatment of trauma, and discussions of the problems of thermal and vascular trauma and of infection. The later chapters are limited mainly to a rationalization of treatment predicated upon a reconciliation of these fundamentals with the characteristic features, effects, and requisites of specific injuries.

Consideration of traumas of the specific regions is prefaced by a brief outline of the special features of surgical anatomy which may influence the choice and technique of treatment or predispose to complications in the management of common injuries. Uncommon injuries are also discussed in sufficient detail to forewarn the unwary of imminent pitfalls in their management and to suggest measures for their avoidance.

Trauma cuts across all branches of medicine with a superb disdain for the man-made boundaries of the different specialties. For this reason a small amount of duplication has been intentionally retained so that the reader may obtain information about certain injuries from multiple sources having different viewpoints and approaches. Fractures in and about the base of the skull, for example, are discussed in various chapters from the viewpoints of the neurosurgeon, the otolaryngologist, the ophthalmologist, and the maxillofacial surgeon.

The discussion of fracture treatment is inescapably dogmatic in appropriate situations. This should be interpreted not as reflecting the only, or even the best, solution of the problem at hand, but merely as presenting one form of treatment which has been employed widely and which, even when used with variable technical competence, has proved as efficient as and safer than others. An effort has been made to avoid the orthodox textbook approach to the treatment of fractures, which by categorical classification so oversimplifies this problem that the inexperienced practitioner soon is led to believe that a fracture is merely a broken bone, and that a roentgenogram and a book of instructions are the sole requisites for successful treatment.

Modern medical literature dealing with trauma, especially in the field of fracture treatment, is often so empirical as to mislead, and at times so controversial as to confuse any but an experienced surgeon. For this reason, and in keeping with the fundamental level which the authors have attempted to maintain, bibliographic citations have, for the most part, been omitted.

My sincere gratitude and appreciation are tendered to all the authors for their splendid contributions; to my good friend, Doctor Preston A. Wade, for his valuable suggestions and criticisms; to Miss Clara Barry, who typed the manuscript and prepared the text, and without whom this work could not have been completed; and to Mr. Alfred Feinberg, who has taken my amateur cartoons and made them into legible illustrations. The unflagging cooperation, assistance, and, above all, the patience of the publishers are acknowledged with thanks.

HARRISON L. MCLAUGHLIN, M.D.

CONTENTS

Part I. GENERAL CONSIDERATIONS

Chapter 1. The Response to Injury 3
By HARRISON L. McLAUGHLIN

Chapter 2. General Principles in the Treatment of Trauma . . 32
By HARRISON L. McLAUGHLIN

Chapter 3. Infection and Antibacterial Agents in Trauma . . . 69
By DAVID V. HABIF

Chapter 4. Thermal Trauma 79
By ROBERT H. E. ELLIOTT, Jr.

Chapter 5. Vascular Injuries 98
By JERE W. LORD, Jr.

Part II. THE UPPER EXTREMITY

Chapter 6. Injuries of the Hand 113
By THOMAS W. STEVENSON† and HARRISON L. McLAUGHLIN

Chapter 7. Injuries of the Wrist 140
By HARRISON L. McLAUGHLIN

Chapter 8. Injuries of the Forearm 179
By HARRISON L. McLAUGHLIN

† Deceased.

Chapter 9. INJURIES OF THE ELBOW 201

By HARRISON L. McLAUGHLIN and BARBARA B. STIMSON

Chapter 10. INJURIES OF THE SHOULDER AND ARM 233

By HARRISON L. McLAUGHLIN

Part III. THE LOWER EXTREMITY

Chapter 11. INJURIES OF THE FOOT 299

By FREDERICK S. CRAIG and HARRISON L. McLAUGHLIN

Chapter 12. INJURIES OF THE ANKLE 333

By HARRISON L. McLAUGHLIN

Chapter 13. INJURIES OF THE LEG 363

By HARRISON L. McLAUGHLIN

Chapter 14. INJURIES OF THE KNEE AND THIGH 383

By HARRISON L. McLAUGHLIN

Chapter 15. INJURIES OF THE HIP 419

By CHARLES S. NEER, II

Part IV. THE TRUNK

Chapter 16. INJURIES OF THE PELVIS 477

By HARRISON L. McLAUGHLIN

Chapter 17. INJURIES OF THE ABDOMEN 495

By LAWRENCE W. SLOAN

Chapter 18. CHEST INJURIES 540

By ROBERT H. WYLIE and NORMAN B. THOMSON, Jr.

Chapter 19. Injuries of the Vertebral Column 558

By FREDERICK M. SMITH

Chapter 20. Injuries of the Cervical Spinal Cord and Adnexa .. 598

By EDWARD B. SCHLESINGER and JUAN M. TAVERAS

Chapter 21. Injuries to the Low-Back Mechanism 618

Low-Back Pain Due to Other Than Intervertebral Disc Injuries 618

By SAWNIE R. GASTON

Injuries of the Intervertebral Discs 639

By EDWARD B. SCHLESINGER

Part V. THE HEAD AND SPECIAL SENSES

Chapter 22. Injuries of the Skull and Brain 651

By LESTER A. MOUNT

Chapter 23. Injuries to Auditory Apparatus, Nose and Paranasal Sinuses, Larynx and Trachea 691

By FRANZ ALTMANN

Chapter 24. Maxillofacial Injuries 715

Fractures of the Mandible 715

By MAURICE J. HICKEY

Fractures of the Facial Bones 726

By STANLEY L. LANE

Chapter 25. Injuries to the Eye 740

By J. VINCENT FLACK

INDEX 759

Part I

GENERAL CONSIDERATIONS

CHAPTER 1

THE RESPONSE TO INJURY

By HARRISON L. McLAUGHLIN, M.D.

REPAIR

An injury damages and kills tissue cells. The resulting gap in the tissue is filled by blood which extravasates along all communicating tissue planes, often for a considerable distance. Repair commences almost at once and is marked by an orderly train of events, many of which may occur almost simultaneously, and each of which is somewhat dependent upon the others for consummation. The morphological aspects of these phenomena are demonstrable, but their biochemical interrelationships, especially in the case of bone repair, are not yet entirely clear.

Injury, Inflammation, and Repair

These three are inseparable, except in the case of avascular tissues, such as the cornea and hyaline cartilage, where injury is followed by neither inflammation nor repair unless the damaged tissues become vascularized. In all other tissues injury not only mobilizes the defense reaction of inflammation for the evacuation of cellular casualties, but also initiates a process of cellular proliferation for their replacement. In the early stages following injury the signs of inflammation prevail, but repair is proceeding apace. As time passes the evidences of healing become predominant, but a subsiding residuum of inflammation remains until repair is complete. The surgeon must recognize that inflammation and repair are coincident and not successive processes.

The Protein Cesspool

Suspended throughout the hematoma that occupies the tissue gap caused by the injury are red blood cells and dead and damaged tissue cells. The ensuing clot bridges the gap by a meshwork of fibrin strands in the interstices of which are these doomed cellular products of tissue damage. This refuse does not remain indefinitely, but must be catabolized, evacuated, and replaced by living cells. Its autolysis commences at once, and progressive decomposition produces a liquefying accumulation of the end-products of protein disintegration. The systemic effects of intestinal obstruction are illustrative of the toxic properties of some of these protein catabolites, but it has become increasingly evident that others serve a useful purpose in the healing process, possibly as building blocks for the reparative matrix which follows. It is logical, therefore, that the treatment of trauma should, among other things, be designed to minimize the total tissue damage and facilitate evacuation of its noxious products.

Concomitants of Cell Death

The permeability of the local capillaries is increased and, augmented by the markedly increased protein concentration of the extracellular fluids in the damaged area, results in an escape of fluid through their walls to produce edema.

Many tissue cells of the region become distorted by changes in both cytoplasm and nuclei. Edema and cell distention progressively obliterate the elasticity of all the regional structures so that they soon become internal splints which, augmented by rapid proliferation of fibrous tissue, effectively maintain displacement, or assist in the maintenance of reduction of the structures distorted by the injury. Early reduction of displaced tendon or bone fragments is, therefore, facilitated by elasticity of the regional structures, and their subsequent rigidity is a mechanical aid to whatever form of fixation is employed. By the same token delayed reduction becomes progressively more difficult as time passes, and its accomplishment entails considerable additional damage to the "jelled" regional musculature.

Margination of polymorphonuclear leukocytes along the walls of the capillaries in steadily increasing numbers is soon followed by their migration through the walls of the vessels into the area from which debris must be removed. These are the scavengers of the undigested protein refuse which cannot be evacuated by diffusion. Many of the leukocytes are destroyed by the toxic properties of the materials they ingest, and their decomposition releases additional enzymes which aid in the digestion of the tissue debris.

The pH of the tissue fluids drops sharply as the injured area becomes saturated in an acid bath by the total products of cell death mixed with serum, lymph, and extracellular fluid.

Local vasodilatation, due to liberated histamine and other products elaborated by dying cells, rapidly supersedes the primary but transient reflex vasospasm caused by the injury. Despite this constant reaction, it seems improbable that there is an increased flow of blood through the injured area. Undoubtedly there is an increased quantity of blood per tissue volume unit, but the equally constant regional vascular effects of an injury (page 9) militate for a state of engorgement and passive congestion rather than to increased blood flow at the injured area.

Local decalcification is peculiar to this state of vasodilatation and passive congestion when bone is involved by the injury or is adjacent to the area involved by the ensuing inflammatory process. The surgeon, as he watches the pathologist decalcify bone specimens by acidification, is tempted to speculate that the acidity of the fluids bathing a fractured bone may contribute to this phenomenon. The calcium apatite emigrates from the bone fragments and diffuses throughout the liquefying ooze of the surrounding hematoma. Formerly it was thought to remain until it was redeposited in the bone-forming process, but recent tracer studies indicate that it enters the circulation and is lost in the urine. New calcium from the circulation is deposited and remains suspended within the scaffolding of the fibrin clot until some unknown biochemical reaction either changes it into a salt that can be utilized for new bone formation or elaborates a calcifiable matrix for its reception. There are some indications that both phenomena may occur.

Fibroplasia

Coincident with progressive evacuation of the products of cell death the fibrin clot is invaded from all sides by an army of young cells derived from all viable connective tissues, probably excepting cartilage, at the site of injury. These undifferentiated cells all are capable of eventuating as fibroblasts. Simultaneously, from surrounding blood vessels, sprout solid outgrowths of similar cells, which eventually become canalized and flattened to form a network of new vascular channels generally adhering to the pattern of the original fibrin clot. Gradually the fibrin scaffolding is replaced by collagen fibrils which form a matrix for accommodation of the invading cellular elements.

To recapitulate, certain products of cell death useful to the repair process remain at the site of injury. As the remaining useless and toxic products are removed, their place is filled by a mass of ingrowing young vessels and connective tissue cells, which adapts itself to the original fibrin scaffolding, and this in turn is dissolved and gradually replaced by a collagenous matrix. This is repair by granulation tissue as it occurs in wounds of all vascular tissues. In the absence of what, for want of a better term, might be described as a specific stimulus, the end-result is a mass of fibrous tissue. In the healing of a fracture it is clear that some influence produces a metaplasia into cartilage and bone as well as into fibrous tissue.

LOCAL EVENTS IN FRACTURE REPAIR

A working knowledge of the orderly sequences of bone repair is necessary to good fracture treatment, but the surgeon must realize that the factors pertinent to a fracture problem are not limited to the injured area. Secondary regional and systemic concomitants and products of the injury must be anticipated and reconciled with local factors before the best plan of treatment can be determined. Above all, the surgeon's concept of a fracture, the problems it presents, and his ultimate goal of treatment must remain in clear clinical focus.

Clinical Definition of a Fracture

A fracture is more than a broken bone, and its outmoded definition as "a solution in the continuity of a bone," which has been accepted by most past and by some contemporary surgeons, is incompatible with modern surgical philosophy. It was this false concept that engendered the equally fallacious dictum that the treatment of a fracture consisted of "reduction and immobilization until the bone healed."

The results of trauma are never limited to bone. A fracture involves primarily all the soft tissues in the injured area as well as the bone; secondarily, all the undamaged structures of the injured region; and, finally, the physical, economic, and emotional state of the injured person. Identical fractures cannot produce identical problems if for no other reason than that they occur in different persons. Consequently fractures should not be categorized as other medical and surgical lesions are, nor can fracture treatment be learned by rote. On the contrary, it must remain adaptable in detail and method to many factors, including the age, size, sex, occupation, and various other characteristics of the patient; the vulnerability of the uninjured regional structures to the penalties of disuse; a priority rating of the functional demands to be satisfied by the injured part after healing occurs; and, finally, the specific features of the local injury. To be of clinical significance the definition of a fracture must be stated as *a localized area of soft tissue and bone damage attended by secondary harmful effects upon adjacent regional structures and upon the patient as a whole.*

Theories of Bone Repair

The process of new bone formation remains an enigma. Confusion is increased by three popular theories purporting to explain the mystery. The advocates of each contrive to rationalize one concept at the expense of the others, but clinical common sense suggests a modicum of truth and error in all three.

The periosteal theory, which envisions periosteum and endosteum as the sole specific source of bone-forming cells, is impugned by the frequent formation of histologically normal bone in tissues devoid of periosteum. It is obvious to the surgeon that periosteum has both beneficial and detrimental effects upon the repair of fractures—beneficial in its shaping and confining influence upon reparative callus, but harmful when it is interposed between bone fragments or when it has been avulsed from its soft-part connections and insulates the bone from extra-osseous circulation. It is clear that cells derived from living periosteum participate in fracture healing, but only in concert with other cells derived from all adjacent mesodermal sources.

The osteoblast theory is also vulnerable to criticism. Its proponents have postulated that extra-skeletal new bone formation results from the activity of "wandering" or "resting" osteoblasts which, before becoming recognizable as such, cannot be differentiated from young connective tissue cells. On the other hand, microscopy reveals forming bone trabeculae to be surrounded by a peripheral layer of cells which are very similar to the osteoblasts of the embryo.

The theory of pluripotentiality of the mesenchyme is consonant with embryonal development, clinical and microscopical observations, and the present state of biochemical knowledge. This theory envisions that, prior to a change in type or potential, an adult cell must be destroyed and replaced, or revert to its primitive state; that metaplasia is peculiar only to young undifferentiated cells; that osteogenesis depends upon reparative tissue matrix and some unknown biochemical influence, rather than upon the intrinsic ability of a specific cell to secrete bone; and that coincident with new bone formation undifferentiated mesenchymal cells undergo metaplasia to eventuate as osteocytes, even as in the embryo.

These and other theories may be allowed to tickle the intellectual curiosity of the fracture surgeon, but they will prove to be suitable mortar for his therapeutic bricks only so long as they remain in complete harmony with clinical events.

The Facts of Bone Repair

Bone heals by the same process as other vascular tissues, except for the superimposed enigma of osteogenesis. As stated earlier, it is clear only that some unknown factor or factors influence the process of repair by granulations to cause a metaplasia into cartilage and bone, as well as into fibrous tissue.

Chondroplasia. In the healing fracture nests of young cartilage cells are to be observed throughout the reparative mass of granulation tissue, and especially in the gap between the bone ends. Possibly the elaboration of these cells, most pronounced at the fracture gap, reflects a response of nature to motion, even as cartilage is elaborated at the bone ends in the embryo. Clinically there is no doubt that excessive mobility of certain fractured bones over too long a period may be an important factor, but not necessarily the sole factor, in a failure of bony union and the production of a primitive joint with cartilage-covered bone ends enclosed within a fibrous capsule.

Normally chondroplasia is a transient phenomenon. Cartilage cells, like their fibroblastic counterparts, disappear and eventually are replaced by bone. It seems unlikely that a direct transformation of chondrocyte into osteocyte takes place; it seems more likely that all cartilage is resorbed or reverts to its primitive mesenchymal form prior to or coincident with replacement by bone.

Calcium and calcification. The composition of the calcium salt in bone is unknown, and the dynamics of its removal and deposition remain a mystery. The inflammatory phase of bone repair is marked primarily by a movement of calcium ions from the local bone into the cavity to be obliterated by the healing process. Possibly at this stage either the calcium is in a form unsuitable for redeposition, or the matrix of the granulation tissue is as yet unprepared for its reception, or both. At any rate, there is evidence that the calcium enters the circulation and most of it is lost in the urine.

Phosphatase, which rapidly accumulates as a result of osteoblastic activity, appears to have an important, but as yet undetermined, influence upon this suspended calcium. Possibly the liberation of phosphorus by this enzyme, with the consequent formation of calcium phosphate, constitutes the first step in a chain of chemical events resulting eventually in a calcium salt harmonious with redeposition.

Calcium withdrawn from the circulation is seen to be enmeshed in the invading granulations within a few days after injury. Microscopy reveals its disposition in a pattern somewhat suggestive of the trabeculae which form later. At first each trabecula appears to be nothing more than a dense area in the young granulation tissue, but as more and more calcium is taken up by the matrix a single layer of cells resembling the osteoblasts of the embryo appears at the periphery of the condensing area. Whether these are true osteoblasts, "resting" osteoblasts derived from the periosteum, or adapted fibroblasts which by metaplasia have attained some osteogenic potency is academic to the clinician, and an unsettled question among those interested in basic research. Sufficient to the surgeon is the comprehension that the advocates of all three theories of bone repair refer to the same cell, and that such a cell having apparent osteogenic potency is elaborated as a normal step in the process of bone healing.

This stage of trabecular development corresponds to the commencement of clinical union by osteoid or pre-osseous tissue. Within the trabeculae are engulfed not only the undifferentiated fibroblasts of the antecedent granulation tissue but also their osteoblastic counterparts. The trabecular network is soft and flexible, and the degree of calcification is quite variable throughout the reparative tissue mass, which feels considerably larger than is indicated by roentgenogram, and on clinical examination the fracture is "sticky."

Progressively, as calcification becomes complete, the intratrabecular cellular elements become sparse and assume the appearance of osteocytes, the rigidity of each trabecula and of the entire callus mass is increased, and examination of the fracture eventually indicates the presence of "clinical union." At this time the callus mass still feels larger and more bony than is indicated by roentgenogram, but true clinical union does not exist until the fracture site is neither tender to pressure nor painful when subjected to leverage and shearing forces.

Clinical union is provided by callus, an unorganized meshwork of "woven bone," built upon the pattern of the original fibrin clot. Like its precursor, granulation tissue, callus is also but a transient phase of the bone healing process. Final consolidation by mature bone commences only after continuity and rigidity have been provided by callus. From then on osteoclasis of callus proceeds simultaneously with the deposition in layers of hard adult bone. As in the growth of a tree, this bone is laid down in quantity where the functional stress is greatest, for example, in the concavity of an angular deformity; and osteoclasis is maximum where strength is least necessary. Often the entire callus mass, including that which plugged the medullary canal, disappears with the restitution of cortical continuity by lamellar bone. This is the final stage of bone repair, which does not occur until many months after clinical union has permitted recovery of function.

REGIONAL FACTORS IN BONE REPAIR

The healing process, and especially the process of bone repair, has often been characterized as the operation of a "closed chemical factory." This inference that regional and systemic factors do not affect the repair process is somewhat of an overstatement. Healing is dependent upon an adequate regional circulation, and injury has an invariable effect upon all the undamaged structures of the region.

Regional Circulation

An adequate circulation is essential to uneventful repair. Useful materials must be delivered by the arterial supply, and the useless and toxic products of cell death evacuated through the venous and lymphatic channels. Every injury is followed by an unwelcome chain of events which reduces the efficiency of both systems. Sympathetic stimulation by the pain of the local injury produces regional vasospasm and a significant decrease in the capacity of the arterial mechanism. Decreased or obliterated mobility of the part due to pain or treatment almost abolishes the muscle pump so essential to venous return. Dependency augments the impediment to venous drainage. Consequently, despite local vasodilatation, the circulation of blood through the damaged area often resembles a stagnant swamp more than a running brook. Unless these factors are recognized and rectified, the repair site will remain in a state of passive congestion for a considerable period as surely as if a partial tourniquet were applied proximal to the injury. The injured part may be elevated to promote gravity drainage, but not so high as to accentuate arterial deficiency. Gentle heat may be used to promote neurovascular, as well as muscular, relaxation, but excessive heat will increase the offending vasospasm. All permissible measures designed to relieve pain and promote normal contractions of the regional muscle bellies, with or without joint motion as the local circumstances may dictate, should be utilized. These are the simplest and most efficient methods for restoration of an efficient regional circulation.

Regional Muscles

The regional muscles, overworked by spasm in the face of a depleted oxygen supply, inevitably deteriorate. Sarcolactic acid and the other end-products of energy combustion are inadequately removed by the sluggish venous system. Primarily the muscles are immobilized by spasm, then by distention, edema, and treatment until finally the muscle mass shrinks from disuse, and cells killed by hypoxia are replaced by fibrous tissue. This common sequence of events perpetuates a chronic state of passive congestion (sometimes termed pathological hyperemia) at and distal to the injured area.

Blood extravasates for some distance along all muscle planes communicating with a fracture. The response to its presence in these areas is identical to that at the fracture site, namely, inflammation and repair by granulations. Immobile muscle planes become obliterated by fibrosis, and joint motion is restricted by fixation of the muscle motors. The surgeon must realize that abolition of muscle function may sometimes be necessary to maintenance of reduction of a fracture but is always a physiological impediment to rehabilitation of the regional circulation and a detriment to the recovery of function.

Regional Joints

Fixation and deterioration of muscle motors is the common primary cause of joint stiffness following injury, but secondary factors usually accentuate this loss of mobility. Prolonged distention of periarticular interstitial spaces by edema is followed by fibrosis and adherence of these moving parts. In certain locations, such as the joints of the fingers, periarticular fibrosis often is the principal offending lesion in the production of a stiff and disabled hand.

Collagen is like leather. With immobility, the molecule loses water and becomes shrunken, stiff, and hard. As with leather or chamois, constant mobility is a prime requisite for maintenance of pliability. This is a generally unrecognized but very important factor in the production of stiff joints and of atrophy and loss of elasticity in muscle.

Intra-articular fibrosis may also contribute to joint stiffness. A joint capsule, in order to fulfill its function as a gliding mechanism, must be loose. Loose synovial folds become obliterated by a plastic exudate in the presence of immobility so that the joint capsule shortens and becomes a checkrein to motion. When capsular contracture is the sole or principal cause of stiffness the joint capsule can usually be stretched and mobility restored by normal muscle motors, except in conditions of long duration. Unfortunately, the post-traumatic stiff joint usually results from a combination of causes: atrophy and fixation of muscle motors, periarticular fibrosis, and synovial adhesions. Once established, each of these complements the effects of the others, to make restoration of function a prolonged and tedious task. It follows that treatment, whenever possible, must be designed to prevent or minimize the establishment of each of these factors in all injuries to the extremities.

Regional Features of the Bone

Cancellous bone fractures progress rapidly to sound union without regard to the type, or presence or absence of treatment. This type of bone is endowed with a rich intra-osseous circulation, and its thin cortical shell is perforated in many places for the entrance of nutrient vessels. Consequently, the promotion of bony union rarely enters into the choice of treatment for a cancellous bone fracture.

Cortical bone fractures, on the other hand, often depend for union upon adequate immobilization. This type of bone resembles a pipe, with thick and virtually avascular cortical walls enclosing a small vascular medullary canal. Repair is slow. Repeated interruptions of the healing process must be prevented by fixation devices until the callus mass has matured. Consequently, the promotion of bone healing is an important factor in the choice of treatment for most shaft fractures of the long bones.

Certain intra-articular fractures will not heal unless adequately treated. These include fractures through the proximal portion of the scaphoid, the proximal portion of the femoral neck, and the proximal portion of the astragalus. Normally the proximal fragment of such fractured bones receives its essential blood supply from the extra-articular fragment. Union can take place only after a growth of granulation tissue from the extra-articular fragment across the fracture gap produces eventual revascularization of the invaded proximal fragment. For this process to culminate in union requires therapeutic maintenance of perfect apposition of the surfaces of the broken bone over a prolonged period.

Double bones are present in forearm and leg. When only one bone is broken the fragments angulate toward the intact bone and, so long as this angulation persists, good apposition of the broken ends is prevented. In this circumstance delayed union is the rule, unless the treatment employed is successful in maintaining a straight alignment of the fractured bone. Even when both bones are broken, one usually heals before the other. The healed bone then may produce distraction of the slower healing fragments of the other bone, to cause delayed union or nonunion. The surgeon must anticipate and prevent these common complications of fractures in the forearm and lower leg.

SYSTEMIC FACTORS AND FALLACIES IN BONE REPAIR

Age

The notion that fractures heal poorly in the aged is fallacious. Age and ability to repair bone are virtually unrelated in the adult. This does not obtain for fractures in children. The nearer a child to his previous embryonic state, the more rapid and certain will be the process of bone repair. Identical fractures of the femur will heal in a newborn child in a matter of days, in the young child in a few weeks, in the adolescent in a few months, but in the adult of any age such a fracture will not heal for many months. Impediments to union, such as distraction of the fragments, soft part interposition, or excessive soft tissue damage or suppuration, commonly fail to prevent union in a child, but are complications of such importance as to dictate the method of treatment for similar fractures in the adolescent or adult.

Diet and Calcium

Except in rare instances of severe avitaminosis, the idea that diet can influence the healing of a fracture is unfounded. The skeleton is the great natural reservoir for calcium storage, and faulty absorption or deficient intake of this mineral is immediately neutralized by its withdrawal from the skeleton in amounts appropriate for maintenance of serum calcium equilibrium. Even in conditions characterized by a chronic calcium imbalance, which predispose to pathological fractures, union is the rule. Only in the presence of a process which destroys bone faster than it can be replaced by repair, such as severe hyperparathyroid states, is control of the systemic cause of the calcium imbalance a prerequisite to union of the collapsed bone.

Neurotrophic Conditions

Certain neurotrophic conditions, such as Charcot's joint, are characterized by progressive degeneration and avascularity of the bone and an absence of pain perception. When fracture occurs through bone of such poor quality, the capabilities for repair are depleted under the best of circumstances. Due to the absence of pain, the feeble ensuing granulation process is disrupted repeatedly by minor unnoticed traumas. Healing is always slow and, except when encouraged by secure and prolonged fixation of the fragments, usually incomplete.

Cortisone

It is a common misconception that the administration of cortisone prevents fracture repair. This is unconfirmed by clinical facts. Cortisone depresses an early phase of the repair process, the elaboration of granulation tissue. With the withdrawal of cortisone healing progresses to completion following this temporary interruption.

SYSTEMIC RESPONSE TO INJURY

METABOLIC EVENTS OF CONVALESCENCE

Injury evokes a systemic response which is set in a pattern as orderly and consistent as are the processes of local inflammation and repair. A working knowledge of this sequence of metabolic events is fully as fundamental to the management of an injured patient as that of fever and leukocytosis is to the care of an infection. The changes which take place represent what is clinically known as convalescence, and may be segregated into three broad successive stages.

Initial protective or "catabolic" phase. The immediate reaction to an injury may be characterized teleologically as a spontaneous defense mechanism. It lasts only a short time after a minor injury. After a major long bone fracture, it usually lasts for a few days to a week; after severe multiple injuries, an extensive burn, or devastating infection, it may persist for a month or more. The patient looks and feels sick; there are fever, leukocytosis, and an elevated erythrocyte sedimentation rate. Anorexia, oliguria, and depressed peristalsis are the rule, and the patient has little interest in what is going on about him. The eosinophil count is reduced, and there is a sharp increase in urinary steroid hormone output. This rapid and spontaneous increase in hormonal activity leaves little room for doubt that the initial response to injury and its attendant metabolic changes are at least a part of what Selye has so aptly termed "the alarm reaction."

Nitrogen and potassium are loosened from the body cells into the circulation. Both are needed, and undoubtedly utilized, for the formation of new tissues at the repair site, but large quantities are also lost through the kidneys. A negative nitrogen balance is rapidly and inevitably established. This does no harm so long as it is not prolonged by starvation for more than a few days. It is difficult or impossible to restore nitrogen balance by hyperalimentation, and forced oral intake usually produces vomiting and a risk of aspiration, for the duration of this initial response. Except in severe injuries justifying anticipation of continuing tissue death or insult, such as massive burns or infections, energetic attempts to restore nitrogen balance in the first week are rarely necessary. In the presence of a continuing injury, however, a high protein intake should be re-established at the earliest possible moment. Similarly, in continuing injuries, especially in the presence of an adequate urine output and absence of oral intake, a serious potassium deficit may accumulate. Potassium should not be administered unless the urine volume is at least 1,000 ml. in 24 hours, but when this quantity is reached a continuing negative potassium balance should be counteracted by the daily administration of small amounts of this electrolyte by slow intravenous drip. One liter of solution containing a mixture of 6 gm. of potassium chloride and 4.25 gm. of sodium chloride per liter of water is an appropriate daily dose until such time as an adequate oral intake has been restored.

Body fat is oxidized, often at a rate that may approximate several hundreds of grams daily. Each 100 grams of oxidized fat provides 900 endogenous calories to satisfy the metabolic requirements of the injured body. Thus the temporary cessation of caloric intake resulting from anorexia and disturbed gastrointestinal function is spontaneously neutralized. Such a consumption of body fat leads to a considerable loss in body weight. Consequently, although fat loss is not commonly of clinical significance in an ordinary injury, severe or continuing injuries require rapid re-establishment of an intake that is high in calories (3,000 daily) as well as rich in protein.

Sodium is resorbed from the glomerular filtrate in quantities sufficient to preserve the total body water volume. In the early stages after injury a rapid reduction in body weight due to fat loss may be incorrectly diagnosed as a manifestation of dehydration. It is important to recognize that the early response to injury is characterized by a retention of body water, and that a patient may be drowned as a result of over-zealous administration of large quantities of fluids.

In short, the normal initial response to injury includes a negative balance of nitrogen and potassium which, if not prolonged, is harmless and which increases the available supply of building blocks for the reparative process; a cessation of caloric intake neutralized by endogenous caloric production through oxidation of body fat which is not harmful unless prolonged; a resorption of sodium which preserves the total body water volume; and evidences of a marked increase in hormonal activity. These changes, except when prolonged, should not be considered to be disorders requiring correction. They are as normal and as intrinsic to the recovery from an injury as fever and leukocytosis are to the recovery from an infection.

Intermediate recuperative or "anabolic" phase. The second stage of convalescence is essentially a reversal of the metabolic changes comprising the initial response. Clinically the patient looks and feels less sick, although he is still wan and weak. The urine output increases and he appears to be drying out. Appetite is restored, and he begins to eat. His interest in the environment is restored, but flags easily. Progressively a normal appetite, interest, and, lastly, strength are recovered and the patient commences to resume his usual daily activities. At the beginning of this phase the previously lowered eosinophil count first returns to normal and then is temporarily raised to a level greatly above normal. At the same time there is a sharp reduction of urinary steroid hormone output. This state, which is similar to that produced by the sudden withdrawal of previously administered steroid hormones, has been termed by Francis D. Moore "the corticoid withdrawal phase."

Nitrogen and potassium are reloaded rapidly into the cells from which they were previously removed, and simultaneously the amount of these electrolytes lost in the urine is steadily reduced. It is as if the body, having provided at its own expense sufficient of these materials to satisfy the requirements of the repair process, immediately sets about to refurbish its depleted cellular stores. Within a short time, except in continuing injuries, there is produced a very strongly positive nitrogen and potassium balance. *Oxidation of body fat* decelerates and gradually ceases as an adequate oral intake of calories is regained and utilized. *Sodium and water* previously retained are unloaded through the kidneys until the sodium balance returns to zero.

In short, during the intermediate period of convalescence the body ceases to burn its own fat for metabolic fuel as appetite and gastrointestinal function are restored to the point where exogenous calories become available; it unloads the previously retained salt and water which is no longer needed to compensate for exigencies of decreased plasma volume subsequent to the injury, and steadily rebuilds the previously depleted muscle cells toward a restoration of strength. Little or no fat is redeposited until a later stage of recovery.

Final recovery phase. The final stage of recovery is a slow process. The patient has returned to his normal activities and is without systemic symptoms. His muscle mass has been rebuilt and the balance of both nitrogen and potassium returned to zero. The sodium and water balances remain normal. The last stage in recovery is marked by a slow but steady replenishment of the depleted fat stores of the body. Restoration of normal weight coincides with complete recovery and a cessation of all metabolic responses to the original injury.

Endocrine Factors in the Response to Injury

Knowledge of the influence of endocrine factors upon the metabolic response to injury is not yet sufficient to be of practical value in the supervision of convalescence. Nevertheless, the hormonal response to injury is attended by metabolic results which fit the pattern of convalescence nicely. This chain-reaction hormonal response includes the release of epinephrine and norepinephrine from the adrenal medulla, a hormone adversely influencing diuresis from the posterior pituitary, ACTH from the anterior pituitary, and deoxycorticosterone and corticosterone from the adrenal cortex. Correlation of their effects with the metabolic pattern of convalescence will emphasize the importance of endocrine factors in the response to injury.

Epinephrine elevates the pulse rate and blood pressure and influences the mobilization of liver glycogen.

Norepinephrine produces peripheral vasoconstriction, diverting the available oxygen supply to more important regions.

ACTH initiates the release of deoxycorticosterone and corticosterone from the adrenal medulla.

Deoxycorticosterone influences the kidney tubules so that sodium is selectively reabsorbed from the glomerular filtrate (with a resultant conservation of body water), but potassium is allowed to pass into the urine.

Posterior pituitary hormone adversely influences diuresis and aids in the conservation of body water.

Corticosterone has multiple effects. Lymphocytes and eosinophils are broken down to increase the available stores of gamma globulin. The proliferation of reparative granulation tissue is depressed. The threshold for passage of fluids through the semipermeable membranes of the body is elevated. The body proteins are catabolized and converted to glucose, glycogen deposition in the liver is accelerated, and the glucose threshold of the kidneys is lowered.

FLUID AND ELECTROLYTE RESPONSES

The body fluids are electrolyte solutions contained within three compartments, separated by semipermeable membranes through which the interchange of water and ions is activated by hydraulic and osmotic pressure gradients. These interchanges are retarded or facilitated by permeability alterations in response to metabolic demands and certain endocrine influences. Water constitutes almost 70 per cent of the body weight, 50 per cent being intracellular, 15 per cent interstitial, and 5 per cent intravascular water. For practical purposes, the electrolyte concentrations in the interstitial and intravascular fluids may be considered as equal, except for protein, and their total volume be considered as contained within a single *extracellular* compartment. Potassium and phosphate are the dominant electrolytes of the intracellular, and sodium and chloride of the extracellular fluid. There is a constant movement of potassium and sodium across the cell membrane and a constant interchange of interstitial and intravascular sodium and chloride (Fig. 1–*1, A*). A major portion of cellular phosphate remains in fairly stable combination with cell protein. Influenced by intake, output, and electrolyte interchange, there is also a constant interchange of water between the intra- and extracellular compartments.

Potassium depletion not infrequently complicates the management of

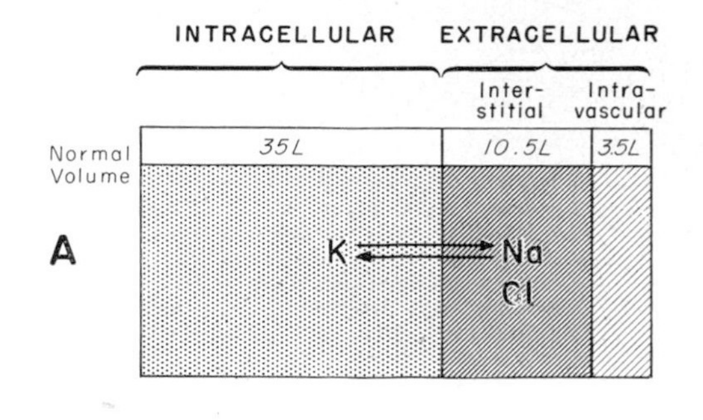

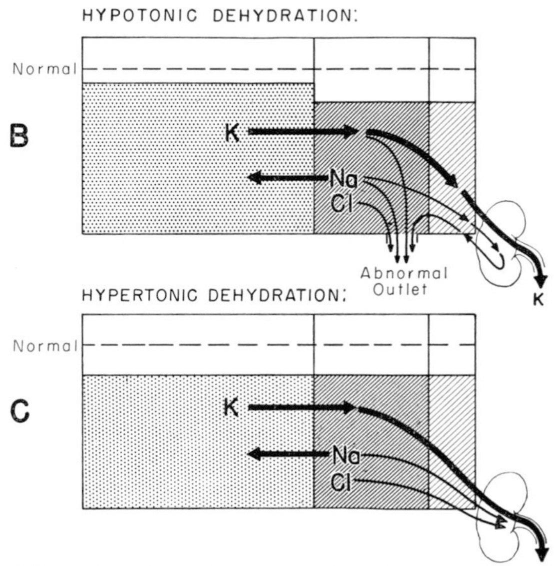

Figure 1–1. Electrolyte disturbances of dehydration.

A. In the healthy animal there is a continuous interchange of sodium, potassium, and water across the cell membrane.

B. Hypotonic dehydration is rapid. Hypotonicity results from a greater loss of salt than of water, usually from an abnormal gastrointestinal outlet. Potassium is drawn from the cells for restoration of osmotic balance, but is promptly lost in the urine (heavy line). Sodium is drawn into the cells to replace potassium so that extracellular hypotonicity is accentuated. Sodium is conserved by the kidney, but all salts are lost through the offending abnormal outlet.

C. Hypertonic dehydration is slow—more water than salt is lost. The extracellular compartment becomes hypertonic, and water, accompanied by potassium, is drawn from the cells in an attempt at compensation. Again the potassium is promptly lost in the urine and replaced by sodium. Osmotic balance is maintained for a time by increased renal excretion of sodium and chloride, but eventually the predominant water loss causes sodium retention and re-establishes a state of extracellular hypertonicity.

an injury. In response to stress, sodium retention and potassium loss are the rule. Hypopotassemia should be suspected when apathy, confusion, and restlessness, or muscular weakness, develop in an injured patient, especially under the following conditions:

(a) absence of intake,
(b) a large amount of tissue damage or necrosis,
(c) large fluid loss,

(d) uncontrolled diabetes.

Almost every type of fluid and electrolyte disturbance influences displacement of potassium from the cell into the extracellular compartment, from which it is promptly lost in the urine. Replacement should not be attempted until a daily urine output of at least 1,000 ml. can be maintained, for extracellular potassium is highly toxic and is apt to produce heart block. In circumstances of advanced potassium depletion, so long as the urine volume is adequate, 2 to 4 gm. of potassium chloride in water may be given by mouth every four hours, or added to at least one liter of replacement solution which then should be infused very slowly. Blood potassium levels, although they conform in general with the manifestations of potassium derangement, may be high when the plasma is transporting potassium (lost from the cells) to the kidney, or low when the cells are reloading potassium from the extracellular fluids.

DEHYDRATION

Under normal conditions a daily water intake of 3,000 ml. is required to counter a loss of water of oxidation from the lungs and sweat from the skin of 1200 ml., a urine output of 1500 ml., and a stool water loss of 300 ml. Under any conditions, including starvation, an insensible daily loss from lungs and skin of 1200 ml. and at least 600 ml. of urine loss (necessary to eliminate the nitrogenous waste products of metabolism) is obligatory. When, as a result of injury or treatment, the intake stops or additional losses are incurred, dehydration is imminent.

Hypotonic (rapid) dehydration (Fig. 1–*1, B*) results from abnormal losses of water and electrolytes, and is especially common to injuries attended by vomiting, diarrhea, a gastrointestinal fistula, or suction drainage. Primarily the extracellular fluid becomes hypotonic from a relatively greater loss of salt than of water. Water and potassium move out of the cells to restore the osmotic balance. Sodium is drawn into the cells to replace potassium. As a result extracellular tonicity is decreased rather than restored to normal, for the potassium gained by the extracellular fluids is promptly lost from the kidneys and the offending gastrointestinal outlet. Eventually the capacity of the kidney to conserve water by a selective reabsorption of sodium (but not of potassium) results in a reduced urine output, but the obligatory and abnormal losses continue.

Symptoms of thirst and potassium depletion occur early and, in the absence of treatment, are followed by a steady diminution of urine output, a decline in blood pressure, and peripheral circulatory collapse. The treatment for dehydration resulting primarily from a loss of salt and water would seem to be replacement of salt and water, but this may do much more harm than good. Administration of sodium chloride overhydrates the extracellular, and to a small extent the cellular, compartment. The excess of salt supplied increases the shift of sodium into the cells and the potassium loss continues. The urine output increases, but usually lags behind the intake. The hematocrit falls owing to increased retention of fluid, and the water-logged tissues become edematous.

Correction of hypotonic dehydration requires replacement of losses with a balanced electrolyte solution of potassium chloride, sodium chloride, and sodium bicarbonate. This replaces all deficits, and an excess of chloride is prevented by the elimination of bicarbonate through the lungs as carbon dioxide. The volume should meet the existing deficit and the continuing obligatory and abnormal losses, and provide sufficient additional fluid to restore and maintain a good urine output.

Hypertonic (slow) dehydration (Fig. 1–*1*, *C*) results from water depletion without a corresponding loss of electrolytes. The usual cause is a combination of absent intake and continued daily obligatory water losses. The extracellular fluid becomes hypertonic and water (accompanied by potassium) is pulled from the cells. Here also the displaced potassium is promptly lost in the urine. An absence of caloric intake usually accompanies water starvation so that the potassium loss is considerably increased by cellular catabolism. In the early stages extracellular hypertonicity is countered by increased renal excretion of sodium and chloride, but this requires additional water loss. The rising water deficit, in turn, is countered by renal reabsorption of sodium in an attempt to conserve the body water volume. At this point extracellular sodium concentration again rises to hypertonic levels, the potassium shift is accelerated, and potassium loss continues despite the reduced urine volume.

In contradistinction to the condition in hypotonic dehydration, thirst and signs of potassium depletion come on slowly, there is no evidence of any abnormal loss of fluids and electrolytes, and the kidneys may fail. Treatment should replace the existing water deficit and provide for obligatory losses and adequate renal output by the parenteral administration of isotonic carbohydrate solutions. The potassium deficit may necessitate the addition of potassium chloride. Treatment by sodium chloride solution alone will serve but to accentuate the offending extracellular hypertonicity and increase the potassium loss.

ACIDOSIS AND ALKALOSIS

Acid-base equilibrium is maintained by the buffering interchange of electrolyte solutes; it is guarded by the ability of the lungs to regulate the excretion of acids as carbon dioxide, and by the ability of the kidneys to regulate the excretion of acids and alkalis in the urine, and to form ammonia to combine with acids. Acidosis may result from an abnormal increase of acids or reduction of alkalis; similarly the reverse, alkalosis, may result from a depletion of acids or an abnormal increase of alkalis. These disorders of acid-base equilibrium may be the product of disturbances in any of the three equilibrating mechanisms, of an abnormal acid or alkali intake, or of the excessive formation of acids by metabolism.

The normal values in the blood of the buffer pair, bicarbonate and carbonic acid, are 27 and 1.35 mEq per liter, respectively, a bicarbonate–carbonic acid ratio of 20 to 1. This ratio is synonymous with a compensated acid-base balance and a normal hydrogen ion concentration (pH 7.4), and any alteration signifies acidosis or alkalosis. There is usually some clinical evidence of a primary respiratory or metabolic cause for an acid-base imbalance in the injured patient. Hyperventilation, by an excessive excretion of carbon dioxide, may induce alkalosis. Of even greater import to the treatment of trauma is that the administration of oxygen in the presence of hypoventilation from any cause, although it may maintain an adequate oxygen content of the blood, may also be attended by an inadequate carbon dioxide output. The resultant respiratory type of acidosis resulting from excessive retention of acid presents grave dangers to the heart. Similarly, surplus of acid may accumulate as a result of kidney shutdown, so that every effort must be made to maintain an adequate urine volume after injury. Acidosis due to alkali depletion may complicate the management of penetrating injuries of the upper abdomen and is peculiar to excessive sodium depletion resulting from loss of fluids from the biliary or pancreatic systems and not infrequently occurs in shock.

Alkalosis most commonly follows chloride depletion due to large or continuous fluid losses from the stomach by vomiting or suction. The onset may be very rapid. This is one of the few electrolyte and fluid disorders that will respond rapidly and well to the simple administration of sodium chloride solution alone. Occasionally, in advanced hypochloremic alkalosis there will be a persistently negative response to the administration of sodium chloride, or even of ammonia chloride. Usually this is the result of excessive displacement of extracellular sodium into the cells for potassium replacement (see Fig. 1–*1*, *B*) and can be corrected only by the administration of potassium.

In general, the correction of acidosis requires supplementation of the alkali stores, not by sodium chloride but rather by a more labile solution of sodium lactate or bicarbonate. The bicarbonate deficit is 0.5 × body weight in kilograms × the bicarbonate deviation from the normal value of 27 mEq per liter. The same number of milliequivalents of sodium lactate or bicarbonate should be provided.

For example:

A 70 kg. patient has a bicarbonate value of 20 mEq per liter, a deviation of minus 7

$$0.5 \times 70 \times 7 = 245$$

The sodium lactate replacement required is 245 mEq, or 1470 ml. of a ⅙ molar lactate solution.

Alkalosis may be countered by administration of acid elements based on similar calculations; 1.76 ml. of 2 per cent ammonium chloride per kilogram of body weight will reduce the bicarbonate value 1 mEq per liter.

For example:

A 70 kg. patient has a bicarbonate value of 37 mEq per liter, an increment of 10

$$1.76 \times 70 \times 10 = 1232$$

Restoration of balance requires 1232 ml. of 2 per cent ammonium chloride solution, which should be diluted with an equal quantity of 5 per cent dextrose to prevent the discomfort occasioned by intravenous infusion of the undiluted solution.

WATER INTOXICATION

As noted in the normal response of convalescence one of the primary defense reactions to injury is conservation of body water by reabsorption of sodium. During the initial phase, while the total sodium content remains normal or slightly elevated, there is often a small reduction in the plasma sodium level. Occasionally, after a severe injury or operation, a significant water shift into the cells is associated with this poorly understood phenomenon. Such cellular hyperhydration may have profound effects, especially on the cells of the brain. The patient may become stuporous or irrational, and muscular incoordination amounting to convulsions may ensue. This syndrome most often results from the enthusiastic but injudicious forced administration of water into an organism already conserving its fluid mass in the early stages following injury.

PROTEIN RESERVE

Protein is an essential constituent of the blood plasma and all the cellular structures of the body. In the plasma *albumin* regulates the osmotic pressure, and *fibrinogen* the clotting mechanism of the blood. *Globulin* functions as a transport for immunizing elements. When the plasma protein level falls from a normal of 7 to 5 gm. or less per 100 ml. albumin depletion results in edema. Hypoproteinemia, resulting in poor healing and general debilitation, is a common complication of trauma and may result from a deficient intake, excessive cell catabolism, excessive cell destruction, excessive loss of plasma (burns), deficient absorption (chronic gastrointestinal disease), or inadequate synthesis (liver disease). Since every injury, by increasing nitrogen catabolism, places a sharply increased demand upon the available proteins, the state of the protein reserve cannot be ignored in treatment. As noted previously, a negative nitrogen balance is not harmful and, in fact, is difficult or impossible to correct in the first few days after injury. In severe or continuing injuries, however, every effort must be made to counter the tendency for an organism to live on its own protein stores by providing an adequate exogenous supply through the oral or parenteral route.

Provision of an adequate oral intake, whenever possible, is the best method for satisfying protein requirements. In health one gram of protein per kilogram of body weight is an average requirement; after a severe injury or during the course of a serious infection, however, several times this amount may be required to maintain a nitrogen balance approximating normal. In the face of a persistent negative nitrogen balance, and inability to provide protein by mouth, other routes must be used. Solutions of pure amino acids or various preparations of protein hydrolysates reinforced with glucose may be given by vein or gastric tube. Whole blood, plasma, and serum albumin temporarily boost the available protein supply, and are useful short-term supportive measures.

Anemia compounds the problem presented by hypoproteinemia. Exogenous nitrogen provided is utilized in the formation of hemoglobin rather than of plasma protein. Anemia, in a patient in negative nitrogen balance, must therefore be corrected by whole blood transfusions before the desired results of protein replacement can be expected.

SHOCK

Shock defies precise definition and remains without a completely satisfactory description. Its effects upon the organism may be reversed spontaneously or by treatment, but, if they are allowed to progress without interruption, often become irreversible and fatal. All states of shock reflect a common denominator of impaired oxygen delivery, which has profound effects upon the organs vital to life (brain, heart, liver, and, to a lesser extent, the kidneys). Consequently the elderly, debilitated, or diseased person usually has a markedly reduced tolerance to shock.

The onset of shock reflects a reduction of the effective circulating blood volume. This usually results from some discrepancy between the capacity of the vascular bed and the volume of intravascular fluid. Obviously, the causes for such discrepancies are not limited to trauma and hemorrhage, or even to the field of surgery, but are numerous and may obtain in any branch of medicine.

Cardiogenic shock frequently follows an acute coronary episode. Oxygen delivery to the tissues and an effective volume of circulating blood are impaired by faulty pumping action of the failing heart. It is not uncommon for a sudden cardiac episode to precipitate an injury. Cardiogenic shock may then be mistaken for traumatic shock, with disastrous results. There is little room for such an error when the potential relationship between a sudden heart attack and an injury is kept in mind. The deranged function of the failing heart is in sharp contrast to the normal heart function common to traumatic shock, and the high venous pressure of cardiac failure is in equally sharp contrast to the low venous pressure common to traumatic shock.

Neurogenic shock may be initiated by various stimuli, including intracranial damage, acute visceral lesions such as a perforated peptic ulcer, certain drugs (especially spinal anesthesia), or operative manipulation of mediastinal structures. The ordinary fainting spell which follows a noxious physical or mental stimulus is such an episode. Through the medium of some unexplained neurological mechanism generalized vasodilatation so increases the capacity of the vascular bed that the existing normal fluid volume fills it only partially. Hypotension and a reduction of effective oxygen transport take place rapidly. This syndrome, formerly known as "primary shock" or syncope, differs from surgical or traumatic shock in that the extremities are warm, pink, and dry owing to vasodilatation, rather than cold, pale, and sweaty owing to the peripheral vasoconstriction of surgical shock. Probably neurogenic shock is but a transient phenomenon because vasoconstriction, so consistently a characteristic of severe shock, is not present.

Vasogenic shock, resulting also from vasodilatation, may attend reactions to histamine, anaphylaxis, and probably certain infections.

Hematogenic shock is of great importance to the surgeon. This category includes the many different types associated with intravascular fluid loss and named for the causative condition, as hemorrhagic shock, wound shock, traumatic shock, surgical shock, hypovolemic shock, burn shock, and the like.

Many theories have been advanced to explain the etiology and pathological dynamics of hematogenic shock, but none explain it completely. It is unlikely that there is a single cause of shock, or that the effect of shock depends upon a single mechanism. Rather, it would appear that multiple causes and effects, by a variety and combination of pathways, eventually produce a common result. Reduced blood volume, for example, can result from a variety of causes:

(a) loss of whole blood, which may be external from a wound, or internal from a ruptured kidney or spleen;
(b) loss of plasma, which may be external from a burn, or internal as in intestinal obstruction and severe peritonitis;
(c) loss of salt and water, as in dehydration states.

THE EFFECTS OF SHOCK

Peripheral vasoconstriction counters reduced blood volume in an attempt to maintain blood pressure. This is most marked in the peripheral circulation of the extremities, and is considered to be a defense reaction which also shunts the available circulating blood to areas in more critical need of oxygen, such as the brain and liver. It offers a logical reason for the cold, clammy, pale condition of the skin surface in the shock patient, and for the frequent absence of serious hypotension with impending shock. As noted above, this is in sharp contrast to the warm, dry skin of neurogenic shock. Coincident with curtailment of the peripheral arterial supply by vasoconstriction, there is a reduction of venous pressure, often leading to venous collapse. This explains the frequent difficulty of venipuncture in the patient in shock, and emphasizes the importance of *early* venipuncture against the subsequent necessity for replenishment of the intravascular fluid volume.

Capillary permeability increases with the continuing hypoxia resulting from prolonged vasoconstriction. In the terminal stages of shock fluid and even the cellular elements of the blood leak into the tissues to further reduce the blood volume.

Sequestration of large quantities of blood in the capillary bed probably occurs. Under normal conditions only a certain number of the total capillaries, precapillary arterioles, and venules function at one time, but in response to stress all channels open simultaneously. The capacity of the capillary bed is markedly increased, and in the presence of a decelerating blood flow a lake of stagnant blood may be trapped in this reservoir, and is essentially by-passed by the *effective* circulation.

Increased heart rate is an attempt by the organism to maintain an effective circulation despite a loss of circulating volume, and clinically this is reflected in an elevated pulse rate. However, in shock due to mixed neurogenic and hematogenic causes, it is possible to find a slow pulse despite reduced blood volume.

Reduced cardiac output occurs despite a functionally intact cardiac mechanism which is pumping at an accelerated rate. Probably the fundamental reason for this phenomenon is an inadequate supply of blood to the heart consequent to the low venous pressure. Owing to the reduced output the pulse feels thready and of poor volume.

Hypotension, although due to increased intravascular capacity in neurogenic shock, is the result of an actual depletion of circulating blood volume in hematogenic shock. The degree of hypotension is a reasonably accurate clinical measure of the severity of existing shock, but is of uncertain value in the diagnosis of impending shock. A pressure below 80, especially when accompanied by a pulse pressure of 25 or less, should be considered as indicative of existing shock; pressure between 80 and 100 should be considered an indication of danger in the injured patient.

Hypoproteinemia may develop as a consequence of shock resulting from a loss of plasma, as in burns, intestinal obstruction, and peritonitis. Loss of plasma protein containing large quantities of serum albumin reduces the osmotic pressure of the circulating blood, augments fluid loss into the tissues, and produces an increased depletion of the effective circulating blood volume.

Tissue anoxia is probably the most important common offending denominator attending the shock syndrome. Its effect on increasing capillary permeability leading to the loss of fluids and proteins into the extravascular areas has been noted. There are indications that increased capillary permeability, if prolonged, may become irreversible. The brain cannot survive more than six minutes of anoxia. In shock it is apparent that brain function is maintained relatively intact until shortly before death. This is consonant with experiments which suggest that the vasomotor response to shock follows a consistent sequence designed to safeguard the brain. Primarily, available circulation is shunted from the superficial and motor-skeletal structures, then from the kidney, and possibly in the terminal stages from the hepaticoportal system, in order to conserve cerebral oxygenation. Hypoxia depresses liver function and creates serious alterations of protein metabolism. Vasoconstriction occurs in the kidneys and eventually the urine output virtually ceases. Myocardial hypoxia eventually interferes with heart function, and may result in sudden death. At what point in shock the altered capillary permeability, deranged liver and kidney function, and the myocardial and brain damage become irreversible is unknown, but it probably bears a close relationship to the onset of irreversibility of the over-all shock syndrome.

THE CLINICAL PICTURE

The patient is pale and cold, and sweats profusely. Respirations are usually unimpressive, but the rate may be fast in severe shock and in acidosis due to depletion of the alkali reserve, and serious hemorrhage may be characterized by air hunger. The sensorium is depressed, but unconsciousness due to shock, per se, is uncommon. The patient is relatively insensitive to pain and oblivious to his surroundings, but occasionally periods of restlessness may supervene. Thirst is common, but oral intake may be precluded by vomiting. The pulse is rapid and weak, and the blood and pulse pressures are reduced. The venous pressure is low, and the veins are collapsed. The oxygen content of venous blood is sharply reduced. An obvious outlet for the loss of blood or fluid may or may not be apparent.

TREATMENT

It is the responsibility of the surgeon to prevent shock when it is impending, and to forestall irreversibility when it is present. This requires the staunching of circulatory losses, whether internal or external, and restoration of an effective circulating blood volume. These matters brook no delay for, among other factors, the risk of irreversible shock is directly proportional to the duration of the untreated shock syndrome.

Prevention of Shock

Early or impending shock may be difficult to recognize. On the other hand, when a patient has suffered a serious injury or a large hemorrhage impending shock must be assumed, even though condition of the patient appears to be good. Pulse and blood pressure changes are the *results* of shock, and are of little value to the diagnosis of impending shock. Nevertheless, readings should be taken frequently, at regular intervals, and any trend toward a fall in blood pressure, an increased pulse rate, or a deterioration of the pulse quality is a warning that shock is imminent. Hematocrit determinations, when available, herald the advent of shock in advance of clinical signs.

Prophylactic measures designed to counter the common contributing causes of shock may tip the balance in favor of the patient. These are appropriate to most injuries, whether or not shock is feared:

Recumbence in a comfortable horizontal position.

Relief of pain and prevention of further trauma to soft tissues by temporary splinting of injured parts.

Minimum narcosis, especially by morphine, because of its depressor effect upon the vital centers; secure stabilization by splints usually provides adequate relief of pain.

Barbiturates and verbal reassurance for anxiety and restlessness.

Preservation of normal body temperature by covers and removal of wet clothes, etc.; heat is to be avoided.

Insertion of a needle into a vein and commencement of a slow saline or glucose drip (whenever shock is a possibility), and coincident removal of blood for typing and cross-matching, hematocrit, or other pertinent tests.

Control of external hemorrhage by a pressure dressing and elevation of the part. A tourniquet is almost never necessary, and sudden shock is often precipitated by the removal of a tourniquet already in place. (See Toxic Factors in Shock, p. 28.)

Gentle handling and moving of the patient at all times. Rapid movements or rough handling may precipitate shock.

An open airway must be maintained.

Drainage of mucus from the upper respiratory tract must be accomplished by suction or gravity.

Supplemental oxygen should be administered by mask or tube in event of hypoventilation from any cause.

Fluid infusion should be accelerated immediately to counter deterioration of the blood pressure or pulse, and a more lasting replacement with plasma or whole blood should be started as soon as possible.

To omit or defer these measures in the early care of a seriously injured patient is to present an invitation that is rarely declined by the progressive chain reaction of the shock syndrome.

The intentional trauma of an operation, especially if prolonged or attended by considerable blood loss or by rough handling of tissues, is as competent a cause of shock as is accidental injury. Conversely, after some injuries, the operative control of hemorrhage or fixation of damaged structures may be the most important single measure that can be carried out for the prevention of shock. It is the joint responsibility of the surgeon and the anesthetist to see that such a procedure is productive of maximum benefits at a minimum physiological cost. Observance of the following principles goes far in assuring such results:

The operation should not start until the general condition of the patient is stabilized (except as a life-saving measure for the control of gross hemorrhage, or restoration of intrathoracic pressure).

Supportive measures, as needed, should continue uninterrupted throughout and after operation.

All moving and handling of the patient must be slow and gentle, even under anesthesia.

The surgeon should work with precision, but also with dispatch, for the recently injured patient is intolerant of a prolonged or leisurely procedure.

The surgeon must be especially vigilant in his watch over blood and fluid losses, and over the force with which retractors are manipulated. He must be quick to note even a mild increasing cyanotic tinge to the blood, and he must handle all the tissues, including bone, with gentle respect.

The anesthetist must be constantly aware of the patient's condition. The depth of anesthesia should be the minimum necessary to the operation. Blood pressure and pulse should be recorded much more frequently than in an uninjured patient who has been prepared for an elective operation. The anesthetist must be astute in his assessment of alterations in the quality of the pulse. He must watch for signs of increased sweating and reduced skin temperature, and maintain the effective circulating volume on an even keel by regulation of infusions and transfusions. Stability of blood volume, however, is not enough. He must also make sure of a constant open airway, of adequate oxygen supplementation, and adequate pulmonary ventilation. Finally, he must be quick to recognize reduced requirements of his anesthetic agents as a sign of danger. It may be said that these are the important duties of the anesthetist in any operation. They are doubly important when the patient is in danger of shock.

Treatment of Shock

The essence of shock treatment is speed. Untreated severe shock progresses inexorably toward irreversibility. Corrective measures, which will be successful if carried out quickly, often are useless when delayed. All the preventive measures listed above are pertinent to treatment, but some of them assume roles essential to recovery when severe shock is established, namely, control of hemorrhage, replenishment and maintenance of blood volume, and an adequate supply of oxygen.

Control of hemorrhage from a wound usually can be accomplished temporarily by a pressure dressing and, when in an extremity, by elevation. Complete division of a major vessel such as the popliteal or brachial artery is followed by retraction and constriction of the proximal open end, and a marked spontaneous diminution in the rate of blood loss. Incomplete division precludes retraction, which mechanically impairs the capacity of the vessel to reduce its lumen, and a corresponding diminution of blood loss is less likely. In the latter circumstance a tourniquet may be required to staunch the hemorrhage until definitive treatment can be carried out. Internal hemorrhage is often sudden, large in amount, rapidly followed by severe shock, and controllable only after laparotomy. A large and continuing internal hemorrhage may not respond to the most heroic supportive therapy. Operation for control of such a hemorrhage may be mandatory despite profound shock. The decision to operate often cannot await the mature judgment of the senior surgeon, but must be made and implemented by his junior associate in the receiving room.

Blood volume must be restored and maintained. The veins may be collapsed so that venipuncture is difficult or impossible. In this event one or more veins should be cut down upon immediately. Needles or cannulae, sufficiently large to permit the rapid infusion of large quantities of fluid, should be placed in position. The benefits of arterial transfusion remain open to some doubts. The reduced cardiac output in shock is largely a reflection of a depleted venous return, and it is probable that volume replacement should be infused by vein, whenever possible.

Water may sometimes be given by mouth, but this is not often possible or wise in severe shock. Any benefits derived from hypodermoclysis will almost certainly be too little and too late. Intravenous crystalloid solutions temporarily raise the blood pressure, dilute the already depleted plasma proteins, and are soon lost into the tissues, following which the pressure drops to a level lower than before. Ringer's, glucose, and sodium chloride solutions, therefore, are useful only for temporary support of the blood volume pending the availability of more durable and efficient replacement materials.

Plasma, serum albumin, and the various plasma expander solutions available provide more lasting support than crystalloid solutions, and are of great benefit when the principal loss has been of plasma, as in burns and peritonitis. In addition, no grouping or cross-matching is required, and such preparations are more likely to be available quickly and in larger amounts than whole blood. The risk of homologous serum jaundice after administration of pooled plasma has been greatly reduced by modern storing techniques. In shock due to loss of whole blood support of reduced volume by plasma alone is not completely satisfactory. Whole blood lost should be replaced by whole blood. In the treatment of shock resulting from hemorrhage, plasma and its substitutes remain temporary supports for maintenance of volume until whole blood arrives.

Severe shock from any cause cannot often be treated satisfactorily without blood transfusion. Rapid administration of whole blood through one or several intravenous inlets, until the blood pressure rises to an arbitrary level around 80 and becomes stabilized, and the other signs and symptoms of shock commence to abate, is the best and usually the only good method for correcting severe shock. As the blood pressure becomes stabilized the rate of infusion may be decelerated. The volume of blood transfused and rapidity of transfusion should always be proportionate to the amount of loss from hemorrhage and the rate at which it occurred, or to the depth of the existing shock syndrome. Overtransfusion and overloading of the heart is a very remote possibility in the face of the depleted cardiac intake and output consequent to the lowered blood volume. The amount of replaced blood should equal or, if necessary, exceed the estimated loss. It may not be possible to estimate the approximate loss. Whether or not this is the case, the surgeon's most reliable measure of his efforts at replacement is the elevation of blood pressure and its stabilization at an adequate level. The amount of blood required to reach this goal may eventually exceed the total normal volume. If fish are carried in a leaking pail a constant replacement of water equal to the leak is necessary to their continued life, until the leak has been repaired. The same is no less true of shock.

Oxygen deficiency is the fundamental factor common to shock from all causes, and the basic objective of all shock measures is to increase the amount of oxygen available for use by the body tissues. The administration of pure oxygen increases the oxygen content of arterial blood by a significant amount, and is of real value in the treatment of shock.

Drugs are of little value, being poorly absorbed from the tissues in the presence of shock, and they may be harmful. An optimal response to shock treatment requires top-flight performance of the brain centers, which are depressed by morphine. The shock patient usually is hyposensitive to pain, so that the use of morphine should be avoided or minimized. In clinical practice the use of Demerol combined with adequate temporary splints provides very satisfactory relief of pain. Various vasoconstricting drugs have been used in an attempt to check the increasing discrepancy between blood volume and intravascular capacity. Norepinephrine may be useful to temporarily retard the shock cycle while adequate replacement is prepared. As a rule, the blood pressure may rise a small amount following the use of these drugs, but it almost invariably drops quickly to a level lower than ever unless, in the meantime, replenishment of blood volume has been started.

Posture has been thought to affect shock by its influence upon cerebral blood supply. A mild head-down posture should aid cephalad circulation by gravity. Too much head-down posture neutralizes this benefit as the weight of the abdominal contents impairs the diaphragmatic contribution to respirations. The foot of the bed or litter should probably be raised a little, but not more than 6 inches. High elevation of the legs may dump as much as 500 ml. of blood into the remainder of the circulation in the healthy patient. This expedient may occasionally be of help in delaying the onset of shock immediately after a sudden large hemorrhage. A little later, after vasoconstriction has already shunted the extremity circulation to more vital areas, this maneuver will be fruitless.

TOXIC FACTORS IN SHOCK

The effects of crushing injuries, of a forgotten tourniquet, or of necrotic undebrided tissues leave little room for doubt that some toxic factor plays a part in the shock syndrome. Shock resulting from any condition attended by absorption of the products of extensive tissue autolysis may not respond completely to supportive measures which correct hypovolemia by plasma replacement alone. That damaged muscle produces some substance toxic to the kidneys, probably myohemoglobin, seems clear.

Crushing injuries produce hypovolemic shock owing to a loss of blood and plasma into the damaged area *after* decompression. For the duration of crushing the circulation can neither lose volume into nor evacuate toxic substances from the compressed area. The amount of fluid loss may be reduced by the application of compression bandages to the crushed extremity immediately after extrication of the patient. Heat to the injured area should be avoided, and some cooling may be beneficial. Shock treatment is that for correction of the hypovolemia. Even when the initial shock responds satisfactorily, serious renal complications (crush syndrome) are to be anticipated within a few days. Urinalysis reveals blood, albumin, and casts. Oliguresis is common, and in severe injuries the kidney output may cease and the patient may die in uremia. Renal damage is related to the precipitation of myohemoglobin in the kidney tubules. Alkalinization of the urine with large doses of sodium citrate and sodium carbonate, in an attempt to keep myohemoglobin in solution, should be carried out. Progressive renal failure, despite these measures, may require amputation of the extremity to save life.

The removal of a neglected tourniquet initiates a reaction similar to the crush syndrome. Whether the tourniquet was applied initially to control hemorrhage from a wound or to facilitate an operative procedure makes little difference to the outpouring of blood and plasma into, and the absorption of toxic products of cell death from, the extremity, when it is eventually removed. Subcutaneous fat necrosis and peripheral nerve injury have been largely eliminated, but ischemia and tissue anoxia remain unaffected by modern pneumatic tourniquets. In the emergency treatment of injuries it is certain that more lives and limbs have been lost through the unnecessary use of a tourniquet than have been saved by its proper usage. It is equally clear that the use of a tourniquet in operations is often a procedure of convenience rather than necessity. The moral, however, is clear and unequivocal. A tourniquet should be used only when necessary and for as short a time as possible; it should be released intermittently for short periods whenever prolonged usage is necessary; and its constant supervision should remain the specific responsibility of one person until it is finally removed.

EMOTIONAL RESPONSE TO INJURY

To diagnose a patient as "psychosomatic" is a refuge of the diagnostically destitute. The body and soul are one. The soul is reflected in a personality which responds to stress fully as much as the physical unit. The body may be young or old, fat or thin, healthy or unhealthy; and the net of such physical characteristics will influence its response to injury. The personality may be mature or immature, stoical or excitable, introvert or extrovert; and the net of such basic traits as these will influence the emotional response. Personality remains adjusted to environment by a buffer system of hopes and fears, triumphs and defeats, aims and frustrations. These emotional electrolytes must be maintained in balance for the preservation of pride, dignity, and an acceptable measure of self-respect. A normally unstable or precarious balance may be disturbed profoundly by an insignificant injury, whereas a mature and stable personality may take the consequences of a serious injury in stride.

Disturbances of emotional equilibrium following injury often are manifested by somatic signs and symptoms which are without any recognizable organic basis. Are these abnormal? Is the patient imagining the symptoms, or prevaricating the signs? An affirmative answer to these questions must indict the majority of all injured persons, who sooner or later complain of bad weather pain at the site of their healed injury, and the more than 50 per cent of all persons involved in automobile accidents who react neurotically in one way or another. The surgeon, before he dismisses a complaint as "psychosomatic," "functional," or "malingering," should recall his first public address, and the increased pulse rate, dysphonia, anorexia, and cessation of salivary gland function which preceded it. Let him recall whether the symptoms resulting from these physiological phenomena were any less real for lack of an organic cause. Let him speculate whether they would have subsided or persisted had the stress which preceded his first public address lasted for weeks or months. He will then hesitate before advising a patient to forget about complaints for which he can educe no organic cause with a brusque admonition "they are all in your mind." He will realize that there are physiological and symptomatic responses to an emotional disturbance which may be as consistent, if not as well understood, as those which attend disturbances of fluid and electrolyte balance; that a pain arising from such a cause is, to the patient, as real as the pain from a broken leg, and that to dismiss it without sympathy and reassurance is but to accentuate its severity. Such complaints are far too common to be classified as abnormal. Their primary etiology is emotional stress; contributing factors include anxiety, suggestion, iatrogenic factors, and, especially following an injury, litigation.

Anxiety is a potent source of emotional stress. An accidental injury often engenders a complex nightmare filled with fears of permanent disability, incomplete recovery, complications of healing, loss of work and earning capacity, hardship in the home, and innumerable other worries which may or may not be apparent to the surgeon. The wise surgeon dispels or minimizes such specters, whether or not they are apparent on the surface. This should be done at the earliest possible moment in order to eliminate uncertainty, which is the most fertile source of anxiety. It should be done in all injuries, for severity alone is not a reliable index of stress potential. A crushed finger is apt to have as profound an emotional impact upon a musician as the loss of a leg upon a laborer.

Chronic neglected anxiety, whether obscure or obvious, soon begets feelings of inadequacy and guilt, a subconscious desire for revenge, and various other compensatory emotional reactions. The well-stabilized personality sooner or later regains emotional balance, and adjusts his life to the effects of injury. Certain individuals overcompensate and go on to greater things as a result of adversity. The unstable personality often is overwhelmed, and must resort to some form of escape mechanism. In any circumstances some form of compensation is necessary to the subjective preservation of personality and self-esteem. In this process distorted emotions often are sublimated into an exaggeration of existing symptoms, the production of symptoms for which no organic cause can be found, and gross personality changes. These emotional responses should not be considered as psychoses, for existing psychotic conditions are not often altered appreciably as a result of injury. They are psychological responses to the stress produced by trauma and its after-effects, and, although they do not conform to as consistent a response pattern as injured physical mechanisms, they represent as innate a response to injury as inflammation and repair. They cannot be identified by any laboratory test, but only by the intuition and understanding of a physician who is truly interested in his patient as a person. They are impervious to the science but easily controlled by the art of medicine, without which a surgeon is little more than a skilled technician.

Suggestion is also a potent source of emotional turmoil. It is impossible for a person voluntarily to perspire, to raise his pulse rate and blood pressure, or to cause goose flesh to appear and the hair to stand on end. The writer experienced all these phenomena while walking through an uninhabited area one dark night, although previously he had traversed the same deserted stretch many nights without a qualm. On the night in question the police were searching the region for a maniacal murderer, and to the writer every dark shadow contained the fugitive. The reactions listed above were due to suggestion, yet they were quite as physiological and unpleasant as if they had been due to some organic cause. If suggestion can have such an effect upon a normal healthy individual, how much more potent will be the effects of suggestion by a surgeon upon an injured patient! It is not necessary to bankrupt the remaining emotional reserve of a patient who is worried about numbness following a knee operation by the blunt statement "the nerve to your knee was cut," or to tell the laborer with a fractured transverse process "your back is broken." As much as physical factors, suggestions such as these are the things of which catastrophes are made.

Iatrogenic reactions are psychological effects produced by the physician and by therapy. They should be beneficial, but may prove to be additional insults superimposed upon an already overtaxed emotional equilibrium. Any unguarded remark within earshot of a patient, if left unexplained or uncorrected, may by virtue of anxiety or suggestion precipitate an obstinate neurosis. To tell a patient, "This is the worst case I have ever seen," manifests a psychological quirk in the surgeon and may produce one in the patient. The unadorned injunction, "you must take it easy," may tip the scales against recovery, and produce a chronic emotional and physical invalid. The indefinite continuance of some empirical or palliative measure for want of something better to do, or for a less laudable reason, is not only poor practice but almost quackery, and represents one of the most common and important causes currently productive of neurotic conditions. To tell the patient nothing is worst of all, for anxiety is bred of uncertainty. The surgeon must bear constantly in his mind that his every word and action are absorbed and interpreted by the patient. The iatrogenic results are his reward or his ignominy.

Litigation is an extremely common impediment to rehabilitation. The primary desire of every injured person is to recover as soon as possible. But modern society is such that most injured patients also anticipate monetary compensation for what has happened to them, from one source or another. Almost from the start they are beset by a sequence of psychological forces, each predisposing to submerge the desire for rapid and complete recovery under the waters of avarice. The first may be a casual or deliberate magnification of the injury and its sequelae by the physician. Following in rapid succession may come suggestions from friends, relatives, union representatives, lawyers, and others that the patient must magnify his troubles in order to recover as large a settlement as possible. Before long the intransigence of the insurance adjuster may transform these incubating suggestions into a determination on the part of the patient "not to let anyone put anything over on me." The desire to recover becomes subservient to a conviction that persistent symptoms and disability are necessary to a defense of his legal position until the argument is adjudicated. Preconceived malingering is rare. Exaggerated incapacity which persists beyond all normal expectations without organic substantiation must be accepted as a normal response to our scheme of society which, in practice, recompenses injury and disability solely by "the gold cure." Litigation cannot be prevented, but its deleterious effects upon recovery from injury usually can be ameliorated by the surgeon.

CHAPTER 2

GENERAL PRINCIPLES IN THE TREATMENT OF TRAUMA

By HARRISON L. McLAUGHLIN, M.D.

CARDINAL PRINCIPLES OF FRACTURE TREATMENT

"Hypothetically, the ideal treatment for any fracture would be to 'wish' the fragments into place, hold them there by 'moral suasion,' and send the patient on about his business while the fracture heals."

CLAY RAY MURRAY

CLAY RAY MURRAY's favorite aphorism epitomized the philosophy of modern fracture treatment. It re-emphasizes that a fracture must not be considered and treated as a broken bone, but rather that the object of treatment is an injured individual. Only the first stipulation of his tripartite hypothesis is directed solely to the injured part; the others take equal cognizance of the local problem, the injured region, and the individual as a whole.

"To 'wish' the fragments into place" stipulates recognition that the primary tissue damage caused by the injury may be multiplied several times by secondary damage resulting from reduction maneuvers; that the rate and quality of recovery are inversely proportional to the total amount of tissue damage; and that reduction, regardless of method, must be designed and carried out in such a manner that its inevitable secondary tissue insult will be minimized.

To "hold them there by 'moral suasion' " is to recognize that all surgical forms of fracture fixation are injurious to physiology and detrimental to function, delay recovery, and increase disability; that some carry more severe penalties than others; and that, of the multiple methods available for most fractures, the best is that which, in addition to providing fixation, interferes least with continuing function of the uninjured regional structures.

To "send the patient on about his business while the fracture heals" is to recognize that a fracture problem is the problem of an injured person. To the soldier with a fracture of the scaphoid a year or more in a plaster dressing, out of the fighting and in warm and comfortable quarters at full pay, may represent a pleasant interlude, but to the mechanic who must work to feed his family the same treatment would be likely to produce emotional and economic bankruptcy. It is not necessary to make a fracture fit a favorite treatment. There are numerous methods available for the treatment of most fractures. These can and should be adapted to fit the needs of the patient as well as the fracture, so that ordinary daily activities are interrupted as little as possible, and full activities restored as soon as possible.

The preceding statements represent established fundamental principles that have remained unchallenged and unchanged for many years. The methods for their implementation are numerous and ever changing. The best method for any fracture remains that which most nearly approaches the hypothetical ideal proposed by Clay Ray Murray, and leads directly to the ultimate goal of both surgeon and patient.

GOAL OF FRACTURE TREATMENT

The fracture result marked by sound union, normal anatomy, full strength, complete joint motion, and an absence of symptoms is perfect, but rare. All of these features are desirable, but more often than not some must be compromised in order to obtain others. The best treatment obtains the features most important to a good result, if necessary at the expense of the remainder. The surgeon who treats all fractures as broken bones, by reduction and immobilization, will produce many roentgen triumphs that are dismal clinical failures. At the other extreme, the enthusiast for "early mobilization" will produce many functionally successful results at an unnecessary cost of pain, weakness, and deformity. Neither is a good surgeon. There is no best method of fracture treatment, but there is a best method of treatment for each individual patient. It is that which will achieve the ultimate goal in the treatment of all traumas—*a return to usual activities as soon and to as nearly normal an extent as possible.*

INITIAL CARE AND TRANSPORTATION

The injured must be transported to the surgeon. The period immediately after injury is pregnant with events which may vitiate the best of treatment and jeopardize the quality of the result. It is all too common for the man with an injured back to be doubled up into the seat of a car which speeds him to a hospital, but produces a paraplegia en route; for the man with an injured leg to be helped to his feet, and a cracked tibia to buckle and pierce the skin; for the man with a broken neck to be killed when some kindly bystander lifts his head so he can take a sip of water; for the unconscious patient to drown in his own secretions; or for hemorrhage, staunched by an amateur tourniquet, to eventuate in gangrene and loss of limb. Similar, if less spectacular, complications are superimposed upon many injuries before any definitive treatment can be done. Simple fractures with excellent prognoses are transformed into complex problems with a bleak outlook. Soft tissues, including nerves and vessels, are mangled by the sharp points of unstabilized fracture fragments. These are the common results of absent or faulty first-aid care of the injured. The surgeon may shrug his shoulders and turn away, but he cannot repudiate responsibility for such defections. Who else has the knowledge, obligation, and opportunity to educate the community in this very important phase of the treatment of trauma?

Care of an injured person until he reaches a doctor must rest in the hands of the laity. Therefore, it must be limited to certain fundamental measures necessary to the preservation of life and the prevention of further damage. These may be listed as follows:

(1) keep the airway open;
(2) keep the unconscious person on his side;
(3) control hemorrhage;
(4) prevent motion of the injured back or neck;
(5) stabilize (splint) injured extremities;
(6) cover wounds with clean cloth;
(7) keep all movements and manipulations slow and gentle;
(8) maintain normal body temperature;
(9) keep sympathy subservient to reason;
(10) transport comfortably rather than rapidly.

Patency of the airway is a matter of life or death. Cyanosis or dyspnea should receive primary consideration, for the brain can survive only a few minutes without oxygen. The tongue must be pulled forward past the teeth if it has fallen backward and blocked the airway. If it will not stay in position it must be held, or the patient rolled on his side so that the tongue hangs forward due to gravity. When the airway is blocked by blood and mucus, attempts to wipe away these secretions are usually ineffectual. The patient should be placed in the lateral or prone position so that gravity aids drainage of the fluid.

The unconscious person must be presumed to have suffered a brain injury. He should be kept on his side if at all possible; otherwise retroversion of the tongue is very likely to block the intake of oxygen and exit of secretions.

Hemorrhage is spectacular, but not often a vital issue. A tourniquet is almost always unnecessary, and likely to do more harm than good. More limbs have been lost due to improper application than to omission of a tourniquet. Application of pressure over certain points, even by an expert anatomist, is of little value. Moderate elevation and the application of a firm pressure dressing to the wound will control the hemorrhage from virtually all injuries in the extremities.

The injured back must not be flexed. Of all motions, extension is least likely to be harmful. Therefore, whenever possible, the patient should be kept in a prone position. Spinal cord damage may result from emergency transportation in the lateral, supine, or seated position, and the risk far outweighs any temporary discomfort produced by the prone position.

When adequate transportation is not available, the patient with back injury *must* be moved in the prone position, for most attempts to carry a supine individual (except by trained attendants) result in flexion of the

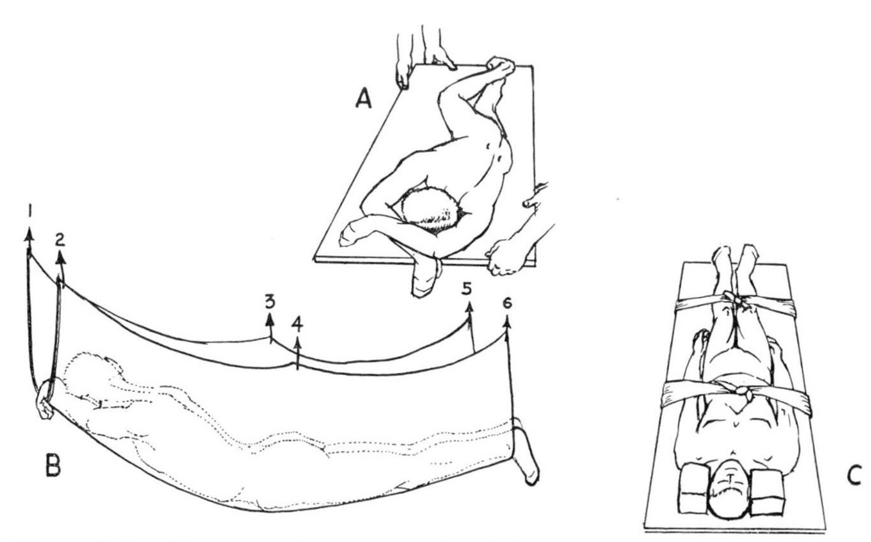

Figure 2–1. Transport of patients with spinal injury.

A. The best method for transporting a patient with a back injury is in the prone position upon a rigid device, e.g., a door, litter, or wide board.

B. When a rigid litter cannot be obtained, the patient with a back injury may be rolled like a log into a prone position upon a doubled blanket spread on the ground beside him. If the blanket is then carried at points 1 to 6, any sag of the spine will be into slight extension.

C. The patient with an injured neck should be transported supine. All neck motion must be prevented by manual or mechanical stabilization of the head.

spine. When a prone patient is lifted the sag of gravity extends the spine. Preferably, the patient should be rolled gently, like a log, on to a litter, door, or wide board (Fig. 2–*1, A*). When a rigid device is not available, the second choice is a doubled blanket (Fig. 2–*1, B*). Above all, the patient with an injured back *never* should be transported in a seated position.

Injury to the neck interdicts transportation in a prone position. The patient should remain supine and be moved in such a way that the neck cannot move in any direction (Fig. 2–*1, C*). This requires constant supervision, for a single unguarded motion of the head on the shoulders may mean the difference between survival and death.

Extremity injuries dictate stabilization by some form of splints or dressings. For injuries proximal to the elbow, the upper extremity may be suspended in a sling, and bound firmly but gently to the thorax (Fig. 2–2, *A*). When the injury is distal to the elbow the forearm and hand should also be bound to some form of splint (Fig. 2–2, *B*). When the elbow is injured the arm should be stabilized by a sling or splint in accordance with the existing degree of flexion or extension, and no attempt should be made to alter this position. Mechanical devices designed to produce a point of countertraction in the axilla should not be used.

Injuries in the lower extremities often require traction in addition to stabilization. The foot should be grasped, and steady manual traction

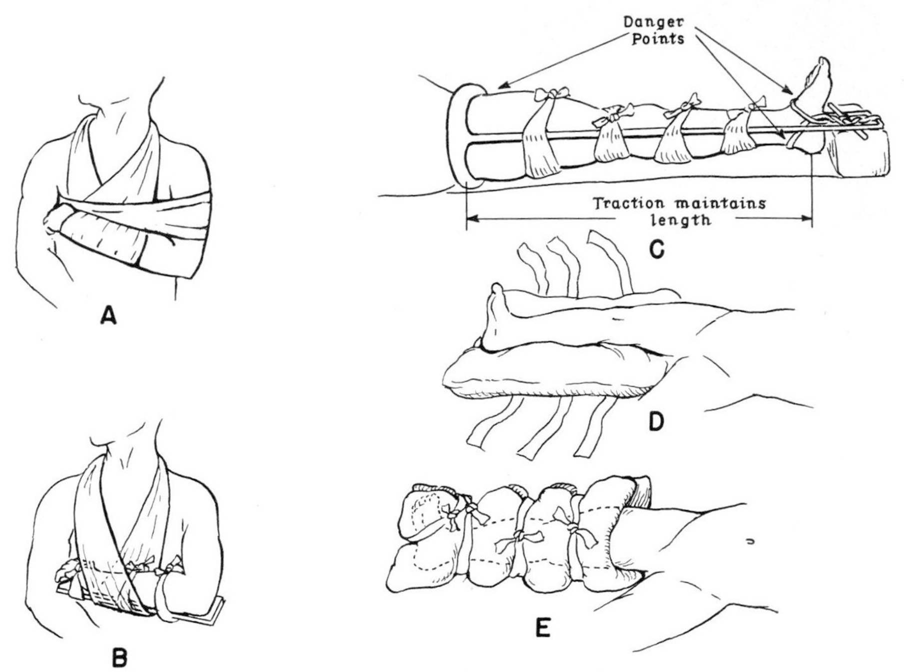

Figure 2–2. Transport of patients with extremity injuries.

A. When the injury is proximal to the elbow, the arm should be placed in a sling and swathe.

B. When the injury is distal to the elbow, the arm should be placed in a sling and some form of splint.

C. Immobilization combined with fixed traction should be used when the injury is proximal to the ankle. Undue pressure at the perineum and at the point of traction should be avoided.

D, E. A pillow splint, with or without a board or magazine incorporated for stiffness, is a simple and efficient dressing for transportation of patients with injuries at the ankle and foot.

applied in the long axis of the limb. If the limb is crooked, it is permissible and proper to restore alignment in this manner. Splints which provide both fixation and traction are appropriate for all injuries proximal to the ankle (Fig. 2–2, *C*). Stabilizing splints without traction (Fig. 2–2, *D* and *E*) should be used to support injuries at the ankle.

The fragment of bone which protrudes through an open wound presents a dilemma. Should the bystander or first-aid attendant splint such an extremity without traction and leave the bone protruding, or should he straighten the deformed limb by traction and carry additional contamination into the depths of the wound as the protruding fragment is replaced in more normal position? There can be no firm answer to this question which demands mature surgical judgment in each case, for a surgeon is rarely present at the scene of an accident. Probably more good than harm would be done if traction were applied in all cases, provided definitive care is available within a short time, and the surgeon is notified that the bone was originally protruding through the skin.

All wounds are contaminated. They should be covered with a dressing of the cleanest cloth available, and thereafter left undisturbed. Disinfectants and cleansing solutions should not be used. Pressure may be applied to the dressing for control of profuse bleeding.

Gentleness must dominate every phase of first-aid care. Neither the patient nor any injured part should be subjected to a rapid or unexpected motion. Good first-aid care promotes comfort. Everything that is done must be done slowly and gently enough to remain within the limits of pain.

Body temperature should be maintained. Covering with a blanket is usually adequate. It is more harmful than beneficial to bundle up the injured patient in many blankets, or to apply heat to the extent that body fluids are lost by sweating.

Emotions must be governed by reason. To the bystander, it may seem callous to leave an injured person lying on the roadside while arrangements are made for splints and transportation, to deny him a drink of water, to force him to lie face down, or to prevent him from arising to test his injured leg. It is frequently from indulgence of such human impulses that catastrophes result.

The speeding ambulance is unnecessary and harmful. Transportation should be as smooth and comfortable as all other first-aid measures. Bells, sirens, and speed have become the universal trademark of the ambulance driver, but a recent study by Dr. Sydney Lyttle, of Flint, Michigan, of 2500 consecutive ambulance runs failed to reveal that speed was necessary, or contributed measurably to the welfare of the patient, except in one instance.

PREPARATION FOR TREATMENT

The injured part may or may not have been splinted prior to arrival of the patient. Additional tissue damage can and does occur during preparations for treatment, almost as easily as at the scene of the accident or in transport. Therefore, unsplinted injuries should be splinted, even for the short trip to and from the x-ray department, for adequate films will require manipulation of the injured part by the x-ray technician. The patient who has had splints applied prior to arrival should be examined immediately to make sure they are comfortable, efficient, and non-constricting. Emergency splints are often applied at the scene of the accident with more enthusiasm than skill, and swelling increases throughout the transportation period. Any constricting dressings should be loosened immediately, but a tourniquet should not be removed until anti-shock treatment has been started. Adequate splints rarely should be removed for a detailed assessment of the injury prior to roentgen examination, but inspection should be sufficient to rule out the presence of an open wound. A review of the roentgenograms makes unnecessary any extensive clinical manipulations of the fracture until the stage has been set for definitive treatment.

The condition of the peripheral nerves and circulation distal to every extremity injury should be evaluated and recorded at the first examination.

A detailed neurological examination is unnecessary. If the patient can flex and extend his toes, even a tiny amount, the major nerves of the lower extremity are grossly intact; if he can spread and flex his fingers and extend his thumb, even if only with a flicker of motion, functional integrity of the major nerves of the upper limb is indicated. Absence of the ability to carry out these motor functions warrants a more detailed examination and, if this is done and a nerve injury is recognized at the start, it will be unnecessary for the patient and surgeon to speculate later whether such injury was produced by trauma or by the treatment.

An obvious injury is apt to captivate the attention of a casual examiner to the exclusion of less apparent concomitant lesions. Only too often has a fracture of the femoral shaft thus camouflaged an associated dislocation of the hip; a fracture of the os calcis, a concomitant spine fracture; fractured ribs, a ruptured spleen; and the crushed pelvis, a serious genitourinary tract injury. These are but a few of the pitfalls that await the unwary surgeon who allows his attention to remain focused upon the obvious. The examination of every injury should include a rapid survey of the entire patient.

An elaborate history is sometimes impossible and is rarely necessary. The time, place, and details of the accident, and a description of intervening events should be recorded. Inquiries into the cardiovascular, renal, and respiratory status of the patient must be complemented by sufficient clinical and laboratory examinations to determine the anesthetic risk, and the agent of choice. The time of the last food intake must be ascertained. The important interval is that between food intake and accident, not between intake and anesthesia. Cessation of gastrointestinal function is among the early responses to injury, and the stomach may not empty for many hours following even a minor painful injury. Unless the stomach is empty there is a risk that vomitus may be aspirated during inhalation anesthesia.

Emotional stress, as well as physical discomfort, must be alleviated as much as possible. Palliative or preanesthetic medication should be administered early, but not before the injured person has been apprised of the facts of the injury and the implications of the projected plan of treatment. A frank discussion, which dispels uncertainties and answers as many questions as possible, promotes the patient's confidence in his doctor, and quickly establishes them as a team with a single goal and a mutually acceptable program.

REDUCTION OF FRACTURES

Difficulty in the reduction of a fracture usually is a reflection of some surgical mistake.

Hypothetically, the ideal reduction would be "to 'wish' the fragments into place," which implies relocation of the fragments without additional tissue damage. Translated into practical terms, the best reduction for any fracture is that which most clearly approaches the hypothetical ideal. The amount of additional tissue damage inflicted by a reduction is proportional to the force necessary for its accomplishment. Force is unnecessary to the early reduction of a fracture, and represents compensation for an error in technique, or an attempt to overpower some anatomical obstruction, which more often than not is unrecognized. Bone fragments which are forced back into position seldom remain in place satisfactorily; those which are relocated easily and without force usually remain reduced. Several factors will determine whether a fracture reduction will prove to be easy (atraumatic), or difficult (traumatic):

(1) the time;
(2) the anesthesia;
(3) the displacing forces;
(4) the choice of method;
(5) the technique;
(6) the criteria of satisfactory reduction.

The Timing of Reduction

To say that a fracture may be reduced any time during the first few days after injury is analogous to saying that suppuration may be drained any time during the first few days after it has become localized. It is true that both procedures usually can be deferred for a few days without destroying the prospects for an eventually successful result. It is equally true that the earlier the procedure is carried out in each instance, the easier it is to do, the less is the attendant morbidity, and the more rapid, certain, and satisfactory the result. To advocate delayed reduction for reasons of convenience or expediency is to repudiate all that has been learned about the pathology of injury and repair.

Muscle spasm is the single impediment common to early reduction. Thereafter the soft tissues become swollen, hard, inelastic, and contracted, as discussed in consideration of the local response to injury in the preceding chapter. When reduction has been done prior to or in the early stages of this response, the "jelled" soft tissues become auxiliary splints which augment the fixation provided by surgical devices. Fixation and inelasticity of all the tissues, which increase inexorably in direct proportion to the interval following the injury, are the impediments common to delayed reduction. When they are "jelled" in malposition these soft tissues, which aid in the maintenance of an early reduction, must then be torn apart by force, and traumatized to an astonishing degree before delayed reduction can be accomplished.

A fracture should be considered a surgical emergency. The facts that the type and urgency of treatment vary, and that the penalties of delayed reductions are minor or catastrophic, do not prejudice this axiom. The supracondylar fracture with a cold white hand is an emergency to be measured in minutes, if the permanent crippling effects of ischemic paralysis are to be avoided; the dislocated elbow with a fracture of the radial head must be repaired not only in a specific manner but also within a specified number of hours if a 50 per cent incidence of myositis ossificans is to be avoided; if the fractured ankle is not reduced within the first 12 hours after injury active treatment may often be precluded for a week or more by soft part swelling and skin blebs; and the incidence and severity of complications is doubled when the fractured hip of an elderly patient is left unreduced for more than 24 hours after injury. The optimal time for reduction of any fracture is as soon as possible after the injury.

Delayed reduction is sometimes necessary in a fracture that has been allowed to remain unreduced for several days or longer. One glance will tell even the inexperienced surgeon that here are damaged tissues which are hard, contracted, bloated by edema and old hemorrhage to or past the point of skin blisters, hypoxic, and depleted of resistance against infection. Swelling and edema make it difficult or impossible to feel the bone fragments, much less grasp and reduce them into proper position. The inelastic adherence of the contracted soft tissues resists replacement of the bone ends until they are forcibly disrupted. When, by chance, these difficulties are overcome and the fracture reduced, the severely swollen soft tissues militate against secure fixation by any form of external dressing. Operative reduction through such devitalized tissues is always an invitation to infection, with results producing a much more severe penalty than the original injury.

Reduction by any method is a mistake under such circumstances. The injured part should be stabilized by a plaster splint over which is bound a smooth and even constant pressure dressing, which must extend distally to the bases of the fingers or toes. The extremity is elevated and the patient exhorted to move the fingers or toes at frequent intervals. Procaine hydrochloride injection of the lumbar or stellate ganglion usually produces an appreciable reduction of discomfort, but little or no measurable increase in the circulation of the injured limb. Reduction should be delayed for several days to a week until swelling subsides and the soft tissues recover sufficiently to withstand the insult of a second (manipulative) injury. Unfortunately, during this waiting period increasing organization, adherence, and inelasticity of all the soft structures mount up and make the eventual reduction procedure more difficult. This is "waiting for the swelling to go down," as it should be practiced, but such a program is justifiable only if, when the patient is first seen, the amount of swelling is severe enough to prevent satisfactory reduction or fixation of the fracture.

Anesthesia

Reduction requires adequate anesthesia; in the early stages following injury, for the obliteration of pain and muscle spasm; and, when treatment has been delayed, to make possible a forcible disruption of the organized soft tissues. The surgeon who attempts to reduce a fracture with inadequate anesthesia or without anesthesia is almost always doomed to defeat, except in the replacement of certain dislocated bones, notably, in anterior dislocation of the humerus from the glenoid. Modern methods of anesthesia can circumvent almost every contraindication formerly advanced to justify delayed reduction of fractures, except inconvenience to the surgeon. The multiplicity of agents and techniques now available make it possible to reduce fractures immediately, or within a few hours, without undue jeopardy to the brain, heart, lungs, kidneys, liver, or full stomach—wherever the risk may lie.

Regional anesthesia, although not so consistently satisfactory as inhalation methods, is eminently suitable for fracture treatment when a general anesthetic is unavailable or contraindicated. Adequate caudal or spinal anesthesia, or a brachial or peripheral nerve trunk block provides the surgeon with as much time and relaxation as is necessary to do his job, and at a minimum of risk. In addition, regional anesthesia wears off gradually over the several hours which, following a general anesthetic, represent the most painful and trying period for the patient.

Local anesthesia is suitable for the reduction of a selected group of fractures, but if used indiscriminately will give disappointing results. It should be reserved for lesions where the area of damaged tissue to be anesthetized is small and contains fluid; that is to say, in the early hours following small bone fractures. Attempts to anesthetize large areas of damaged tissue at the site of a fracture of a large bone, or to anesthetize the site of any fracture after its hematoma has commenced to clot, are seldom completely satisfactory. It is also difficult to obtain satisfactory local anesthesia when bone fragments must be disimpacted, and in children who are too frightened to cooperate.

One or 2 per cent procaine hydrochloride may be used. The patient should always be premedicated with a barbiturate, at least 30 minutes before anesthesia, to counteract the occasional sensitivity reaction that may be encountered. The skin is shaved, cleansed, and prepared, as if for operation, and a wheal is made on the skin over the apex of the fracture hematoma. It is an invitation to infection to pass the injecting needle through intact skin into a fracture site. A small nick is made in the skin with the point of a scalpel and its edges are separated for passage of the needle. Most of the blood is aspirated from the hematoma, and this is replaced with procaine hydrochloride until mild tension (measured by pain) has been re-established. It is then important to do nothing for at least 15 minutes, after which the anesthetic fluid will have pervaded throughout the damaged cavity and produced a maximum effect. Early manipulation or testing to see if the anesthetic is effective may reduce or vitiate its ultimate effect.

The aged patient often is denied the benefits of early reduction of a fracture because of fear of the dangers of anesthesia, or of a desire to do a detailed and time-consuming medical work-up. Local and regional anesthetic techniques often nullify these excuses for delay, but at times a general anesthesia is required. It is probable that the risk to a geriatric patient from a well-conceived and well-administered anesthetic is not so great as that produced by over-all immobility due to pain. Aged patients tolerate general anesthesia, within certain limitations, almost as well as do younger patients; in fact, if they were not endowed with essential organs of good quality, they would not be aged. With the exception of diabetic acidosis and cardiac failure, few of the medical complications of old age can be improved promptly enough by therapy to warrant postponement of a necessary anesthetic.

The agent employed is not as important as the manner of its administration. *Small* doses of Demerol and scopolamine are suitable for premedication. Morphine should not be used, for even a small dose is apt to depress the respiratory rate below 10 per minute for several hours. The induction must be slow and gentle. Hypotensive agents (including spinal anesthesia) are to be avoided. A clear airway, abundant oxygen, and an adequate respiratory exchange at all times are mandatory. Blood loss must be replaced promptly, but other parenteral fluids should be given slowly and with caution. No more than the minimal amount of anesthetic drug required to do the job at hand should be used. In the words of E. H. Rink, in advising those contemplating anesthesia on the aged, "When faced with a wet and slippery road on a dark night, a first-class driver does not alter his techniques in any essential way. He merely redoubles his safeguards and precautions. He avoids rapid acceleration and braking, but he reaches his destination very nearly as quickly and safely as he does under good conditions."

The Displacing Forces

Except when a bone fragment has been avulsed by a ligamentous or muscular tug, primary displacement is in accordance with the mechanical forces of the injury. Because of this, classifications of fractures predicated upon the deduced directions of their injuring forces have come and gone. Currently it is popular practice to classify, and even treat, certain fractures of the shoulder, hip, and ankle, according to whether they were caused by abduction or adduction of the joint involved. This is an oversimplification of the problem which, although facilitating education by rote, is not always accurate (Fig. 2–3). It suggests to the novice that fractures resulting from identical forces are pathologically and therapeutically identical (which is not true), and ignores the basic fact that fractures are primarily injuries to persons, each with individual problems and requirements. Such regimentation cannot help but foster in the mind of the student a false concept that bone fragments remain in the displaced position, produced by the injury, as if inanimate and devoid of muscular attachments, and that the sole problem in reduction is to reverse the mechanical forces of the original injury.

The deformity to be corrected in the reduction of a fracture is the resultant of many forces, including the direction of the injury, the manipulations of initial care, and splinting, or the uncontrolled mobility of the unsplinted bone fragments, the strength and direction of the muscles attached to each fragment, the presence or absence of loose bone fragments wedged across the main fracture gap, and the influence of soft tissues penetrated by or interposed between the bone fragments. Consequently, a classification of fractures based solely upon the mechanics of injury, although it may be useful to an orderly concept of fracture pathodynamics in the mind of the student and of more than passing interest to the expert, is of little value, and often productive of misinformation in the detailed planning of treatment. The surgeon should assess and prorate the im-

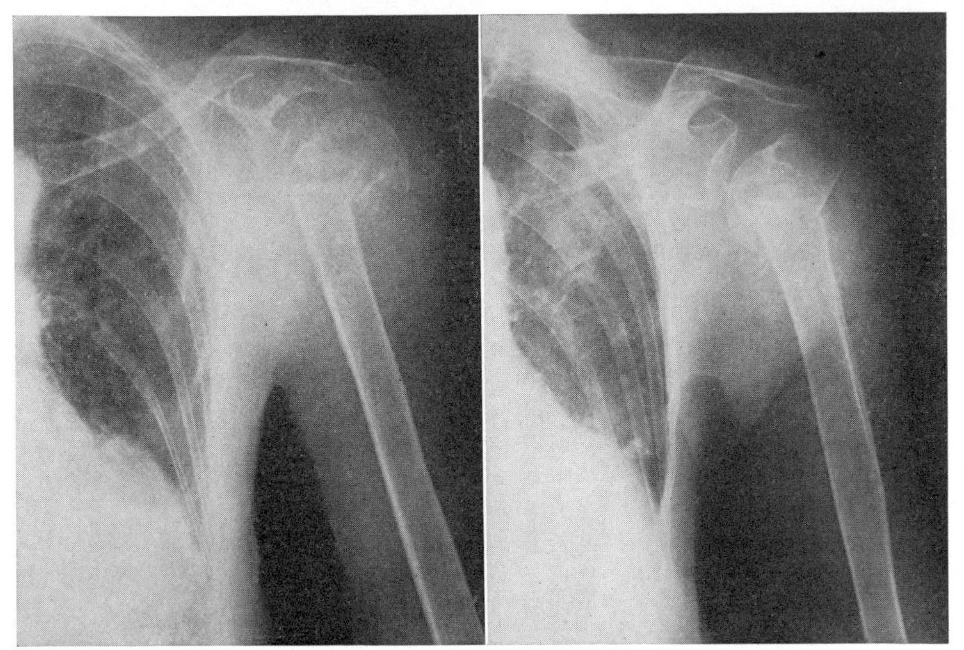

Figure 2–3. Roentgenograms showing the fallacy of treatment predicated purely upon deformity. Films in internal (left) and external (right) rotation disclose this lesion to be both an "abduction" and an "adduction" fracture of the humeral neck.

portance of all overt and occult displacing forces prior to electing a method of reduction and proceeding with its implementation.

The Choice of Method

Manipulation is the simplest, but not always the best, method of fracture reduction. Simplicity is not consistently synonymous with safety or with a good result, and sometimes manipulation produces nothing but harm. It is the height of futility and, in fact, it greatly increases the severity of the injury to manipulate a fracture which cannot be reduced by this method. Such a mishap is more than bad luck; it is an error in judgment.

The fracture which cannot be reduced by manipulation is recognizable or suspect. But if the surgeon's concept of fracture pathology is limited to some system of classification, and his treatment dependent upon the position in this system occupied by the problem at hand, his only recourse is trial and error. When manipulation is unsuccessful he tries again, sometimes several times. After repeated failures the specialist eventually consulted may try once more, unless the necessity for operative reduction is unequivocal. All the tissues in the region of the injury become so damaged and devitalized by repeated manipulative insults that the prospects for success by any method of treatment are greatly reduced, and usually the final method is falsely indicted as the cause of the inevitable poor result. Unless some anatomical obstruction is present, a technically adequate manipulative reduction should be successful and, except when failure has been the result of faulty technique, each repeated manipulation is less likely to succeed than its predecessor. Manipulation, if unsuccessful, should not be repeated until the problem has been re-evaluated, the cause of failure determined, and the plan of treatment altered accordingly. Certain fractures are not amenable to manipulation and must be reduced by operative methods. Operation, when required, should be the *primary* procedure.

The Technique of Manipulative Reduction

The essential preliminary step in reduction of a fracture by manipulation is restoration of length of the broken bone. No matter how small the amount of shortening, or whether it is due to spasm, contracture, or impaction, length must be re-established before any attempt is made to re-appose the fragments. This is done by firm and steady traction and countertraction in the long axis of the limb. The few exceptions to this rule, such as in the reduction of metacarpophalangeal dislocations, are described in detail in subsequent chapters. In certain impacted fractures gentle rocking through a small arc should accompany application of traction, in order to disengage the telescoped fragments. As a rule it is advisable to replace the distal fragment in apposition to the proximal. When the path of displacement has been deduced correctly, and the muscular and other forces to be overcome have been assessed correctly, it is a simple matter to guide the distal fragment back into normal position, but only if normal length is simultaneously maintained by continuance of the preliminary traction. Without traction, manipulative reduction is usually a lost cause. Rotatory deformity should be corrected just before and angulation deformity just after apposition of the bone ends has been accomplished. Strong force, except in the application of traction, is seldom necessary. The problem differs in delayed reduction, which with time becomes progressively more difficult and requires progressively more forceful manipulations. It is an axiom of fracture treatment that a technically adequate early manipulative reduction is usually accomplished with ease, whereas a delayed reduction, by comparison, is never easy.

The Criteria of Satisfactory Reduction

In adults. An anatomically perfect reduction is desirable, seldom essential, and rarely obtained, except when the fragments are seen and replaced exactly at operation. The essential objective of a manipulative reduction is adequate anatomical and perfect functional replacement of the fracture fragments. Success or failure is measured by subsequent roentgenograms, but every surgeon with operative experience in the treatment of fractures soon appreciates that the great majority of reductions are not as good as they appear to be in these films.

The criteria of a satisfactory reduction are not constant; on the contrary, they must vary according to the characteristics of the fracture, the region involved, and the individual. A satisfactory reduction of a finger fracture in a desk worker might be quite unsatisfactory in a musician; that suitable for an elbow which requires mobility, even at some expense in comfort and strength, might be quite unsuitable for a similar injury to the knee which, above all, should be stable and comfortable; and that which would suffice for a comminuted fracture requiring traction for maintenance of axis and length might well prove inadequate for a fracture where maintenance of position depends on secure engagement of the bone ends. Anatomical perfection may be important to the healing process, as in fractures of the femoral neck and of the carpal navicular; to function, as in fractures of the forearm, elbow, and wrist; or to the cosmetic result, as in fractures of the clavicle in women. But it is not always important to the healing of trochanteric fractures immediately adjacent to the femoral neck, or to eventual function in upper extremity fractures in a young child, or to appearance following fracture of the clavicle in a boy. The surgeon should strive, but not blindly or to the exclusion of all else, for anatomical perfection in reduction. He should individualize the criteria for a satisfactory reduction, bearing in mind that many imperfections of reduction are innocent of significant functional or cosmetic sequelae, and cannot be corrected except at a cost of considerable additional tissue damage.

Rotatory deformity must be corrected completely. Especially in fractures of the proximal radius and femur, gross rotation of one fragment on the other may pass unnoticed and produce severe disability. Angulation should always be corrected, particularly in fractures of the lower leg, forearm, or fingers, where the penalties of this deformity are greatest. Considerable latitude is permissible in the correction of displacement. Apposition of the fragments sufficient to make secure fixation mechanically feasible must be obtained or the reduction will slip, but complete apposition is not always necessary if it can be obtained only by great force and extensive additional insult to the tissues. This does not mean that the surgeon should be happy or satisfied with a sloppy, incomplete reduction, but rather that, having done his best, he will be well advised to pause and speculate whether or not a small improvement in the reduction already obtained is worth the additional damage necessary to its accomplishment.

In children. Nature exhibits a remarkable ability to correct residual fracture deformity in a growing bone. This is most marked in the very young and diminishes progressively with each passing year, so that while gross deformities may be obliterated spontaneously after fractures in children below six years of age, progressively less correction can be expected after fractures which occur in children between six and twelve years of age. The criteria for reduction of fractures in the teenage group are similar to those for adults. Rotation is the only deformity unaffected by growth: angulation is reduced and, when it accentuates a normal bony curve, often obliterated, and displacement is frequently obliterated completely. Bone growth is stimulated temporarily by a metaphyseal fracture so that even shortening may be corrected and, in fact, certain fractures of the shaft of the femur in young children have a more normal result if immobilized with the fragments unapposed and overriding. Consequently, although derotation is imperative, and correction of angular deformities desirable in all cases, restoration of normal length and apposition of the broken ends of the bone assume significance in the criteria for reduction only in proportion to the age of the child.

A displaced epiphysis should be manipulated with great care. In contrast to the temporary acceleration of growth stimulated by a metaphyseal fracture, epiphyseal injuries may result in temporary retardation or complete cessation of growth. The penalties of these complications are greatest in the very young, and diminish in severity with increasing age. Certain types of epiphyseal injuries are thought to be more conducive to subsequent growth disturbance than others, but any mechanical classification is an undependable index of the risk involved in an individual case. Frequently an epiphyseal injury, quite without displacement, will be followed by some growth disturbance. In all epiphyseal injuries, the parents of the child should be warned of the possibility of later growth disturbance, reassured that corrective measures are available, and urged to return for roentgen examinations at appropriate intervals for the following two years.

The risk of growth disturbance is largely proportional to the total damage inflicted upon the epiphyseal plate by the displacing injury and the corrective manipulations. Operative reduction and direct handling of the cartilaginous epiphyseal plate is almost always followed by premature epiphyseal closure. This is not always an indictment of operative reduction, per se, since this method is not often used except after repeated unsuccessful (and traumatic) manipulations. Nevertheless, operative reduction is strongly contraindicated, except when the advantages to be gained are sufficiently important to counterbalance the disadvantages of premature epiphyseal closure. On the other hand, in children under eight years of age gross residual displacement of an injured epiphysis is to be preferred to some improvement in position gained by force. Gradual, and virtually complete, spontaneous correction can be expected during the following two years, even if the fragments are left with 50 per cent or less apposition. With each additional year of age thereafter, the necessity for anatomical reduction increases and the penalty of growth disturbance progressively decreases.

In short, the risk and severity of deformity and malfunction due to growth disturbance resulting from accidental and therapeutic damage to the epiphyseal plate is greater than that resulting from incomplete reduction of a displaced epiphysis below the age of six to eight years. Thereafter, this risk ratio is progressively reversed, so that after the age of twelve years epiphyseal involvement seldom should influence fracture treatment. The standard of reduction in a young child is the best position that can be obtained without force; with increasing age anatomical perfection progressively becomes a dominant criterion of reduction.

EXTERNAL FIXATION

To immobilize is to make immobile or immovable. The most efficient external splint produces only relative immobility of the fracture or intact skeleton.

It is an almost universal misconception that when a limb is fixed in splints or circular plaster of paris dressings the bones or bone fragments are immobilized. This is not true. The involved bones, joints, or bone fragments continue to move in response to their muscle motors, through a range roughly proportional to the thickness of flesh between the supposedly immobilized skeleton and the external dressing. Those who may be skeptical that this is true need but to wear a snug circular plaster dressing for 24 hours to be convinced. Therefore, the surgeon must accept that what he clinically calls "external immobilization" provides merely a relative immobility of the bone fragments.

The foregoing misconception is compatible with another common misconception, that immobility of the fracture fragments is necessary to the process of bone repair. It is clear that an injured bone heals by the same process as any other wound, except for the superimposed phenomena of osteogenesis. It is equally clear that motion, within certain limits, does not deter and may increase new bone formation. Virtually all clinical studies of wound healing have been carried out on wounds of the abdominal wall, which moves with each respiration. From the viewpoint of healing, the patient with a belly wound must be allowed to breathe, but should be prevented from coughing or sneezing; the tissues at a fracture site should also be allowed to breathe and carry on with stress-free physiological functions, but they must be protected from motions sudden or extensive enough to disrupt the healing process. In clinical practice absolute immobility has seemed to be essential to the bone healing process only in a few specific fractures: notably, certain fractures of the femoral neck, scaphoid, and astragalus. In short, the repair of fractures in man is no more dependent upon absolute immobility than it is in the remainder of the animal world. Nature will not be denied. The great majority of fractures would unite spontaneously without treatment, but history reveals that such unions are attended by gross deformities and functional defects due to malposition of the fragments.

Undoubtedly the relative immobility provided by a plaster of paris dressing is beneficial to tissue healing by prevention of motions which might disrupt the orderly process of repair by granulations, frequently essential to maintenance of a reduced position of the fracture fragments until healing has occurred, but such immobility is invariably harmful to healing by perpetuation of vascular stasis, and to the uninjured regional structures by obliteration or reduction of their normal functions. Plaster of paris dressings serve many purposes: Traction, as in the "hanging plaster" treatment of humeral shaft fractures; protection against re-injury, as in recently healed long bone fractures in an active child; rest and comfort, as in certain soft tissue injuries; psychological and economic occupation, through enabling the patient to return to work, as by use of a walking plaster boot for incompletely healed fractures of the ankle and leg; fixation, to promote bone healing in selected fractures; and maintenance of adequate functional position of the fracture fragments during the healing process. The treatment of a reduced fracture, therefore, is not merely "to wrap the limb in a plaster of paris encasement and leave it there until healed," which in many instances would produce more disastrous results than complete neglect of the original injury. External fixation should not be used unless the surgeon first determines that it will do more good than harm, and then it should be used only in such a way that it will do the most good and the least harm. This means that he must decide first *why* a plaster dressing is needed; second, if the benefits to be derived are sufficient to counterbalance the deleterious effects of abolition of function; third, the minimum extent of the plaster dressing compatible with the objectives in view; and, fourth, the earliest date at which he will probably be able safely to begin reducing the invariable disadvantages of this method of treatment. The old adage that both the joint above and that below a fracture must be immobilized is, more often than not, invalid; the optimum extent of a plaster dressing is that which will accomplish its necessary objectives with a minimum of interference with continued function of the uninjured regional structures.

Plaster of Paris Fixation

Bandages impregnated with plaster of paris are the materials almost universally used for the external fixation of fractures. Dressings of any size or shape can be applied and molded to the contours of the injured area while the plaster is wet. The plaster dries and hardens within minutes and, if properly constructed, will then remain rigid. There are four common technical variants in the use of plaster for fracture treatment: With or without padding, and as a splint or a circular encasement.

The use of padding under a plaster dressing leaves room for swelling, reduces the necessity for precise molding of the plaster to the contours of the body, somewhat reduces the risk of pressure sores at bony prominences, and increases the thickness of compressible elements between the bone and the plaster. In other words, a padded plaster can be applied with a minimum of skill and precision, gives the surgeon a sense of security against an increase in swelling, does not touch, much less hold firmly and securely, the injured part, and, when swelling subsides, becomes even more loose and ineffectual. Yet such a dressing is often termed "immobilization"!

An unpadded plaster must be applied with precision, and be molded accurately to every detail of the body contour. It is skin tight and, therefore, must present a smooth and even surface against the skin. It leaves no room for increased swelling and must be carefully supervised. But, despite the necessity that it must be applied with skill and watched carefully until the risk of swelling has passed, an unpadded plaster provides the maximum fracture fixation possible by any form of external dressing. It may be applied directly to the skin or over a layer of stockinet, after all bony prominences have been adequately protected (Fig. 2–*4*).

A circular plaster encases the injured part completely, allows no latitude for an increase or subsidence of swelling, is stronger and more enduring than splints, requires minimum supervision after the danger from swelling has passed, and must be removed completely or not at all. Small angular deformities can be corrected by cutting and bending the plaster cylinder in the desired direction, and then repairing the defect with an additional wipe of plaster, but other alterations of reduction cannot be

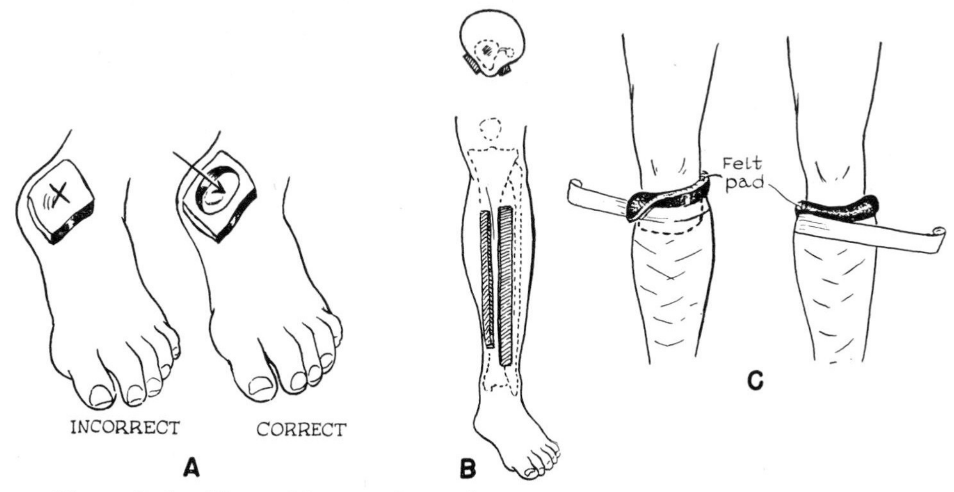

Figure 2–4. The padding of plaster dressings.

A. Pointed bony prominences cannot be effectively protected by a solid pad, which does not alter the production of maximum pressure over the point of the prominence. The pad should be cut out to prevent pressure over this point.

B. Subcutaneous bony ridges should be protected by a long pad applied at either side of the bone edge.

C. The proximal and distal ends of a plaster dressing should be covered by a smooth pad.

made unless the plaster encasement is completely removed and a new one applied. Immediately after application a circular plaster should be cut longitudinally from end to end, so that it may be spread open easily and quickly at the first sign of circulatory embarrassment. Skin should be visible throughout the entire length of this split. Consequently, the surgeon who elects to use a circular plaster following reduction of a fracture treads on very thin ice. Constant surveillance of the circulation distal to the plaster is mandatory until swelling subsides, and he may have to remove the plaster and start treatment anew for a variety of reasons.

Plaster splints provide external fixation almost equal in security to that provided by circular plaster dressings for extremity fractures distal to the knee and shoulder. A splint is not as strong nor will it stand as much abuse as a circular plaster dressing. However, a splint can be loosened or tightened easily and quickly to compensate for an increase or subsidence of swelling, and can be removed and replaced with a minimum risk of losing the reduction obtained. Moreover, after swelling has subsided, the cloth bandages which bind a splint in place can be replaced by wet plaster of paris bandages, which changes the splint fixation to a circular plaster encasement, without the injured area being handled directly, or the risk of loss of reduction being incurred.

Unpadded plaster dressings provide maximum comfort and fixation, and should be used in all phases of fracture treatment. The circulation distal to all plaster dressings of any type must be assessed at frequent intervals until the reaction of swelling has passed. The trauma of manipulative reduction superimposed upon that produced by the injury invariably results in increased swelling at the injured area after fixation dressings have been applied. For this reason a circular plaster encasement is a precarious device until the size of the injured area becomes fairly stationary. Early fixation by adequate plaster splints, molded to the limb and bound in place by cloth or elastic bandages, is safe and equally secure. Subsequent swelling which increases the size of the limb is accommodated by rebandaging in accordance with the increase in swelling. As swelling eventually commences to subside, the bandages are tightened. Meanwhile the plaster splint or splints have remained in place. Fixation is thus maintained coincident with accommodation for the inevitable increase and decrease in circumference of the injured area. When the stage of swelling has passed it is permissible and safe to transform the splints into a circular plaster encasement by rewrapping with plaster of paris bandages.

CONTINUOUS TRACTION

When a fracture is transverse or the fragments can be engaged securely, traction may safely be released after the bone ends are replaced in apposition, but when the fracture is oblique or comminuted continuous traction is necessary to preserve the reduction. Skin traction (Fig. 2–5) should be reserved for situations where not more than a few pounds of pulling force are required and, with few exceptions, is unsatisfactory for the treatment of fractures of large long bones. Continuous traction in excess of 5 pounds should be applied through the bones. The traction force may

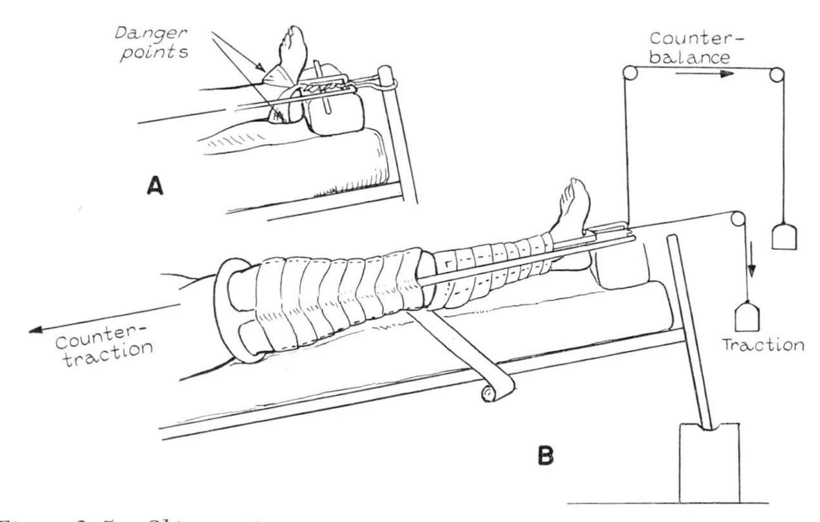

Figure 2–5. Skin traction.

A. Temporary skin traction may be provided by fastening the windlass to the foot of the bed or litter, which is then raised sufficiently so that body weight, pulling to the head of the bed, maintains a constant pull.

B. Permanent skin traction should be used only when not more than 5 pounds of pull is required. The stabilizing splint may be suspended by a counterbalance or rested upon a block. Countertraction is by gravity. The heel must be kept off the bed.

then be adjusted according to the strength of the muscles to be overcome, without risk to the skin or the apparatus. Normal bone length regained at the time of reduction may thus be maintained, but concomitant rotation, angulation, and displacement deformities must be managed simultaneously by other devices. Continuous traction is an adjuvant to the maintenance of an unstable reduction, *is not a method of reduction,* and serves but three purposes in the treatment of fractures:

(1) reduction of pain and muscle spasm;
(2) restoration of length;
(3) maintenance of length.

Reduction of pain and muscle spasm is important during the interval between admission of the patient and reduction of a long bone fracture. Control of pain is desirable in all cases. Release of spasm is especially important when the long muscles spanning a fracture have decreased the length of the bone. Spasm subsides steadily, and often disappears as the muscles tire and stretch in submission to continuous steady traction. Concurrently, relief of pain more potent and lasting than can be obtained by narcotics is the rule, overriding or telescoping of the bone fragments is reduced, the eventual reduction is facilitated, and the total tissue insult is minimized. Whenever the reduction of a spiral, comminuted, or overriding long bone fracture must be delayed for more than a short time some form of temporary continuous traction (Fig. 2–5) should be used in conjunction with stabilizing splints.

Restoration of length is an essential step preliminary to reduction. Delayed reduction finds a fractured long bone shortened. The primary cause was muscle spasm, but secondary fixation by organization of all the contracted soft tissues soon supervenes. Length cannot be restored by manual traction and manipulation without inflicting considerable additional damage upon these "jelled" tissues. Under such circumstances, since the benefits of an early reduction have already been lost, it is often advisable to apply continuous skeletal traction (Fig 2–6) for a period of 36 to 60 hours in an effort to stretch the contracted soft parts gradually before manipulation is carried out.

Maintenance of length is necessary to the integrity of the reduction in most spiral, comminuted, and unstable fractures. A skeletal traction device should be applied prior to manipulation, and activated immediately following reduction. How many pounds of force should be applied? The muscle forces to be overcome can only be estimated. Excessive traction is a factor commonly associated with nonunion. Paradoxically, underestimation of the traction force required is the most common error attending this form of treatment, and leads to a stereotyped sequence of mishaps. Roentgenograms reveal incomplete bone length, so the inadequate traction force is increased and new films are ordered for the next day. These show a little improvement and the traction is again increased. Bit by bit, as the days pass, the traction force is increased until it approaches proportions threatening to pull the patient out of the bed, but bone length is still incomplete. Organization of the tissues has kept pace with and nullified the effects of gradually increased traction, and the remaining alternatives

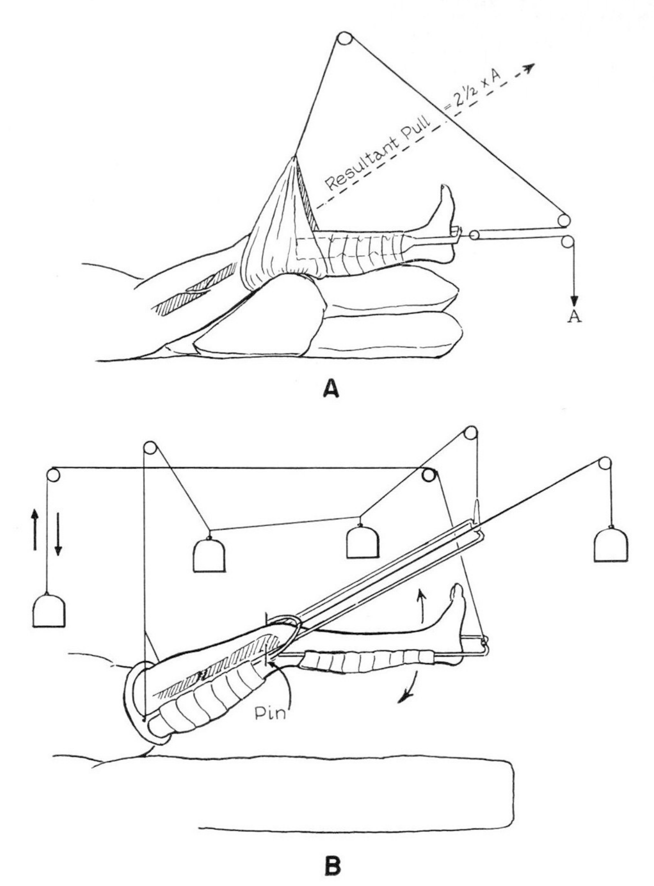

Figure 2–6. Other methods of traction.

A. Russell traction. A useful method for stabilization and maintenance of length and alignment of a lower extremity with a fracture of the femur when skeletal traction is contraindicated or undesirable.

B. Skeletal traction. The leg is suspended in the hammock formed by a Thomas splint and a Pearson low-leg attachment. Traction is applied through a pin transfixing the lower end of the femur. Some knee motion can be maintained.

are limited to an acceptance of malunion or operative intervention. The primary traction force applied should be generously in excess of that estimated to be necessary. Roentgen examination should be done *immediately,* after which the traction is reduced sufficiently to eliminate any distraction of the fragments revealed in the films. When roentgenography and subsequent reduction of traction is delayed until the next day, or longer, distraction is likely to persist, and delayed or fibrous union of the fracture may be feared.

FIXED SKELETAL TRACTION

Technically adequate fixed traction produces true immobility of a fracture. Impugning the concept that immobility is necessary to good fracture healing, and that mobility is the essential culprit in nonunion, it is an interesting clinical fact that a failure of union is no more uncommon to this method of treatment than to any other, whether or not the fragments are distracted by the traction.

The bone is transfixed with stiff stainless steel pins or Kirschner wires, proximal and distal to the fracture. Their eventual immobilizing effect is maximal when the main fracture fragments are transfixed, but when the injury is close to a joint it is necessary to utilize some more distant intact bone as a point of traction (Fig. 2–7). The projecting ends of these pins are virtual external "handles," by which the fragments can be manipulated, and the length of the bone restored manually during reduction and maintained exactly thereafter by incorporating the projecting pins into a circular plaster of paris case (Fig. 2–7, *D*).

Various mechanical pin-holding devices have been designed to substitute for plaster of paris in the treatment of fractures by external pin fixation. None are as safe, simple, or secure as plaster of paris.

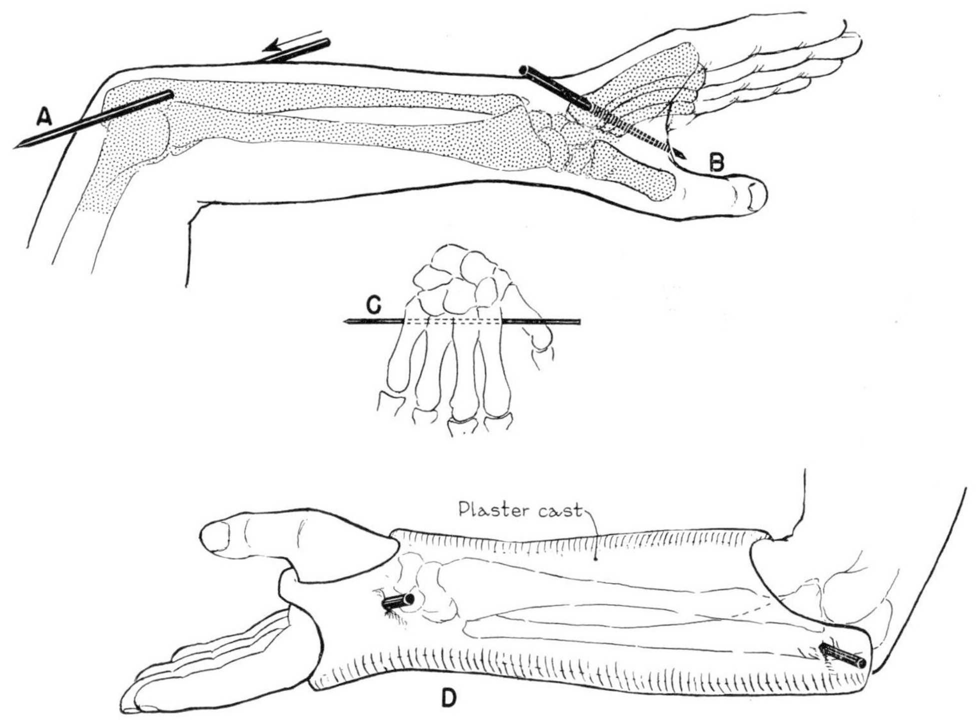

Figure 2–7. Fixed traction.

A. One pin is inserted through the olecranon from the medial side (with care not to injure the ulnar nerve).

B. A second pin is inserted through the metacarpal bases from metacarpal 2 through 5.

C. The distal pin must pass through the metacarpal bases, and not the shafts. In this way the intermetacarpal structures are not jeopardized, and insertion of the pin is simplified.

D. After the fracture is reduced the transfixion pins are incorporated in a circular plaster dressing. A fixed length between the pins prevents collapse of unstable fractures within the plaster dressing.

OPEN REDUCTION AND INTERNAL FIXATION

Every surgeon uses the internal fixation of the soft tissues when treating a fracture. The "fallacies" of implanted internal fixation are not of the method, but of the surgeon who abuses it.

The question of operative fixation of fractures has remained fraught with more dogmatism and controversy than almost any other surgical procedure. That the process of bone repair is still an enigma precluding certain substantiation or rebuttal of adverse postulates creates a fertile field for dogmatism, and most of the common controversies have been illusional or without common grounds for dispute.

The Materials of Internal Fixation

The ideal material for internal fixation will be completely inert to the chemistry of the body fluids, light in weight and small in volume, strong and tough, yet possessed of a resilience to resist prolonged fatigue strain. It is not yet available. The alloy Vitallium, and 18 and 8 SMO stainless steel are in common use. The alloy is chemically more inert, but by clinical comparison it is neither as tough nor as resilient as stainless steel. Both are satisfactory, except when misused. The two complications commonly ascribed to the materials of internal fixation, breakage and tissue reaction, depend much more upon the technique of application than upon metallurgical considerations. The screw that is not plumb or is overtightened until the bone thread is stripped, the plate poorly fitted to the contour of the bone or too short for its intended task, the tight wire suture that produces necrosis, the loose intramedullary device, or any of the innumerable other technical defects which promote concentration rather than dispersion of stress are the usual causes for breakage of fixation and absorption of bone. Electrolytic destruction of bone is an insignificant clinical factor when Vitallium or 18 and 8 SMO stainless steel internal fixation devices are applied with precision and the load to be carried is adequately distributed.

The Amount of Internal Fixation: "Internal Suture or Rigid Fixation"

Should the amount of internal fixation be the least that will approximate the bone ends until a plaster of paris dressing can be applied, or enough to obviate or minimize the need for supplemental external immobilization? The truth of the matter is that there is a very definite place for each method in the internal fixation of fractures.

Internal fixation by necessity is "to make the best of a bad job that could not be done at all by other methods." Secure internal fixation may be impossible, and supplemental external immobilization is then mandatory. Under these conditions necessity demands acceptance of both the operative risk and the penalties of immobilization, and it would be illogical to implant more than the least amount of fixation necessary to appose the bone ends. But no such double jeopardy is justified in the fracture that is internally fixed by election. Elective internal fixation accepts the calculated operative risk in return for a reduction of morbidity and disability time. In these circumstances a sufficient amount of fixation to obviate or minimize the need for external splints is a good clinical bargain because, unless function can be maintained throughout the healing period, such an operation is a failure. There is no doubt that secure and rigid internal fixation most closely approaches the hypothetical ideal of fracture treatment, but it is equally clear that when secure internal fixation cannot be obtained, the less foreign material implanted the better.

The selection of the type and amount of internal fixation to be used must depend upon the mechanical problems presented by the fracture and the objectives of the surgeon. A decision between "rigid fixation" and "internal suture" must be made. Internal suture should generally be elected, except when it appears possible to obtain fixation rigid and secure enough to obviate or minimize the need for supplemental external immobilization. An adequate internal suture is the least amount of internal fixation that will maintain apposition of the bone ends until a plaster dressing has been applied. Thereafter the internal fixation supplements the external immobilization. Adequate rigid fixation entails the insertion of as much internal fixation as is necessary to obviate the need for supplemental external immobilization. The surgeon cannot occupy a middle ground between the two without courting disaster—his internal fixation must be one or the other.

Contact Compression and the Slotted Plate

Distraction is detrimental to bone repair. Is compression beneficial? A small amount of compression augments engagement and approximation of the bone ends. Eggers found that membranous bone in rats healed more rapidly when influenced by elastic compression forces. Charnley reported accelerated union of human cancellous bone under controlled turnbuckle compression. The case for any influence of compression on cortical bone repair has not been documented. Nevertheless these conclusions from spongy bone experiments have been widely applied to the internal fixation of long (cortical) bone fractures. Slotted plates are utilized to accommodate a concept that, unless internal fixation allows the bone ends to remain compressible by muscle tone, a gap due to bone absorption, and becoming the equivalent of distraction, will develop at the fracture site. The use of a plate is usually justified only in an attempt to secure rigid fixation. When a slotted plate is molded to the contour of a bone and fastened securely in place with screws no further compression by muscle forces is possible; or, if it is fastened loosely enough to permit compression, the fixation is loose and insecure. There are but three common causes for a gap between the fragments of an internally fixed fractured bone—infection, motion at the fracture, and fixation in distraction. Success or failure depends not on the type of plate but upon the manner of its application.

Reconciliation of Internal Fixation and Basic Principles

Fundamentally, open reduction and internal fixation is consonant with the principles of fracture treatment. Carried out with gentle and precise dissection operative reduction inflicts much less additional tissue damage than any form of manipulation; internal fixation provides more certain and secure support of the fractured bone than any external device; and a maximum maintenance of function is made possible throughout the healing period. But these postulates are valid only when the case is properly selected and the treatment is well done, and the penalties of an error in judgment, of a defect in technique, or of infection following the operation are so great that stringent limitations are placed upon the use of this method of treatment; it should be employed only by an experienced and competent surgeon, in an immaculate surgical environment, and when the indications are unassailable.

Indications for Internal Fixation

Internal fixation is warranted in only a small percentage of all fractures. The indications are clear and simple. Open reduction and internal fixation may be required by absolute necessity, justified by relative necessity, or occasionally be permissible as a method of choice.

Absolute necessity exists only to save life, or when reduction cannot be obtained or maintained by any other method.

Relative necessity applies when this method promises a more rapid, certain, or better result than seems possible by any other method, obviates some serious disadvantage of other methods, or facilitates necessary treatment of concomitant injuries or disease.

As a method of choice operative fixation may be permissible when, as a calculated risk under ideal circumstances, it promises a reduction of morbidity and disability time sufficient to neutralize the risk involved.

Conditions Necessary to Open Reduction

To be safe and satisfactory, the operative treatment of fractures must be a strict and specialized discipline, for the penalties of failure are much more serious than those of no treatment at all. The implantation of foreign fixation material is always potentially harmful, and results in a net benefit only when applied with precision and mechanical perfection. Natural defenses against infection, such as are operative in surgical procedures on organs in the peritoneal or pleural cavities or on undamaged tissues with a normal circulation, do not exist. The tissues at the site of a fracture are dead or damaged and, if viable, are depleted in resistance by circulatory stagnation and hypoxia. The surgeon who dares to inoculate such an ideal bacterial pabulum must, indeed, have a good reason for doing so, and then must proceed only under stringent conditions. These require the following:

Maturity of surgical judgment to select quickly and with certainty the fractures which require operation. To attempt several other methods of treatment unsuccessfully and finally turn to operation as a last resort indicates one of two conditions—either failure to recognize primarily the necessity for operation, or admission of a risk from operation in the hands of the surgeon involved sufficient to mandate exhaustion of all possible nonoperative methods prior to its acceptance. Either alternative reflects surgical circumstances unfitted for the most exacting, difficult, and dangerous of all methods of treatment. The need for operation is recognizable immediately, or at least after the first failure of nonoperative treatment. Repeated failures and delays inevitably and progressively reduce the prospects for a successful result by any final method of treatment.

Surgical adaptability, so that the surgeon may, at a moment's notice, alter his plans and procedure to fit unexpected mechanical and anatomical problems. The exposure of a displaced fracture is not an exercise that can be learned by rote, for the anatomical structures are in bizarre and distorted positions. The preoperative roentgenograms tell only a part of the story of a fracture, and the surgeon must be prepared to deal with unexpected mechanical problems rather than persist in some rigidly preconceived plan of procedure. Above all, he should not attempt to make the fracture fit a favorite form of internal fixation but, conversely, he should tailor the fixation to the individual mechanical requirements of the problem at hand.

Surgical competence and a mechanical bent. Surgical skill is not enough. In all humility the great majority of surgeons must realize that, except for the surgical technique required, any good carpenter would do a much better job of internal fixation than is ordinarily accomplished.

An armamentarium of specialized tools for holding and immobilizing bone fragments. The carpenter can leave his job until he obtains the special tool necessary to meeting an unexpected problem, but the surgeon must complete his task as best he can with what he has. The result of a missing tool is invariably a makeshift job, less well done than it could have been. To operate upon a fractured bone without an adequate assortment of bone instruments is as inexcusable as attempting to do an arterial anastomosis without rubber-shod clamps.

Inviolate aseptic technique by the operating team, with equal care exercised in the packing and sterilization of the drapes, sponges, and sutures, or the preparation of the theater for operation. Defects in these disciplines may carry penalties as great as defects in the operation itself. Consequently, open reduction of a fracture is unjustifiable, except in a surgical environment that is beyond reproach in every detail. Adequate surgical and nursing assistance is important, but the surgical technique promulgated by Arbuthnot Lane, in which none of the surgical team ever touched the tissues or any portion of an instrument that entered the wound, is outmoded by the facts of current surgical life. This technique was designed to promote the utmost in asepsis, and was an important factor in reducing the incidence of infections in an era when surgical technique and asepsis were in their infancy. Great advances have been made since the time of Lane, and there are now few instructors qualified in his discipline, fewer hospitals where it is practiced, and almost no surgeons who spend enough continuous training time in the surgery of trauma to become proficient in its use. Ordinary surgical technique which measures up to modern standards is adequate for the operative treatment of fractures. Surgical skill and competence are but two of the factors essential to success. Unless all the preceding requirements can be satisfied fully, open reduction and internal fixation cannot be justified, except by urgent and absolute necessity.

The Timing of Open Reduction

The tissues at a fracture site are in optimal condition to withstand the insult of an operation at the moment of injury, and deteriorate inexorably for several days thereafter. They are at their worst between the third and the sixth day following injury. Operation should be carried out as soon as possible, or deferred until the tissue tension and acute inflammatory reaction have subsided. That delay is sometimes unavoidable does not detract from the import of these facts, and there can be no valid excuse for any unnecessary delay. Multiple preparations of the skin may cleanse more thoroughly than one, but consume a period during which the tissues become tense, edematous, devitalized, hypoxic, and progressively depleted of their natural resistance against infection. Delay, pending resuscitation from profound shock or the management of concomitant, more critical injuries, is often necessary, but reduction and fixation of a fracture is often the single measure most effective for the control of impending or established shock. At times the indications for operative reduction are not recognizable until after an unsuccessful manipulation. Otherwise, given an adequate anesthetic risk, skin that can be cleansed, and shock that can be controlled, open reduction and internal fixation, when indicated, should be carried out at the earliest possible moment.

Technique of Open Reduction and Internal Fixation

Fundamental surgical principles apply to this, as to any other operation—precise dissection, gentle handling of all tissues including the bone, complete hemostasis, excision of dead tissue, avoidance of dead space, and closure without tension. Only the first two principles, however, can be followed consistently. Blood will ooze from every lacerated surface so that complete hemostasis is impossible. Dead and damaged tissue abounds throughout the entire fracture region, and not more than a small portion of the total amount can be removed. Accumulating hemorrhagic ooze and tissue fluid create a dead space filled with hematoma at every point where tissues were separated from bone by the injury or by the surgeon. Wound closure without tension is possible only prior to the onset of swelling, after which tension supervenes in any event. A snug layer-by-layer closure suitable for a surgical wound of healthy tissues should not be done lest increasing tension develop within the deep tissue planes and cause expansion at the expense of all compressible tissues. Tissue layers and skin edges should be approximated, but loosely enough to allow the escape of blood and tissue fluids during the critical hours following operation. The temptation to carry out a snug cell-to-cell closure of tissue layers and skin over a fracture must be tempered by the realization that virtually all infections in clean fracture surgery commence in the nidus of a locked-in hematoma.

AFTERCARE OF FRACTURES

The first week after fracture reduction is a period of increasing swelling, during which the danger from loss of position and soft tissue complications is most pronounced. Immediately after reaction from anesthesia has occurred, the integrity of the circulation and peripheral nerves distal to the immobilizing dressing should be verified. Roentgenograms confirming the reduction should be taken after recovery from the anesthetic reactivates the tone of the muscles in the injured region. The use of a circular plaster dressing, or any uncertainty concerning the circulatory status of the injured part, requires that the patient be kept under close surveillance for several days, or until the dangers from circulatory embarrassment no longer exist. When splints are applied the original gauze bandages used to bind them in place must be removed and replaced after the plaster has set. Otherwise the first bandages, wet by the spillage of plaster from the splints which they encircle, harden and become the equivalent of a circular plaster.

No patient should be allowed out of sight, even overnight, without specific instructions to return immediately at the first indication of white, blue, cold, or insensitive fingers or toes distal to the immobilizing dressing. He should also be instructed to return if severe and intractable pain supervenes, for a well reduced and immobilized fracture should not produce severe symptoms, and non-localized increasing pain usually signals increased tissue tension worthy of release. A constant and localized burning pain usually is indicative of a pressure point under the plaster dressing or by a constrictive bandage. It should be investigated and decompressed immediately because, once the over-compressed tissues commence to necrose, they also become relatively insensitive. A large and deep "pressure sore" may then develop silently and remain unrecognized until its telltale exudate seeps through and stains the plaster.

Advice concerning elevation of the injured part should be coupled with detailed instructions in finger or toe exercises to be carried out for short periods at frequent intervals. It should be explained in simple language that swelling constitutes the immediate danger; that the cause of swelling is an accumulation of fluid which flows best down hill, and hence the rationale for elevation; that, with each motion of the fingers or toes, muscles pump some of this fluid back where it belongs; and that failure to reactivate these muscle pumps will retard the rate of recovery and jeopardize the final result. It may also be threatened, and with justification, that undue delay in muscle reactivation will allow the accumulated blood and fluid to clot and jell, and to create adhesions between moving structures that may require many months of tedious stretching exercises before motion can be regained. This is the surgeon's opportunity to establish and explain his treatment. He should outline the projected plan of treatment, explain its rationale and objectives, delineate the patient's responsibilities and emphasize their importance, and establish a rapport ensuring mutual confidence and cooperation.

The site of injury should be re-examined the day after reduction, and the immobilizing dressing checked for comfort, efficiency, and absence of constriction or unwanted pressure. From time to time, until tissue swelling has passed its peak, splints may have to be rebandaged less tightly, or the longitudinal split in a circular cast spread open for decompression of the tissues. As swelling recedes splints should be rebandaged more securely, or a loose circular splint be replaced for continued efficiency of fixation. The frequency of re-examination must be dictated by circumstances, and the injury never should be allowed to remain unchecked except for periods during which the surgeon is sure that all will remain in order.

Progressively, with subsidence of pain, exercises and as much normal use as is safe and possible should be encouraged for all unencumbered joints. The treatment of a Colles fracture may be carried out to local perfection, but unless the unimmobilized joints of the limb are kept mobile during the period of active treatment, subsequent intractable pain and stiffness in the shoulder may produce a disability that will make the wrist injury seem trivial by comparison.

Roentgen examinations must be carried out at appropriate intervals; during the early stages to document the integrity of the reduction, and later, the state of repair. Roentgenograms, however, often give false evidence concerning the strength of union. Especially in long bone (cortical) fractures, roentgen evidence of complete consolidation lags many months behind clinical union adequate for a resumption of function. The complete absence of tenderness on pressure and of pain on leverage, shearing, and torque stresses at a fracture is evidence of sound clinical union. Assessment of the progress of repair should be based upon combined roentgen and clinical evidence, and that of the roentgenograms should not be allowed to outweigh common sense and sound clinical judgment. Above all, roentgenographic appearance cannot be accepted as the sole reason for indefinite continuance of plaster immobilization, as in one patient with fracture of the tibia encountered by the writer, who had remained in a groin-high circular plaster dressing, reapplied every few months to maintain efficiency, for more than seven years. The surgeon who ruined this patient emotionally, economically, and physically, had been taught that fractures must be firmly immobilized until they were healed, and that the cause of nonunion was too early cessation of immobilization. He had learned his lesson so well that common sense was obliterated by dogma.

Fractures heal rapidly in children, who are virtually impervious to the penalties of immobilization; such injuries heal more slowly in adults, who must also pay heavy penalties for a temporary abolition of function. As a general rule, therefore, the long bone fracture in a child may be immobilized until abundant callus is present, and then for a generous additional period during which the union becomes seasoned and strong. If splints are removed as soon as roentgen evidence of union is present, childhood proclivities to re-injury frequently result in refracture. The average adult, on the other hand, usually can be delegated responsibility to spare and voluntarily protect his injured part. As his repair progresses there is often a steady reduction in the extent of immobilization necessary to adequate stabilization of the healing fracture. When these circumstances obtain, the extent of the external immobilization should be reduced at intervals, in accord with the increasing stability provided by continuing repair. Immobilizing casts often may be replaced by removable protective splints, and a gradual resumption of gentle motion and function commenced prior to the advent of complete consolidation of the fracture. The recovery of function in a child bears little relation to the duration of immobilization, but the rate and quality of recovery in an adult is constantly and inversely proportional to the amount and duration of abolition of function.

REHABILITATION

What a tormented and abused word is rehabilitation! Webster defines it as "to restore to former capacity." The goal of fracture treatment has been defined earlier in this chapter as "a return to usual activities as soon and to as nearly normal an extent as possible." Obviously, treatment and rehabilitation are synonymous, yet the latter has been so clothed in trite slogans as to suggest that the two are separate divisions of medicine. It is time for the surgeon to realize that the development of specialized physiatrists and of formal rehabilitation centers was necessitated by his own therapeutic inadequacies. Except for vocational retraining and reeducation aimed at compensation for the loss of some physical structure or physiological function, the principal problem of modern physiatry is to overcome unnecessary therapeutic errors of omission or commission, and the patients in most large rehabilitation institutes constitute in large part a sad commentary upon current standards in the treatment of trauma. The circumstances peculiar to military medicine may justify mass rehabilitation of injured personnel as a separate effort but, with few exceptions, the civilian fracture patient who requires a separate rehabilitation program before he recovers either has been mistreated or overtreated, or has a doctor who is no longer interested in his problem. Rehabilitation should be the responsibility of the surgeon; retraining, the responsibility of the physiatrist.

Recovery after treatment of an uncomplicated fracture by the family physician may not be quite as perfect as could be obtained by a specialist, but the patient seldom requires formal rehabilitation by a separate agency. The family physician has many advantages over the specialist. He is not only a doctor, but a friend—a friend who knows the patient, his temperament, his job, his weaknesses and strengths, his family, his problems, and often his innermost hopes and fears; in addition, the family physician is unencumbered by a burden of specialized scientific knowledge that may limit his horizon to the joint above the fracture. The patient comes to the specialist as a stranger to a strange place, to entrust his paramount problems to a stranger. If the specialist is first a doctor, and second a skilled technician, he will at once take steps to obtain all pertinent information, and integrate therapy with the problems of the individual, as well as of the fracture. But many a specialist has never learned to be a doctor, and to his ilk the patient and his problems may be little more than a bothersome appendage to an interesting scientific problem. Ignorance in the art of medicine shares equally with defective treatment in the production of candidates for separate rehabilitation therapy after the completion of active treatment. Watson-Jones aptly and succinctly epitomized this unfortunate fact by a quotation from Plato which is truly germane to the modern practice of surgery: "This is the greatest error in the treatment of sickness, that there are physicians for the body and physicians for the soul, and yet the two are one and indivisible."

PRINCIPLES OF TREATMENT OF OPEN FRACTURES

An open (formerly called "compound") fracture is distinguished from its closed (formerly "simple") counterpart by a wound through which the fracture site communicates with the skin surface. This situation is attended by peculiar clinical implications unrelated to the size or cause of the break in the skin. Normal skin is host to a multitude of organisms, but is also an impenetrable barrier against their entry into the deeper tissues. A fracture associated with any break in this barrier is contaminated or infected. Treatment is complicated by the simultaneous and sometimes conflicting demands of shock, infection, and fracture. Shock requires supportive treatment and may dictate a delay in other active measures. Potential or established infection cries for early wound excision or drainage. The fracture needs reduction and fixation. All these measures must be provided, but each in a way that will not jeopardize a successful outcome of the others.

During the first few hours after injury an open fracture is contaminated. Organisms have entered through the wound to infest the fracture hematoma and settle on the lacerated tissue surfaces. In this environment, nurtured by an ideal pabulum, they multiply rapidly and, within a few hours after injury, commence to invade the tissues. During the contaminated phase the wound can be cleansed, but after tissue invasion commences the wound is infected. Surgical removal of invasive infection is impossible, and each stroke of a scalpel or manipulation of the bone fragments opens many new channels for the invading organisms. During the contaminated phase, invasive infection can be prevented and the fracture reduced simultaneously, but the onset of invasive infection interdicts fracture reduction and permits only the provision of adequate drainage. The duration of the contaminated phase depends upon many variables, and in the average civilian open fracture is superseded by infection between 8 and 12 hours after injury. This is the "golden period" during which shock must be stabilized, infection prevented, and the fracture reduced. *Chemotherapy and antibiotic agents will not delay the onset of invasive infection.* Operative prevention of infection by wound excision must be done early, or not at all; and fracture reduction must be done early, or delayed until the infection has subsided completely.

Wound Treatment

Debridement. The objective of debridement is to prevent infection from occurring in a contaminated wound. Obviously all bacteria cannot be removed. But, surgical wounds heal per primam even though the great majority of them house organisms that entered during the course of the operation. Primary healing occurs in these wounds because implanted organisms are destroyed before they can gain a foothold, by tissues that are viable, virile, and vascular, dry and devoid of dead spaces. Debridement prevents infection by transforming an accidental into the equivalent of a surgical wound.

The skin of the wounded region should be cleansed widely, and as scrupulously as for a clean operation. The edges of the surface wound are excised back to healthy bleeding skin. The location of the wound may dictate placement of the incision, but its size is not an index of the deep exposure required. The skin incision must be long enough to lay open the full extent of the deep tissue lacerations. Similarly, all fascial envelopes must be opened widely enough for exposure of the depths of the wound, from end to end. All dead and devitalized *unessential* tissues are ablated. All foreign bodies, with the exception of certain embedded or inaccessible missile fragments, are removed. All bleeding points are caught and ligated. The electrocautery, which produces small islands of dead tissue, should not be used for hemostasis. Lacerated fascia and muscle may be widely excised. Muscle which does not bleed when cut or twitch when pinched with a forceps is dead, and should be removed. Muscle which bleeds, but does not twitch when pinched, is alive, but should be trimmed of all lacerated ends and separated fibers. Essential structures—nerves, tendons, large vessels, and ligaments—should be cleansed mechanically; frayed areas should be trimmed economically, and the structures should be left in place. Bone fragments completely free of soft parts may be removed if they are few and small. Many small fragments, as in a shattered fracture caused by a high velocity missile, should be left in place, as well as larger fragments with some remaining soft part attachments. Decision as to the amount of bone that should be removed is often difficult. Bone is an essential structure, but a loose bone fragment becomes a sequestrum to perpetuate any infection that may occur. In general, it is better to err on the side of removing too little rather than too much. Dirty bone ends must be thoroughly cleansed, if necessary by a brush or by a curet, removing the surface from which embedded dirt cannot be removed. Adult periosteum is composed predominantly of fibrous tissue and should not be considered an essential structure. Surgical excision of the wound leaves behind many small separated particles of tissue which cannot be recognized, much less picked out and removed. The debrided wound cavity should be flushed clean by a mechanical lavage, from the depths outward, with warm saline or water.

Antibacterial measures. Tetanus antitoxin should be administered unless the patient was immunized within the preceding four years, in which event a booster dose of 1 ml. of toxoid should be given. Gas gangrene antitoxin is useful for treatment, but not for prevention of clostridial myositis. (See Chapter 3.)

Antibiotic agents do not prevent wound sepsis. They have no effect upon progressive tissue necrosis due to proteolytic enzymes, or upon the decomposition of hematoma and dead tissue into what Oscar Hampton has so aptly termed "the pabulum of sepsis." Neither can they sterilize the dead tissue in a wound. These precursors of local infection must be eradicated by wound surgery. Antibiotic therapy limits invasive infection and protects against septicemia. That it is commonly used from the start as a defense against the spread of an impending infection does not alter these facts, but this practice has done considerable harm in encouraging a widespread misconception that modern wound surgery is less important and exacting for the prevention of local infection than it was in former years. The inadequately excised wound is prone to sepsis with or without ancillary antibiotic therapy, and if a false sense of security has prompted closure of such a wound suppuration is apt to progress quietly under well-healed skin. The antibiotic protection will then limit the spread of the infection, depress the systemic signs of suppuration, and may save life; however, when a bag of pus finally becomes apparent several weeks after wounding, the limb may be lost. The prevention of wound sepsis depends upon wound treatment; control of infection upon adequate drainage supplemented by antibiotic therapy.

Fracture Treatment

The fracture fragments, which have been completely exposed in the course of wound treatment, should be reduced gently under direct vision. Fixation should be determined according to the mechanical problems of the injury and, if the wound is in satisfactory condition, should not be influenced by the possibility of sepsis. Internal fixation may be used if it is needed. This requires the implantation of foreign materials into a contaminated wound. The wound, however, already contains some unexcised dead tissues, and the ends of the bone fragments are partly dead. These are foreign bodies. It is frequently advisable to accept the theoretical disadvantages of implanting an additional, but sterile, foreign body in return for the great practical advantages of obtaining stability for those already in the wound.

Aftercare of the Wound

To close or not to close the incision is the final question requiring a decision after wound and fracture treatment has been carried out. The dangers from sepsis in a closed wound are great; in an open wound, small. An open wound, however, results in rapid death and slough of almost all exposed tissue surfaces, except fat and muscle. Antibiotic therapy does not prevent sepsis in a closed wound. Therefore, primary closure is only permissible under ideal conditions. These require a lapse of only a few hours between injury and operation, minimal tissue damage, minimal contamination, adequate wound excision, secure fracture fixation, good hemostasis, an absence of dead space, and a skin incision which can be closed without tension. Secondary, or delayed wound closure is safer and advisable in the great majority of cases. Sutures are placed at operation.

but the wound is packed open. Between the fourth and the sixth day after operation the wound is dressed under anesthesia. If sepsis is evident, the wound is left open. If the wound is healthy, the skin edges are approximated and the sutures are tied. Secondary closure prior to the fourth day after operation is unsafe, and later than the sixth or seventh day is made difficult by tissue organization. Whenever operation has been delayed more than 12 hours, or tissue damage is severe, or contamination extensive, the wound should not be closed primarily, but should be left open and closed secondarily, or allowed to granulate pending revision or coverage by skin grafts at a much later date after all damage from sepsis has abated.

Aftercare of an open fracture following wound healing should be similar to that for a closed fracture.

PRINCIPLES AND PRIORITIES IN MULTIPLE INJURIES

Accidents are steadily increasing in number, severity, and multiplicity, but with improved transportation the time lag between injury and treatment is steadily diminishing. A progressively increasing number of patients with multiple injuries are surviving the trip to a hospital, where they present the most exacting demands upon its facilities and upon the judgment, competence, and cooperation of its staff. The problem is to provide the precisely planned and integrated sequence of diversified, and sometimes conflicting, treatments necessary to survival of the patient with several severe injuries. Adequate treatment requires the services of several surgeons. They must be a harmonious team, with all members prepared to play their assigned roles under direction, for without someone to hold the reins their efforts will be conflicting and futile. Specialists may assume temporary control when and while the immediate problem falls within their respective jurisdictions, but the authority and responsibility for the over-all continuity of care should be invested in one individual.

Oxygen Supply: The Airway and the Pulmonary Pump

The airway must remain patent. A lateral recumbent position, with the head slightly lowered and turned to the side, usually prevents blockage by retroversion of the tongue or aspiration of vomitus. The constant attention of a nurse, and availability of an automatic suction device, is usually necessary for the removal of mucus as it accumulates. The time to do a tracheostomy, especially in the presence of a maxillofacial injury, is as soon as it is thought that this *may* be necessary. (See Chapter 18.)

A clear airway is not enough. Oxygen must be pumped into the pulmonary alveoli before it can be taken into the blood. Thoracic trauma may influence this transport of air adversely in a number of ways. Extensive pneumothorax or hemothorax may necessitate aspiration of the fluid. The flail chest wall with paradoxical breathing should be stabilized by traction or some form of support. The sucking wound of the chest wall must be sealed. Pain from fractured ribs sufficient to abolish respiratory excursion should be relieved by intercostal nerve block rather than by morphine, which depresses the respiratory center. Optimal posture is that in which respirations are least distressed and, in the presence of shock, the head-down position should be discontinued if it is seen to make respirations more difficult.

Oxygen Transport: Shock

The patient with multiple injuries, when first seen, is in established or impending shock. Needles should be inserted quickly into one or several veins before peripheral circulatory collapse supervenes. Dextrose in saline solution, followed by plasma and, as soon as it can be obtained, compatible whole blood should be infused continuously. All other measures adjuvant to the general management of shock (see page 24) should be carried out without delay.

Despite adequate supply and transport, oxygen may not be utilized adequately by brain tissue, due to extensive intracranial damage or decelerated cerebral blood flow. Nevertheless, an oxygen deficit from any cause warrants the supplemental administration of pure oxygen by mask or rubber catheter.

Examinations

All clothing should be cut away or removed so that a complete inspection of the entire body is possible. Clinical examination should be complete but, above all, gentle. The unmolested patient with multiple injuries may remain in apparently good condition for a long period, only to be precipitated into profound shock by some sudden manipulation or change in position. Similar gentleness and caution should be exercised during roentgen examinations. Films necessary to the clarification of all urgent problems should be obtained, but the patient should remain on one litter throughout. Whenever possible use of a portable machine is preferable to moving the patient, even though the films may be of inferior technical quality. Films in the erect position, three-position films of the abdomen, a complete series of skull films, and other roentgen examinations requiring alterations of posture should be deferred until shock has been stabilized.

The unconscious patient with multiple injuries presents a foreboding problem. Brain injury must be presumed, profound shock must be considered, and, in the absence of a reliable history, the possibility of drug toxicity cannot be overlooked. The effects of insulin, narcotics, barbiturates, alcohol, an acute cardiac episode, or a pulmonary embolus may simulate or accentuate shock due to trauma. All such possibilities must be weighed in assessment of the unconscious patient lest the improper use of shock therapy produce fatal results.

Therapeutic Priorities in Multiple Injuries

It is possible, if improbable, for a patient with serious injuries involving each of the major systems of the body to survive transportation to a hospital. He would be in shock. Examination might disclose a depressed fracture of the skull, a maxillofacial injury, a thoracic wound with a tension pneumothorax, an abdominal injury, a pelvic injury with a ruptured urethra or bladder, multiple soft tissue lacerations, and fractures of the large bones of the legs. Each surgical specialist would be impressed by the urgency of his respective problem. Without one individual in charge of continuity of care the result would be conflict, chaos, and complete failure.

First priority must be allocated to the demands of the tissues for oxygen. The airway must be opened, and the facial injury by-passed by the insertion of a metal or plastic airway or by tracheostomy. Thereafter the supported or diverted air channel must be kept clear of mucus and blood, and pure oxygen administered through a rubber catheter. But a patent airway, insufflated with oxygen, is of little benefit in the absence of intrathoracic pressure. The chest wound must be closed, or at least sealed, at once. Neither procedure brooks any delay. Both must be carried out immediately, regardless of existing shock. Only with a clear airway, supplemental oxygen intake, and restored intrathoracic pressure, can shock be stabilized.

Control of massive hemorrhage also rates high priority. However, except with imminent exsanguination from a ruptured spleen or from hemorrhage of one of the major branches of the aorta, a period of replacement therapy and some stabilization is usually advisable, and likely to incur less risk than a heroic operation carried out in the face of steadily increasing untreated shock. Except when one of the great vessels is open, the rate of blood loss will diminish as the blood pressure falls. Under any circumstances, the procedures necessary to restoration of an adequate alveolar concentration of oxygen, and to stabilization of the circulating blood volume, take precedence over all others in the management of multiple injuries. Vigorous supportive therapy should then continue until the next operation is permissible.

Determination of the order in which subsequent procedures should be carried out demands the utmost in clinical judgment. The skull fracture is producing increased intracranial pressure; the abdominal injury is producing hemorrhage and soilage of the peritoneal cavity; and the extravasation of urine into the tissues has a devastating effect. Leakage of bile, however, may be equally devastating, and no schedule of priority can be consistently correct. In general, laparotomy should take precedence only in the presence of massive hemorrhage constituting an immediate risk to life and, as pointed out above, this may occasionally be required in certain splenic injuries even before the general condition can be stabilized. The brain should be decompressed before anything else is done, if the intracranial pressure is rising rapidly. If intracranial pressure remains reasonably stable, however, the next step in treatment should be a suprapubic cystostomy and diversion of the urinary stream. Pertinent to assessment of the urgency of this procedure is the fact that in youth the urine is clear and clean and that, as the years pass, the volume and virulence of the urinary flora increase.

Once the intracranial pressure has been stabilized, and the urine stream diverted, the abdominal injury must receive attention. The nature and extent of intra-abdominal damage is often difficult to determine and, by the same token, the duration and impact of the operation is uncertain. Consequently, laparotomy should be deferred until the shock has been stabilized and an ample supply of blood placed in reserve.

Meanwhile the soft tissue wounds and the extremity fractures should not have been neglected. Priority of their treatment is low, in comparison with the life-saving procedures which enjoy therapeutic precedence, but splintage of the fractures and control of hemorrhage from minor wounds, from the beginning, are measures essential to the management of the shock and the prevention of additional tissue damage.

CHAPTER 3

INFECTIONS AND ANTIBACTERIAL AGENTS IN TRAUMA

By DAVID V. HABIF, M.D.

THE PRINCIPLES of management of accidental wounds are essentially the same as those for elective civilian surgery. Accidental wounds differ in that there may be more damage to and loss of tissues, a higher degree of contamination with bacterial organisms of greater variety, and delay in treatment for a variety of reasons. When surgical care is delayed or inadequate, such wounds usually become infected regardless of the type, route, and amount of antibacterial therapy. Systemic administration of antibiotics is indicated primarily to prevent or minimize invasive infection from the wound into the surrounding normal tissues or the blood stream. Thus, the sine qua non to prevention of wound infections in the traumatized as well as in the civilian surgical patient is adequate surgical debridement and wound care. The traumatized wound infected with pyogenic microorganisms is treated in the same manner as an elective surgical wound.

Infection in the burned patient is frequently difficult to prevent and, at times, more difficult to treat, particularly in persons with extensive second and third degree burns. Many traumatized wounds are contaminated with clostridial organisms, but proper treatment should prevent the development of clostridial cellulitis and myositis (gas gangrene). The epitome of adequate treatment is surgical debridement which results in a clean wound having no necrotic or devitalized tissue. Tetanus could probably be eradicated if active immunization with toxoid were routinely practiced. Since many who are not so immunized sustain trauma, both prophylaxis and therapy of tetanus must be considered.

CIVILIAN SURGERY

Elective civilian surgery should have a wound infection rate of no more than 2 per cent for clean and clean-contaminated cases. This record can result only with Halstedian surgical technique in an immaculate surgical environment.

Analysis of the wound infection rate at the Presbyterian Hospital in New York City for 1955 through 1957, including the services of general surgery, orthopedics, gynecology, neurosurgery, plastic surgery, and otolaryngology, disclosed an incidence of less than 2 per cent following surgery in clean and clean-contaminated cases. From a review of the causes of these infections, it was apparent that there was almost always some break in technique resulting in hematoma, tension with compromised blood supply, or implantation of foreign body such as too heavy silk, metal, or plastic material. It is an interesting fact that the rate was essentially the same over the last twenty or more years, even prior to the use of antibiotics.

On the general surgical service prophylactic systemic antibiotic therapy is routinely given after pulmonary, cardiac, vascular, and gastrointestinal operations, but not in other "clean" cases. The duration of therapy is often longer than necessary. It should not exceed 72 hours, unless there is specific indication, since there is a constant danger of pus formation in the wound, which may be masked by the suppression of cellulitis. Antibiotics so administered have probably decreased the incidence of invasive infection, and the development of septicemia, particularly from Group A beta hemolytic streptococci. This gain, however, must be considered in the light of the toxicity and adverse side-effects from the antibiotics, as well as the appearance of superinfections, staphylococcal enterocolitis, and probably pseudomembranous enterocolitis.

Staphylococcus pyogenes var. *aureus* is the predominant microorganism causing localized wound infections in civilian surgery. It may exist alone in 50 to 75 per cent of such infections, and may be present in an even higher percentage, in combination with other microorganisms. Pathogenic coagulase-positive staphylococci are found in the air, and on the skin and clothing and in the nares of the professional and non-professional staff members of many hospitals. Although there are many carriers of coagulase-positive staphylococci, few persons have been found to harbor phage type 42B/52/81, recovered from the pus of the majority of wounds. The mode of transmission of this phage type remains to be elucidated.

More than 50 per cent of pathogenic staphylococci cultured from in-hospital acquired infections are resistant to penicillin, streptomycin, tetracycline, and erythromycin, particularly when these drugs are used frequently. Among the antibacterial drugs tested and found to show a high percentage of sensitivity are bacitracin, chloramphenicol, novobiocin, and Furadantin. The importance of obtaining cultures initially, and subsequently as indicated, to guide antibiotic therapy cannot be overemphasized. Sensitivity of the bacteria to antibiotics may be rapidly determined by the disc plate method as practiced in the Surgical Bacteriology Laboratory of the College of Physicians and Surgeons of Columbia University. A highly trained technical staff is needed, as well as the use of *moist* discs, owing to the great variability and current lack of standardization of commercially available dry antibiotic discs. Filter paper discs which absorb about 0.1 ml. of solution are kept refrigerated in Petri dishes containing excess solution. The concentrations per milliliter of the various solutions are as follows: penicillin, 20 units; bacitracin, 40 units; streptomycin, 250 micrograms; tetracycline, 100 micrograms; neomycin, 100 micrograms; chloramphenicol,

100 micrograms; erythromycin, 100 micrograms; novobiocin, 100 micrograms; polymyxin, 300 micrograms; and Furadantin, 1,000 micrograms. Antibacterial agents selected on the basis of this method have been found to be clinically effective when given in the doses generally employed.

In view of the prevalence of pathogenic staphylococci in hospitals, care must be exercised to avoid introduction of the microorganism into the wounds of traumatized patients admitted for treatment.

PROPHYLACTIC ANTIBIOTIC THERAPY

All open traumatic wounds are contaminated with microorganisms, the type and virulence of which depend on the terrain where injury was sustained and on the method of production of the wound. Infection may develop if a hematoma or injured muscle is contaminated through damaged skin, or by a bacteremia. Wounds involving the mouth or the respiratory and alimentary tracts are exposed to endogenous, as well as exogenous, contamination. Damaged tissue combined with hematoma, and at times augmented by destruction of blood supply to muscle, serves as an excellent culture medium for bacterial growth.

The bacteria which may be introduced primarily into a wound are of two main types: (1) aerobic or pyogenic, and (2) anaerobic or clostridial, including organisms causing cellulitis, myositis, and tetanus. In the first category, the organisms encountered most frequently are *Staphylococcus pyogenes* var. *aureus*, hemolytic and non-hemolytic streptococci aerobic and anaerobic, and the coliaerogenes group. Proteus and *Pseudomonas aeruginosa* (*pyocyaneus*) are also frequent contaminants which may cause a wound abscess when in pure culture. The organisms introduced include many saprophytes which die easily, or are washed out by wound bleeding or irrigation.

Swab cultures from all open traumatic wounds are indicated and, in addition, cultures of debrided tissue are valuable in defining the existent bacterial flora and determining its sensitivity to various antibiotics.

Open traumatic wounds should be covered with as clean or sterile a cloth as available, and be carefully protected at all times from secondary bacterial contamination, because newly introduced organisms may be more pathogenic and resistant to antibiotic therapy than the primary invaders. Local antiseptics, by and large, are tissue irritants, and should not be used. The instillation of sulfonamide powder in wounds at the time of injury as practiced years ago in military and civilian casualties was subsequently shown to be of little value in preventing local wound suppuration. These drugs, however, minimized the spread of infection into the general circulation.

More important than the use of antibacterial agents in the wound at the time of injury is early debridement and irrigation by saline (0.9 per cent) solution, which will remove the major portion of contaminating bacteria. Attempts have been made to further decrease the remaining bacterial population by irrigation, subsequent to debridement, with a combination of non-allergenic bactericidal antibiotics in solution, such as bacitracin (1:500), neomycin (0.5 per cent), and polymyxin (0.1 per cent). There is no clear-cut evidence, however, that the added irrigation of the wound with antibiotic solution affords increased protection against local suppuration.

Adequate debridement of a contaminated wound within six to eight hours after injury, prior to the onset of invasive infection, will result in a low (5–10 per cent) incidence of wound infection. Delayed surgery or inadequate debridement carries a higher incidence of local suppuration (20–25 per cent).

Systemic or oral administration of antibiotics is indicated at the time of an injury resulting in major wounds to soft parts, compound fractures, and extensive burns (1) to extend the "golden period" for debridement beyond six hours; (2) to prevent invasive local infection, as well as osteomyelitis, meningitis, peritonitis, empyema, and septicemia; and (3) to decrease the incidence of tetanus and clostridial cellulitis and myositis. Antibiotics are used before and after debridement, for a period of five to seven days, and longer if needed, whether the wound is closed primarily or left open and sutured subsequently in four to five days. They must be chosen empirically before the bacterial flora and sensitivities are known, and be effective against both gram-positive and gram-negative organisms. Agents recommended are penicillin (procaine) 600,000 units, and streptomycin 0.5 gram intramuscularly every 12 hours; tetracycline 100 milligrams intramuscularly, or 250 milligrams by mouth, every 6 hours; and chloramphenicol 0.5 gram every 8 hours intramuscularly or by mouth. After cultures have been made and sensitivities of the bacteria are known, these antibiotics may be continued, or a change may be made. Cultures should be made from open wounds at three- to five-day intervals to aid in determining eradication of the primary flora, development of resistance, or appearance of secondary invaders.

It should go without saying that the antibiotics are administered to help the patient recover from the injury without local suppuration or invasive systemic infection. Above all, they should be used, when indicated, in proper dosages for specific periods of time to avoid the toxicity or side-effects common to all antibiotics. Skin rashes of varying severity, and anaphylactoid reactions, as well as sudden death, may occur from the use of penicillin, so that, where possible, a history of prior use or allergic reaction should be obtained. The otic complications attending administration of both streptomycin and dihydrostreptomycin are well known. Streptomycin is preferred because of equal effectiveness and less chance of serious toxicity, notably irreversible deafness. Tetracycline and related compounds may cause stomatitis and gastrointestinal upsets, including nausea, vomiting, and diarrhea, of varying severity. Certain blood dyscrasias have been associated with administration of chloramphenicol, and, as with the tetracyclines, there may be profound depression of the normal intestinal bacterial flora leading to symptomatic monilial infections. Unless bacitracin and polymyxin are given in accordance with specific instructions, serious nephrotoxicity, as well as neurotoxicity, may result. Skin rashes and gastrointestinal complications may occur with the use of erythromycin and novobiocin. Fulminating diarrhea due to staphylococcal and pseudomembranous enterocolitis, and superinfections may result from the use of broad-spectrum antibiotics, as well as from a combination of penicillin and streptomycin. Finally, the use of antibiotics prophylactically in patients with wounds treated by primary closure may mask the presence of local pus by suppression of cellulitis. This leads to delay in diagnosis and in establishment of drainage which, in many cases, may result in catastrophe.

BURNS

Local and invasive infection, which can rarely be prevented, continues to be a major problem in management of the severely burned patient. Organisms primarily implanted from multiple sources are frequently augmented by secondary invaders.

Local infection leads to pain, metabolic derangements, and delayed healing, as well as an increase in depth of the injury. The burned surface may become infected by one or more types of pyogenic bacteria, which may not be completely abolished unless epithelialization occurs or grafting is accomplished. Group A beta hemolytic streptococci, uniformly sensitive to penicillin, tetracycline, Chloromycetin, erythromycin, novobiocin, and other agents, should be eradicated prior to skin grafting. Other pyogenic organisms should be reduced in numbers and activity by combined local and systemic antibiotic therapy. Although the value of local antibiotic therapy in ointment form to prepare a wound for grafting has not been clearly established, many surgeons have the distinct clinical impression that it decreases the number and activity of those organisms which cause pus formation. Antibiotics used systemically and locally should be selected on the basis of bacterial sensitivity determined by culture and the disc plate method.

Septicemia in the extensively burned patient is a more frequent serious complication than was previously appreciated, and is a major cause of death. *Staphylococcus pyogenes* var. *aureus, Proteus,* and *Pseudomonas* are the most common causes, and frequent blood cultures are necessary to document their existence. Treatment consists of appropriate antibiotic drugs in large doses, selected on the basis of determined sensitivity. Not infrequently septicemia is caused by *Staphylococcus aureus* which is resistant to the majority of commonly used antibiotics but is sensitive to bacitracin. Personal experience by the writer with bacitracin administered systemically in a variety of serious staphylococcal infections confirms the extensive writings of Meleney that this is a safe, potent bactericidal agent. When it is given in doses of 20,000 to 30,000 units intramuscularly every six to eight hours (with 2 per cent procaine as a diluent), and the urine is kept alkaline with a minimum output of 1,000 ml. per 24 hours, nephrotoxicity is a mild reversible finding to be expected, rather than a serious symptomatic toxic reaction to be feared. As much as 300,000 units of the drug per 24 hours has been given to burned patients with staphylococcal septicemia, with apparent success and without significant toxicity. If the daily urine output falls below 600 ml., or the blood urea nitrogen rises above 25 mg. per 100 ml., the drug should be discontinued.

Septicemia caused by Pseudomonas organisms is best treated with polymyxin. The total daily dose is 2.5 mg. per kg. of body weight diluted in 2 per cent procaine, given intramuscularly in three doses at eight-hour intervals. Because of nephrotoxicity, the urinary output should be maintained at 1,000 ml. or more per 24 hours, and the blood urea nitrogen should be determined at three-day intervals. Neurotoxicity manifested by numbness of the nose and digits is a reversible symptom.

Probably-fatal septicemia due to an organism such as Proteus, which is resistant to all antibiotics except neomycin, may be treated with this antibiotic given intramuscularly as a last resort, because of its very serious neuro- (eighth-nerve) and nephrotoxicity. The recommended dose is 0.5 gm. diluted with 2 per cent procaine every 12 hours.

TETANUS

Clostridium tetani is a strict anaerobe commonly found in warm humid soil and is a normal inhabitant of the intestinal tract of the horse. The spores are very hardy. Tetanus is an ever-constant threat in soil-contaminated traumatic wounds, both superficial and deep, but constitutes a greater danger when muscle is damaged.

The remarkable achievement of almost complete prevention of this infection in American soldiers in World War II, when there were only twelve recorded cases of tetanus, one of which was from injury sustained in combat, bears witness to the fact that this eventuality could probably be eradicated through a program of active immunization with tetanus toxoid. Although a very large proportion of the civilian population in the United States has now been protected, such immunization cannot, as yet, be taken for granted.

All patients sustaining traumatic wounds and all persons receiving moderate to severe burns should receive a booster dose of tetanus toxoid at the time of, or shortly after, wounding, if there is a well-documented history of previous immunization, i.e., of three doses of 1 ml. subcutaneously at three-week intervals. At the Presbyterian Hospital in New York 0.5 ml. of tetanus toxoid fluid only is given intramuscularly if the interval since active immunization is four years or less. Tetanus antitoxin is added to this, if the interval is five years or more. If active immunization has not been done, or if the history is uncertain, 1500 to 5,000 units of tetanus antitoxin is given intramuscularly after appropriate testing for sensitivity to horse serum (0.02 ml. of 1:10 dilution of T.A.T. intracutaneously, read in 20 minutes, and/or 1 drop of undiluted T.A.T. into the conjunctival sac). When treatment of a traumatic wound has been delayed in the non-immunized patient, the dose of antitoxin should be 10,000 to 20,000 units, which provides passive immunity for five to ten days. This should be repeated as indicated, with sensitivity to horse serum being tested prior to each injection. All previously non-immunized patients receiving tetanus antitoxin are followed after recovery from their wounds, to be certain they are given a course of toxoid. Wall has recently suggested that a dose of 1500 units of tetanus antitoxin prophylactically for non-immunized patients may be too little, and that consideration be given to raising this to 40,000–100,000 units. In selected cases or when treatment has been delayed, this dose is reasonable.

Clinical tetanus caused by the toxin is a very serious disease, carrying a mortality rate of about 40 per cent, even with excellent hospital care. Charity Hospital in New Orleans has had the greatest experience with the treatment of tetanus in the United States. During the 14-year period beginning with 1943, 558 patients with tetanus were treated. Only one patient had received a full course of toxoid previously, and another patient had received one dose. Neither was given a booster dose of toxoid at the time of injury. A third patient, not actively immunized, received 1500 units of T.A.T. after injury, but developed tetanus. The recommended therapy for tetanus emphasizes good supportive care of the patient as the most important single factor, augmented by the following procedures:

1. Opening the wound widely, or debridement and excision when feasible.
2. T.A.T.—50,000 units intramuscularly, and a like amount intravenously.
3. Sedation and anticonvulsive therapy with mephenesin, barbiturates, and Chlorpromazine.
4. Maintenance of an adequate airway with tracheostomy, if indicated.
5. Antibiotics—namely, penicillin, 300,000 or 400,000 units intramuscularly daily.
6. Gastrostomy for feeding purposes.

Although antibiotics (Terramycin) given in adequate dose shortly after injury will prevent experimental tetanus in animals, such therapy is not effective once the disease has become established.

OTHER CLOSTRIDIAL INFECTIONS

The anaerobic clostridial group of microorganisms has many species in addition to *Cl. tetani*, but *Clostridium welchii, septicum, oedematiens, histolyticum,* and *sordelli* are the most important clinically. Clostridial organisms are found in soil, dust, and the alimentary canal of many animals and man. They may be cultured from 7 to 100 per cent of acute traumatic civilian wounds, depending upon the degree of soilage of the wound, and the time intervening between injury and culture. MacLennon documented the high incidence of anaerobic, as well as aerobic, microorganisms culturable from wounds in Africa during World War II, and emphasized the fact that anaerobic infections are clinical entities.

Clostridial infections do not develop unless the organisms can grow in devitalized tissue. There are two distinct clinical entities—namely, clostridial cellulitis and clostridial myositis.

Clostridial Cellulitis

This is a painful septic disease, due predominantly to *Clostridium welchii,* which involves the subcutaneous and fascial tissues and not living muscle. It progresses from initial swelling of the part to a rapidly spreading cellulitis with crepitation, tissue slough, and abscess formation associated with blood vessel thrombosis and gangrene of the overlying skin. There is a foul, putrid, profuse, brownish seropurulent discharge from the wound, with moderate fever and systemic reaction.

The institution of prompt treatment results in survival of the majority of patients. Operation is indicated to decompress the tissues, drain all pus, and excise all necrotic tissues. Antibiotics in the form of penicillin and a broad-spectrum agent intravenously or intramuscularly are given. Supportive measures, consisting of blood transfusions along with needed fluid and electrolytes, are necessary.

Clostridial Myositis

Clostridial myositis (gas gangrene) is a clinical entity characterized by gangrenous infection of necrotic muscle leading to early pain, toxemia, and death, unless it is promptly treated. Necrotic muscle of the buttocks and legs, especially with compromised blood supply, is most commonly involved, but the infection spreads to involve normal muscle as well, and is usually associated with edema, crepitation, and a slight to profuse watery brown exudate. Radical surgery, consisting of decompressing incisions, excision of all necrotic and dying or infected muscle, or in some instances of amputation of the limb, must be accomplished as soon as the diagnosis is made. Antibiotic therapy, in the form of intravenously administered tetracycline, 500 mg. every 6 to 8 hours, and 1 million units of aqueous crystalline penicillin G intramuscularly every 3 hours, is given.

Antitoxin therapy consisting of four vials of the pentavalent serum is given intravenously as early as possible and repeated, as indicated, in an attempt to help control the toxemia. The patient must be tested for sensitivity to horse serum. Supportive treatment, in the form of continuous maintenance of blood volume, fluid and electrolyte balance, and intestinal decompression, is a most important part of the management of these patients.

Clostridial myositis may be prevented by timely, adequate wound debridement and care. Once it is established, immediate radical surgery becomes mandatory to survival.

GENERAL THERAPEUTIC USE OF ANTIBIOTICS

Antibacterial agents are indicated for the treatment of cellulitis and lymphangitis, including osteomyelitis, pneumonia, cystitis, pyelonephritis, meningitis, and septicemia. On the other hand, the indicated treatment for an abscess is surgical drainage with or without concomitant antibacterial therapy for associated cellulitis. Even in the presence of an abscess, invasive infection may be controlled or prevented with antibiotics to which the organisms are sensitive. After adequate drainage of the pus has been established, antibiotics may not be necessary, depending upon the degree and severity of cellulitis and the type of the organism. Adequately drained abscesses caused by hemolytic staphylococci are less likely to require additional antibiotic therapy than those due to hemolytic streptococci. Certain cases of anaerobic cellulitis involving fascia and muscle require long decompressing incisions, plus excision of all dead or partially devitalized tissue, where possible.

Antibiotics are best selected according to determined bacterial sensitivities, but until the flora is determined empirical therapy should be directed against both gram-positive and gram-negative pyogenic organisms. Treatment should be continued until the cellulitis is resolved, or the temperature has been normal for 48 hours. Individualization of treatment is essential for all wound infections, but acute osteomyelitis requires at least two weeks of treatment, and treatment of severe pneumonias, meningitis, and septicemias should be continued as long as is necessary to achieve a cure.

Cultures of infected open wounds should be repeated at three- to five-day intervals to determine the emergence of resistant microorganisms, or the development of superinfections.

Antibiotics selected empirically for invasive infections should produce a favorable response within 48 to 72 hours. If this does not occur, an abscess or the presence of resistant organisms should be suspected, particularly if the wound is closed. If the former cannot be diagnosed, the latter should be assumed, and the antibiotics administered should be replaced by others rather than given in increased amounts.

It must always be remembered that pus formation may occur and be clinically masked during antibiotic prophylaxis or treatment of cellulitis. These abscesses may be deep, but are usually in the subcutaneous space. Thus, an abscess should be suspected if the temperature rises while prophylactic antibiotic therapy is being given, or if fever continues after the resolution of cellulitis. In addition to inspection of the wound, a search for distant abscesses should be made.

If it is remembered that surgical treatment is indicated for almost all wound infections, except pure cellulitis, lymphangitis, and early acute osteomyelitis, antibiotic therapy will remain in proper focus as an adjuvant to be used in a manner that will result in benefit with a minimum of toxicity.

BIBLIOGRAPHY

Artz, C. P., and Reiss, E.: The Treatment of Burns, Chap. 7, p. 147. Philadelphia, W. B. Saunders Co., 1957.

Caswell, H T., et al.: Bacteriologic and clinical experiences and methods of control of hospital infections due to antibiotic-resistant staphylococci, Surg., Gynec. & Obst. 106:1, 1958.

Creech, O., Jr., Glover, A., and Ochsner, A.: Tetanus; evaluation of treatment at Charity Hospital, New Orleans, Louisiana, Ann. Surg. 146:369, 1957.

Liedberg, N. C.-F., Reiss, E., Kuhn, L. R., Amspacher, W. H., and Artz, C. P.: Infections in burns; evaluation of local use of chloramphenicol ointment and Furacin soluble dressings on granulating surfaces following extensive full thickness burns, Surg., Gynec. & Obst. 100:219, 1955.

MacLennon, J. D.: Anaerobic infections of war wounds in the Middle East, Lancet 2:63, 94, and 123, 1943.

Meleney, F. L.: Statistical analysis of a study of prevention of infection in soft part wounds, compound fractures and burns with special reference to the sulfonamides, Surg., Gynec. & Obst. 80:263, 1945.

Meleney, F. L.: Present status of antibiotics in surgery, Surg. Clin. of North America 36:273, 1956.

Pulaski, E. J.: Prophylaxis and Treatment of Wound Infection, Symposium on Treatment of Trauma in the Armed Forces, October, 1939. Army Medical Service Graduate School, Walter Reed Army Medical Center, Washington, D. C., 1952.

Pulaski, E. J., Meleney, F. L., and Spaeth, W. L. C.: Bacterial flora of acute traumatic wounds, Surg., Gynec. & Obst. 72:982, 1941.

Wall, C. A.: Use and abuse of tetanus antitoxin in acute injuries, Am. J. Surg. 95:664, 1958.

CHAPTER 4

THERMAL TRAUMA

By ROBERT H. E. ELLIOTT, Jr., M.D.

Of the many types of injury which the physician or surgeon may be called upon to treat, the burn is one of the commonest. At the same time it is frequently one of the least understood. Few forms of trauma can be as devastating in their consequences, or demand as much patient, intelligent, painstaking care as severe thermal injury. Such advances as have been made in our knowledge of the treatment of burns in the last thirty years have occurred largely in the field of systemic rather than of local therapy. Although this advancement has been considerable, there is still much to be learned and much that is poorly understood. With regard to local therapy, aside from the employment of antibiotics, comparatively little progress has occurred in the past half century, although considerable knowledge of a negative nature, i.e., of what not to do, has accumulated.

GENERAL CONSIDERATIONS

Nature of Injury

Failure to appreciate the fact that the severe burn is in reality a *wound with loss of substance* has no doubt led to some of the misconceptions about therapy prevalent among medical students and practitioners. Undoubtedly this confusion has been increased somewhat by the fact that the trivial burn heals rapidly with almost any reasonable form of local therapy, whereas patients with severe thermal injury may either die within a short time or be hospitalized for long periods during which impatience and frustration on the part of the physician may result in care of the patient being relegated to the junior staff.

The concept, then, that a burn is essentially a wound with loss of substance is fundamental to intelligent handling of this type of injury, not only from the standpoint of local treatment but also from that of systemic therapy. Unlike certain other forms of trauma, however, where the tissue injury may be reasonably well localized and perhaps even sharply demarcated, a burn diffusely affects the tissues around it and may extend over a wide area. Therefore, while these other forms of trauma may lend themselves to the immediate removal of devitalized tissue or possibly prompt suture or grafting, tissue devitalized by heat cannot generally be handled by these measures. In addition, the full extent of the injury caused by a burn is usually not apparent as early as in injuries produced by other modalities. Nevertheless, the fundamental *factors of wound healing* are essentially the same in all forms of trauma, whatever the mechanism of production, although the therapeutic problems involved may be quite different indeed. Viewed in the light of the foregoing, many important factors in thermal trauma can be more readily understood. With regard to the matter of infection, for example, it becomes quite apparent why a burn of any magnitude, with its adherent, devitalized tissue, is so much more susceptible to bacterial invasion than wounds caused by most other forms of trauma. As a corollary of this, it can also be readily understood why the observance of strict aseptic technique in the handling of the burn wound is of the utmost importance.

Extent of Injury

As in any form of trauma, the seriousness of the injury is directly proportional to its *extent* (surface area involved, in the case of a burn) and its *depth* (penetration). With regard to extent, the total of body area burned is readily calculated by the use of the "Rule of Nines"* (Fig. 4–*1*).

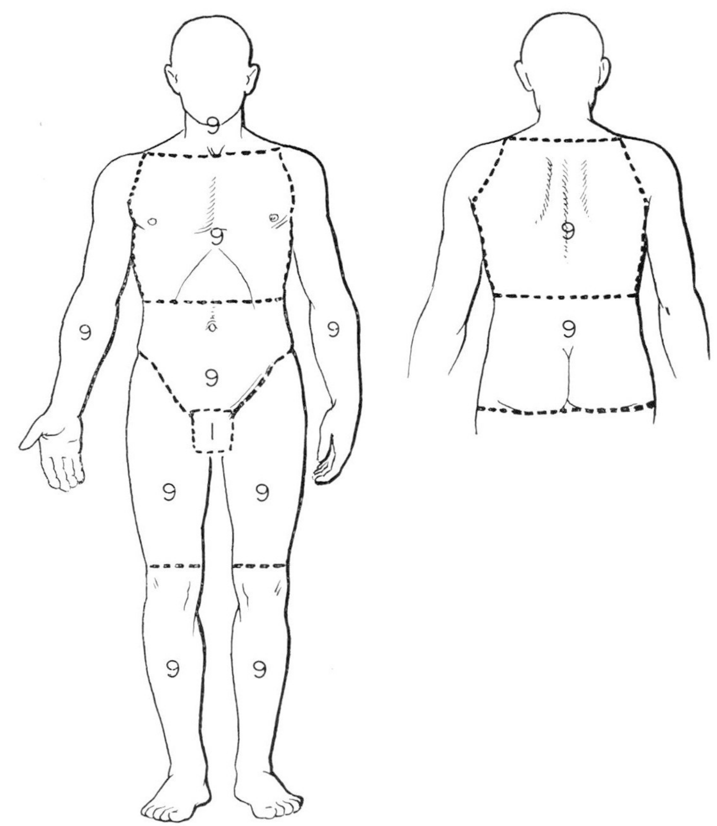

Figure 4–1. The "Rule of Nines," for estimation of extent of burns.

* The "Rule of Nines," in widespread use today, has largely supplanted the older and more exact Berkow scale. It has been found that, for all practical purposes, the slight inaccuracy of this rule is more than offset by the facility with which it can be remembered.

From the diagram it will be observed that each lower leg represents approximately 9 per cent of the total body surface, as does each upper leg. The same value is assigned to the anterior trunk and to the posterior trunk, to the anterior chest and to the posterior chest, to each upper extremity, and to the entire head and neck area. The remaining 1 per cent is allocated to the external genitalia.

In extensive burns, it may be several days or longer before both the extent *and* the depth of the injury can be accurately evaluated. For, although the total surface area of involved *skin* may be rapidly estimated by use of the "Rule of Nines," the amount of concomitant damage to the respiratory tract and lungs (if flame or hot gases have been inhaled) may not become apparent for hours or even days. It is likewise well known that the question of whether a given thermal injury penetrates the full thickness of the skin frequently cannot be ascertained with certainty until the burn eschars commence to separate, a phenomenon which may not take place until several weeks have passed.

Physiology and Anatomy of the Skin

Essential to an understanding of the systemic as well as the local problem in thermal trauma is a knowledge of both the physiology and anatomy of the skin. In brief, the functions of the skin are protective and metabolic. With regard to metabolism, its excretory, absorptive, and heat regulatory roles should be kept in mind. With regard to the anatomy of the skin, it will be appreciated that in this type of trauma its thickness, vascularity, and the number and depth of penetration of its epithelial appendages (hair follicles, and sebaceous and sweat glands) all play a most important role not only in the ability of the integument to resist heat and infection, but also in the rapidity of the healing process. The thickness of the skin of the soles of the feet, of the palms of the hands, of the back, and of the posterior cervical region, for example, is proportionately greater than that elsewhere in the body; likewise the greater vascularity of the face, neck, and fingers, and the presence of the hair follicles of the beard on the face and neck of the male are important considerations in the healing of a burn. In regions of greater vascularity, greater resistance to infection and more rapid healing may be anticipated. Where epithelial appendages penetrate in abundance through the skin, providing a source of reparative epithelium, the deep types of burns are better tolerated from the standpoint of the rapidity of wound healing in general and epithelialization in particular. On the other hand, in areas where the collagenous fibers of the dermis or subcutaneous connective tissues are abundant, the separation of the burn slough may be unduly delayed. This is not infrequently seen in third and deep second degree burns of the back, or of the back of the neck.

Topographical implications. It is thus apparent that, in addition to extent or amount of surface area involved, and depth of penetration of the burn, its *location* and the character of the skin in the involved area must also be taken into consideration. With regard to location, three additional factors arise in connection with the wound healing process: local tissue immunity to infection, as seen in the skin surrounding the body orifices; the problem of motion of the part; and, lastly, the matter of pressure on the part. With regard to the latter two factors it will be realized that healing tends to be retarded over joints and weight-bearing surfaces. If, for example, the back is involved in the burn process, pressure plus infection may convert a second to a third degree injury.

Pathology and Classification of Injury

The essential pathological feature of a burn is necrosis of tissue. Burns are commonly classified in this country in three degrees, depending on the depth of penetration of the injury. When only the most superficial layers of the epidermis are destroyed and no blisters are formed, the burn is classified as first degree. When the burn is of sufficient severity to produce blebs, but destroys only partial thickness of the skin, it is called second degree (Fig. 4–2); and when the full thickness of the integument, together

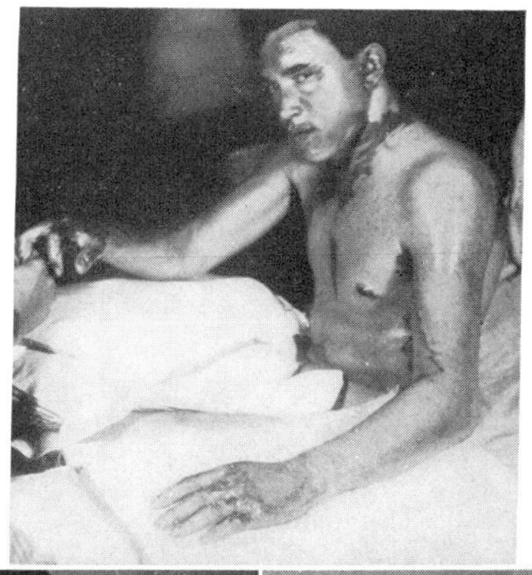

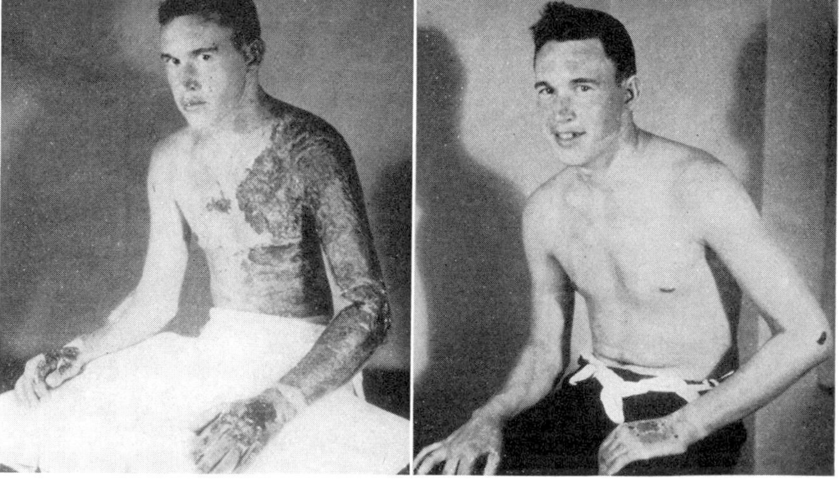

Figure 4–2. Second-degree burn: Immediate, intermediate, and final appearance. (Photographs, courtesy of Curtis P. Artz, M.D., Lt. Col. MC, USA (Ret.).)

with its epithelial appendages, is necrotized, it is called third degree (Fig. 4–3). A still simpler classification is also sometimes encountered. In this, burns are classified in two degrees only, namely: partial thickness, and full thickness.

It will be appreciated that in burns of any magnitude a very large absorptive and transudative surface is created. In extensive thermal trauma, therefore, care must be exercised to apply locally only those medicaments which are known to be neither toxic nor allergenic when absorbed. The vital role played by the absorption of toxins from destroyed tissues, and from bacterial invasion when this occurs, cannot be overemphasized. Furthermore, it will be readily understood that the larger the burn surface, the greater the transudation of fluids, proteins, and electrolytes. Occasion-

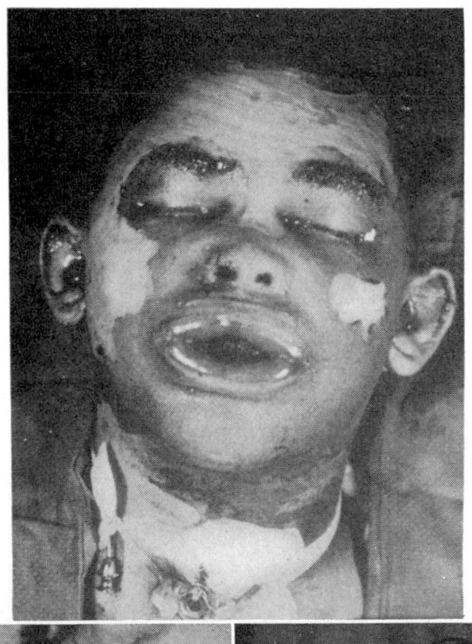

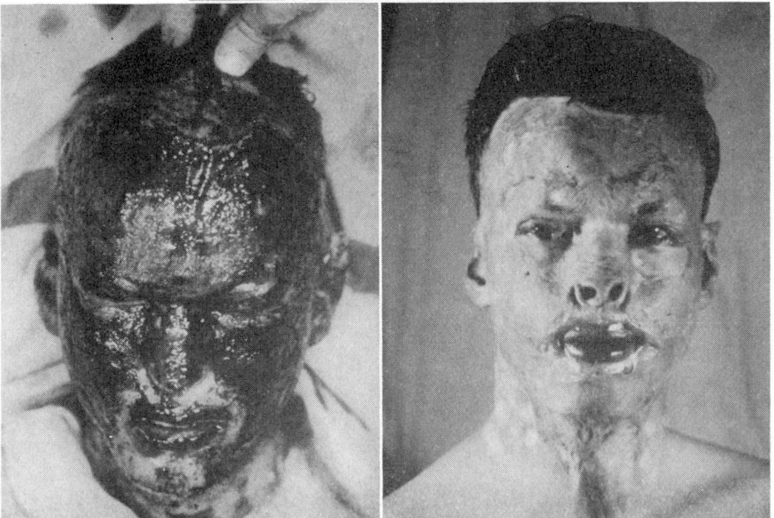

Figure 4–3. Third-degree burn: Immediate (note tracheostomy tube), intermediate, and final appearance. (Photographs, courtesy of Curtis P. Artz, M.D., Lt. Col., MC, USA (Ret.).)

ally, and perhaps more in burns of the extremities than elsewhere, important nerve trunks and blood vessels may be destroyed by the thermal process. This is rare, however, except in instances of deeply penetrating third degree burns.

The effect of these pathological processes on the organism as a whole is in many ways the most important consideration of all. Too often this aspect of the total picture is either overlooked or misjudged. As mentioned earlier, it is principally along these lines that modern investigative work on the burn problem has contributed most.

Causative Agents

By far the commonest causative agent in thermal trauma is flame. Hot or boiling liquids are next in order of frequency. Exposure to hot gases or noxious fumes is also a relatively common modality, although occurring usually only in conjunction with fire burns. Corrosive chemicals (e.g., lye, certain acids and alkalis, etc.) constitute a small but important group of causative agents. From the standpoints of incidence and importance, electricity belongs in this category also. Irradiation and exposure to fission products have become increasingly significant mechanisms, particularly during the last decade.

It should be noted that scalds are almost as common as fire burns among infants and young children. In the adult, serious burns all too frequently result from smoking in bed. This habit, particularly when coupled with over-indulgence in alcohol, accounts for an impressive number of the burns encountered in the emergency rooms of civil hospitals.

Special mechanisms. Among the special mechanisms which are worth re-emphasizing are: (1) the inhalation of flame or hot gases, with resultant burns of the upper respiratory tract and lungs, a type which is frequently overlooked because it is not suspected; (2) contact with chemicals; (3) contact with electricity; (4) exposure to irradiation; and (5) exposure to thermonuclear explosions. These are given special consideration later in the chapter.

Recognition of Injury

As in any other form of acute trauma, the primary objective when a burned patient is first seen is to treat shock (present or threatened) and to relieve pain. Once measures to control and prevent these factors have been initiated, and emergency treatment in general is under way, attention should be directed to the history. Aside from the usual important considerations of duration of injury, circumstances and mechanism of occurrence, and previous treatment, it is essential to inquire concerning the possibility of previous and existing systemic ailments in general, and of diabetes, alcoholism, drug addiction, and epilepsy in particular. Unlike certain other types of severe trauma, the badly burned individual may face many weeks of debilitation as a result of the toxic effects of injury and infection, not to mention the deleterious influences of protracted wound healing. This places a constant and long-continued strain on all of the principal systems of the body, as will be seen from the discussion of complications later in this chapter.

When the patient is inspected for the severity of the injury, the percentage of body surface involved and the depth should be rapidly assessed. As intimated earlier, even the experienced observer may have difficulty in deciding how much of a given burn is partial thickness and how much is full thickness. It should always be remembered that each degree of burn is associated with lesser degrees also. The physical examination should be as complete as circumstances permit, and should include inspection of the nares and upper respiratory passages. This is of special importance when hot gases or flame may have been inhaled, and should therefore be routine in all patients receiving burns of the face. Singed hairs in the nostrils may be the first clue to a burn of the lungs. Examination of the throat may reveal intense erythema. When this is observed it is advisable to attempt also to inspect the larynx and vocal cords. The assessment also of such factors as age and general nutrition, as well as of the cardiovascular and renal systems, is of great importance for the reasons mentioned earlier in this section. The all too common error of concentrating on the local lesion at the expense of the patient as a whole must be avoided at all costs. In suspected burns of the lungs, and whenever the possibility of a chronic lung ailment exists, an immediate chest film should be taken. This will serve as a baseline for future reference. It should be noted here that x-ray indication of thermal trauma to the lungs is often not apparent for several days.

Other essential preliminary determinations are the hematocrit (or, if this is not possible, determination of the hemoglobin), urinalysis, and complete blood count. Blood grouping and cross-matching should be done promptly, against the need for transfusion, which may be immediate or delayed.

LOCAL THERAPY

Before the local treatment of burns is discussed, it must be re-emphasized that the "first thought in burns" is *not* of caring for the injured surfaces, but the treatment of the patient as a whole, with particular reference to present or impending shock. This will be gone into in more detail later in the discussion of Systemic Therapy.

It may next be well to examine the objects to be accomplished by local treatment. Ideally these should include:

(1) relief of pain;
(2) prevention of infection;
(3) protection of the injured tissue;
(4) prevention of damage to remaining islands of uninjured epithelium in the burned area;
(5) prevention, in so far as possible, of the escape of serum from the damaged integument and of plasma loss into the surrounding tissues;
(6) promotion of early skin grafting.

Suffice it to say that as yet no ideal form of local treatment has been devised, as is witnessed by the many forms of therapy available. It can be stated, however, that all forms of treatment fall into one of two categories: closed treatment, in which the burn is wrapped, or encased in a protective covering; and open treatment, in which no bandages or special coverings are used. A combination of the two categories may be used in special areas.

Closed Treatment

This type of local treatment, in addition to a protective encasement of the burned area, generally includes the use of ointments, wet dressings, or special local applications which come into direct contact with the burn surface and which are designed to prevent adherence of the bandages or encasement to the wound. The most popular and widely used form in this category is the pressure dressing in which the ointment or ointment-impregnated gauze is snugly bound in place by a well padded, elastic type of bandage. Once in place, this initial dressing is left undisturbed for at least seven days and, if circumstances permit, for two weeks, unless evidence of supervening infection such as local pain or a septic type of temperature necessitates earlier redressing. In addition to the pressure dressing and modifications thereof, encasement of the extremities in a skin-tight plaster has been employed occasionally. This type of dressing has not been widely accepted, however, because of the skill necessary for its correct application. Paraffin dips and special plastic irrigating bags have also been used. By far the simplest of these methods, however, is the pressure dressing. Properly applied such dressing lends itself to ease of transportation of the patient, and, in general, requires less attention for longer periods of time than do other methods. The pressure, which must be evenly and not too forcefully applied, is designed to minimize the escape of serum from the wound surface and of plasma into the surrounding tissues. A more detailed description of this technique is given under admission treatment (p. 89).

With regard to the ointments used, these generally have a petrolatum base, and may or may not include medicaments to prevent pain and combat infection. Antibiotics have been incorporated in some of these ointments, but it must be remembered, as mentioned earlier, that sensitization and toxic drug reactions can supervene, particularly if the burn surface is large. Petrolatum-impregnated fine-mesh gauze is perhaps the simplest, safest, and most widely used of these agents.

Wet dressings of saline and the like find their greatest usefulness in cleaning up local infection and in preparing burned areas for skin grafting.

Open Treatment

Escharotics. In the past, the open method of treating burns has relied largely upon the use of escharotics to cause rapid pellicle formation on burned surfaces. Tannic acid and tannic acid in combination with silver nitrate were among the earliest of these agents. Triple dye (crystal violet, brilliant green, neutral acriflavine), picric acid, triethanolamine, and other chemicals, applied by spray or wet dressing, were also popular at one time. Some, notably tannic acid, were found to have toxic properties and in some instances to be capable of destroying residual epithelium. This, plus the higher incidence of infection among burns treated in this manner and the masking action of the eschar as regards both depth of injury and the presence of infection, led to general abandonment of their use.

More recently, in some of the larger treatment centers of the country, this form of treatment has been revived, with the important difference that no escharotic agent is employed. The burn surface is exposed to the air and allowed to form its own protective pellicle of dried clotted serum. In addition, where feasible, the use of Kirschner wires with balanced suspension has occasionally been advocated. Although this type of local treatment has much to recommend it from the point of view of necessitating a minimum of care once it has been properly set up, it must be remembered that it is intended as a definitive form of therapy and is not to be recommended when early transportation or evacuation of the injured patient from one hospital to another is contemplated.

Special Treatment of Certain Areas

Certain areas of the body lend themselves to various types of local therapy and it is therefore not infrequently desirable to combine both the open and closed techniques in the same patient. Burns of the face, the genitalia, and the perineal and perianal areas, for example, are frequently best handled by the open method of treatment. These so-called "critical" areas are subject to soilage—from food and nasal secretion in the case of the face, and from excrement in the case of the genitalia, perineum, and perianal region.

Burns of the face, head, and neck. Within 24 hours after thermal trauma to the face, massive edema may appear which is particularly evident about the eyes and jowls. This gives rise to the aptly named "pumpkin face" appearance. These burns do well if left open and if lightly coated with petrolatum or other suitable ointment. Should a covering which is easy to change seem advisable, a helmet can be fashioned from wide, sterile stockinet. Apertures are cut for the eyes, nose, mouth, and ears, and the cephalic extremity of the dressing is closed off with a simple tie of cotton tape. Irrespective of the type of surface treatment, the patient's head and shoulders should be kept highly elevated on a Gatch bed until all edema has subsided.

Burns of the genitalia. These are best left open or lightly smeared with ointment. It is of the utmost importance to insert an indwelling catheter into the bladder as soon as possible after injury. If this is not promptly carried out, edema may close off the urethra within a matter of a few hours, making subsequent catheterization difficult and painful.

Burns of the perineum and perianal area. Burns of these areas are among the most difficult to keep clean, and are best handled by the open method. The use of a Bradford frame (Fig. 4–4) or similar apparatus is

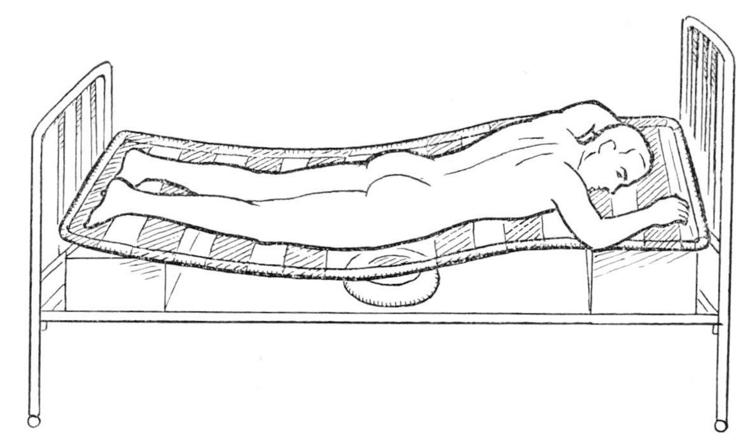

Figure 4–4. Bradford frame, with bedpan in position beneath patient.

often helpful in this regard. With the buttocks exposed, fecal material can be gently flushed or sponged away with saline solution and the injured perineum or perianal area in this way kept free of soilage.

Burns of the respiratory tract. If burns of the respiratory tract are suspected, a baseline x-ray film of the chest should be taken as soon as possible and the patient placed in an oxygen tent. A tracheostomy set should be kept in readiness nearby and the trachea opened promptly at the first sign of respiratory obstruction due to laryngeal edema. The danger of the development of this formidable complication is very real during the period of the accumulation of edema and should be watched for closely during the first 72 hours. It is of course of special importance to institute prophylactic antibiotic therapy in all patients with suspected burns of the respiratory tract.

Burns of extremities and trunk. Burns of the extremities and the trunk and chest can be adequately handled by either the open or the closed method. A notable exception to this is burns of the hands, which are best treated by wrapping. In dealing with the extremities, it is well to remember that the part must be elevated, maintained in a position of function, and early active motion should be encouraged. This will minimize edema and help prevent the development of contractures and foot or wrist drop.

PREPARATION FOR GRAFTING

As mentioned previously, one of the main considerations in the local care of a burn is facilitation of *early* skin grafting. It is worth while briefly to bring up here a few points concerning preparation for grafting from both the local and systemic standpoints. If local infection is suspected, the involved area should be immediately inspected and trapped exudate released. This may be accomplished by gentle local debridement and wet dressings. Cultures should be made from the exudate to determine the antibiotic sensitivities of the offending organisms, after which appropriate therapy, both *local* and general, should be instituted.

By the end of the second week after injury, most superficial burns will have healed, and the areas of third degree and deep second degree burns will have become apparent. When granulations appear, they may be cleansed and freshened in preparation for a graft by the simple expedient of the wet-dressing technique. Not infrequently it is advisable to attack the involved areas directly by surgery,* excising under anesthesia devitalized tissue and cutting back exuberant granulations with the immediate application of a split-thickness or other form of skin graft. In burns which are old and have been heavily infected, the so-called postage-stamp type of graft may be preferable. Before grafting is attempted, as will be emphasized later under Systemic Therapy, measures to ensure adequate blood replacement and satisfactory protein and electrolyte levels should be instituted.

STANDARD TECHNIQUES OF IMMEDIATE TREATMENT

Minor Burns

In general, it may be said that minor or trivial burns (mild second degree or less, and limited to a small surface area) do well with almost any reasonable form of local treatment which has as its object the protection of the damaged area and the prevention of infection. Thus, any form of sterile covering over some form of ointment (to prevent adherence of the dressing) is usually adequate. Many types of "burn ointments" are available on the market, no one of them at present enjoying any great superiority over the others.

Major Burns

Immediate (or "on the spot") local treatment of major burns will to some extent depend on the time and distance involved in the evacuation of the patient to the treatment center. For all practical purposes, covering the exposed areas with clean linen (freshly laundered towels or sheets) will suffice. Adherent clothing should *not* be removed at this time. This should await the arrival of the patient at the hospital. Use of ointments, butter, lard, pastes, etc., should also be avoided as these will in all probability only have to be removed at the hospital by the individual undertaking definitive therapy, thus causing unnecessary pain to the patient and delay in the ultimate cleaning up of the burn. If it is deemed advisable to administer an immediate opiate for the relief of pain, the dosage, type of drug, and time of administration should be written down and this information sent with the patient to the hospital.

ADMISSION TREATMENT

As in the initial management of all acute trauma, the primary objectives in the admission treatment should be (1) to treat shock, (2) to re-

* At this juncture, and frequently somewhat earlier, debridement by chemical or enzymatic agents is sometimes attempted. It should be noted, however, that this method of debridement is still under investigation and has not as yet received wide acceptance.

lieve pain, (3) to prevent infection, and (4), in the case of major burns, to minimize fluid loss. A number of suggestions for facilitating attainment of these objectives are listed below. These suggestions are not intended as a formal plan of treatment. Rather is it hoped that they may prove helpful to the uninitiated in expediting the admission treatment of the severely burned.

1. The patient should be taken without delay to a suitable treatment or operating room. In hospitals where burn casualties are seen frequently, it is wise to set aside one such room for this purpose and to maintain it in a constant state of readiness by continually restocking it with appropriate supplies.
2. Every person in this room while treatment is in progress, including the patient, should wear a cap and a mask.
3. The dressers scrub as for a standard surgical operation and don sterile gowns and gloves.
4. Morphine (or one of its equivalent drugs), intravenously or intramuscularly, provides satisfactory analgesia in the great majority of cases. Inhalation anesthesia should rarely be necessary.
5. Blood for typing, cross-matching, and hematocrit determinations is drawn immediately, and an intravenous drip of 5 per cent dextrose in water is started through the same needle. If, as frequently happens in extensive burns, difficulty with venipuncture is experienced, a suitable vein should be exposed surgically without delay and cannulated under direct vision.
6. An indwelling catheter is inserted into the bladder, if this seems indicated.
7. While blood hematocrit, grouping, and cross-matching are being determined, adherent clothing is removed, loose skin trimmed away, and the burned surface gently cleansed, if indicated, with a detergent and sterile water or saline solution. Intact blisters are best left unruptured.
8. If a *pressure dressing* is to be applied, it may be prepared in the following manner: A sterile 12-inch absorbent gauze and cotton roll of the "Acme" or "Dakins" type* is cut into appropriate lengths and laid out on a table with the absorbent surface uppermost. On top of this is placed a layer of plain flat gauze and on top of this, in turn, a layer of fine-mesh gauze impregnated with ointment. This dressing is then applied *in toto* to the burned areas and snugly bound in place with a cotton-elastic bandage. Care should be exercised to keep the pressure even and not excessive, particularly over joints where a dressing which is too tight or inadequately padded may become thinned by motion and exert a tourniquet-like effect.
9. By the time the initial dressing has been completed, the hema-

* Sterile mechanic's waste may be substituted for the gauze and cotton roll. This material, however, suffers from two disadvantages: it is more difficult to apply than the ready-made roll, and suitable grades of waste are often difficult to obtain.

tocrit and blood-typing determinations should be available and plans for appropriate initial systemic therapy can be drawn up.

10. In the event that the *open method* of surface treatment is elected, the patient's bed should be prepared while the burns are being attended to as described under Paragraph 7. This involves the setting up of cradles or frames over the bed, when indicated, to keep the bed clothing off the burned areas. Sterile sheets are best used under these circumstances, and apparatus for heating the cradles or frames should be provided as needed.
11. Efforts should be made to segregate burned patients during their convalescence, in view of the fact that most serious infections occurring in these patients are of hospital origin. Also with this in mind, the masking of all visitors and attendants should be rigidly enforced during this period.
12. Prophylactic broad-spectrum antibiotic therapy is advisable in all burns of any magnitude. Although authorities differ on the advisability of the routine use of tetanus toxoid or antitoxin in these cases, this writer is of the opinion that as a matter of general principle one or the other of these agents should be used in patients with third degree and deep second degree burns.

Burn Team

Mention should be made here of the "burn team"—an organization of the staff widely used in many hospitals, both military and civilian, during World War II. This team should consist of a general surgeon who is interested in the problem of infection, a plastic surgeon, a physician thoroughly familiar with problems of nutrition and fluid and electrolyte balance, and, of equal importance, a group of nurses and orderlies selected, when possible, for their familiarity with this type of casualty and the trying and exacting care it entails. This type of organization, in centers where serious burns are frequently handled, has proved, in matters of patient care, to be vastly superior to the casual hospital group. Obviously, during peacetime and especially in smaller centers, such an organization may be neither feasible nor practical. It is advisable, however, to have this organizational set-up in mind when the occurrence of multiple casualties of this nature appears to be a possibility. At a minimum, the general surgeon should bear in mind that the plastic surgeon should see these patients at the earliest possible moment, and, whenever possible, at the time of admission to the hospital. Only in this way can early, adequate reconstructive surgery be intelligently planned for.

SYSTEMIC THERAPY

It is well known that the importance of treating shock and maintaining body fluids equals or exceeds that of the handling of the local lesion in burns. It has been mentioned earlier that the loss of serum from burned surfaces is a characteristic feature of this form of trauma and in severe cases may well be the deciding factor in the death of the patient. It is therefore of the utmost importance, from the outset, not only to treat shock but to keep pace with and to anticipate when possible the loss of body fluids. Needless to say it is impossible to go into this aspect of therapy in any great detail. Much has yet to be learned about the fine points of this form of treatment and much that has been written in the literature is still controversial. It will suffice here to point out the more important objectives to be attained.

The problem, in brief, is to treat shock and to prevent or keep pace with the subsequent loss of body fluids and electrolytes. Primary shock is best handled by immediate administration of intravenous glucose or glucose in saline solutions. When there has been a marked fall in blood pressure, the early transfusion of blood or blood substitutes is indicated. Plasma infusions were employed extensively during World War II, and ideally plasma should be one of the most important therapeutic agents. Unfortunately, in the recent past the high incidence of hepatitis following the use of pooled plasma has largely interdicted its employment except under the most desperate circumstances. At the present time, however, methods of ensuring the sterility of plasma are being developed which give promise of restoring the therapeutic usefulness of this important agent. Should the sterility of plasma be open to question, plasma expanders such as solutions of gelatin or dextran may prove useful in its place, not to mention the administration of electrolytes, whole blood, and, when available, albumin.

Among the most important yardsticks for ascertaining the fluid and electrolyte requirements of the patient are the hematocrit with falling-drop protein determination and measurement of the urinary output. These determinations are essential. Of equal importance, but not always immediately available, are facilities for determining, at a minimum, the following constituents of the plasma: chlorides, CO_2, Na, and K, and protein partition. It goes without saying that during the early treatment of the severely burned patient an accurate record of the 24-hour intake and output, as well as of the foregoing values, should be kept on a separate "fluid balance" sheet in the patient's chart. When this is done, at any given moment the exact status of the fluid and electrolyte balance can be seen at a glance.

It is not unusual, in extensive burns, for the fluid requirements during the first 24 hours to reach between 4 and 8 liters. Various formulas for computing these requirements have been devised. That described by Cope and Moore is representative and worth quoting:

> In the average sized adult for each 1 per cent of the body surface burned, 75 cc. of plasma[*] and 75 cc. of non-colloid-containing isotonic electrolyte fluid are given in the first 24 hours. . . . One-half of the calculated amount of plasma and electrolyte fluid is given in the first eight hours and the second half in the subsequent 16 hours, ... the plan includes for the second 24 hours a fluid ration equal to one-half that given in the first 24 hours.
>
> In addition to the above, 2,000 cc. of fluid is given in each 24-hour period to main-

[*] As noted previously, the use of pooled plasma at the present time may carry with it a risk of infectious hepatitis. It is suggested, therefore, that substitutes such as dextran or dextran and albumin, plus blood transfusions, be used instead, unless the sterility of the available plasma is unquestioned.

tain urine flow. . . . The fluid is given preferably by mouth and consists of palatable liquids; those containing sugar and potassium, such as fresh fruit juices, being offered freely. If the fluid has to be given intravenously, glucose in water is used. The volumes of each of these three fluids [i.e. plasma, electrolytes, and additional fluid just mentioned] are subject to alteration according to the exigencies of the case, the continued presence of hemoconcentration or cessation of renal output indicating the need for accelerated intake.*

A valuable rule of thumb is to maintain a total intake sufficient to ensure a 24-hour urinary output of at least 1,000 ml. In this connection, it should be remembered that overhydration, especially in elderly patients and cardiacs, can be as serious an error as underhydration. It should also be re-emphasized that, whenever possible, the oral route of administering fluids is preferable to the parenteral. To this end it may occasionally be advisable to administer fluids by gavage, using a nasogastric catheter and a continuous slow drip of appropriate fluids. If this is carried out, however, caution must be exercised not to overload the stomach.

After the initial phase of therapy is over and the patient is sufficiently recovered to handle the greater portion of his fluids by the oral route, supportive treatment should be aimed at maintaining nutrition and, in third degree burns, readying the patient for skin grafting. As has been stressed previously, this should be undertaken as soon as possible, although it should be pointed out that in the more severe grades of injury this will usually not be possible before the third or perhaps the fourth week. Of the utmost importance, in this connection, is the maintenance of adequate protein levels. As suggested previously, albumin and the transfusion of whole blood and plasma may well be necessary, in addition to high protein nourishment. Because of the coexistence of toxemia and local infection, severe anemia with hypovolemia is common and must be corrected by transfusion before grafting can be undertaken.

In the later phases of convalescence and until the burned areas are healed, continued vigilance against anemia and hypoproteinemia must be maintained. The protracted convalescence of the severely burned patient also necessitates that constant attention be given to bolstering the morale of the patient, particularly if the injuries seem destined to result in cosmetic disfigurement or crippling loss of function of the extremities. Much can be done along these lines with properly directed occupational and physical therapy.

Mistakes in Systemic Therapy

Perhaps the commonest mistake in systemic therapy is to initially underestimate the severity of the thermal injury. This may lead to inadequate handling of shock, and this, in turn, to increasing failure to keep pace with the patient's fluid and electrolyte requirements.

An almost equally common mistake, particularly when frank shock does not develop, is to underestimate replacement therapy during the early phase of treatment, with resultant renal shut down or profound debilitation.

* Cope, O., and Moore, F. D.: The Redistribution of Body Water and the Fluid Therapy of the Burned Patient. Annals of Surgery, Vol. 126, p. 1014, 1947.

Conversely, the error of overhydration, as previously mentioned, must be avoided, especially in elderly individuals and in patients with cardiovascular or renal disease.

Another not uncommon error occurs when skin grafting is attempted before the patient is in proper condition to withstand the procedure. This may result in severe shock, particularly if extensive grafts are taken under general anesthesia.

PROGNOSIS IN MAJOR BURNS

It can be said in general that recovery from a severe burn is dependent upon the same factors which govern recovery from any other type of trauma, namely, extent and severity of the injury, state of health at the time of the injury, and the age of the patient.

Extent of the injury. Although no hard and fast rule can be laid down, it can safely be said that if over 50 per cent of the body surface is involved in second and third degree burns the prognosis is poor and that, at best, a difficult and protracted struggle lies ahead. The presence of lung burn adds greatly to the gravity of the outlook. Nor should it be forgotten that extensive second degree burns (50 per cent or more) are frequently fatal. In this connection, it should be noted that "pink plasma" is of poor prognostic import. This sign, referring to the color of the plasma as seen, for example, in the hematocrit tube following centrifugation, indicates that the thermal trauma has been sufficiently severe to cause partial hemolysis of the patient's red cells. When present, it is found immediately after injury. Its intensity and persistence are roughly proportional to the magnitude of the burn.

State of health at time of injury. Needless to say, individuals debilitated from whatever cause tolerate even minor thermal injury poorly. Patients suffering from chronic alcoholism, with or without associated liver disease, or from cardiovascular or renal disorders fall into this category. Concomitant trauma, whether of a crushing or penetrating variety, will obviously also add to the gravity of the prognosis.

Age. Infants and old people withstand thermal trauma poorly. Burns or scalds of relatively minor proportions, especially of the head and neck, not infrequently cause serious convulsions in very young children. The reason for this is obscure. In any event, the development of this complication usually indicates a grave prognosis.

COMPLICATIONS

Local Complications

The most serious early local complication is the development of infection. It is agreed by most authorities that all severe burns become infected to a greater or lesser extent. These infections may become evident before the end of the first week or may not become apparent until slough begins to separate or is cut away. Bacteremia with concomitant metastatic abscesses (usually to the lungs) was not infrequently seen before the advent of the antibiotics. The writer well remembers an instance in which an abscess of this nature developed in the eye of a severely burned patient, leading to panophthalmitis and necessitating enucleation of the affected globe. This type of complication, however, is usually late and may be preterminal. In deep burns of the extremities, thrombosis, either arterial or venous or both, must be watched for, a constant check being kept on the state of the circulation of the part. The later complications to be looked for in the healing stage include contractures and the development of keloid or other cicatricial deformities. Although local infection and delayed grafting are the commonest causes of these difficulties, faulty blood supply or improper positioning and omission of prophylactic exercises, active or passive, may also be responsible. Decubitus ulcers are quite common in the long-term patient.

General Complications

As intimated in an earlier section, the principal systems in the body may both individually and collectively be subjected to severe stress in major burns. It frequently happens that none escapes completely, and therefore the general complications of this form of trauma are many and varied. Because of this, only the most significant can be mentioned. They will be dealt with briefly and according to system.

Respiratory. As mentioned previously, respiratory obstruction due to *laryngeal edema* occurs early and may be rapidly fatal unless relieved by tracheostomy. *Pulmonary edema, atelectasis, pneumonia, and lung abscess* are seen either alone or in various combinations as a result of thermal trauma to the lungs. More often, however, these complications are the *indirect* result of external burns of major proportions. Pulmonary edema, for example, may be precipitated by overloading the circulation with parenteral fluids or by their otherwise injudicious use. Pneumonia is a constant threat, particularly in infancy and old age, just as it is in any other severe and debilitating ailment. Lung abscess, likewise, may be metastatic in origin from infected surface burns. *Pulmonary infarction* is generally the result of embolization from a peripheral phlebitis.

Cardiovascular. *Cardiac arrhythmias, coronary thrombosis, and heart failure* are not uncommon, particularly in the aged. *Septicemia* may result from uncontrolled local infection. *Peripheral thrombosis,* as intimated previously, may be seen in deep burns. *Thrombophlebitis* is quite common, particularly among patients who must be confined to bed for long periods.

Gastrointestinal. *Anorexia, nausea, and vomiting* are frequently seen during the first few days. *Gastric dilatation* must be watched for during this period also. Later, *ulceration of the stomach or duodenum* (Curling's ulcer) has been observed. In the very severely burned, a *hemorrhagic enteritis* may develop. *Jaundice* may appear fairly early in the course of therapy as the result of a *toxic hepatitis.* Infectious hepatitis should not be confused with this because of its considerably more delayed onset. Anorexia and *malnutrition* with concomitant dependent edema, common to all severe burns, should be mentioned. *Hypoproteinemia,* it should be remembered, may be seen late as well as early. When seen late, it is principally a nutritional phenomenon in contradistinction to the early variety, which is due to loss of plasma through the burn. *Anemia,* likewise, may be seen late as well as early. When seen early, as mentioned previously, it is usually the direct result of the destruction of red cells by heat. Later on it may be due to malnutrition, infection, or both.

Renal. *Renal shutdown* with oliguria or anuria may be an early and ominous complication. Later, *lower nephron disease* may ensue. Ascending infection of the urinary tract frequently occurs, especially when catheterization has been employed. Under these circumstances, *cystitis, pyelitis, and pyelonephritis,* any one alone or all three in combination, may be encountered.

Adrenal. Adrenal failure with an Addisonian-like picture may be an early or late phenomenon. This is one of the most serious and most classic of all of the many complications due to thermal trauma. It is also one of the most common causes of death.

Central nervous system. Hyperpyrexia with *delirium* (toxic psychosis) is common in the early phase of the treatment of the severely burned patients, as is *delirium tremens* among alcoholics. Later in the convalescent period *anxiety states, depressions,* and *overt psychoses* are occasionally encountered.

BURNS RESULTING FROM OTHER MECHANISMS

Chemical burns. From a strictly pathological viewpoint, burns due to acids, alkalis, and corrosive solutions do not differ from those due to flame, in that the fundamental process is destruction of tissue. Immediate first-aid treatment calls for prompt flushing of the area with copious quantities of water or an appropriate weak neutralizing agent in dilute solution. This type of injury, if circumscribed and deep, may be handled by immediate excision and grafting. Later, cicatricial deformities are common and usually require reconstructive measures or plastic surgery.

Electrical burns. These fall into two categories: flash burns, and burns from passage of current through the body. The former, in its purest variety, is due to the flash (heat) produced by a short circuit. Inasmuch as this is usually of brief duration and intensity, this type of burn is far less severe than that due to passage of current through the body. It is also considerably more common than the latter. To the patient, it may be extremely frightening, for a film of soot may be deposited upon the affected surface. When this has been washed away, it is usually discovered that the burn is no worse than second degree and frequently only first degree. It must be understood, however, that a flash burn can ignite clothing and under these circumstances the result may be extremely serious. Treatment is the same as for any other burn.

Burns due to passage of current through the body, if the patient survives, are severe indeed. In their purest form they are third degree and may pass through the entire thickness of the body. It should be remembered that such injury may be accompanied by flash burns and burns due to clothing which has been ignited by the flash.

A point of entrance of the current as well as a point of exit may be observable. These usually present a dead-white or baked appearance and may be well circumscribed. It is frequently found that the tissue has been cooked right down to bone, depending on the amount of current received. If the part has become caught against the source of the current, it may become charred or present a mummified appearance, and frequently early amputation may be necessary. If the patient has been "thrown away" from the source of the current, as sometimes happens, other injuries, in addition to burns, should be looked for.

Radiation burns. Burns due to exposure to x-rays or radium are uncommon today because of the newer techniques developed to safeguard both doctor and patient. It occasionally happens, however, that such burns occur either because of the injudicious use of these agents, with resultant overdosage, or because heavy irradiation has been employed in a deliberate attempt to control malignancy. The immediate result is not unlike a moderate second degree thermal burn in that it may lead to extensive desquamation and a raw, weeping epithelial surface. As these burns are generally restricted to a small area of body surface, the constitutional effects are minimal. Pain, however, may be severe. They can be treated as any mild second degree burn with an ointment and a sterile covering. It should be noted, however, that healing is usually delayed and may not be complete for a month to six weeks. The late effects of this type of burn are really of more consequence than the early, in that epitheliomas may develop in the injured areas many years later. Permanent tanning and loss of hair with telangiectasia generally result.

Burns due to thermonuclear explosions. Space does not permit more than the most cursory mention of this type of injury. It should be pointed out that, in addition to the thermal burn, there may also be general trauma (due to the force of the explosion) and radiation sickness. The degree of injury is of course proportional to the proximity of the individual to the point at which the explosion occurred.

Reports from Hiroshima and Nagasaki indicate that all three degrees of injury were incurred on exposed surfaces. This type of burn has also been referred to as a flash burn, but differs markedly from the previously described electrical variety not only in the amount of heat produced but also in its composition. The heat produced comes from the entire spectrum of light, from ultraviolet to infrared. Clothing, if not extremely light, was found to afford good protection unless, of course, it became ignited. Although electrical flash burns as seen in civilian practice are seldom serious, it was estimated that approximately one fourth of the fatalities in the Japanese explosions were due to this type of burn, as distinguished from flame burns. The treatment of these burns does not differ per se from that of the latter variety. As indicated previously, space does not permit discussion of radiation sickness except to indicate the obvious, that where present it vastly complicates all aspects of general therapy and obscures the prognosis.

CHAPTER 5

VASCULAR INJURIES

By JERE W. LORD, Jr., M.D.

Of the three components of the vascular system, in regards to injuries, the arteries are by far the most important in terms of tissue damage and loss of functional capacity. With certain exceptions trauma to the venous system is less serious and the complications are more easily managed. Finally, injury to the lymphatic component, usually as the result of surgical trauma in special areas of the body, may be clinically significant.

ACUTE ARTERIAL INJURIES

If rewards of a political and social nature are skimpy following major wars, such is not true of arterial trauma. World War I focused attention on the devastating effect upon the extremity of interruption of arterial blood flow, and inspired surgeons to study vascular injuries and to attempt to restore blood flow through damaged arterial trunks. Early in World War II Gordon-Taylor and his associates stated: "The main indication for amputation is irreparable interference with blood supply. No matter how severe the destruction of skin, comminution of bones, or contamination of tissues, if the main blood vessels are not destroyed, the limb can usually be saved." Several careful reports of small groups of patients sustaining injuries to the major arteries were made during and after World War II. Gangrene necessitating amputation varied widely with the location of the artery and also in the experience of different authors. However, a most complete study was made by DeBakey and Simeone, who noted the incidence of gangrene subsequent to injury of a major artery to be as follows:

Brachial artery above profunda	55.7 per cent
Brachial artery below profunda	25.8 per cent
Femoral artery above profunda	81.1 per cent
Femoral artery below profunda	54.8 per cent
Popliteal artery	72.5 per cent

Unfortunately, attempts to restore arterial continuity either by non-suture vein graft or by direct suture methods failed to lessen significantly the incidence of gangrene observed after simple ligation of the artery.

It is of great moment, therefore, to note the remarkable results obtained by Jahnke and Seeley in Korea during a four-month period in 1952. Of 33 patients in whom major arteries were repaired, only three lost a limb, an incidence of 9 per cent. Later in this section the reasons for this profound advance will be analyzed.

In acute arterial injury caused by a small penetrating object such as a bullet, ice pick, or knife, there is little associated injury to the adjacent soft parts, and the point of entrance (and occasionally of exit) is small. On the other hand, the trauma may be caused by a piece of shrapnel or an automobile accident, resulting in badly displaced fragments of fractured bone or dislocation of a knee, elbow, or shoulder joint, with associated damage to the soft parts. The status of the collateral circulation will depend to a great extent on the type of trauma sustained.

A second consideration is the manner in which the artery may be injured. A partial tangential laceration of an artery may produce a gaping hole which cannot close spontaneously and from which bleeding will cease only if the pressure of the blood in the surrounding tissues equals that within the artery, an unlikely occurrence if the soft part wound has a large opening to the outside. However, if the artery has been completely severed, the ends can retract and the adventitial coat of loose fibrous filaments will close over the open end, which is narrowed as vasoconstriction takes place. Thrombosis usually ensues and hemorrhage ceases. Both general and local factors influencing the occurrence of hemorrhage from a traumatized artery are listed in Table 5–*1*.

An artery may be traumatized directly by a blunt force or indirectly from violence in a neighboring area. In the latter there may be merely spasm with temporary (or occasionally permanent) cessation of blood flow through the involved segment. If contusion of the wall has occurred, the damage may involve all coats of the artery including the endothelial lining. This may lead to occlusion by thrombus.

The effects of disruption in the flow of blood through a major artery to an extremity depend on the extent and integrity of the collateral circulation. For example, there is a poor collateral circulation at the level of the external iliac artery, whereas the collateral circulation is excellent

TABLE 5–*1*. FACTORS INFLUENCING OCCURRENCE OF HEMORRHAGE FROM TRAUMATIZED ARTERY.

Favoring Cessation	*Favoring Continuation*
General	
Hypotension	Hypertension
Normal clotting mechanism	Abnormality of clotting mechanism
Reflex vasoconstriction	Anemia
Local	
Complete division of artery	Partial division of artery
Closed soft parts	Gaping soft part wound
Muscle mass–tissue juices rich in thromboplastin	
Local vasoconstriction	

in the region of the superficial femoral artery in the mid-thigh. However, a large cavitational wound involving marked loss of the soft parts in the mid-thigh region plus severance of the superficial femoral artery could so damage the collateral circulation that ligation of the femoral artery would be followed by gangrene of the extremity. The writer treated one patient who sustained a small penetrating injury which resulted in contusion with thrombosis of the superficial and deep femoral arteries. The associated soft part injury was not great, but gangrene of the leg would have followed if blood flow had not been restored through a vein graft sutured to the healthy ends of the superficial femoral artery.

Loss of tissue does not always follow the interruption of a major artery. Usually, however, there is some functional impairment when exercise demands a rapid inflow of oxygenated arterial blood. Occasionally conservative therapeutic measures will lead in time to the development of a rich arterial collateral circulation which is adequate for all functional needs.

Complications of Arterial Injury

Two important complications of an arterial injury may occur, depending on the type of injury and the kind of early treatment applied.

Traumatic arteriovenous fistula. If the concomitant vein has been lacerated simultaneously with the artery, a short circuit in the form of an arteriovenous fistula may develop. This is usually a self-perpetuating lesion which only occasionally closes spontaneously. The blood on the arterial side under high pressure finds ready access into the low-pressure venous channel and is rapidly returned to the heart. The chances for the development of such a fistula are enhanced when the external wound is small. Locally the hematoma absorbs, the skin wound heals, and the lesion may go unrecognized unless it is carefully sought for. The effects of an arteriovenous fistula vary. The local changes usually include: dilatation of the veins of the extremity, increase of the arterial collateral circulation, dilatation of the artery proximal to the fistula with narrowing of it distally, increased warmth and bone growth (in the young), and a continuous thrill and bruit over the fistula. General physiological changes in the cardiovascular system include: increase in blood volume, increase in the venous return to the heart, increase in the cardiac output, tachycardia, widening of the pulse pressure, left ventricular hypertrophy, and eventually cardiac failure. Digital closure of the fistula slows the heart and elevates the diastolic pressure (Branham's sign). The magnitude of the systemic changes depends on several factors, namely, the size of the fistula, the size of the artery and the vein, and the relative proximity of the fistula to the heart.

False arterial aneurysm. The second important complication of an arterial injury in which there is gross hemorrhage into the soft parts and the escape of blood is prevented by small size of the external wound is the false arterial aneurysm. This lesion develops from a pulsating hematoma, the walls of which organize into a false sac which may be clinically indistinguishable from a true aneurysm characterized by the presence of one or more of the coats of the arterial wall. A false aneurysm rarely will develop when the external wound is large or when arterial continuity has been promptly restored. The false aneurysm presents as a pulsating mass with an expansile quality; it may be detected by placing the index fingers, one on each side of the mass, and observing their further separation with each pulse wave. There is usually a systolic bruit without a diastolic component, and the pulses in the distal part of the extremity are readily palpable. There may or may not be concomitant venous changes, depending on whether there is pressure on the concomitant vein by the aneurysmal sac. Also, pain may be present if contiguous nerves are pressed on or have been injured. There are no systemic circulatory effects from this lesion.

Surgical Trauma

Trauma to an artery may also occur in the operating room, either accidentally during an operative procedure having nothing per se to do with the arterial tree, for example, hernioplasty, bowel resection, or radical lymph node removal in the cervical, axillary, or inguinal region. Further, with the recent trend toward radicalism in the surgical approach to the eradication of cancer, neoplasms formerly deemed inoperable because of encroachment on or encirclement of an artery have more recently been handled by resection of the artery in continuity and restoration of blood flow by venous or arterial grafts.

Diagnosis of Arterial Injury

The diagnosis of an acute arterial injury is readily made if shock is not profound. First, in the absence of shock, pulsations should be present in the extremity beyond the point of injury. If they are absent and the distal part of the extremity is cold and anesthetic, then major arterial occlusion has occurred. Locally, marked hemorrhage usually follows a major arterial injury unless the skin wound is small, whereupon examination might reveal a pulsating hematoma. If contusion with thrombosis has occurred, then hemorrhage would be of smaller moment unless a large vein had been severed. Finally, marked spasm alone without serious bleeding is sometimes responsible for the local changes observed in the distal part of the extremity.

Treatment of Arterial Injury

In most injuries to a major artery, hemorrhage is marked and, if it is uncontrolled, death may rapidly ensue. The best method for the control of hemorrhage from either a small or a large wound of the soft parts associated with the arterial injury is by a pressure dressing. Such a dressing should be firmly applied and when traction of the extremity is possible (by Thomas splint) the combination will control hemorrhage in the vast majority of cases. A tourniquet should never be applied unless the extremity is so badly mutilated as to eliminate all consideration of arterial repair and the need for immediate amputation is clear. The only exception to this principle is presented when an effective pressure dressing cannot be applied. Control of hemorrhage should be paralleled by immediate restoration of the circulating blood volume by whole blood transfusion. Only when blood is not available should plasma and plasma substitutes be used. Finally, as a poor but temporary stopgap until blood has been made available, normal saline solution may be used. Although shock may not be evident, whole blood should be available and administered if it is thought that blood loss has been significant. Some authors have used intra-arterial transfusion of blood in severely shocked patients, but recent experimental studies suggest that rapid intravenous transfusion is equally efficient in restoring blood volume, improving cardiac output, and relieving tissue anoxia, and is certainly safer in that gangrene of an extremity is an occasional sequela of intra-arterial transfusion, even in experienced hands. Further clinical experience will be necessary to establish the best method for widespread use.

The patient in shock should have the head placed lower than the rest of the body in the absence of severe cranial or thoracic injuries. Heat in general should not be applied, and under no circumstances should heat be applied to the cold extremity with an arterial injury. Morphine must be given with great caution to the patient in shock unless pain is severe.

Certain principles are basic to the successful care of arterial injuries, and these have been shown to prevail both in military and in civilian patients. First, there must be a firm intent on the part of the surgeon to repair the injured artery in every case in which ligation alone might possibly be followed by gangrene. Common sense would dictate the simple ligation of the radial artery when the ulnar is patent and the five fingers exhibit an adequate circulation. Similarly, a single injury to the profunda brachialis, profunda femoris, or anterior or posterior tibial artery does not require repair when the associated soft part injury is not severe. Second, as has been repeatedly pointed out, a few useful instruments safe for temporary closure of an artery without trauma to the wall are essential. Although there are many instruments suitable for such a purpose, the Potts multitooth clamp is by far the best and can replace all of the rubber-shod variety. In their absence, the Blakemore-Crump, the Blalock, and other similar rubber-shod clamps function well. Finally, a fine braided arterial silk, 5-0 in size, swedged on a minimal-trauma curved needle, is essential. Fine neurosurgical thumb forceps without teeth, needle holders which are not crushing, and petrolatum or mineral oil round out the basic and important armamentarium for arterial repair. Third, only a surgeon who has had the opportunity to perform vascular suture should undertake the management of arterial injuries. Fortunately, the tremendous volume of clinical and experimental cardiovascular surgery has led to the training of many young surgeons capable of the careful technique necessary for good vascular anastomosis.

The timing of arterial repair. One of the most critical factors in the successful management of an arterial injury is the time-lag between the moment of injury and the performance of repair. In general, the first six hours have been termed the "golden period" for arterial repair. Thrombosis in the smaller peripheral arteries and arterioles takes place shortly thereafter. Further, when ischemia is marked, irreversible changes in the muscles may develop in spite of restoration of a pulsatile arterial blood flow. DeBakey and Simeone reported an incidence of amputation following arterial wounds treated within 10 hours of 36.7 per cent, in those treated within 10 to 20 hours 48.8 per cent, and in those treated after 20 hours 63 per cent. In spite of the opinions and data cited above based on World War II experiences, Jahnke and Seeley found from personal experience in Korea that following repair of all arterial injuries of major arteries no amputation was necessary when the time-lag was less than 9 hours; amputation was required in 28.5 per cent of those treated 9 to 12 hours after injury, and in only 25 per cent of those treated 12 to 15 hours after injury. The important lessons to be learned are (1) the great emergency with which arterial injuries must be dealt, and (2) the necessity of surgical repair even when delay has been unavoidable, unless irreversible changes have taken place in the extremity.

Infection and antibiotics in arterial repair. Another factor of considerable importance in the management of arterial injuries is the problem of contamination and infection. When the vessel has been injured during a clean operative procedure, this factor is of little consequence. On the other hand, when there is a huge cavitational wound full of contaminated foreign material, then infection may be a significant factor in spite of a thorough debridement and the use of antibiotics. Nevertheless, arterial repair should be performed unless the patient has sustained more critical injuries elsewhere. Jahnke and Seeley pointed out that the addition of an arterial repair in trained hands added little to the patient's difficulties and did not interfere with appropriate treatment for the concomitant injuries. However, when gross infection ensues, the arterial anastomosis may undergo thrombosis, secondary hemorrhage, or aneurysmal formation.

Antibiotics have been of immense help in the control of infection and should be employed routinely in arterial repair unless a contraindication to their use exists. However, sound surgical principles and delicate blood vessel technique, brought out so clearly by Carrel, remain the important factors in the successful management of arterial injuries.

Anticoagulation and arterial repair. The role of anticoagulants in the postoperative management of arterial injuries is a difficult one on which to take a firm stand. The writer has more or less followed Shumacker's philosophy that anticoagulants are of no value in maintaining the patency of a poor vascular anastomosis, are not needed following a good one, but may be of value in the borderline group. The trials and tribulations caused by postoperative hemorrhage resulting from the use of heparin, including the occasional fatality resulting from its misuse, led Jahnke and Seeley to abandon its use after arterial repair. Their extraordinarily low incidence of thrombosis (approximately 1 per cent) is strong evidence that anticoagulants are not necessary postoperatively.

When arterial continuity cannot be re-established, for whatever reason, and hemostasis is satisfactory, then anticoagulant therapy is justified and will probably save some extremities which would otherwise be lost owing to a complicating venous thrombosis associated with a sluggish collateral arterial blood flow. Herrmann has pointed out that heparin is usually safe to administer beginning six hours postoperatively.

Technique of Arterial Repair

The techniques of arterial suture have been clearly described and illustrated by Shumacker, and are generally standardized. The following points should be mentioned: (1) All traumatized artery should be resected, along with one centimeter of each end beyond the evident limit of gross injury (this holds only for contused and severely traumatized arteries). (2) The adventitia should be excised to prevent strands of this filmy fibrous layer from entering the lumen of the anastomosis and stimulating thrombosis. (3) The endothelium of the intima should be guarded by keeping it moist with physiological saline solution. (4) The ends of the vessel should be handled carefully with thumb forceps so that the endothelium will not be injured. (5) The intimal layers of the two ends of the vessel should be carefully coapted by means of two everting mattress stay sutures, the anastomosis being completed by an over-and-over suture. (6) The anastomosis should be completely covered with muscle or fascia. (7) Longitudinal tension greater than the physiological recoil which normal arteries exhibit should be avoided. Mild tension due to loss of only a short segment of an artery can be readily overcome by mobilization of the ends of the artery for several centimeters in each direction. If necessary, small branches can be tied flush with the artery and divided for added mobility. However, if a greater loss of substance is found and mobilization of the arterial ends does not suffice to overcome longitudinal tension, then recourse to a vessel graft is indicated.

Vessel grafts and prostheses. There are at present three types of "grafts" available to bridge gaps in an artery. The most desirable one is the autologous vein graft which functions well, remains viable, and after a few months thickens to resemble an artery. Eventually these grafts may undergo calcification, but this change does not interfere with their function. The saphenous and cephalic veins are usually adequate as donor vessels, but where neither is satisfactory, as will occasionally be the case, then the superficial femoral vein in the middle third of the thigh will do. A transplanted segment of vein must have its direction reversed so that valves, if present, will not impede arterial blood flow through the graft.

Vein grafts are suitable, however, only in arteries of the extremities when the surrounding tissue can be used for support. Within the thorax and abdomen, arterial defects should be bridged either by arterial grafts or by prosthetic devices. Homologous arterial grafts preserved by any one of a variety of methods will be useful. These grafts serve simply as struts or conduits which are gradually covered by the host's endothelium and invested with the host's fibrous tissue. A viable graft which will live permanently in its new environment would be highly desirable, but at present has not been developed.

Recent studies by Voorhees, Jaretski, and Blakemore, and by Hufnagel suggest that plastic materials such as Vinyon "N" cloth and Orlon fashioned into tubes function beautifully as permanent conduits of arterial blood and hence may ultimately become the ideal "graft" to bridge gaps in the aorta and other large arteries within the thoracic and abdominal cavities. Studies in our laboratory suggest that Dacron may be the most suitable plastic.

The techniques of suturing grafts are identical to those of suturing arterial anastomoses. The grafts should be under "physiological" tension and not be permitted to angulate or buckle. Excessive longitudinal tension must be avoided. All authorities agree that the grafts should be carefully covered by pleura or peritoneum.

Conservative Measures

In the occasional case of arterial injury wherein restoration of continuity is not possible for any of several reasons, then so-called conservative or medical measures may be of considerable value in developing an adequate collateral circulation to save the extremity. The proper use of gravity is extremely important in the management of the limb which must survive on its collateral arterial circulation. The blood pressure is usually low in these small vessels, and elevation of the foot or hand 12 inches above heart level may render it ischemic. On the other hand, by placing the foot or hand 6 inches *below* heart level, the collateral flow readily fills the capillaries and veins. The most satisfactory way to elevate the bed is by placing 6-inch blocks under the posts at the head and allowing the patient one pillow. A position such as "high Fowler's" is deleterious since the venous pressure is elevated to such an extent that the poor arterial flow will be further hampered. Bending of the hips and knees in a Gatch bed also interferes with arterial and venous flow.

Abolition of vasomotor tone is most helpful in improving the collateral arterial blood flow. Tobacco is completely forbidden because of its constricting effect on the small blood vessels. Reflex vasodilation is valuable and is encouraged by placing an electric pad or warm water bottle on the abdomen either continuously or for one hour four times a day. No heat in any form is applied to the extremity, a cradle is used to prevent trauma from the bed clothes, and the foot or hand is wrapped in cotton for protection, for the containment of whatever warmth the part may have and, finally, for avoidance of the vasoconstricting effect of chilling drafts.

Anticoagulant therapy may be of genuine value in the conservative management of an arterial injury. There is a threefold purpose in lessening the tendency of the blood to clot, namely, the avoidance of thrombosis in the small arterial collateral vessels, as well as in the main artery proximal and distal to the site of occlusion, and, finally, to avoid the devastating effect of a deep venous thrombosis which is prone to occur when the arterial flow is sluggish. Heparin, Tromexan, and Dicumarol, alone or in combination, may be employed, depending on the facilities available for their careful control.

Vasodilating drugs, such as Priscoline, papaverine, Etamon, alcohol, and a host of other agents, are worth very little. Our experience with the intra-arterial use of histamine and Priscoline has been disappointing for the most part.

In summary, the important factors in the conservative management of arterial injuries are (1) the proper use of gravity, (2) the elimination of vasomotor tone, and (3) the judicious use of anticoagulant therapy.

ARTERIAL EMBOLIC OCCLUSION

An arterial embolus may arise from a mural thrombus in a fibrillating left auricle, from a mural thrombus in the left ventricle subsequent to a myocardial infarction, from a thrombus within an aortic aneurysm, and, finally, from a thrombus loosely adherent to an ulcerated arteriosclerotic plaque in the aorta.

The effect of an embolus is proportional to the size of the artery occluded (characteristically at the point of its bifurcation) and the magnitude of the collateral circulation. When the embolus lodges at the terminal aorta, most of the arterial supply to both lower extremities is lost. Not only may gangrene of the legs follow, but life itself is in jeopardy. On the other hand, a small embolus to the anterior tibial artery may cause only a few days of discomfort in the leg.

The collateral circulation is stimulated by partial gradual narrowing of a main arterial channel, hence if complete occlusion then occurs suddenly as a result of an embolus, the extremity may survive handily. This point is of some value in the consideration of operative intervention in the elderly arteriosclerotic.

Diagnosis

The sudden onset of pain in an extremity which becomes cold, numb, and weak characterizes a block in a major artery. Objectively, there will be an absence of pulsation below the site of obstruction. Coldness usually is noted 6 to 12 inches below the level of the block, and loss of sensation of the foot or hand may be demonstrated. Precisely the same symptoms and signs may be associated with a sudden thrombotic occlusion as with one of embolic origin. Differential diagnosis rests on the demonstration of a likely site of origin of an embolus. If there is none, and the patient is in his forties or older, then an arteriosclerotic thrombotic occlusion is likely.

Treatment

Recent thinking expressed in the literature tends toward operative intervention in the majority of patients whether the obstruction is thrombotic or embolic in origin. Certainly all good- and fair-risk patients with an occlusion of the axillary or brachial artery or iliac or femoral artery should be operated upon promptly. In more peripheral blocks and poor-risk patients the situation should be carefully analyzed before surgical intervention is imposed. In conjunction with Dr. Irving S. Wright and Dr. A. Wilbur Duryee, the writer has observed a considerable number of patients with embolic and thrombotic arterial occlusions who not only have survived but also have later developed a collateral circulation adequate for the functional needs of the extremity. Such patients have been selected for the conservative medical measures outlined under acute arterial injuries because of their poor risk status, because of the delayed arrival at the hospital, or, finally, because of the obvious successful tolerance of the occlusion prior to the adoption of medical measures.

The position outlined above does not apply to sudden embolic occlusion of the terminal aorta, the common or external iliac, or the common femoral artery. In these instances prompt embolectomy is performed.

The comprehensive management of the patient with an embolism not only includes the care of the local problem surgically but also requires the most diligent effort by appropriate surgical and anticoagulant therapy to prevent the occurrence of further embolic episodes.

REFLEX VASOMOTOR DYSTROPHY

Following many types of injury the sympathetic nervous system to the involved extremity may become overactive and lead to disability out of proportion to the magnitude of the original trauma. For instance, a man falls a few feet from a ladder and sprains his ankle only mildly but tends to favor the injured part by avoiding use of it. Disuse atrophy may set in rapidly because motion is painful. X-rays show demineralization. The sympathetic nervous system is triggered into overactivity, which results in edema, sweating, and greater pain. These findings are noted often in emotionally unstable individuals and present a particularly difficult problem when compensation is involved. If untreated, the hand or foot may undergo far-advanced changes associated with fibrosis of the periarticular tissues, subluxations, profound atrophy of the soft parts, and a useless extremity.

Treatment is directed toward active use of the part, and abolition of sympathetic tone by chemical blocks, or occasionally by sympathectomy. In some patients psychotherapy is valuable. The best therapy is preventive and is based on correct early management of the injured part and on early active motion and use of the extremity. If signs of sympathetic overactivity appear, appropriate measures should be instituted to control the efferent outflow of the sympathetic nervous system.

In addition to minor sprains and fractures, injuries to a major nerve may be followed by burning pain in the extremity which is sometimes disabling. Causalgia, as this type of reflex vascular dystrophy is called, responds to the same therapeutic approach.

The study by Shumacker and Abramson is classical and should be reviewed by all who are interested in this aspect of trauma.

INJURIES TO VEINS

There are three significant complications which may follow trauma to a vein. First, there may be a laceration such as an accidental tear in the inferior vena cava during excision of an arteriosclerotic aneurysm of the abdominal aorta. If one recalls that the pressure in this large vein is usually less than 10 mm. of mercury, the concept of digital control above and below the point of injury, of clearing of the blood by aspiration and irrigation, and of careful approximation of the edges of the vein with an everting mattress suture of 5-0 braided silk is relatively simple and yet ideal. The continuity of the vein is maintained and hemorrhage controlled.

If a varicose vein in the lower leg is struck by a sharp object and begins to hemorrhage externally, this can be a most terrifying event to the patient; it is, however, easily managed by having the patient lie down, combined with elevation of the foot and digital pressure over the bleeding point. A light pressure dressing followed by application of an Ace bandage from toes to knee will be useful.

The second complication which sometimes follows trauma to a vein is thrombosis with, occasionally, embolic phenomena. If no contraindication exists, then anticoagulant therapy is valuable in conjunction with bed rest and massive warm compresses with rapid control of the thrombotic process. When pain and tenderness have cleared, ambulation with an Ace bandage, later to be replaced by a custom-made elastic stocking, will prevent the development of post-thrombotic edema.

The third complication, although rare, is the development of air embolus through a partially lacerated vein in the neck or thorax. Each inspiration draws in air and only small amounts may lead to difficulty. The lungs will filter out a moderate amount of air, but, if a patent foramen ovale exists, air in the coronary arteries or brain may rapidly cause death. Therapy is based on immediate closure of the hole in the vein either by pressure or by clamping. Once air is in the heart, a remedy sometimes useful is to place the patient in the head-down position to protect the brain.

TRAUMA TO THE LYMPHATICS

For practical purposes there is only one site where trauma to the lymphatic system may cause serious trouble of an acute nature, namely, the thoracic duct. During surgical procedures in the thorax, laceration of the thoracic duct may occur. The writer has inadvertently divided the duct high in the left chest on three occasions, twice during the performance of end-to-side subclavian pulmonic anastomosis in children with tetralogy of Fallot, and once in the excision of a coarctation of the aorta followed by end-to-end anastomosis. In each instance the opening in the duct was closed by transfixion sutures and an uneventful recovery followed. The complication of chylothorax develops only if the injured duct is not sutured. The therapy of this complication is considered in Chapter 18.

Chronic difficulties following trauma to the lymphatic system are encountered in the group of patients who develop lymphedema of the arm after radical mastectomy or lymphedema of the leg after radical groin dissection. It is generally accepted that infection of some degree must have been present postoperatively to explain the development of edema. Therapy for post-traumatic lymphedema includes elevation of the arm or leg, compression by a properly fitted elastic sleeve or stocking, and the control of fungus infection of the digits. Usually, moderate to marked improvement will follow.

BIBLIOGRAPHY

DeBakey, M. E., and Simeone, F. A.: Battle injuries of the arteries in World War II, Ann. Surg. 123:534, 1946.

Fairbank, H. H. T., Gordon-Taylor, G., and Page, C. Max: Emergency amputations, War Med. 2:147, 1942.

Jahnke, E. J., Jr., and Seeley, S. F.: Acute vascular injuries in the Korean War; analysis of 77 consecutive cases, Ann. Surg. 138:158, 1953.

Lord, J. W., Jr.: Traumatic lesions of the arteries, Surg. Clin. North America 30:377, 1950.

Lord, J. W., Jr., and Burke, G.: The comprehensive surgical management of aortic saddle emboli, Surgery 33:294, 1953.

Lord, J. W., Jr., and Schetlin, C. F.: Trauma to major arteries in the course of cancer surgery, Am. J. Surg. 87:209, 1954.

Report of a Committee on Blood Vessel Banks: Recommendations for the establishment and maintenance of a blood vessel bank, Circulation 13:270, 1956.

Shumacker, H. B., Jr.: The problem of maintaining the continuity of the artery in the surgery of aneurysms and arteriovenous fistulae; notes on the development and clinical application of methods of arterial suture, Ann. Surg. 127:207, 1948.

Shumacker, H. B., Jr., and Abramson, D. I.: Post-traumatic vasomotor disorders; with particular reference to late manifestations and treatment, Surg., Gynec. & Obst. 88:417, 1949.

Shumacker, H. B., Jr., Abramson, D. I., and Lampert, H. H.: The use of anticoagulants in the surgery of aneurysms and arteriovenous fistulas; with particular reference to Dicumarol, Surgery 22:910, 1947.

Part II

THE UPPER EXTREMITY

CHAPTER 6

INJURIES OF THE HAND

By THOMAS W. STEVENSON, M.D.†

and HARRISON L. McLAUGHLIN, M.D.

THE HUMAN HAND is an incomparable instrument which, considered in the light of its precisely balanced attachment to the forearm, approaches the ultimate in mechanical perfection. The mechanical devices with which man has surrounded himself cannot replace the hand, but greatly increase the likelihood of its accidental injury. All available knowledge pertinent to tissue salvation must be utilized in the care of an injured hand and should be implemented not only in conformity with the principles of tissue care common to all fields of surgery, but also with special attention to certain anatomical and physiological features peculiar to the hand.

ANATOMICAL FEATURES OF THE HAND

The Nails

Each finger is adorned with a nail (Fig. 6–*1*), which is of the same general derivation as hair. The nails originate from a level much closer to the distal interphalangeal joint than is apparent on casual inspection. For this reason complete surgical removal of a nail may prove difficult, and an apparently complete accidental avulsion may be followed by a surprisingly satisfactory regrowth of a new nail.

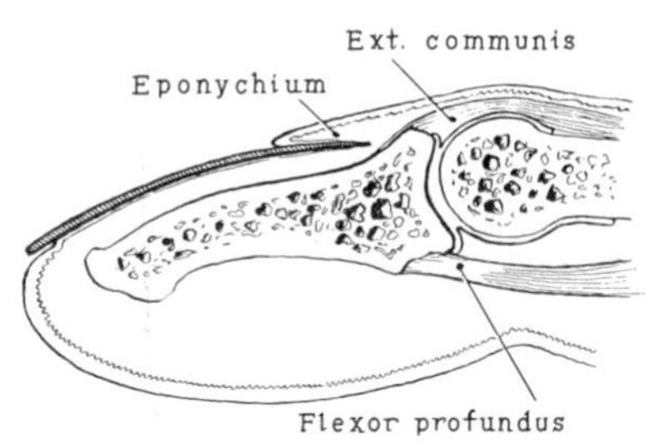

Figure 6–1. Sagittal section of finger showing arrangement of the nail and its eponychium, with the extensor and flexor tendon insertions. The nail is usually found closely applied to the bone and is practically inseparable from the periosteum of the bone

† Deceased.

The normal nail has a projecting distal edge which is the only instrument with which a small object, such as a pin, can be picked up from a smooth surface. Each lateral nail margin is recessed within a cutaneous fold, the paronychium, and the base of the nail rests beneath a similar fold, the eponychium. The exposed nail surface is curved from side to side so that its concave surface conforms to the dorsal surface of the distal phalanx of the finger. Longitudinal nail growth takes place from a broad proximal segment of nail bed which extends distalward to the visible crescentic lunula. Distal to this point the nail may increase slightly in width, but not in thickness. Deep to the nail is a rich capillary bed which, in its response to compression, constitutes a reliable index of the terminal circulation of the extremity.

The Skin and Fat

The skin is applied to the hand and fingers with a much more perfect fit than could be obtained with a rubber glove. If a glove fits well in extension, it constricts in flexion; if it fits well in flexion, it is loose in extension. Multiple transverse ridges in the skin ensure a good fit in all positions. The dorsal skin is thin and, by virtue of loose subcutaneous fat and areolar tissue, quite mobile and elastic. The palmar skin is thick, quite tough and inelastic, fixed and relatively immobile in places, and yet adequately provided with creases and folds to allow free mobility at the joints. The proximity of the palmar skin creases to the underlying tendons and joints increases the vulnerability of these structures to trauma. Between the creases is a specialized layer of subcutaneous fat which is compressed by a dense fibrous stroma arranged somewhat in the fashion of the springs in an innerspring mattress. These flexor areas are designed to withstand pressure, and their dorsal counterparts are but sparsely provided with any similar protective mechanism.

The Fascia

The fascial layers of the hand and fingers converge to subdivide the deep palmar spaces and to separate incompletely certain of the dorsal areas of the fingers from their corresponding flexor spaces. The palmar fascia (Fig. 6–2) is a greatly condensed structure which protects the deep contents of the palm from direct trauma, and also seems to function somewhat as a guy-wire designed to prevent undue hyperextension of the hand-finger unit.

The Tendons and Their Sheaths

Deep to the palmar fascia is a complex mass of structures arranged in an amazingly orderly manner. The long flexor tendons and their sheaths are the most easily discernible structures and, because of their size, firmness, and fixation, most vulnerable to injury (Fig. 6–3). Between them, one pair for each finger, lie the short flexor muscles and neurovascular

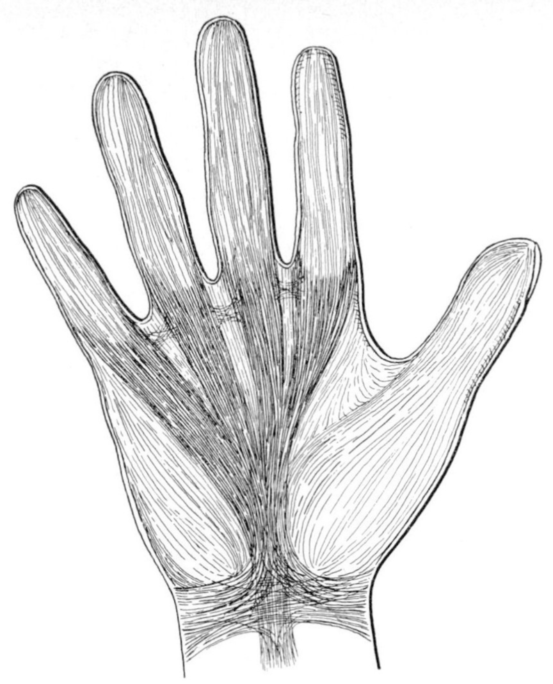

Figure 6–2. The palmar fascia.

Because of the frequency with which bands are seen running from the wrist up the radial side of the thumb, from the thumb to the base of the index finger, and up the ulnar side of the hand, the palmar fascia suggests a glove rather than four separate fascial bands as it is generally illustrated. It is true that in some hands very little evidence of fascia can be seen.

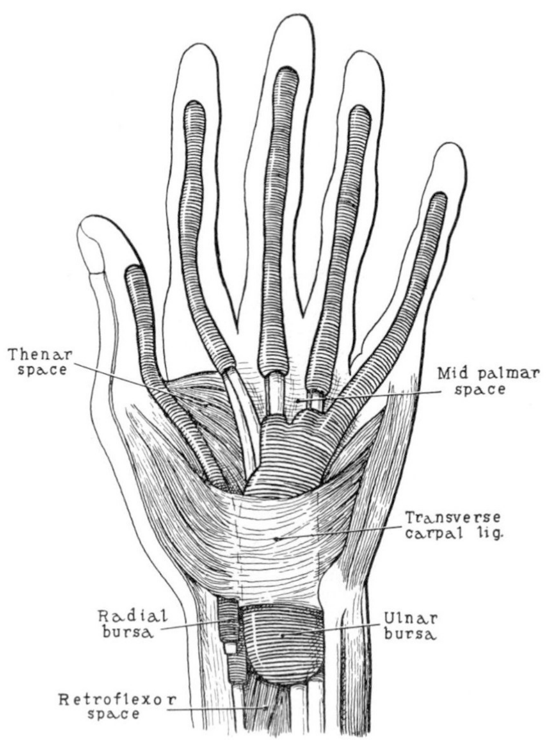

Figure 6–3. Flexor surface of palm with usual arrangement of sheaths, all of them distended. Note that the communication between the fifth finger sheath and the thumb is hidden by the transverse carpal ligament.

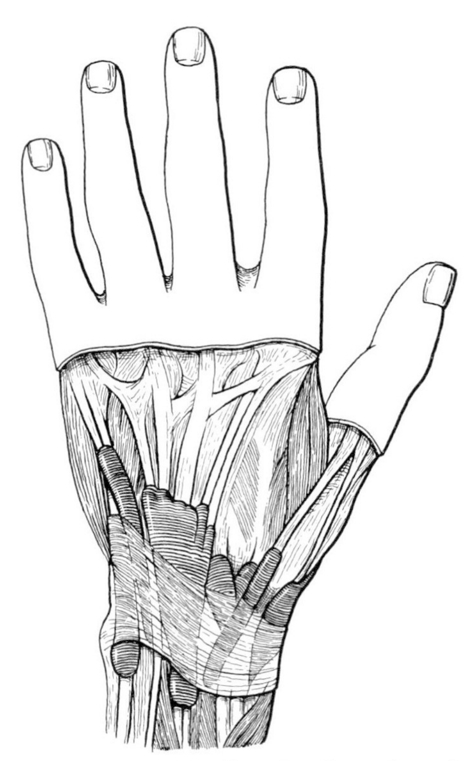

Figure 6–4. Average arrangement of tendon sheaths and tendons on dorsum of hand—all sheaths distended. Tendon sheaths are seldom found as distinct as this.

bundles. In the palm all tendons are invested with synovial sheaths which facilitate their movement under the constricting volar carpal ligament. As a rule, these sheaths extend distalward to enclose the entire lengths of the long flexor tendons to the thumb and fifth finger, and communicate under the volar carpal ligament, while the continuity of the palmar and digital portions of the remaining tendon sheaths is interrupted just proximal to the metacarpophalangeal joints (Fig. 6–3). All sheaths are composed of thin serous tubular membranes, arranged in visceral and parietal layers which remain in mobile contact to form a gliding mechanism somewhat similar to that of the conjunctiva of the eye. The extensor tendons are devoid of sheaths, except at the level of the wrist (Fig. 6–4).

The blood supply to a sheathed tendon comes from the two ends and via the vinculum tendinum. There are no demonstrable blood vessels within the substance of a tendon, but there is a wide superficial plexus of vessels just deep to the visceral synovial membrane. Unsheathed tendons are surrounded by areolar tissue. Consequently they are less apt to suffer from vascular privation following any type of injury, or to retract as far as do their sheathed counterparts when divided.

The function of a tendon is to transmit power from a muscle to a bone. This prerequires a strong inelastic structure which can be directed around a corner and prevented from prolapsing into a bowstring. The thumb has a single long flexor tendon of maximum caliber. Each finger has two flexor tendons, a sublimis which divides and inserts into each side of the middle phalanx, and a profundus which inserts into and motivates the distal phalanx (see Figure 6–6). Annular ligaments hold the flexor tendons against the phalanges to prevent their prolapse in the position of flexion.

Bones, Joints, and Ligaments

The bones of the hand and fingers are hung together by joint capsules and ligaments which permit appropriate and defend against excessive motions. The middle metacarpal is almost rigid, whereas the remainder, especially the first and fifth, are mobile. The resting hand forms a long arch from wrist to finger tips, and a short arch across the metacarpal heads, both concave toward the volar surface. In the position of grasp the lateral axes of the forearm and first metacarpal coincide, and all fingers point

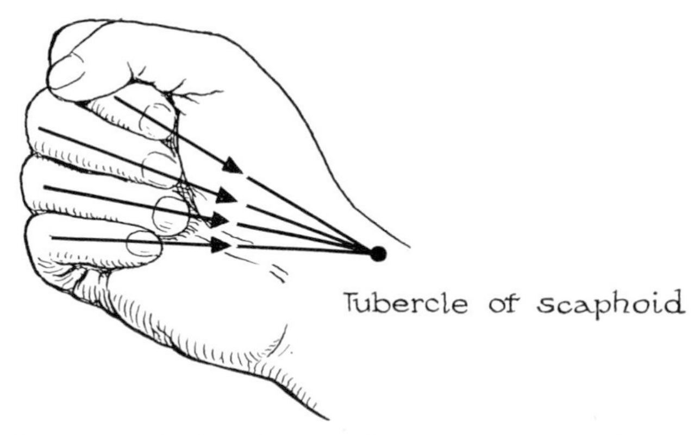

Figure 6–5. Axes of the flexed fingers do not correspond to those of the metacarpal or forearm bones, but converge on the tubercle of the scaphoid. Finger traction should be made in this direction.

toward the tubercle of the scaphoid bone (Fig. 6–5). With rare exceptions this is the position in which the immobilized hand must be maintained if maximal function is to be retained.

SOFT TISSUE INJURIES

Hand trauma takes so many forms and may involve such a diversity of tissues that the final deforming effect cannot often be foretold immediately after an injury. Most minute injuries pass without more than momentary notice, but may lead to serious damage. Conversely, seemingly devastating trauma may be followed by a good result. The capricious benevolence of nature is not as important a factor in these variable results as the technical grace by which the injured member is managed by the surgeon. The functional responsibilities of the hand and the complexity of its anatomy place a greater than average demand upon the judgment and art of the surgeon, and yet the essentials of good hand treatment are but the fundamental principles of all surgery.

Lacerations

A linear cut predisposes to the formation of cicatricial bands which limit motion, especially if it crosses a flexion crease. An excessively curved laceration may eventuate in necrosis or retraction of the skin flap. A laceration of any depth is likely to injure the underlying tendons, nerves, or vessels. Sharp amputation is quite a different problem from amputation by crushing or avulsion. Fingertip injuries are most commonly seen in the child who has caught his finger in a door, and if the finger is withdrawn before the door is opened, the flesh is avulsed. Press punch injuries may crush several fingers or the entire hand. Avulsion of the bony insertion of the extensor, and less commonly the flexor, tendons from the distal phalanx is not infrequent, but except for the extensor pollicis longus (p. 155) the tendons of the wrist and hand seldom rupture through their substance.

IMMEDIATE TREATMENT

Every hand injury, regardless of apparent severity, warrants special attention for the patient's livelihood may hang in the balance. Definitive treatment is often required as urgently as for a perforated gastric ulcer. Control of bleeding by compression over a sterile, or at least a clean, dressing should be accomplished at the scene of the accident. A tourniquet is almost never necessary. After a sterile dressing has been applied to the wound it is copiously covered with soft fluffy material which is bandaged in place with moderate pressure, with the wrist slightly dorsiflexed and the fingers semiflexed. The total dressing should be sufficiently firm and bulky to provide relative immobility of the hand.

Shock and pain may require treatment, but sedation should not be excessive, for a detailed history and examination will be required before treatment is commenced. Roentgen examination for the localization of bone injuries or embedded foreign bodies should be done. The hand is then inspected and, in so far as possible, the nature and extent of the tissue damage is appraised before final disposition is determined.

Safety and wisdom dictate that even a simple and benign-appearing wound should be regarded as serious in preference to accepting the risk of overlooking a severed nerve or tendon, or the risk of infection. In general, all patients with injuries in which any doubt is possible deserve hospital admission for observation, and prompt discharge as soon as the doubt has been dispelled. Included in this doubtful category are all wounds in which the tissues show color changes suggestive of a jeopardized blood supply, most wounds attended by visible deformity, and many wounds containing foreign material.

Sensation must be assessed in the light of knowledge that the sensory patterns of the ulnar, median, and radial nerves do not always adhere to as constant a distribution as is suggested in most anatomical texts. The shortcomings of sensory tests in infants, frightened children, and adults suffering from alcoholism or other reductions of sensorium must be taken into account. All tests should include response to pin prick, light touch with a cotton swab and, for the most accurate results, these tests should be done out of sight of the patient.

A divided tendon should be suspected in the absence of voluntary joint motion, except when motion is interdicted by pain. Palpation is permissible, except at the wound area, and may reveal bone deformities otherwise camouflaged by swelling. Crepitus, a traditional sign of fracture, should not be elicited intentionally. In the absence of a pulse at the wrist the circulatory status of each finger may be determined by compressing the nail bed.

In short, based upon what can be seen, felt, and tested, the patient should be hospitalized for definitive treatment, or allowed to go home. In the latter circumstance the wound should be cleansed, dressed, and the hand elevated as scrupulously as if the patient remained in the hospital. Full and clear orders must be given. It is natural for the ambulatory patient to consider that if a wound does not hurt all is well and he may use the hand as he wishes. Without precise orders the surgeon must not be surprised if a child obtains satisfaction from sucking a bandaged thumb, or playing with toys in a toilet bowl. Orders should commence with instructions to keep the hand clean, dry, quiet, and elevated. Special instructions are necessary when moist applications are in order. Above all, the patient must be persuaded of the benefits of rest and elevation in militating for rapid and sound wound healing.

The hospitalized patient should be apprised not only of the nature and potential of his hand injury but also of the projected treatment program, and of the great importance of his cooperation. It is fair tactics to warn him of the dire consequences of any infractions of the therapeutic rules. Otherwise a perfect tendon repair may be disrupted soon after the patient leaves the supervision of the hospital environment.

OPERATIVE TREATMENT

Anesthesia

Local infiltration with 1 or 2 per cent procaine hydrochloride may suffice for procedures that are minor and of short duration. It is ordinarily contraindicated when infection is present, and when it may further compromise an already embarrassed tissue nutrition. Local anesthesia should not be used for time-consuming procedures for, although the operative field can be re-infiltrated, a much greater tissue burden and a reduced anesthetic effect is the inevitable result.

Regional brachial block anesthesia obviates the discomfort of tourniquet pressure, and is a very appropriate anesthetic for hand operations of intermediate duration. The technique is exacting and not without pitfalls and complications. Except in expert hands, a brachial hematoma, pneumothorax, or anesthetic failure is not uncommon.

Many patients require or prefer general anesthesia, which facilitates the technical task of the surgeon, makes the duration of the operation a matter of no vital significance, and produces a minimal emotional impact upon the patient.

Skin Preparation

Wide variations in methods of skin preparation exist. Many surgeons are content with thorough cleansing by soap and water alone, but a multitude of antiseptic solutions are also in common use. The skin should always be shaved over a wide field surrounding the wound. Prolonged gentle washing with some soap solution is the best method for cleansing the skin, and a small amount of hydrogen peroxide mixed with liquid soap provides an improved lather. It is logical to follow a soap and water surface cleansing with an ether rinse, in order to dissolve residual soap and fatty substances from the skin. A final washing with alcohol or some other clear antiseptic may have a beneficial effect, but the use of a colored solution, such as tincture of merthiolate, often makes it very difficult to assess the relative viability of the skin in the vicinity of the wound.

Tourniquet

Preparations for the use of a pneumatic tourniquet should be made in advance of the operation. A few turns of soft gauze or sheet wadding are bandaged loosely around the arm, midway between shoulder and elbow. A pneumatic cuff, *at least 3 to 4 inches wide,* is applied over this padding. A pressure dial should be attached to the cuff, which should be inflated to, but not in excess of, 300 mm. of mercury. It is not only physiologically sound but also conducive to a completely bloodless operative field to express all blood from the extremity by the application of a rubber bandage to the elevated extremity immediately prior to inflation of the tourniquet.

Prior to the advent of pneumatic tourniquets, neurological, vascular, and local complications were constant potentialities of bloodless operations; even with properly applied modern pneumatic devices and controlled pressure, similar complications may occur. Consequently, once a tourniquet has been applied, the operation should be carried out with all precision and dispatch compatible with safety. Although the potential penalties of operation upon an injured hand through a bloody field greatly overshadow those of the modern tourniquet, nevertheless no extremity should be maintained in an exsanguinated state any longer than is necessary.

Inspection and Cleansing of the Wound

The edges of the wound are raised gently with small hooks, and its cavity inspected. Coincident irrigation with sterile water or saline cleanses by lavage floats loose tissue fragments to the surface, and facilitates identification of devitalized tabs of attached tissues suitable for removal. Overtly necrotic skin margins should be trimmed by sharp dissection. All foreign material must be removed. When the immediately visible wound cavity has been cleansed and trimmed, the deeper reaches of the cavity should be explored. The findings will dictate whether or not the accidental wound should be extended by additional incisions.

Wound Extension and the Location of Divided Tendons

When a tendon has been divided, some extensions of the accidental wound, or additional incisions, are usually necessary. Knowledge of the position of the hand when the cut was inflicted will prove to be useful. A cut on the flexor surface of the closed fingers justifies anticipation that the distal cut end of the tendon will be found a considerable distance distal to the wound, as the finger is explored in the extended position, and the proximal cut end will be found only a short distance proximal to the wound. Such a history provides information indicating the necessity for distal extension of the wound. The reverse is true when a volar cut has been inflicted with the fingers extended. Under such circumstances the distal cut end of the tendon often can be delivered into the wound by flexion of the finger, and the proximal fragment sometimes recovered by flexion of the wrist. When the latter maneuver fails the surgeon should not grope blindly for the retracted tendon fragment. This invites unnecessary damage to tendon sheath, nerves, and vessels. A separate incision (Fig. 6–6) should be made at the level of the metacarpal head proximal to which the index, middle, and ring finger tendons rarely retract. The tendons to the thumb and fifth finger often retract a considerable distance, and a more proximal incision at the level of the wrist (Fig. 6–6) may be necessary for their recovery.

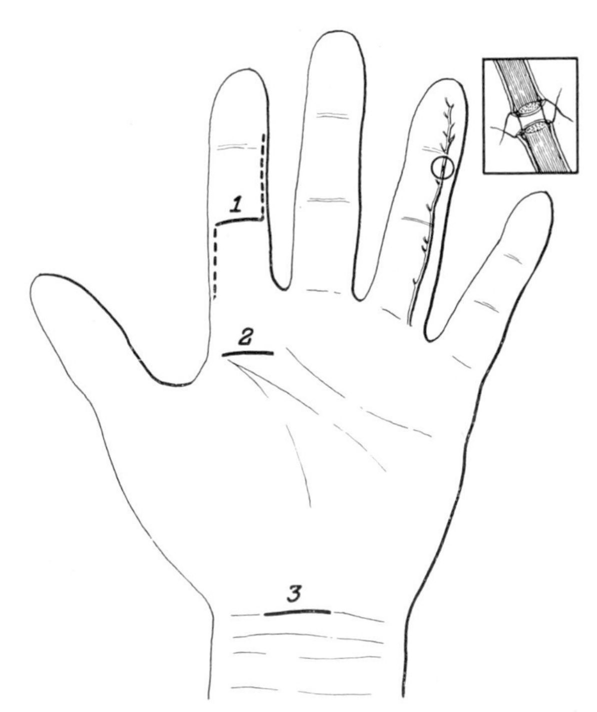

Figure 6–6. Methods of wound extension and placement of additional incisions useful in recovering a divided tendon. Insert illustrates technique of nerve repair. When the tendon has been severed at 1, *the retracted proximal fragment can be found at* 2. *In injuries to the thumb and fifth finger the proximal fragment may retract to* 3.

Tissue Conservation

Tissues with compromised circulation should be assessed and the areas to be excised mapped out and marked prior to the application of a tourniquet, after which estimation of skin viability is undependable. Any error in the excision of damaged tissues should be on the side of economy. Skin which is obviously and irreversibly damaged warrants excision and replacement by skin graft, but as a general rule, if damaged skin is badly needed, it should be left in place. Suture material should be restricted to the minimal amount necessary for hemostasis in wounds of more than six hours' duration, even if this requires that deep structures be left without repair. The skin wound should be repaired as precisely as possible, except in event of gross contamination. Grossly contaminated wounds of more than a few hours' duration usually should not be closed. A repaired tendon should be covered not by a free skin graft, but rather by a pedicle flap of skin from an adjacent area. The donor site of the pedicle may be covered by a free partial-thickness skin graft.

REPAIR OF INJURED STRUCTURES

Pairing of Cut Tendons

The surgeon repairing a complex hand injury may be unduly comforted by the presence of a standard textbook on anatomy, forgetting that its author probably never saw or dissected a hand in disrepair through a bloody field. A better guide than a knowledge of normal anatomy may be required in order to identify and re-approximate multiple cut tendon fragments with accuracy. Every tendon lies at a specified depth beneath the skin. The palmaris longus is subcutaneous; its cut ends are easily located, marked with sutures, and turned out of the wound. The sublimis tendons occupy the next deeper tissue stratum. They are not often cut transversely by an accidental laceration. Each cut tendon end may, therefore, be matched to its mate, marked, and turned aside. The profundus tendons occupy the deepest layer. No two are identical in caliber, and usually no two cuts are at exactly the same angle. The cut ends of these tendons may likewise be matched with reasonable accuracy.

Tendon Repair

Tendon repair should be accomplished with a single, buried, nonabsorbable suture. One of the numerous methods in common use is illustrated in Figure 6–7. The suture enters the cut end of the proximal fragment and, after several convolutions through the tendon substance, emerges close to its point of entrance. With a needle on each, the free ends of the suture are then inserted into the cut end of the distal fragment. After the first convolution the suture is snugged up until the tendon ends are approximated. Several more convolutions are then taken in the distal fragment, and the two ends of the suture are tied at a common point of exit. There should be no "bunching" of the tendon fragments, nor should any gap remain between their cut ends. When both the sublimis and profundus

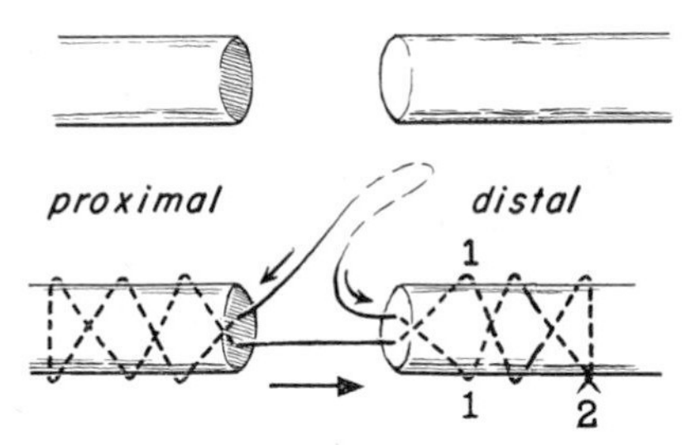

Figure 6–7. Tendon repair by a single buried suture.

The suture is woven into the proximal fragment, entering and emerging from the cut end. With a needle on each end of the suture, one convolution is then made in the distal fragment to 1. The tendon ends are then snugged up and just approximated. Several more convolutions are then made through the distal fragment, and the suture ends are tied at a common point of exit (2).

tendons have been severed in the digital flexor canal, the profundus only should be repaired, and the sublimis removed. Attempts to suture both tendons will result in failure. The tendon sheath may be repaired with very fine catgut, but is often excised to leave the tendon repair covered by fat and areolar tissues. If the carpal ligaments or fibrous tendon sheath has been divided by the injury or the operation, secure repair is necessary to prevent subsequent tendon prolapse.

Primary tendon repair should not be done in the absence of good equipment, good light, ample time, and technical competence. Except under ideal circumstances, the course of wisdom and safety is to cleanse and excise the wound, close the skin, and plan for later reconstruction of the damaged tendons. Late reconstruction is followed by results which are comparable to those of successful primary repair, but with much less risk of complications.

Nerve Repair

Laceration of a nerve almost always accompanies tendon laceration. Certain rules are important to successful nerve repair. The sutures should be fine and small, and placed in the perineurium rather than in the substance of the nerve (see Figure 6–6). A nerve should not be sutured until all tendon damage has been repaired. Otherwise, the delicate and weak nerve repair may be disrupted. The digital nerves, contrary to a widespread misconception, are almost as large as the lead in a pencil, and should be repaired whenever possible. In the absence of repair, nerve regeneration will not bridge a gap of any kind, nor will the nerve on the other side of the finger compensate for loss of sensation by division of its mate.

EMBEDDED FOREIGN BODIES

Foreign bodies in the hand are common and potentially serious problems. Wood or glass often cannot be located by roentgenogram. All radiopaque bodies should be localized before any attempt is made to remove them. Two fine wires, such as are used to clean hypodermic needles, are crossed at right angles on the skin over the suspected area. Additional wires are arranged at 1 cm. intervals in both directions. A roentgenogram will then localize the embedded body in relation to the surface wires, and the exact spot is marked on the skin with methylene blue. If the hand is then explored in exactly the same position as when the roentgenogram was taken, the incision should be precisely over the foreign body.

PENETRATING WOUNDS AND INFECTIONS

Puncture wounds by small sharp objects often seem trivial at the time. They may sever a deep structure, but their most dangerous sequel is infection. Puncture by a human tooth is usually attended by a specially virulent and rapid infection. Bullet wounds, which in most areas must be reported, are another kind of puncture wound. Small bullets may stop in the hand, but larger missiles pass through, leaving a small wound of entrance, a large gaping wound of exit, and devastation to all intervening structures. Particles of lead, glass, wood, stone, grease, or indelible lead may be introduced through a small puncture wound, leaving a traumatic tattoo after the wound heals. The foreign material must be removed immediately if this complication is to be prevented. The removal of grease, especially as in injury by a service station grease gun, may prove impossible.

Felon

Puncture of the pulp of a finger tip may result in an infection of the anterior closed space (Fig. 6–8). The pulp of the finger becomes hard,

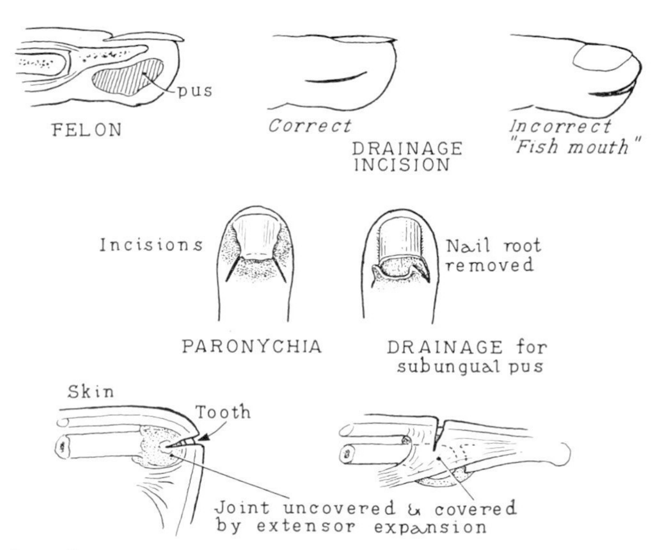

Figure 6–8. Placement of incisions for drainage of felons (above) and paronychia (middle). Below, a tooth wound at the metacarpophalangeal joint is almost always incurred when the joint is flexed, and both the extensor expansion and the joint capsule are penetrated. When such a wound is examined with the joint extended the wound of the capsule is hidden.

tense, and exquisitely tender. The original site of puncture may or may not be apparent. Delay in decompression of the abscess invites extension of the infection to produce osteomyelitis of the distal bone phalanx. Incision for drainage should be placed over the lateral border of the distal phalanx. The tip of the finger should not be opened to produce a "fish-mouth" aperture, which usually eventuates in a painful scar.

Paronychia

Infection of the cutaneous recesses which house the nail should be drained quickly lest it extend to undermine the nail. When the infection has invaded the subungual region a flap of eponychium should be elevated, and the root of the nail removed to allow free egress of the subungual pus (Fig. 6–8). When this procedure has been early and adequate, satisfactory regrowth of the nail may be anticipated.

Tendon Sheath Infection

More often than not infections of tendon sheaths result from puncture wounds which were, at first, considered insignificant. Gradually the finger swells, assumes a position of semiflexion, becomes exquisitely tender except on the dorsal surface, and cannot be extended at all without severe pain. Early drainage by an appropriate incision (Fig. 6–9) should be done. When the tendon sheath to the thumb is involved the infection may extend to the wrist, and into the sheath to the fifth finger via the carpal communication between the radial and ulnar bursae (see Figure 6–3). Conversely, infection may also travel from the fifth finger to the thumb. Adequate drainage usually requires incision into the retroflexor compartment at the wrist (Fig. 6–9).

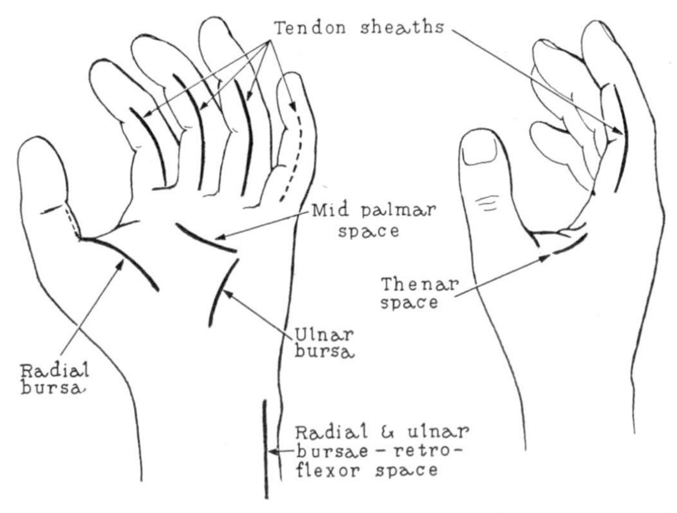

Figure 6–9. Incisions for drainage of infections in tendon sheaths and spaces of the hand. (After Kanavel and Mason.)

Middle Palmar and Thenar Space Infections

The middle palmar space (see Figure 6–3) may be infected by a penetrating wound, or by extension of pus from the digital tendon sheaths of the middle or ring finger. The hollow of the palm becomes convex and tender, and the entire hand is swollen. The abscess is located between the unsheathed segments of the flexor tendons to the ring and middle fingers. In a similar fashion the thenar space may be infected by penetration from without, or by pus from the digital tendon sheath to the index finger. The abscess forms anterior to the thumb adductor muscles. The thumb assumes a position of abduction, and the web space between it and the index metacarpal becomes greatly swollen and tender. Appropriate incisions for drainage of infections in these areas are indicated in Figure 6–9.

Human Bites

These injuries are most commonly located on the presenting prominence of the metacarpophalangeal joint where the closed fist came into contact with a tooth. Frequently treatment is not sought until considerable time has elapsed, and a virulent infection has become well established.

Failure to recognize metacarpophalangeal joint involvement is a common mistake. At the moment of injury the fist was clenched, and this joint unprotected by the fibrous expansion of the extensor tendons; at examination with the hand in a position of rest the lacerated joint is covered by the extensor expansions which present an apparently intact surface to inspection through the wound (see Figure 6–8). The surgeon must examine and explore such wounds with the fingers clenched. Bite wounds should not be sutured; rather, they should be drained well, rested, splinted, elevated, treated by antibiotics and antitetanus serum, and allowed to close by secondary intent. Extension of such joint infections into metacarpals and phalanges, and along the lumbrical tunnels into the intermetacarpal spaces is not uncommon.

BURNS OF THE HAND

Burns comprise a substantial proportion of injured hands, and vary in severity from a tiny spot burned by a drop of hot grease to deep electrical burns involving all soft tissues and bones. Many chemicals burn, especially when combined with heat, and these injuries are encountered with increasing frequency in the plastics industries. Hot plastic material may be injected through the palm under high pressure and come to rest under the skin on the dorsum of the hand where the final damage is done by heat until this large foreign body cools.

Roentgen rays produce a sinister burn, which is most often incurred by physicians, veterinarians, and scientists, but may result from accidental over-exposure in a patient. In contrast to thermal burns, wherein the cause and effect are immediately apparent, the roentgen burn has a delayed effect which may not become obvious for days or years. An acute roentgen burn at first resembles sunburn, commencing with redness and soon followed by blisters and necrosis. A painful indolent ulcer requiring block excision and pedicle graft coverage of the defect is often the end-result. Repeated exposure to small doses may not produce an acute burn. Instead, the skin subsequently becomes atrophic, pigmented, telangiectatic, and host to multiple keratoses which often manifest epitheliomatous changes requiring amputation or, when superficial, excision and replacement by partial-thickness skin grafts.

Treatment of Thermal Burns

The principles for treatment of the burned hand have been described in Chapter 4, Thermal Trauma (p. 79). Except for small and well-circumscribed areas of deep burn, there is seldom any need for immediate excision and skin graft of the burned area. Early replacement of irreparably burned skin is always a great time saver, but, as a rule, it is difficult and often impossible to recognize and delineate the burned areas appropriate for eventual skin replacement in the early period after injury. Excision and replacement, therefore, should generally be deferred until a firm decision becomes possible.

The burned skin should be thoroughly but gently cleansed, and all particles of foreign matter removed from the surface. Tags of loose skin and open blisters should be removed, but closed blisters should remain unmolested. With the hand in the position of maximum function a pressure dressing should be applied over sterile fine-mesh petrolatum gauze, and the extremity elevated and put at rest on a splint. Barring indications of infection, this dressing should remain undisturbed for seven to ten days. Many of the burned areas at first thought to need grafting will heal. Areas of deeper burn will demarcate within two or three weeks, after which excision and replacement may be carried out with safety and confidence.

ATTRITIONAL TRAUMA AND DEGENERATIVE CONDITIONS

Tenosynovitis

Irritative and inflammatory penalties of excessive mechanical wear and tear may become manifest at any point of friction in the tendon–tendon sheath system. Acute synovitis may result from a single period of overuse. Often this condition commences with nothing more than soft crepitus on motion, which may be followed by a tense effusion into the tendon sheath cavity. Abolition of the offending motion and rest usually are followed by rapid recovery.

de Quervain's stenosing tenosynovitis involves the thumb tendons at the radial styloid process, is usually of occupational cause, and results from frequently repeated wrist motions coincident with tension of these tendons. The clinical picture follows a consistent pattern. Often there is a visible and tender prominence at the radial styloid. The thumb tendons are tender at this area. Resisted abduction or forced passive ulnar deviation of the thumb metacarpal produces or accentuates the patient's presenting complaint. Immediate relief is provided by incision of the constricting fibrous tendon sheaths which bind the thumb tendons to the radial styloid.

Trigger finger is a descriptive term which denotes a small localized area of tenosynovitis in the flexor tendon–tendon sheath mechanism, usually located at about the level of the metacarpal head. A small area of tendon sheath becomes irritated. The tendon just distal to this constricted area becomes swollen. As this small swollen area snaps back and forth through the constricted tendon sheath the finger also snaps into flexion, extension, or both, in the manner of a trigger. The degree of snapping is quite variable in different patients. The trigger area is tender. Usually if the finger does not snap visibly, the lump in the tendon can be felt to snap back and forth under its constricting band. Incision of the constricted tendon sheath produces immediate relief.

Calcium deposits may develop in any of the tendons of the hand. Their pathology and life cycle correspond to that described in detail in the discussion of similar deposits in the shoulder (p. 281), but chronic painful symptoms are almost unknown. In the hand an acute episode of short duration is the rule. The resultant acute synovitis of the tendon sheath involved may be differentiated from a suppurative lesion by a marked discrepancy between the acute clinical picture and the mild and insignificant systemic response. Operative treatment is rarely necessary. If the acute symptoms of this self-limiting painful condition are controlled for 48 to 72 hours, full recovery will occur spontaneously.

Ganglion is the most common tumor of the hand. This lesion may occur in relation to any joint, but is usually encountered as a cystic, elastic, nontender mass which presents on the dorsum of the wrist. It should be differentiated from a tendon sheath effusion, which may present a similar appearance but can be milked back and forth under the dorsal transverse ligament at the wrist (Fig. 6–*10*). The traditional treatment of ganglion by striking and rupturing the soft lump with a book is usually followed by recurrence. Aspiration of the contents of the cystic cavity, with or without

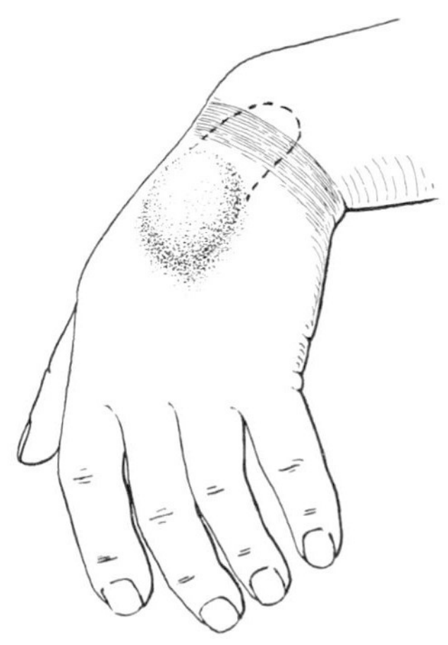

Figure 6–10. Large ganglia and tendon-sheath effusions on dorsum of wrist can be differentiated. Pressure on a synovial effusion distal to the annular ligament (see Figure 6–4) forces the fluid under the ligament to form a new lump more proximally. This is not true of a ganglion.

the use of sclerosing fluids, is attended by a high incidence of failure. The tumor should be removed or ignored. The risk of malignant change is negligible.

Dupuytren's contracture of the palmar fascia (see Figure 6–2) remains an etiological enigma, occurring in about 1.5 per cent of the white male population, and being about equally common in laborers and in sedentary workers. It is not caused by trauma, for it is usually bilateral, and the plantar as well as the palmar fascia is often involved. Trauma to the palm may aggravate an existing fascial lesion and create temporary symptoms of pain.

The essential pathological change is thickening and contracture of the fascial bands in the palm, which appear first as a small, hard, non-tender lump, with dimpling of the skin of the palm opposite the fourth metacarpal head. Gradually the fourth finger is pulled into flexion. In advanced cases acute and intractable flexion deformities may develop in any or all of the fingers, and occasionally in the thumb. The condition is slowly but inexorably progressive, quite benign, but sometimes difficult to distinguish histologically from well-differentiated fibrosarcoma. When treatment is necessitated by disability consequent to contracture, the palmar fascia, including its extensions to the fingers, should be removed completely.

INJURIES OF THE FINGERS

Subungual Hematoma

Contusion or crushing of a nail results in subungual hemorrhage. The blue hematoma is visible through the nail. The area is exquisitely tender and painful. Immediate relief results from decompression of the hematoma by drilling a small hole through the nail.

Crushed Fingertip

The fingertip is caught in a closing door. All tissues are crushed, and the phalanx may be broken. Subungual hemorrhage occurs, but often is decompressed spontaneously through fractures in the phalanx. The nail should not be opened. Even when the phalanx has been fragmented this injury should be treated not as a fracture but in accord with the dictates of the soft part damage. No form of treatment can alter the position of bony fragments of the distal phalanx, which are stabilized securely by soft part attachments. Warm soaks, rest, elevation, and protection against injury should be applied until the symptoms subside.

Traumatic Amputation

Forcible withdrawal of a finger which has been caught and crushed in a door may produce a traumatic amputation. This is a much more serious problem than a clean-cut amputation by a sharp edge, where the only problem is coverage or closure of a viable stump. When the amputation has been produced by a crushing injury the viability of the stump tissues

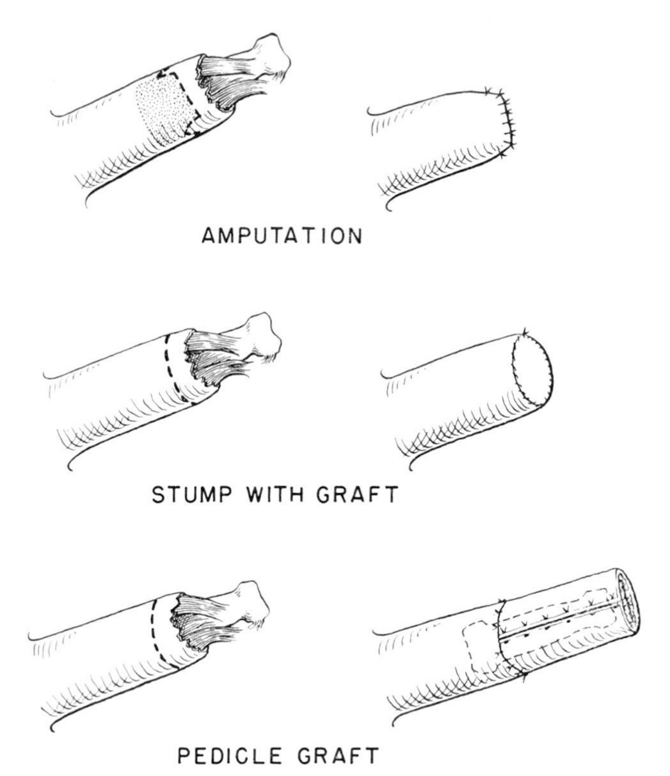

Figure 6–11. Methods of repair for traumatic amputation.

This injury is repaired most easily by amputating the bone at a level proximal to that of the soft tissues, which are then fashioned into flaps and closed by suture. This is not often justifiable in the thumb. When shortening is contraindicated, the stump may be closed by a free full-thickness graft. In thumb injuries and ring avulsions characterized by loss of tissue and preservation of bone, the bone may be surrounded with a pedicle graft.

is always uncertain, and there is a constant consequent risk of infection or circumscribed gangrene.

The wound must be closed. When the tissues are permitted to heal by granulations a painful and sensitive stump is almost inevitable. Bone which projects a small distance beyond the amputated soft tissues may be shortened a little in order to facilitate skin closure (Fig. 6–*11*), but *the thumb should not be shortened or amputated as a primary procedure.* Digital nerves, which present in the wound, should be pulled down and divided as far proximal to the stump as possible lest their ends become caught in the scar. Hemostasis should be complete. All devitalized tabs should be trimmed back to viable tissue. It is poor practice to suture the flexor and extensor tendons to each other over the end of the bone stump, for this impedes motion and is almost always productive of disability. The skin must never be sutured under tension.

When the wound cannot be closed by suture without undue shortening of the bone, closure may be accomplished by covering the stump-end with a free full-thickness skin graft (Fig. 6–*11*). This may be cut from the abdomen, or, when a recently amputated finger tip has been carried in with the patient, its skin may be cleansed, separated from all subcutaneous tissues, and re-applied as a graft.

Ring avulsions, resulting from the forcible avulsion of a ring from the finger along with much of the flesh and skin, and amputations of the thumb characterized by the loss of much more soft tissues than of bone, often deserve coverage with a pedicle graft (Fig. 6–*11*). Such a procedure is of particular importance for the treatment of appropriate thumb injuries where all possible length must be preserved, and in which unnecessary shortening may well be catastrophic. The trimmed and cleansed stump is buried under a pedicle of skin and subcutaneous tissue in the abdominal wall. The pedicle may be separated and a tubular covering fashioned for the stump after about three weeks.

FINGER FRACTURES AND JOINT INJURIES

Injuries to the bones and joints of the fingers, probably because the tissue damage appears small and localized, are very often productive of prolonged incapacity and followed by a poor result due to neglect; however, disastrous results are as easily and almost as often produced by over-treatment or poor treatment. Deformity is the chief penalty of neglect; stiffness, of over-treatment; and both are likely to result from poor treatment.

The most common causes of deformity are malunion of a phalangeal fracture and chronic subluxation of an interphalangeal joint. Chronic joint subluxation usually follows dislocation with avulsion or rupture of one collateral ligament. Following reduction the phalanx continues to deviate away from the unsupported side, and normal alignment must be maintained by splints. This complication should be suspected when roentgenograms disclose a chip of bone (representing the ligament attachment) to be avulsed from the base of the dislocated phalanx.

Malunion of a fractured phalanx in the anteroposterior plane interferes with flexion and extension. This deformity is usually caused by neglect or immobilization in extension. Malunion in the lateral or rotatory plane results in deviation of the finger, which then overlaps or underlaps the other fingers, and obstructs their motion when the hand is used as a unit. These deformities may result from neglect, but more often are produced by immobilization or traction applied to the finger in the long axis of its metacarpal rather than in a line centering upon the tubercle of the scaphoid bone (see Figure 6–5).

Unstable fractures should be immobilized in flexion. Only the injured finger should be immobilized. The remaining fingers must have their mobility maintained. Passive stretching of a stiff joint is harmful and increases stiffness. Prolonged edema promotes fibrosis and stiffness, and must be counteracted by elevation. Adherence to these principles will minimize, but not prevent, results which are less than satisfactory. The finger mechanism is composed almost completely of connective tissues which are so intricate, functionally interdependent, and delicate that the mere superimposition of nothing more than the normal fibrosis of repair may produce a substantial reduction of joint mobility. This is well illustrated by a simple sprain of a finger joint which, with or without treatment, is prone to remain stiff, swollen, and painful for months.

Mallet Finger

The end of the extended finger is struck by a ball, or the terminal phalanx is forced into sudden flexion by some other mechanism, against coincident extensor contraction. The extensor tendon is avulsed from the terminal phalanx, usually accompanied by a small chip of bone representing its bony attachment. The terminal phalanx droops in a semiflexed position and cannot be actively extended.

The avulsed fragment cannot be reduced and held in proper position except when the middle interphalangeal joint is flexed enough to neutralize

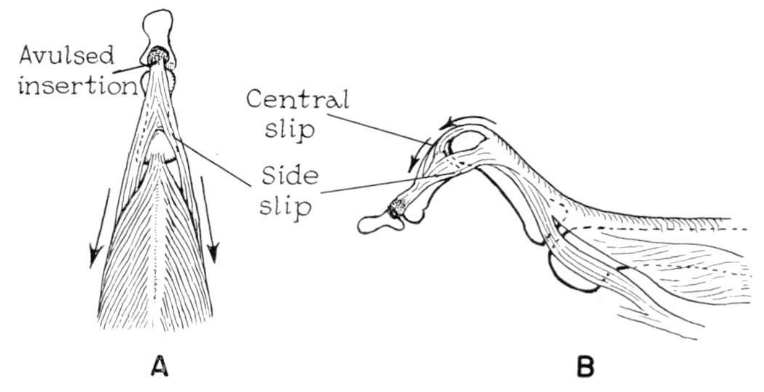

Figure 6–12. Avulsion of extensor tendon.

A. The side slips of the extensor mechanism exert the retracting force applied to the avulsed terminal tendon attachment.

B. Flexion of the proximal interphalangeal joint, by pulling the central slip distalward, neutralizes the retracting force of the side slips. Flexion of this joint and extension of the distal joint are necessary to replacement and maintenance of replacement of an avulsion of the terminal extensor attachment (mallet finger).

the retracting force of the extensor mechanism (Fig. 6–*12*). Coincidentally, the terminal joint is immobilized in full extension. Efficient splints are not easy to apply; they are difficult to maintain effectively; and few patients will tolerate an efficient splint for a long enough period to ensure sound healing. Eventual fibrous union, attended by some loss or weakness of extension of the distal phalanx, is the rule. Fortunately, the consequent functional defect is usually unimportant.

Fracture of the Middle Phalanx

A fracture of the middle phalanx caused by crushing, or by a direct blow, is apt to be quite stable. A simple splint in the semiflexed position will prevent loss of position of the bone fragments, which remain well stabilized by intact soft part attachments. Under such circumstances prolonged immobilization is an invitation to stiffness. Soaks and gentle progressive resumption of active motion usually are permissible within two or three weeks after injury.

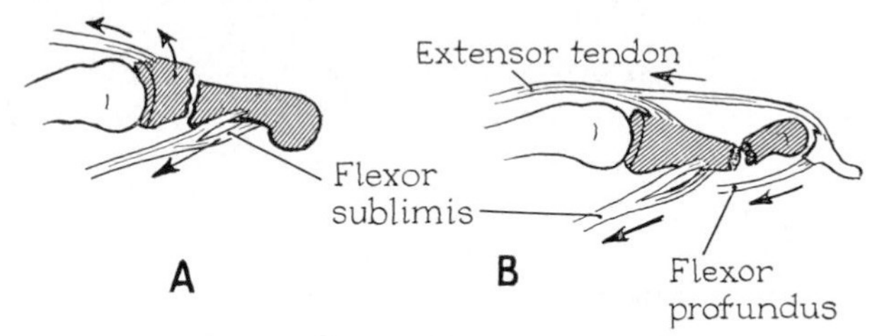

Figure 6–13. Fractures of middle phalanx.

A. The small proximal fragment of a fracture of the middle phalanx proximal to the sublimis insertion is extended by the central slip of the extensor mechanism. The distal fragment must be re-aligned with this uncontrollable fragment.

B. Both fragments of the middle phalanx are controllable when the fracture is distal to the sublimis insertion. Immobilize in flexion.

Unstable fractures of the middle phalanx assume a fairly consistent displacement pattern, which depends upon the location of the injury. When the fracture is proximal to the sublimis insertion (Fig. 6–*13, A*) the small proximal fragment is extended by the central slip of the extensor tendon, and the distal fragment is depressed and flexed by the flexor tendons. The distal fragment must be realigned with the small and uncontrollable proximal fragment, and maintenance of reduction may require immobilization of the finger in the extended position. When the fracture is distal to the sublimis insertion (Fig. 6–*13, B*) the proximal fragment is flexed, and the distal fragment is extended. This displacement should be reduced and the finger immobilized in the flexed position.

Fracture of the Proximal Phalanx

The majority of finger fractures involve the proximal phalanx. The deformity pattern is usually characterized by angulation with an anterior

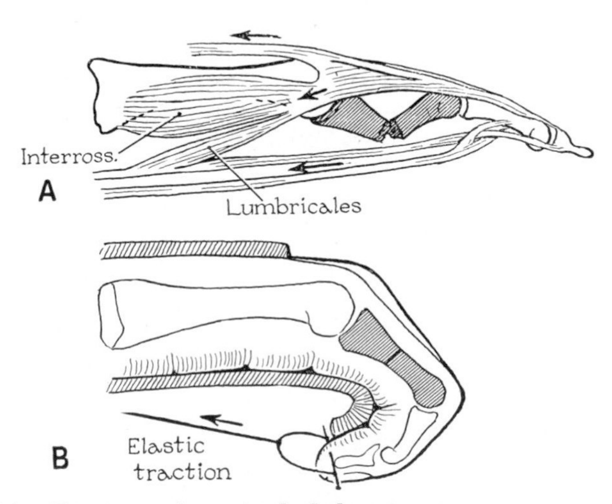

Figure 6–14. Fractures of proximal phalanx.

A. All the muscle forces acting upon a fracture of the proximal phalanx collaborate to produce an angular deformity, apex forward.

B. Proximal phalanx fractures must be immobilized by well-fitting splints with the finger flexed. Unstable fractures may require supplemental traction.

apex (Fig. 6–*14, A*). These fractures are reduced with ease, but must be immobilized in flexion, for the deformity will recur if the finger is extended. In certain unstable or oblique fractures immobilization in flexion must be supplemented by light elastic traction (Fig. 6–*14, B*) before reduction can be maintained. Reduction and secure fixation of these fractures is important. Malunion with residual angulation implicates the flexor canal and its tendons in a mass of healing tissues to produce a finger that is not only deformed, but stiff.

Dislocation and Fracture-Dislocation of Finger Joints

Dislocation of an interphalangeal joint results from hyperextension and is reduced by traction and flexion. Maintenance of reduction requires maintenance of flexion. As a rule, progressive motion and use may be commenced within two weeks after injury.

When the base of a phalanx, or the condyle of a phalangeal head, is fractured coincident with dislocation, the reduction is unstable. Redislocation may not occur, but subluxation is common. A subluxed interphalangeal joint is synonymous with a stiff finger, and when loss of position cannot be prevented by immobilization, prolonged traction and, at times, operative repair may be required for a good result. Neither of these procedures should be approached casually for each, in its own right, is liable to produce a stiff finger.

DISLOCATION OF METACARPOPHALANGEAL JOINTS

The metacarpophalangeal joints differ from the interphalangeal joints not only in size but also by virtue of an additional structure, the tough, strong palmar ligament, which is incorporated into the volar capsule (Fig. 6–*15, A*). In these joints, also, dislocation is produced by hyperextension, but *should never be reduced by traction.* In a simple metacarpophalangeal dislocation the dislocated phalanx is hyperextended at right angles to the metacarpal (Fig. 6–*15, B*). If the finger is pulled, in an attempt at reduction, the phalanx is apt to pivot on the intact collateral ligaments and drag the tongue of avulsed palmar ligament into a position of interposition (Fig. 6–*15, C*). The dislocation then is made complex; open reduction is usually required for extrication of the palmar ligament, and the prognosis for a good result is greatly jeopardized. A simple metacarpophalangeal dislocation should be reduced by *pushing* the dislocated phalanx into normal position (Fig. 6–*15, B*).

Complex dislocation should always be suspected when the long axes of the dislocated bones are parallel rather than at right angles. Repeated attempts to obtain reduction of such a dislocation by force are doomed to failure and accomplish nothing, except additional tissue damage. Immobilization of an incomplete reduction is even worse, and ensures an eventually stiff and painful joint. When reduction without force cannot be obtained by manipulation, operative extrication of the interposed palmar ligament should be done at once.

In the metacarpophalangeal joints of the index and middle fingers

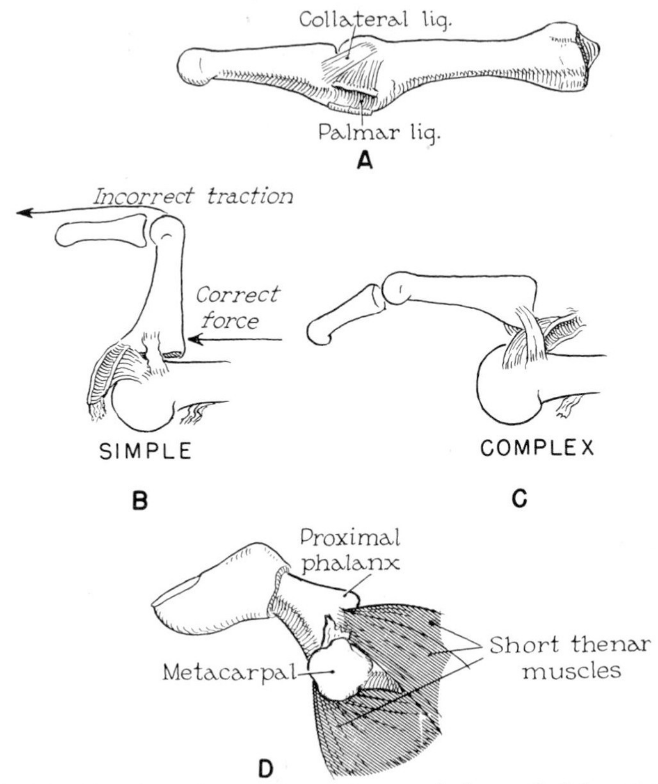

Figure 6–15. Simple and complex metacarpophalangeal dislocation.

A. The volar aspect of a metacarpophalangeal joint capsule is reinforced with a palmar ligament or fibrocartilage.

B. In a simple dislocation the phalanx is hyperextended and the palmar ligament hangs like a curtain over the metacarpal head. Traction may pivot the phalanx on the intact collateral ligaments and interpose the palmar ligament between the bones. The phalanx should be pushed into place.

C. The finger is not hyperextended on, but more nearly parallel to, the metacarpal in a complex dislocation. The volar joint capsule and palmar ligament are interposed, and usually prevent reduction by manipulation.

D. In the metacarpophalangeal joint of the thumb the short thenar muscles augment the pivot force predisposing to complex dislocation.

most complex dislocations are produced by wrongfully attempted reduction of a simple dislocation by traction. At the metacarpophalangeal joint of the thumb the short thenar muscles insert into the base of the phalanx. Subsequent to or coincident with dislocation, even without the help of improper manipulation, these may produce the pivot force necessary to buttonhole the metacarpal head through the joint capsule and interpose the palmar ligament between the dislocated bones (Fig. 6–*15, D*). Open reduction is almost always required.

Bennett's Fracture

Despite the wide variety of episodes described by patients to explain the etiology of this fracture, the great majority of such injuries are in-

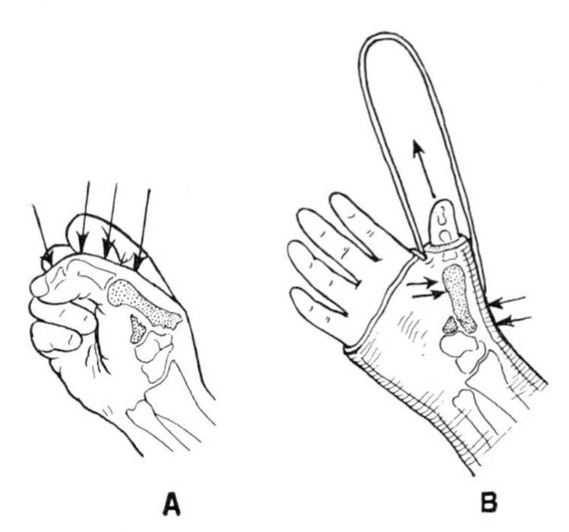

Figure 6–16. Bennett's fracture.

A. Bennett's fracture is produced by a blow against the dorsal surface of the clenched thumb. The small inner triangular fragment articulates normally; the remainder of the metacarpal subluxes, due to muscle pull.

B. Maintenance of reduction requires continuous traction, outward pressure against the distal and inward pressure against the proximal end of the thumb metacarpal. An excellent traction outrigger may be fashioned from a wire coat hanger.

curred in a fist fight. The query, "How does the other fellow look?," will usually produce a sheepish grin and the truth. An opponent's head or jaw is struck by the flexed and adducted thumb instead of the knuckles (Fig. *6–16, A*). A triangular fragment of bone is broken from the inner aspect of the base of the thumb metacarpal, and remains in apposition to the greater multangular (trapezium), while the remainder of the metacarpal subluxes as far as intact capsule and ligaments permit. The base of the thumb is swollen, tender, and painful, and the thumb metacarpal appears shortened.

Reduction is accomplished without difficulty by traction on the thumb and inward pressure against its subluxed base, but these forces must remain in continuous operation if reduction is to be maintained. This requires a plaster of paris gauntlet, well molded to the contours of the thumb metacarpal, and continuous traction in the long axis of the thumb (Fig. *6–16, B*). This is a clumsy apparatus requiring the utmost in patient cooperation for continued efficiency. Herein lies the problem, for cooperation cannot be counted upon from a patient who engages in brawls, and it is folly to obtain reduction and fixation, the effects of which will be vitiated quickly by neglect or wilful disobedience. In selected patients, therefore, the most practical management of this injury consists of symptomatic treatment and acceptance of malunion from the start.

Malunion following Bennett's fracture is reflected in deformity, but there is little or no pain or significant functional defect. This is illustrated in one or both hands of most professional boxers who have plied their trade for more than a few years. The thumb metacarpal is short, and its base broad and prominent. Thumb abduction is somewhat limited and might inconvenience a pianist, but this defect is seldom noticed by the type of patient to whom this injury is indigenous.

Fractures of Finger Metacarpals

Fracture through the base of a finger metacarpal rarely displaces, except when it accompanies a carpometacarpal dislocation, remains securely fixed in good position by intact ligament attachments, and requires only symptomatic treatment. The majority of metacarpal fractures involve the shaft or neck of the bone. The displacement is constant, and consists of an angular deformity with a dorsal apex (Fig. 6–*17*, *B*, *C*) and a consequent depression of the metacarpal head into the palm. The arch of the knuckle

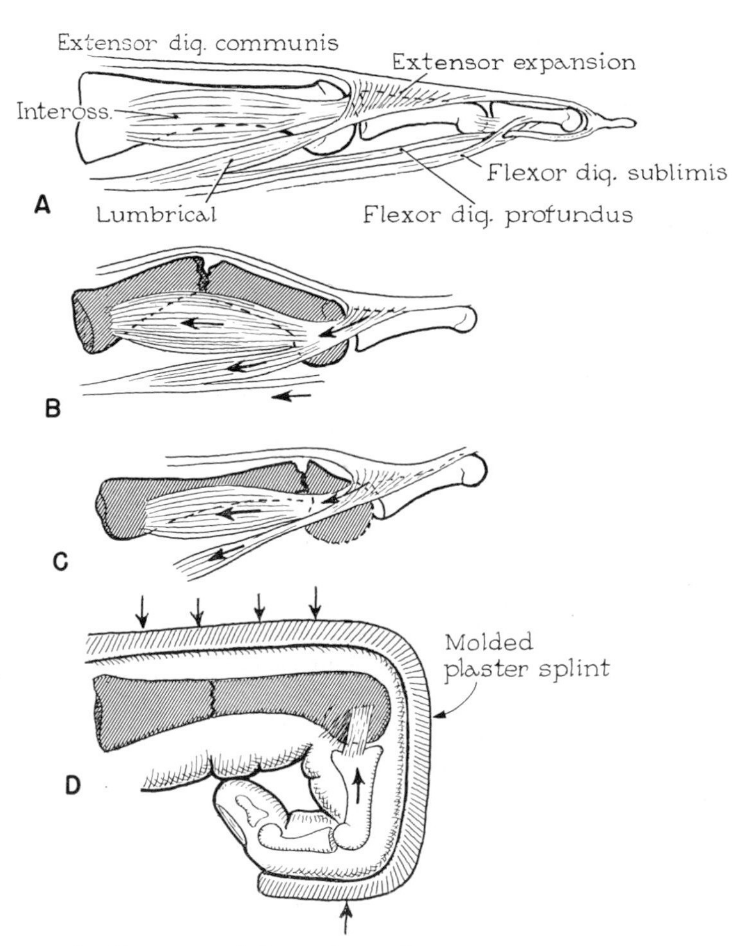

Figure 6–17. Fractures of the metacarpals.
A. Normal finger motors.
B, C. The consistent deformity of metacarpal fractures resulting from muscle pull.
D. Correction of deformity requires pressure downward against the apex of the deformity, and upward under the metacarpal head. Pressure points by splint (arrows) must be watched closely for skin damage.

line is distorted, but rarely enough to create a significant cosmetic defect. When the head of the relatively immobile third metacarpal remains depressed it becomes painful when grasping handles, such as a hammer; but a similar malunion in the other more mobile metacarpals seldom produces significant symptoms.

Stable transverse fracture of a metacarpal shaft or neck can be reduced and fixed securely only by downward pressure upon the dorsal aspect of the angular deformity and upward pressure against the metacarpal head (Fig. 6–*17, D*). Splints used to implement these requirements must be watched closely for pressure points on the skin.

Stable spiral fractures of a metacarpal shaft shorten slightly, but this deformity creates neither a functional nor a significant cosmetic defect. Traction is contraindicated by the inevitable prolonged finger stiffness which it produces. A snug dorsal splint and maintenance of gentle finger motion is the treatment of choice.

Unstable metacarpal fractures, productive of gross deformity, especially in the index and middle fingers, should be treated by continuous traction until healed. The inevitable penalty of this form of treatment is

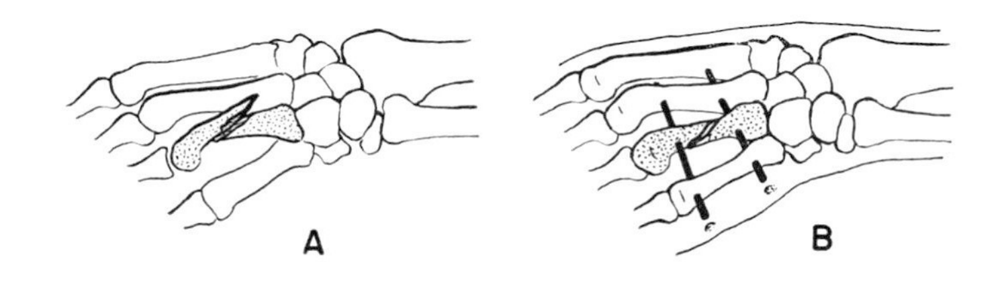

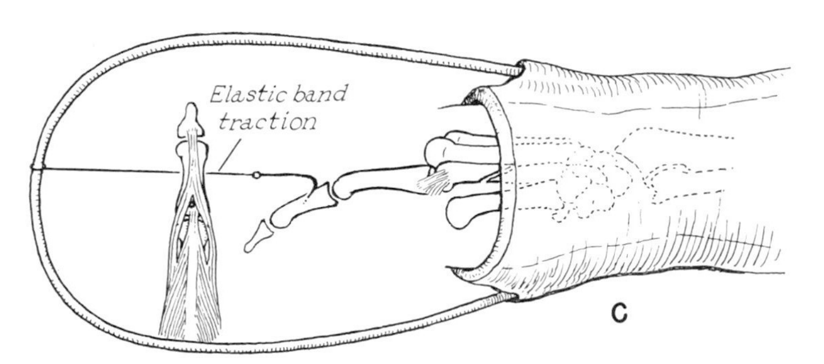

Figure 6–18. Fractures of the metacarpals.

A. Unstable metacarpal fractures with gross deformity require traction or internal fixation.

B. In the third and fourth metacarpals the fracture may be transfixed in such a way as to utilize the adjacent intact bones as splints.

C. Traction by a barbless fishhook, inserted into a hole bored in the dorsal surface of the middle phalanx just distal to the insertion of the central slip of the extensor mechanism, implicates nothing but skin and bone. This is preferable to and less damaging than traction through a pin which transfixes the motors of the finger.

prolonged stiffness of the finger and, for this reason, traction should not be employed unless the indications are clear and unequivocal. In selected cases open reduction and internal fixation by some medullary device, or by transfixion pins (Fig. 6–*18*) may be justified in an attempt to maintain mobility of the fingers during the healing period.

CHAPTER 7

INJURIES OF THE WRIST

By HARRISON L. McLAUGHLIN, M.D.

GENERAL CONSIDERATIONS

THE REMARKABLE FLEXIBILITY of the wrist joint results from skeletal architecture and muscle motors designed to facilitate mobility of the hand in every plane. Stability, in the face of such mobility, is necessarily dependent upon the muscles crossing the joint, but is augmented to a surprising degree by a complicated but precise connection of the hand to the forearm by the carpal mechanism.

The Carpal Mechanism

Seven small carpal bones of irregular sizes and shapes occupy the interval between the metacarpal and the forearm bones. They are packed

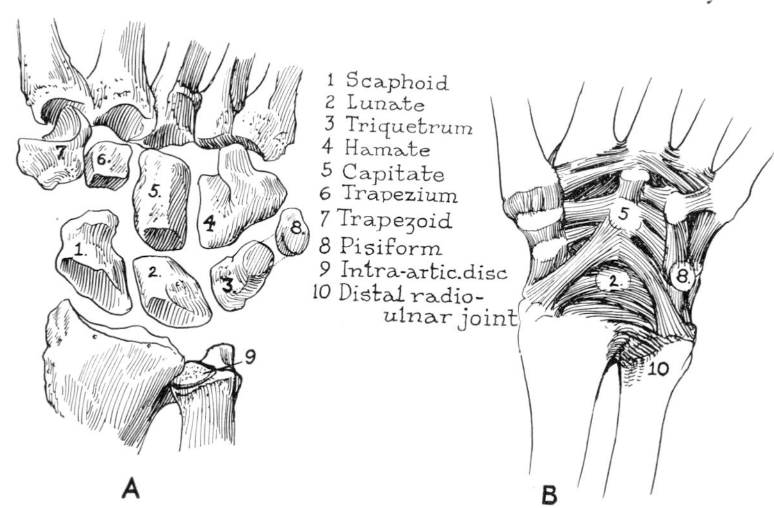

Figure 7–1. Structure of the wrist joint.

A. The bones of the carpal mechanism, opened on their volar surfaces, are irregular in size and shape but fit perfectly like the pieces of a jigsaw puzzle (after Grant).

B. Many strong ligaments hold the carpal bones firmly in place, connecting their volar surfaces to the radius, the metacarpals, and to each other.

The intra-articular disc separates the wrist joint from the distal radio-ulnar joint, and acts as a soft-part hinge upon which the radius swings around the ulnar head in supination and pronation.

tightly together in two rows, like ball-bearings in a machine; but, owing to their irregularity in shape and size, the resulting pattern of intercarpal articulations appears as complicated as a jigsaw puzzle (Fig. 7–*1*, *A*). Many strong ligaments support the volar surface of these joints (Fig. 7–*1*, *B*), but the corresponding ligamentous support to their dorsal surfaces is weak and vulnerable to injury. The ligaments allow only a small amount of mobility between any two carpal bones, but are arranged to permit considerable motion at the midcarpal and radiocarpal joints.

The Volar Carpal Canal

Spanning the gap between the pisiform and the tubercle of the scaphoid proximally, and the hook of the lunate and a ridge on the trapezium distally, is the broad and strong volar carpal ligament (see Figure 7–5, *B*). This forms the roof of the volar carpal canal which contains the median nerve and the eight tendons of the flexor muscles to the fingers. Any decrease in the capacity of this tunnel may be reflected in signs and symptoms of damage to the median nerve, which is by far the most compressible of its contents.

The Midcarpal Joint

The pisiform is a sesamoid in the flexor carpi-ulnaris tendon and is virtually excluded from the functional mechanics of the carpus. The proximal carpal row contains the scaphoid, lunate, and triquetrum. The trapezium, trapezoid, capitate, and hamate comprise the distal carpal row. The intervening midcarpal joint has a range of motion which, although small and difficult to measure clinically, serves to provide considerable resilience to the carpus as a unit (Fig. 7–2).

The scaphoid bone (Fig. 7–3) is located in the proximal carpal row, and also projects into the distal row. In effect, this bone bridges the midcarpal joint. Forcible wrist extension finds the scaphoid attempting to adjust its long axis to the positional plane of both carpal rows. The degree to which this is possible is sharply limited and, as a consequence of this functional incongruity, damage to and about the scaphoid is the injury most commonly encountered in the carpal mechanism.

The Radiocarpal Joint

A major portion of all wrist motion, except rotation, takes place at the radiocarpal joint (see Fig. 7–2). The articular surface of the radius is indented by two shallow concavities which accommodate the scaphoid and the lunate in the resting position. The triquetrum articulates with an intra-articular disc which bridges the gap between the radius and the styloid process of the ulna (Fig. 7–3), and excludes the distal end of the ulna from the wrist joint cavity.

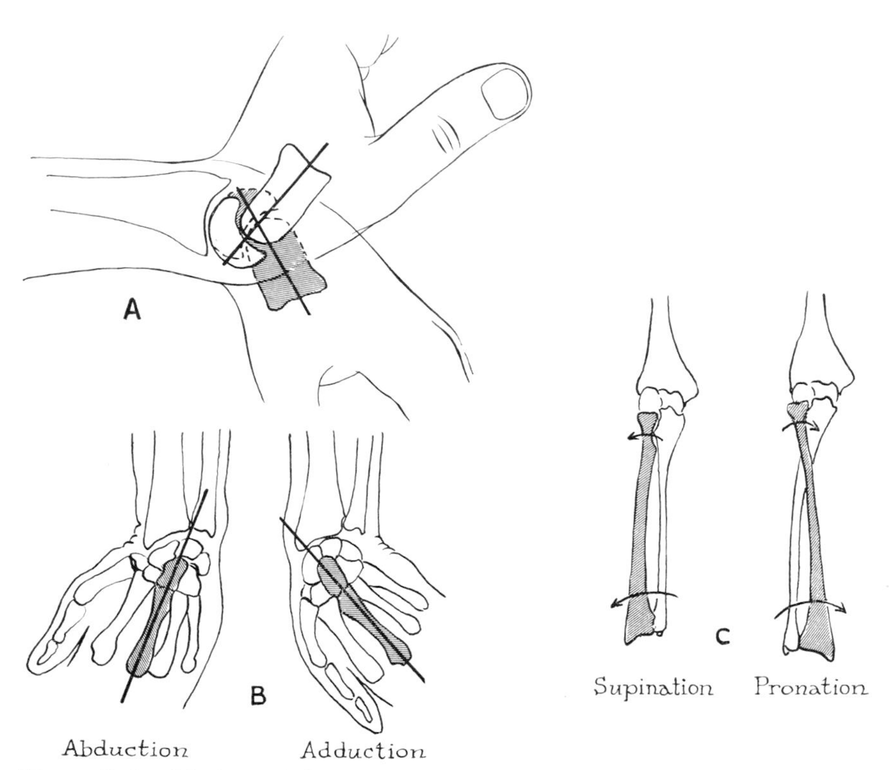

Figure 7–2. Motions of the wrist joint.

A. Flexion and extension are mainly products of radiocarpal motion. The axis of the capitate bone changes much more in relation to the radius than to the lunate.

B. Abduction and adduction are mainly products of radiocarpal motion. Here also the axis of the capitate bone changes little in relation to the proximal carpal row, but mainly in relation to the radius. The midcarpal joint, therefore, contributes only a small amount of motion to flexion, extension, abduction, and adduction.

C. Pronation and supination of right forearm, viewed from in front. The radial head rotates around a fixed pivot point. The forearm bones are parallel in supination, and crossed in pronation. The distal end of the radius swings like a gate around the ulnar post on the hinge provided by the intra-articular disc and its supporting ligaments (Fig. 7–1).

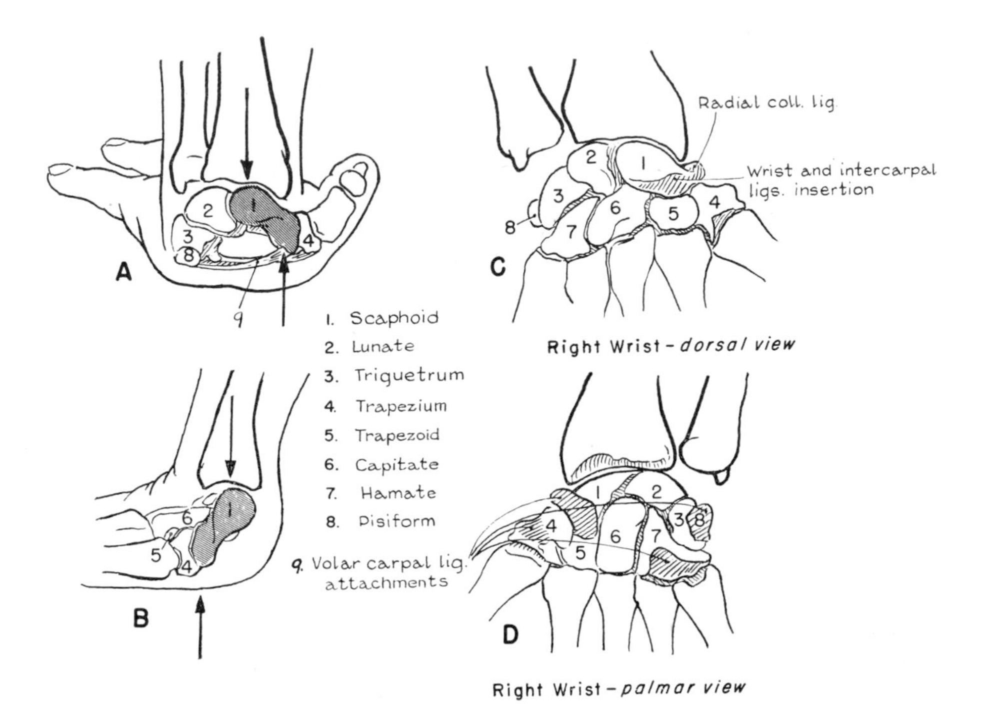

Figure 7–3. Mechanism of wrist injury.

A. The volar carpal ligament and canal in cross section. When a person falls on the fully extended hand, the force of the impact (arrows) is primarily accepted by the waist of the scaphoid.

B. Lateral view of carpal bones. A fall on the fully extended hand also centers the force of the impact (arrows) at the narrow mid-portion of the scaphoid. Since this bone cannot adjust itself simultaneously to the plane of both the proximal and the distal carpal row, such an injury is a common cause of fracture of the scaphoid.

C, D. Dorsal and palmar views of carpal bones. The soft-part attachments of the scaphoid are illustrated. The remaining (unshaded) surfaces are intra-articular. When the intra- and extra-articular portions are separated by a fracture, the intra-articular portion is also separated from its blood supply. Note, in the palmar view, how the scaphoid projects into the distal row.

The Distal Radio-ulnar Joint

The pivot of rotation is the ulnar insertion of the intra-articular disc (Fig. 7–*1*), but the radiohumeral and proximal radio-ulnar joints must also participate in all rotatory motions (Fig. 7–*2*). In effect, the intra-articular disc and its ligamentous supports act as the hinge upon which the radial gate swings around the ulnar post. The ulna does not rotate, but swings toward the midline in supination, and away from the midline in pronation. Most communications between the radiocarpal and distal radio-ulnar joint are products of trauma, or attrition of the intra-articular disc, and are of little clinical significance except in the spread of a local infection.

SPRAIN OF THE WRIST

This injury does not occur in children. The distal epiphyseal plate of the radius gives way before the wrist ligaments rupture. Epiphyseal injuries without displacement are commonly misdiagnosed as sprains. When, after 7 to 10 days, the pain and tenderness of an injury to the wrist in a child is less diffuse but remains circumferentially restricted to the area of the radial epiphysis, and the roentgenogram remains negative, the correct diagnosis is an injury to the epiphyseal plate. The parents should be warned of the remote possibility of subsequent growth disturbance. The wrist should be splinted until symptoms have disappeared.

A true sprain of the wrist is uncommon in the adult. It is not produced by the usual mechanism of ligament injury by overstretch. The trauma is forcible hyperextension of the wrist, yet the volar (stretched) ligaments are uninjured, and all evidences of damage are restricted to the dorsal (relaxed) ligaments. The explanation of this apparent paradox is that the dorsal ligaments are injured by an incomplete and self-reducing subluxation of the carpals. Fracture of the scaphoid, some form of carpal dislocation, or a fracture of the radius is much more common than a pure injury of the dorsal ligaments of the wrist. An undisplaced fracture of the scaphoid is the lesion most frequently misdiagnosed as a sprain of the wrist. A clinical differential diagnosis between these two lesions is usually impossible in the early period after injury. Scaphoid fracture often cannot be seen by roentgenogram until after some decalcification has occurred at the fracture line.

Treatment of "Wrist Sprain"

The apparently sprained wrist should be treated as a scaphoid fracture for at least two weeks. A plaster gauntlet is applied and indeed, if the injury proves to be a sprain, this is excellent treatment. After two weeks the gauntlet is removed and additional roentgenograms are obtained. Only after the presence of a fracture has been excluded with certainty in this way does the diagnosis of sprain become valid. Immobilization is then

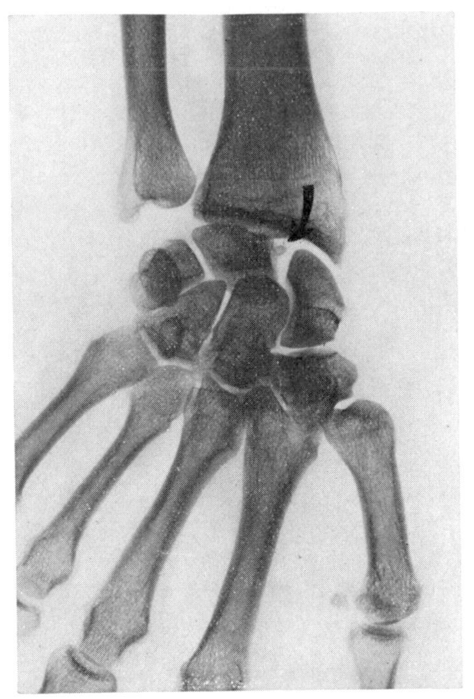

Figure 7–4. *"Sprain" of the wrist, followed by two years of unremitting pain on use. The tiny ossicle (arrow) and increased space between lunate and scaphoid reveal the true lesion to have been rupture of the intercarpal ligaments between these bones. Pain resulted from continued scaphoid instability, and was controlled by use of a molded leather gauntlet. (Courtesy of Mr. Carl Nissen.)*

continued or not according to the dictates of the subsiding symptoms. Occasionally wrist pain on strenuous use will persist. Films with the hand in various positions of stress should then be obtained. Persistent pain, in the absence of fracture, often results from hypermobility of one carpal on another, consequent to disruption of intercarpal ligaments (Fig. 7–4).

TENDON DEPOSITS

Deposits of tissue debris impregnated with calcium salts have been encountered in every tendon of the wrist and hand, but most commonly occur just proximal to the pisiform bone in the tendon of the flexor carpi ulnaris. In pathomechanics and behavior these deposits are similar to those occurring in the intrinsic tendons of the shoulder (see Chapter 10, Injuries of the Shoulder and Arm, page 281). Painful symptoms often follow soon after a mild injury. The inflammatory response to the deposit material implicates the appropriate tubular tendon sheath and often simulates an acute suppurative tenosynovitis. Suppuration is excluded by the great disproportion between the acute local reaction and the mild or absent systemic response. Identification of the deposit in the roentgenogram indicts it as the offending lesion.

Treatment of Painful Calcium Deposits

Spontaneous disappearance of both the deposit and the pain can be expected within a few days, with or without treatment. Acute pain justifies complete rest of the painful member in a plaster splint and the use of other palliative measures. Decompression of the chemical furuncle by needle accelerates the subsidence of pain, and occasionally operative incision of the inflamed deposit may be required. The efficacy of radiotherapy, as in all other similar episodes which subside rapidly, regardless of treatment, cannot be measured.

COLLES' FRACTURE

A Colles fracture does not occur in a child. Instead, the lower radial epiphysis is displaced, or the proximal radial shaft is fractured. The implication of each is far different from that of a Colles fracture, which occurs only through the cancellous bone at the distal end of the radius in an adult. The injury is caused by a fall on the outstretched hand (see Fig. 7–6, *A*), and the clinical characteristics of the fracture depend upon the force of the fall and the exact position of the hand at the moment of impact.

DIAGNOSIS

Normally the radial styloid lies at a level about 1 cm. distal to that of the ulna to produce an ulnar deviation of about 10 degrees in the resting hand. The long axis of the third metacarpal meets that of the forearm at the level of the wrist joint, regardless of the position of the hand. The volar curve and the flat dorsal surface of the distal radius are visible and palpable. The uninjured wrist is available for comparison of these anatomical features, adequate evaluation of which can disclose almost as much information about a Colles fracture as the roentgenogram.

When the distal fracture fragment is angulated backward the volar curve is reduced or reversed. Dorsal displacement of this fragment produces a palpable ridge across the flat dorsal surface of the radius. Radial displacement distorts the axial relations of the third metacarpal. Radial angulation reduces or reverses ulnar deviation of the hand in proportion to the bony deformity. Impaction, or any other deformity decreasing the length of the radius, has a measurable effect upon the relations of the styloid processes.

Usually, in a Colles fracture, the small distal fragment is driven backward so that the flexor tendons and the median nerve are stretched over the apex of the angular deformity (Fig. 7–5). The functional status of the median nerve should always be tested and recorded before and after reduction of the fracture. The radial and ulnar arteries may become compressed or injured, and frequently swelling and deformity may preclude evaluation of the pulse at the wrist. Nevertheless intact terminal circulation in the fingers must be confirmed throughout all phases of treatment. This may be done by compressing the nail beds and comparing their rate of refilling with that on the uninjured side.

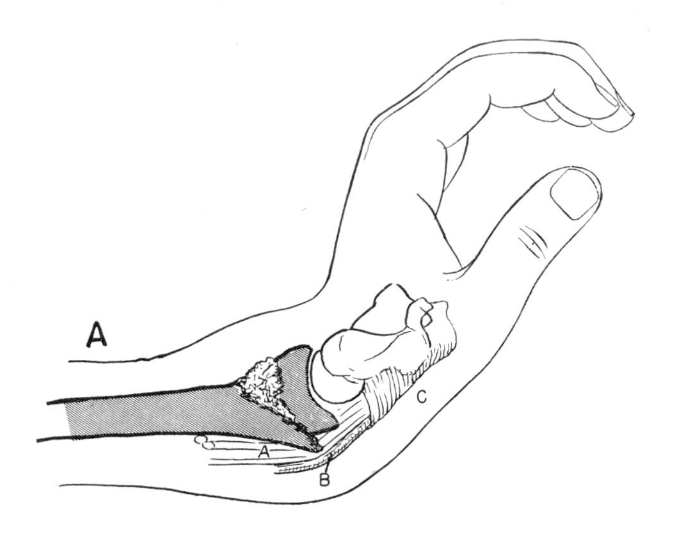

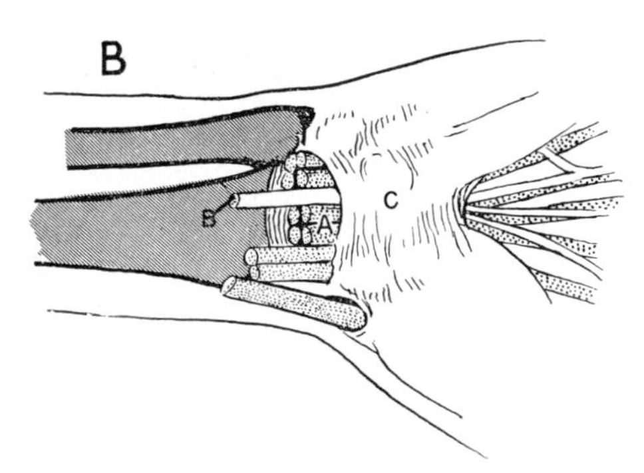

Figure 7–5. Volar carpal canal.

A. The usual dorsal displacement of a Colles fracture stretches the flexor tendons and median nerve over the apex of the bone deformity.

B. Normal anatomy and contents of the volar carpal canal.

GENERAL PRINCIPLES OF TREATMENT

There is no single or best method of reduction or fixation, nor is there any standard period of immobilization for a Colles fracture. Acceptance and use of any routine treatment program is synonymous with a misconception that all such fractures are alike. The details of treatment must be predicated upon the characteristics of the individual problem.

Reduction (Figs. 7–6, 7–7) should be carried out in accordance with the deformities to be corrected. Traction, accompanied by a gentle rocking

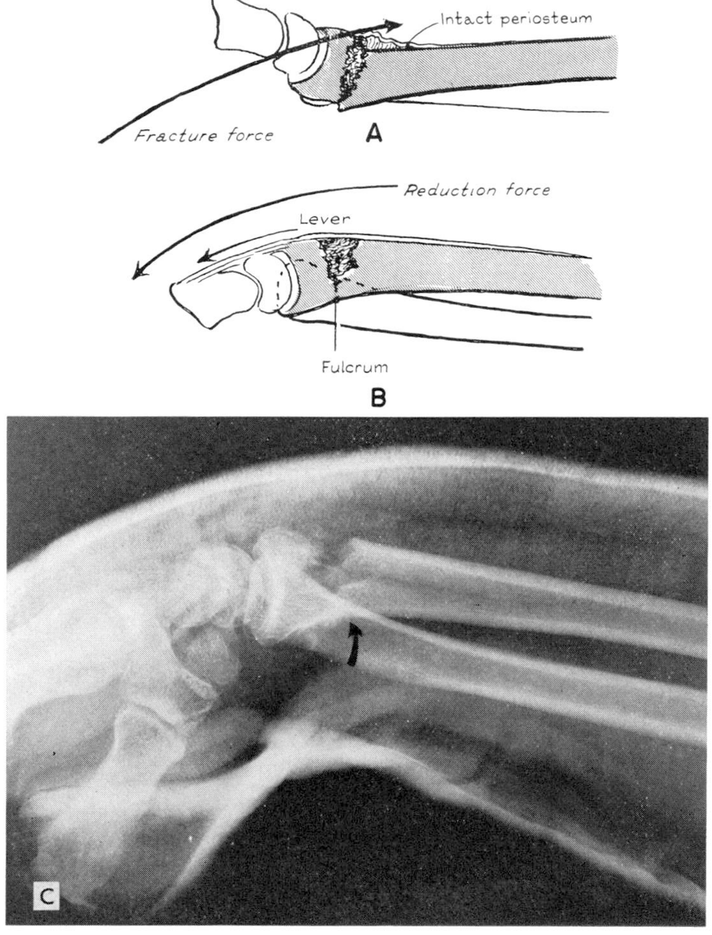

Figure 7–6. Forces of production and reduction of a Colles fracture (lateral view).

A. A fall on the outstretched hand angulates and displaces the hand, carpus, and distal fragment of radius dorsalward. The dorsal periosteum remains intact.

B. Reduction requires reversal of these forces. The distal fragment is pushed volarward. Flexion of the wrist utilizes the intact volar cortex as a fulcrum, and intact dorsal soft parts as a lever for correction of the angular deformity.

C. Roentgenogram illustrating dorsal defect due to comminution. Plaster maintains reduction only by virtue of the flexion lever provided by plaster splints, and the fulcrum (arrow) provided by the intact volar cortex of the radius.

of the fragments, is necessary to release impaction, should precede all other manipulations, and should be maintained continuously until the reduction is completed. Restoration of length of the radius is confirmed when the relationship of the styloid levels has been returned to normal. Existing displacements are corrected by replacement of the distal in apposition to the proximal bone fragment. The normal volar inclination of

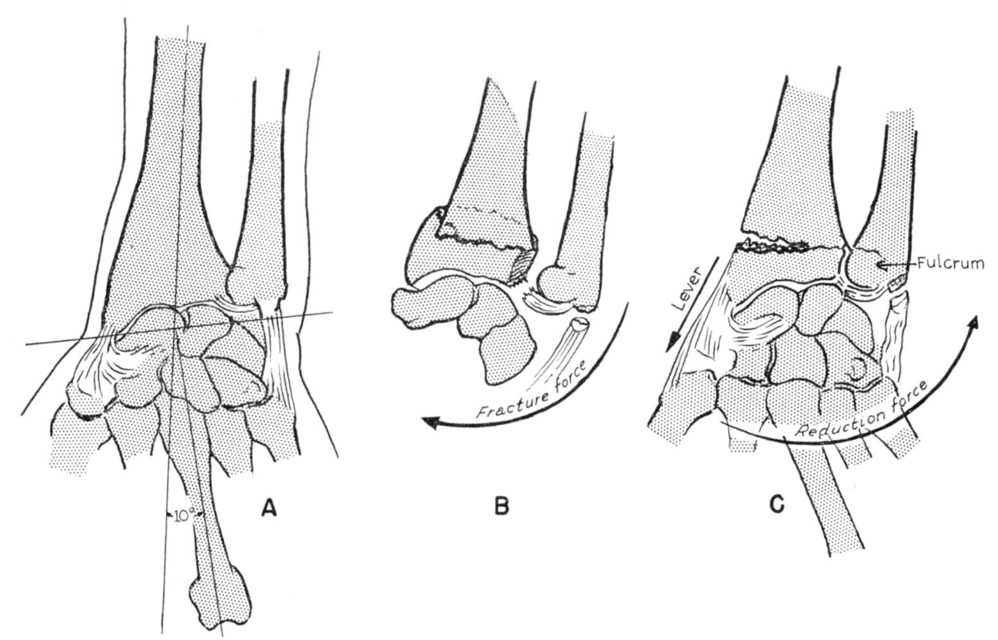

Figure 7–7. Forces of production and reduction of a Colles fracture (anteroposterior view).

A. Normal alignment. The carpals deviate slightly toward the ulnar side due to the plane of the wrist joint.

B. Coincident with forcible extension, the wrist is driven into radial deviation (arrow) by a fall on the outstretched hand. The distal fragment of radius is carried radialward with the carpus and hand, and the ulnar styloid is avulsed.

C. Correction of this displacement is by reversal of the forces in B. Ulnar deviation utilizes the ulnar head as a fulcrum, and the radial collateral ligament as a lever, to replace the distal fragment of radius.

Radial displacement, *when present, must be corrected by manual pressure of the distal fragment toward the ulna.*

the distal radius is restored by strong pressure against the dorsal surface of the distal fragment, augmented, if necessary, by flexion of the wrist. Prior to release of traction, radial length is maintained by strong ulnar deviation of the hand which utilizes the ulnar head as a fulcrum over which the radial collateral ligament exerts traction upon the radial styloid (Fig. 7–7).

Maintenance of reduction is difficult. To hold the reduced fracture in good position during the application and hardening of plaster splints is an exacting and difficult task. Circular plaster dressings, unless supervised closely during the first few days after application, are a constant potential source of circulatory embarrassment, and as swelling subsides they become progressively more loose and inefficient. Carefully molded "sugar tongs" splints (see Chapter 8, Injuries of the Forearm, Figure 8–6), although not so strong, can be fitted to the limb as well as a circular plaster, and may be loosened or tightened by rebandaging without jeopardizing the reduction of the fracture. For general use they are safer than and as efficient as a circular plaster dressing until after swelling subsides, after which they may be replaced by a circular plaster dressing, if desired.

The optimal position and immobilization period for a Colles fracture are discussed later, according to the variable circumstances which govern these aspects of treatment. It is worthy of emphasis that plaster fixation merely maintains a constant relationship between the hand and the forearm and, indirectly, a constant position of the fracture fragments. Maintenance of the reduction of unstable Colles' fractures depends upon two fulcrums—the volar cortex (Fig. 7–6) and the ulnar head (Fig. 7–7). Leverage developed over these two points by the position of immobilization is the essential force which holds the bone fragments in position.

Aftercare. Immobilization devices must permit free interphalangeal and metacarpophalangeal joint motion, and the patient must move these joints from the start. The volar dressing must not extend past the palmar flexion crease; otherwise metacarpophalangeal joint flexion is blocked. The dorsal dressing should extend almost to the knuckle line; otherwise dorsal edema may prevent metacarpophalangeal joint extension. All the unencumbered small joints should be moved frequently, and the hand should remain elevated until swelling no longer is present. A progressive resumption of light use of the fingers should be encouraged. A sponge or soft rubber ball should be carried and squeezed frequently. Above all, the patient must be persuaded that the speed and quality of his recovery will be in direct proportion to the speed and frequency with which finger motions and use are resumed.

The consistency with which a hand is ruined due to neglect of finger motions following a Colles fracture is astonishing, and the resulting disabilities are usually much more severe than would have followed a complete absence of treatment of the fracture. The shoulder joint is almost equally prone to become stiff, painful, and disabled if the limb is placed in a sling and permitted to remain dependent during the treatment of a Colles fracture. The sling should be removed and the shoulder exercised through a full motion range at frequent intervals, if this catastrophe is to be avoided.

DEFINITIVE TREATMENT

The details of treatment of Colles' fracture depend upon the type of the fracture.

An undisplaced Colles fracture is surrounded by essentially intact periosteum and ligaments. Displacement cannot occur unless these structures are disrupted. Intact, they provide more exact fixation than any external splint. This fracture does not need immobilization, but requires protection against re-injury as well as relief of pain and maintenance of function. A volar molded splint is sufficient for protection and comfort. Within a few days this may be removed at frequent intervals for gradually progressive active exercises, warm soaks, and resumption of use within the limits of pain. By the time the bone has healed the soft tissues are ready for full use. A comfortable, useful extremity is present in the third week, and complete recovery takes place rapidly.

A stable Colles fracture, when reduced, becomes the equivalent of an undisplaced lesion, except for the absence of stabilization by surrounding soft tissues. External immobilization must be applied, but, if the reduced fragments are stable, this may be done with the hand in a position of optimal function. The fingers are moved and used from the start, and in the third week after injury healing in and around the fracture is sufficient to permit removal of the splints for supervised exercises, within pain limits, and warm soaks. As bone union strengthens, active motion and use are increased progressively. Splints may be discarded during the fourth week.

An unstable Colles fracture is one in which the dorsal aspect of the radius is comminuted. The degree of instability is proportional to the amount of comminution. Maintenance of reduction is dependent upon the volar fulcrum (Fig. 7–6, *C*), without which external splints are of little use. The wrist must be immobilized in flexion to prevent the distal fragment from tilting backward to collapse the area of dorsal comminution. Immobilization must be continued until the comminuted area consolidates, a period of five to eight weeks, depending on the amount of comminution. But, if the wrist is fully flexed, the fingers cannot be flexed, and unless finger mobility is maintained the result will be a stiff, disabled hand. Consequently, the *minimal amount of flexion necessary to maintain reduction is the optimal position for immobilization.* As healing progresses the splints should be changed, and the amount of wrist flexion reduced every week or two. Finger motion, even if done passively, must be insisted upon from the time of reduction until healing occurs.

A shattered Colles fracture, with extensive comminution and without a solid volar cortex to act as a fulcrum, can be reduced but cannot be held in position by external immobilization. The radius collapses within the best of plaster dressings. Continuous skeletal traction is required to maintain radial length. A stiff steel pin is passed through the bases of the metacarpal bones. At this location pins do not involve the soft tissues in the interosseous spaces, and a straight pin may be passed through all four bones with ease; consequently, the complications and difficulties encountered in attempting to transfix the shafts or necks of the metacarpals are eliminated. Another pin is passed through the olecranon. An assistant restores the normal length of the radius by distraction of the pins, while the surgeon manipulates the fragments into position. A circular plaster dressing, into which both pins are incorporated, is then applied and trimmed enough to allow full motion of the fingers and thumb and flexion and extension of

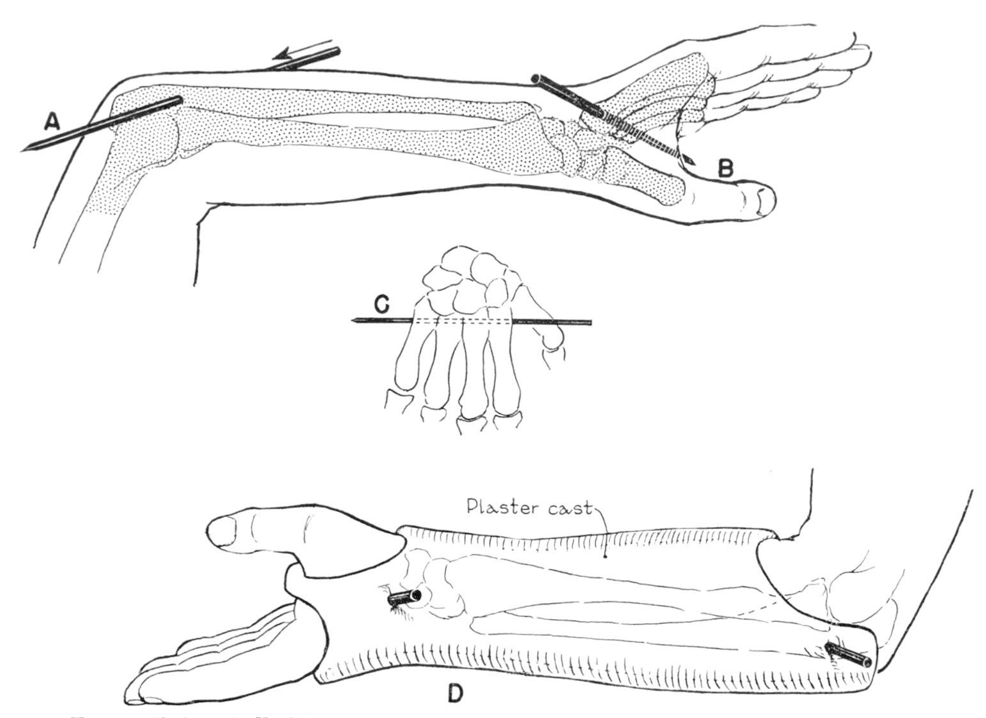

Figure 7–8. Colles' fracture treated by fixed skeletal traction.

Finger motion and use are possible. Flexion and extension of elbow are possible. Fixed traction obviates need for wrist flexion; radial shortening is prevented. Traction must be maintained until sound union occurs.

the elbow. This technique (Fig. 7–8) has proved to be a simple and reasonably safe method for the secure fixation of markedly comminuted Colles' fractures which otherwise would collapse within plaster dressings.

A reverse Colles fracture is marked by anterior displacement of the small distal fragment and accentuation of the volar curve of the radius. Manipulative reduction is identical in principle to that of the usual fracture marked by dorsal displacement, but the maneuvers are reversed. Maintenance of reduction requires immobilization with the wrist extended, but the frequent absence of a good dorsal fulcrum may make fixation by plaster alone very difficult. Skeletal traction is often required, especially in oblique fractures which enter the dorsal aspect of the radial articular surface rather than extend through the dorsal cortex of the bone.

The duration of immobilization for an unstable Colles fracture should be governed by the amount of dorsal comminution. Mild instability and a small amount of comminution justify removal of immobilization in the fourth or fifth week after injury. When the comminution requires considerable wrist flexion to maintain reduction, immobilization should be continued for five to eight weeks. Skeletal traction required in the most comminuted lesions should not be removed before seven or eight weeks. Regardless of the duration of immobilization required by the fracture, the maintenance of finger and thumb functions throughout the entire period remains by far the most important single prerequisite to a satisfactory result.

THE DILEMMA OF COLLES' FRACTURE

Colles' fracture is common to the elderly woman with an arthritic wrist, arthritic finger joints, and osteoporotic bones. Treatment in many such cases by reduction and immobilization results in permanent pain and stiffness despite all possible efforts to maintain mobility. After a few such results most surgeons appreciate and dread the implications of this problem. Many attempt to solve it by reduction and a short immobilization period, in the hope that the wrist can be improved by the reduction and the stiffness escaped by a curtailed immobilization period. The reductions collapse, the fragments return to their original deformities, some harm results from the immobilization, and the results are dismal failures.

The solution is to ignore the deformity and concentrate upon maintenance of function. Malunion with gross deformity is seldom attended by symptoms, limited motion, or disability sufficient to inconvenience the average elderly woman in any serious way. In selected patients of this type the surgeon is amply justified in presenting two therapeutic alternatives. The patient may be assured of obtaining a comfortable, useful, and limber wrist in a short time, if she is willing to accept a cosmetic defect and some mild weakness. This is accomplished by the application of a removable splint and a program of warm soaks, with early active motion and use. As an alternative she may be offered a good-looking wrist following reduction and immobilization, but she should be warned that both hand and wrist may remain stiff and painful after the treatment is completed. Many factors must enter into the decision, but in the experience of the writer the first alternative produces much happier results in a large number of patients who have passed the age of vanity.

OLD UNREDUCED COLLES' FRACTURE

Manual reduction usually can be accomplished fairly easily up until about two weeks after injury. During the third week correction of displacement requires considerable force and manual reduction becomes difficult. After three weeks, refracture by means of some such device as a Thomas wrench is a prerequisite to correction of the deformity. These consistent findings have the following important therapeutic implications:

(1) All reduced Colles' fractures should be checked by x-ray not later than 10 days after reduction. At that time, if the fragments have lost position, manipulative revision can be carried out with reasonable ease and without undue additional trauma.

(2) Stable reduced fractures unite at the same rate, or at a faster rate than unreduced fractures. Considerable manual force is required to alter the position of unreduced fragments during the third week. Therefore,

commencement of a gradually progressive exercise program at that time should be both beneficial and safe for reduced stable fractures. The concept that all Colles' fractures should be subjected to a single immobilization period is illogical and ignores the fundamental principles of fracture treatment.

COMPLICATIONS OF COLLES' FRACTURE

Fracture of Ulnar Styloid Process

The ulnar styloid is avulsed by the ulnar collateral ligament in the majority of displaced Colles' fractures. This is not significant, nor does it require any treatment, except for that accorded the fracture of the radius. Fibrous union without symptoms or disability is the rule.

Derangement of Triangular Fibrocartilage

This structure is expendable. Operative excision of the distal end of the ulna obliterates its normal functions (Fig. 7–9) without ill effects. It is ruptured by moderate or gross displacement of a Colles fracture. Complications may ensue after such a fracture which heals with only mild

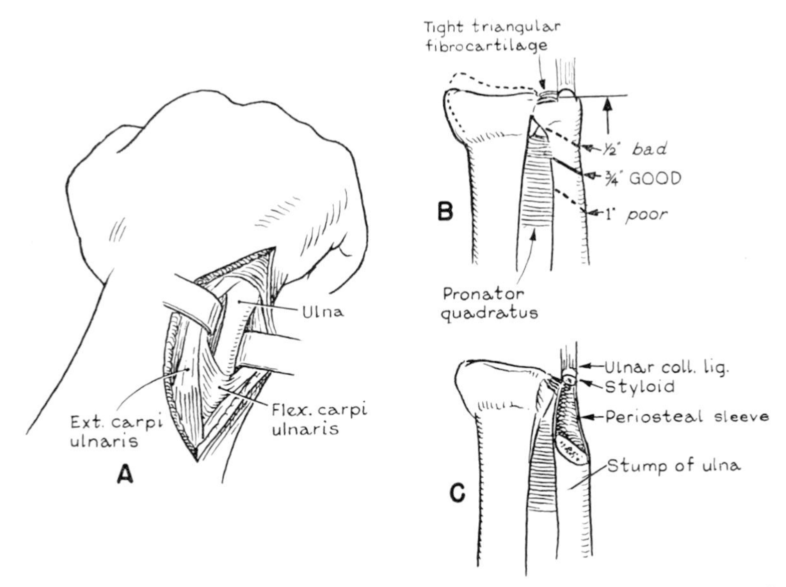

Figure 7–9. Excision of ulnar head for relief of painful inferior radio-ulnar joint.

A. Operative exposure; the ulnar nerve and artery must be avoided in the volar depths of the wound.

B. A painful radio-ulnar joint is caused by a tight triangular fibrocartilage resulting from a small *shortening of the radius after a Colles fracture.* Gross *shortening ruptures the fibrocartilage and is not attended by this syndrome.*

C. The ulnar head should be removed subperiosteally. The bevelled stump should just clear the radial articular surface and be long enough to retain the stabilizing effect of the pronator quadratus.

displacement, *insufficient to rupture the fibrocartilage* (Fig. 7–9, *B*), but enough to place it on the stretch and produce pain at the limits of pronation and supination. The majority of patients who suffer a Colles fracture complain of pain in the region of the ulnar head on rotation of the wrist for about six months after injury. Persistence of pain at the extremes of rotation after this period is indicative of some irreversible derangement of the inferior radio-ulnar joint mechanism. Imperfect apposition of the ulnar head to the radial sigmoid may contribute, but cannot be considered an important factor because gross malunions (in which the fibrocartilage is unquestionably ruptured) are usually free from such symptoms. The simple operation of subperiosteal excision of the lower end of the ulna (Fig. 7–9, *C*) relieves rotation pain efficiently without jeopardizing over-all wrist function.

Trigger Finger

A surprisingly large number of women, but few men, complain of symptoms in the palm of the hand, and are found to be suffering from a trigger phenomenon in one of the long flexor tendons following recovery from a Colles fracture. Whether the preponderance in women is due to the relative softness of the female palm and the lesion due to pressure from the edge of a splint or to the original trauma are undetermined. Probably some such lesions antedated the fracture, but were recognized only after attention became centered on the injured member. Treatment is described in Chapter 6, Injuries of the Hand (p. 128).

Rupture of Extensor Pollicis Longus Tendon

This rare complication has occurred in only 5 of 1341 Colles' fractures in the writer's experience. The time of rupture varied from a few days to several months after the injury. Ruptures which occurred soon after injury were the result of direct tendon injury by displacement of bone fragments, but late ruptures appeared to follow attenuation and progressive fraying of an injured segment of tendon which had undergone localized avascular necrosis. The clinical syndrome of sudden inability to extend the distal phalanx of the thumb, in the absence of a second injury, is uniform and unmistakable. Without operation this condition is permanent, but many simple and ingenious procedures are available for restoration of terminal phalanx extension.

Subluxation of Ulnar Head

The normal mobility of the ulnar head is quite variable. Subluxation from the radial sigmoid at the limits of pronation and supination may occur as a result of forceful rotation (Fig. 7–*10*), or may follow rupture of the inferior radio-ulnar ligaments coincident with a Colles fracture. Frequently

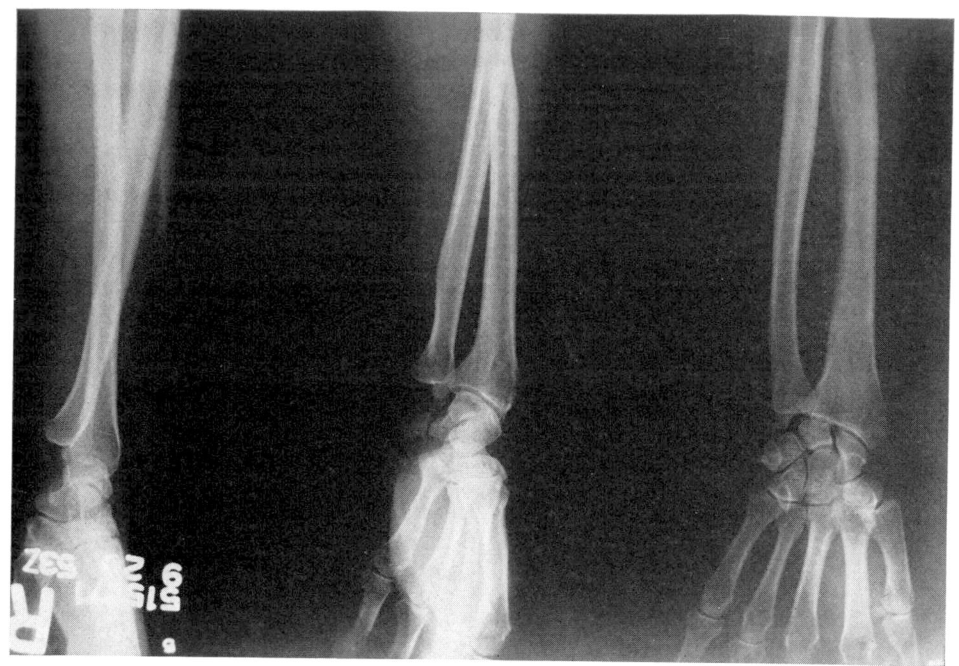

Figure 7–10. Volar dislocation of ulnar head.
A hypersupination injury; reduction should be by direct pressure and pronation.

such a hypermobile ulna is asymptomatic, but occasionally the recurrent subluxations are painful. Ulnar head resection is a simpler and more certain method of relieving such symptoms than any form of ligament reconstruction.

Subluxation of Extensor Carpi Ulnaris Tendon

Occasionally the annular fibers binding this tendon into its groove on the dorsal surface of the ulnar head are stretched or torn when the hand is driven backward and toward the radial side as a Colles fracture occurs. The tendon may snap in and out of the groove with a twinge of pain after wrist motion is resumed. Operative stabilization can be done, but ulnar head excision provides the most rapid and certain relief of these symptoms.

Nonunion of Colles' Fracture

Nonunion following Colles' fracture is an exceedingly rare complication, which probably does not occur except when the process of bone repair has been overwhelmed by infection until fibrous union becomes irreversible. This has obtained in three cases which the writer has encountered. In each case, after complete subsidence of the infection, reconstruction was performed by a technique similar to that illustrated in Figure 7–*11, A*.

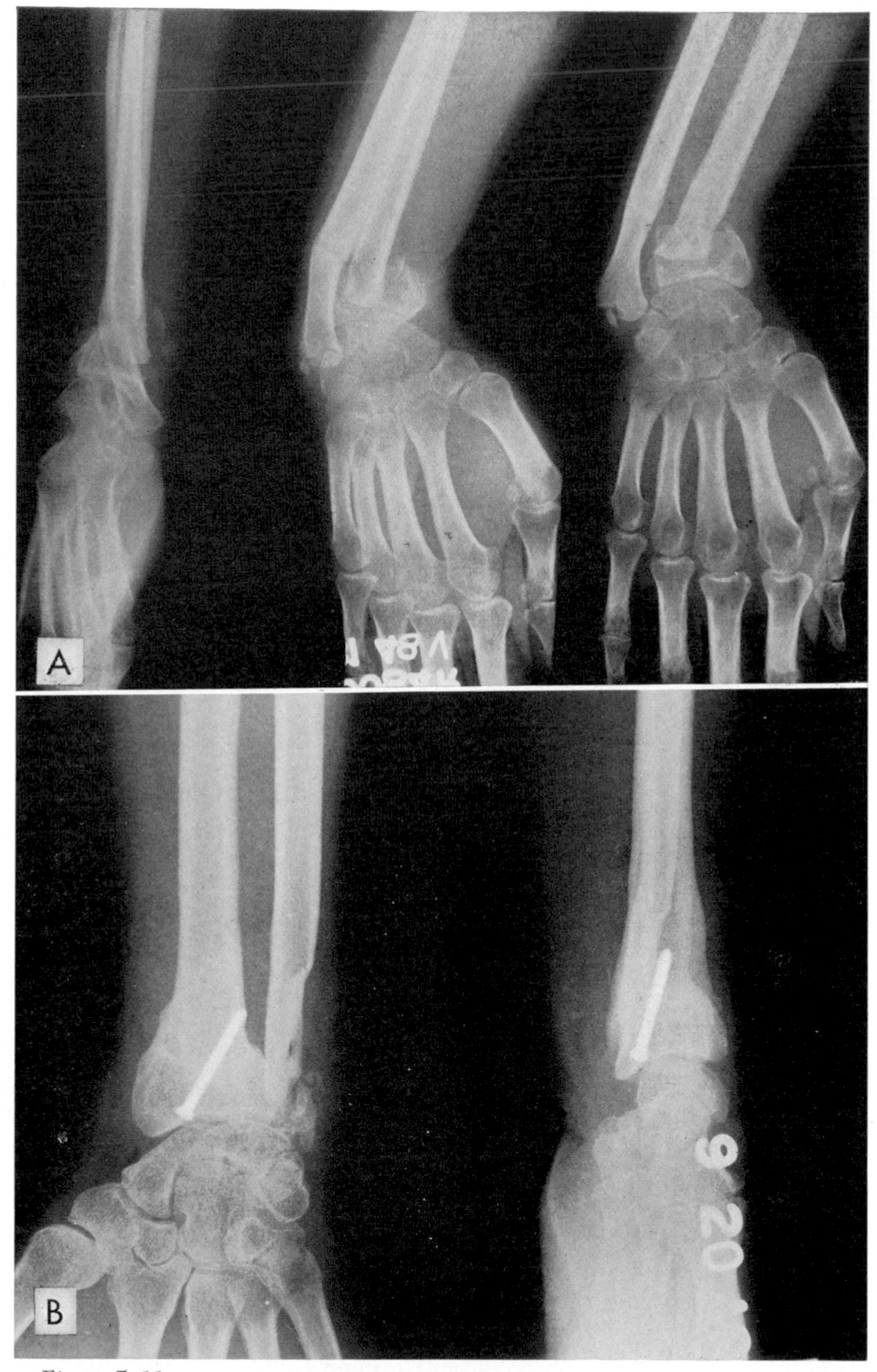

Figure 7–11.

A. Nonunion following Colles' fracture. The ulnar head was excised and used as a bone graft to the reconstructed radius fracture. (Operation by Dr. Frederick M. Smith.)

B. Result after one year.

EPIPHYSEAL INJURIES AT THE WRIST

Injury to the distal radial epiphysis results from a fall on the outstretched hand. The mechanical forces involved and the displacement of the epiphyseal fragment are similar to those of a Colles fracture, except that dorsal comminution of the bone does not occur. Instead, the displaced epiphysis carries with it a triangular fragment from the adjacent metaphysis, which may vary in size from a tiny chip to a large fragment involving almost the full thickness of the bone. That portion of the epiphyseal plate between the metaphyseal fragment and the epiphysis remains uninjured, and may be expected to continue growing at a normal rate. The remainder of the epiphyseal plate is injured and may subsequently undergo a disturbance of growth, depending upon whether the cleavage plane crossed the metaphyseal or the epiphyseal surface of the epiphyseal cartilage. Usually the former is the case, but in 10 to 15 per cent of such epiphyseal displacements subsequent growth disturbance of a temporary or permanent nature indicates the proliferating cartilage cells were damaged. It is only logical that the degree of damage under any circumstances is proportional to the total trauma inflicted upon the epiphyseal plate. Forceful reduction is as damaging as the original injury. Lesions requiring debridement and cleansing of the fracture surfaces are almost invariably, and other closed lesions subjected to repeated or forceful manipulations are likely to be, complicated by subsequent growth disturbance. Excluding these factors, temporary retardation or cessation of growth occurs in 10 to 15 per cent of all cases of injury to the lower radial epiphysis, regardless of the presence, absence, or degree of displacement. More often than not this is a subclinical phenomenon demonstrable only by roentgen comparison with the other wrist, but occasionally the growth of the radius is stopped or retarded sufficiently to produce a visible prominence of the ulnar head and an unsightly radial deviation of the hand.

Treatment

Reduction must above all be gentle. It is impossible to overcorrect the displacement, but insistence upon complete replacement often requires the use of considerable force in manipulations. This incurs an unwarranted risk of secondary injury to the epiphyseal plate. Perfection of reduction is not required. Almost all residual deformities are corrected by growth, except in adolescents approaching the age of epiphyseal closure. Up to the age of 10 to 12 years an incomplete reduction obtained easily is far better than a perfect reduction obtained by force. After this age the penalties of growth disturbance and the ability to correct deformity by growth both lessen, and the desirability of a complete reduction increases progressively with each advancing year. A "sugar tongs" splint is molded to the limb and left in place for three to five weeks. The parents are warned of the small risk of subsequent growth disturbance and urged to have the child examined every six or eight months through the next several years.

Growth Disturbance after Injury to the Distal Radial Epiphysis

This is equally prone to follow an apparent sprain of the child's wrist in which the x-ray is negative, as a grossly displaced epiphysis. Deformity results from retardation or cessation of growth at the distal end of the radius. The distal end of the ulna continues to grow normally, becomes unduly prominent, and the hand swings into radial deviation (Fig. 7–*12*). Other deformities may follow interference with the growth of only a portion of the radial epiphyseal plate while the remainder continues to grow at a normal rate (see Fig. 7–22). Mild deformities of any kind occurring within a year or two after injury should be checked by x-ray and clinical examinations every six months, and operative correction of the deformity should be deferred as long as is consistent with the progression of the deformity. When deformity becomes gross and the necessity for its correction is established beyond question, this should be done before distortion of the associated ulna and surrounding soft parts becomes irreversible. The usual deformity caused by a discrepancy between the lengths of the radius and ulna is most simply rectified by ulnar epiphyseolysis (Fig. 7–*12*), or by excision of the lower end of the ulna, including its epiphyseal plate.

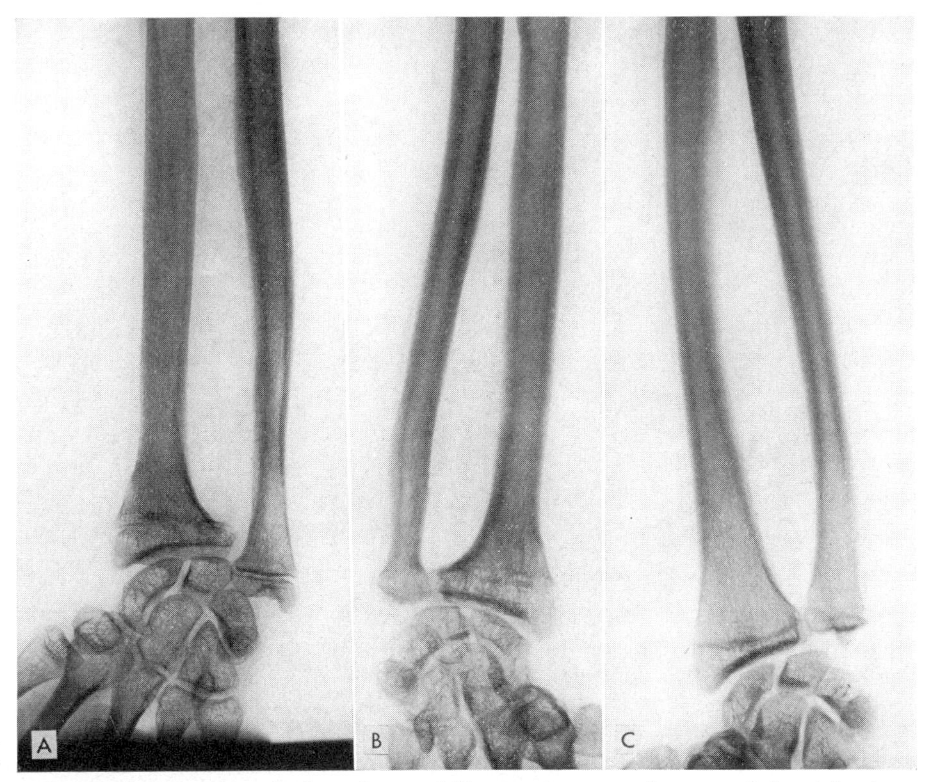

Figure 7–12. Growth disturbance following injury to lower radial epiphysis.

A. At age 11, two years after injury. Note radial deviation of the hand. Ulnar epiphyseolysis was carried out.

B. Result at age 14. Both epiphyses are closed (compare with C).

C. Appearance of normal other wrist.

Occasionally extreme volar or dorsal tilting of the articular surface of the radius, due to growth disturbance of only a portion of the epiphyseal plate, requires correction by osteotomy.

DISLOCATION OF THE LUNATE BONE

The wedge-shaped lunate, situated between the capitate and the radius, may be partially or completely extruded into the volar carpal canal by a fall on the moderately extended hand (Fig. 7–*13*). All except the volar soft-part sources of blood supply to the bone are avulsed so that avascular necrosis is a common late complication of this injury. The intact volar soft parts act as a hinge around which the lunate rotates (usually through 90 degrees, but at times through 180 degrees, or even 270 degrees) into a displaced position. The capitate is pulled against the radius by muscle spasm to obliterate the space formerly occupied by the lunate. The ligamentous connections between lunate and both scaphoid and triquetrum

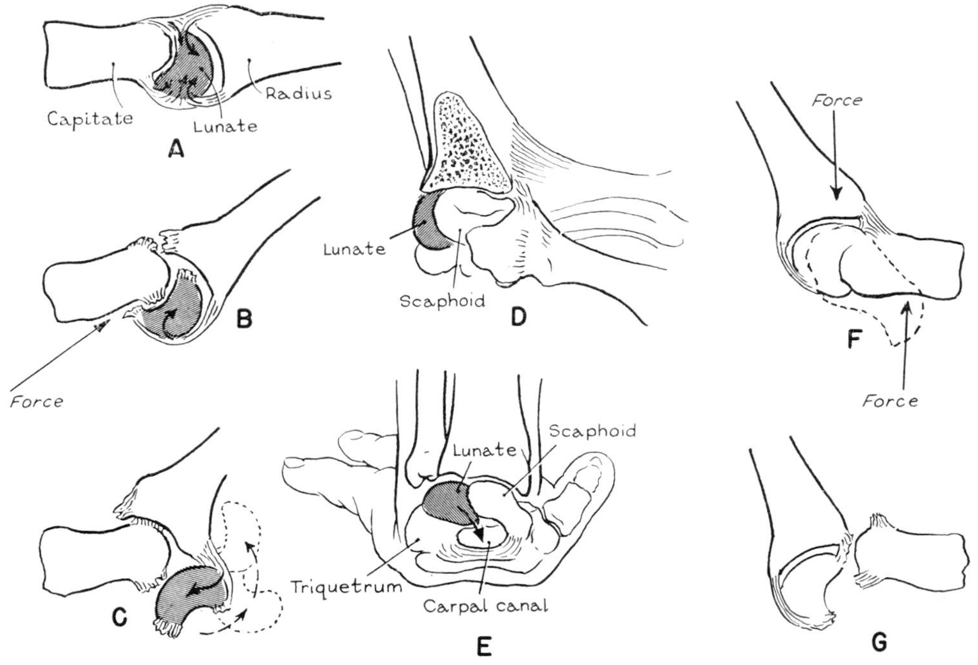

Figure 7–13. Dislocations of and on the lunate.

A. Normal relations, lateral view. Arrows indicate vascular supply to the lunate.

B. An appropriate force, with the wrist moderately extended, may extrude the lunate from between the radius and the capitate bone.

C. The displaced lunate rotates around the volar soft-part hinge, which is its only remaining source of blood supply. The capitate bone is forced against the radius.

D, E. The extruded lunate encroaches upon the flexor tendons and the median nerve in the volar carpal canal.

F, G. An appropriate force to the hyperextended carpus tends to displace the other carpals on the lunate. Impact of the proximal end of the scaphoid against the radius may fracture this bone so that only the distal fragment accompanies the capitate bone into a dislocated position.

are also disrupted, and these two bones are always somewhat displaced. Occasionally these ligaments prove stronger than their attachments, so that a portion or the entire substance of the scaphoid or triquetrum may accompany the lunate into its displaced position.

DIAGNOSIS

Failure of diagnosis is common and usually results from incomplete clinical and from casual roentgen examination. The wrist is swollen and painful, but not deformed, and the dislocated lunate is not palpable. The absence of roentgenographic findings, the films at first glance appearing negative, increases the temptation to diagnose a "sprain of the wrist." However, *the extruded lunate compresses both the median nerve and the flexor tendons of the fingers within the volar carpal canal.* Examination of the hand discloses numbness or hypesthesia of the first three fingers, paralysis or weakness of the small hand muscles supplied by the median nerve, and a distinct to marked weakness of grasping power. Not infrequently the patient seeks advice about a *painless* cigarette burn on a finger a week or two following what he thought was merely a sprain of the wrist. Superimposition of the carpal bones on each other may make roentgen diagnosis of the lesion difficult or impossible, and a true lateral view of the wrist must be obtained (Fig. 7–14). *A wrist sprain accompanied by numb fingers and a weak grasp must be considered a lunate dislocation until proved otherwise.*

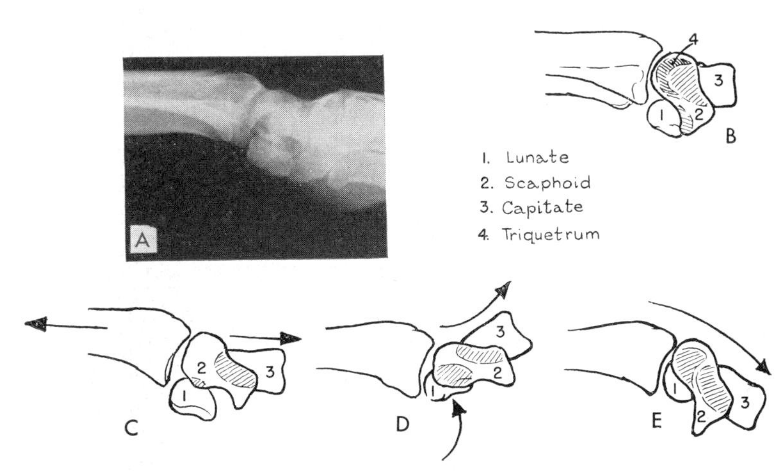

Figure 7–14. Dislocation of the lunate.

A. Lateral view shows the space between capitate and radius to be reduced, and the lunate rotated (in this film 90 degrees) volarward. The films must be technically good, and the projections true, or the diagnosis may be missed.

B. Tracing of the film, showing more clearly the roentgen findings.

C. The traction (arrows) used in reduction must first re-establish sufficient space between capitate and radius to accommodate the lunate.

D. Coincident mild extension of the wrist (upper arrow) further widens this space so that the displaced bone can be pushed into position by finger pressure (lower arrow).

E. Reduction, once obtained, is maintained by moderate wrist flexion.

TREATMENT

Manipulative reduction is usually successful during the first few days after injury, but with further delay becomes increasingly difficult and soon is impossible. The passage of time also depreciates the prognosis progressively by continued compromise of the blood vessels in the volar soft-part hinge. Adequate general or regional anesthesia must precede reduction. Traction is applied to the hand until the capitate is withdrawn from the radius to re-establish a gap sufficient to accommodate the lunate (Fig. 7–*14*, *C*). Moderate coincident wrist extension further widens the volar aspect of this gap through which the lunate must be replaced (Fig. 7–*14, D*). Firm thumb pressure at the volar flexion crease of the wrist forces the displaced bone into its normal position between capitate and radius. The wrist is then flexed about 45 degrees and must be held in this position in order to prevent re-displacement. Successful reduction can be confirmed only by fluoroscopic examination, or a true lateral roentgenogram. Aftercare requires immobilization of the wrist in a flexed position (Fig. 7–*14, E*) for several weeks, and prevention of sudden extension movements for about six weeks after reduction.

The results are uncertain. Recovery of strength and comfort often is retarded or incomplete. The prognosis should be guarded, and the patient should be warned that a painful and weak wrist may result from (1) avascular necrosis of the replaced lunate, or (2) instability of the proximal carpal bones due to faulty healing of the disrupted intercarpal ligaments. Both complications result in a painful arthritis of the wrist.

Open reduction or excision of the lunate should be done for the relief of pressure in the carpal canal when manipulative reduction fails. Within a short time after injury, adhesions and contracture may prevent manual separation of the capitate from the radius, without which the lunate cannot be replaced. More powerful force by skeletal distraction pins through metacarpals and olecranon may succeed, but the results in late cases which require this maneuver are seldom good, and are prone to be complicated by both avascular necrosis and carpal instability.

When manipulative reduction fails the radiocarpal joint should be opened through a *dorsal* exposure. Exposure through the volar aspect of the wrist usually ruins the small remaining blood supply entering the lunate through its soft-tissue hinge. Through the dorsal approach the lunate is lifted into position by small hooks and smooth elevators which are used as "shoe horns." If the bone appears viable, as indicated by healthy and intact soft-part attachments, the wound is closed and aftercare is similar to that used after manipulative reduction. If the lunate is already necrotic or is traumatized by operative insult, it should be removed. Mild permanent weakness and a small defect in motion follow this procedure, but the results are generally very satisfactory, and are characterized by a comfortable and useful hand.

DISLOCATION ON THE LUNATE (PERILUNATE DISLOCATION)

Dislocation *of* the lunate results from a force applied to the palm of the moderately extended hand, but a similar force to the hyperextended

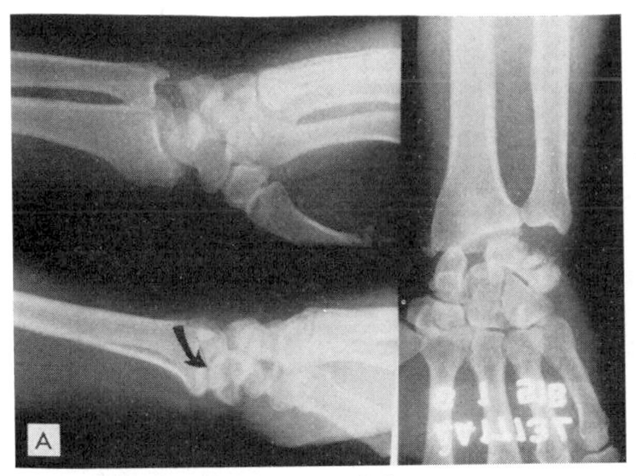

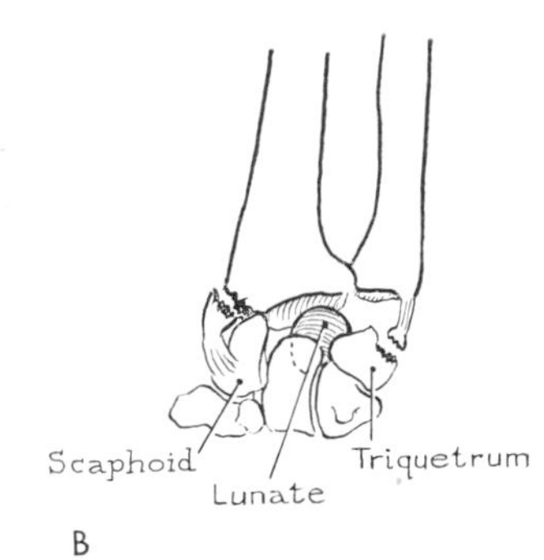

Figure 7–15. Perilunate dislocation.

The displacing scaphoid has fractured the radial styloid instead of the radial collateral ligament. The carpal insertion of the ulnar collateral ligament has been avulsed from the triquetrum. The lunate (arrow) remains in normal apposition to the radius.

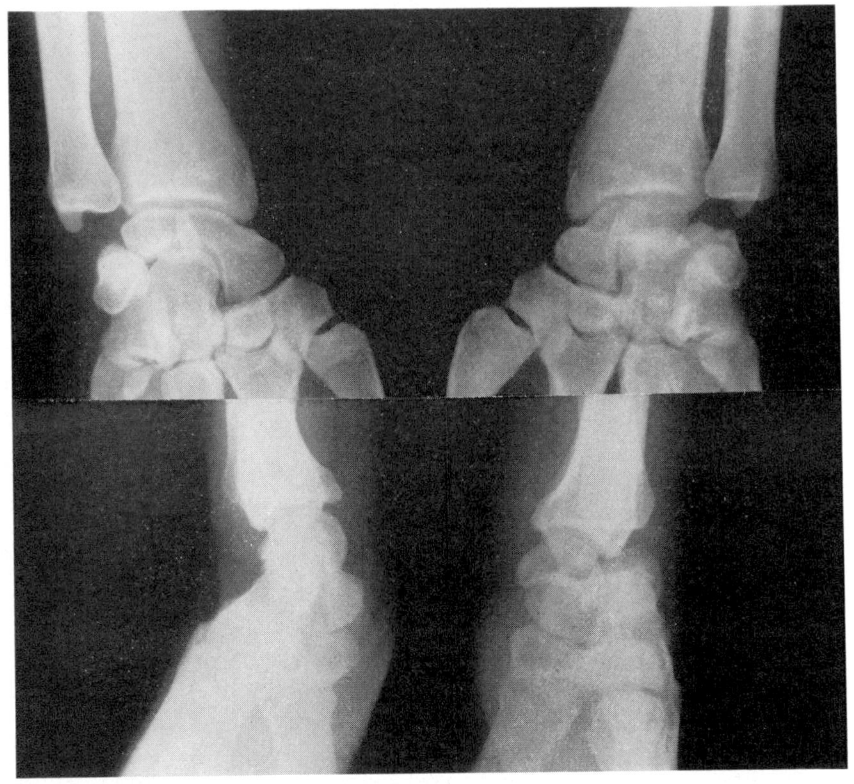

Figure 7–16. Dislocation of remaining carpals on lunate and triquetrum.

Roentgenograms in anteroposterior (upper) and lateral (lower) views contrasting uninjured (left) and injured wrist (right). The triquetrum has remained with the lunate, while the remainder of the carpus has been dislocated backward.

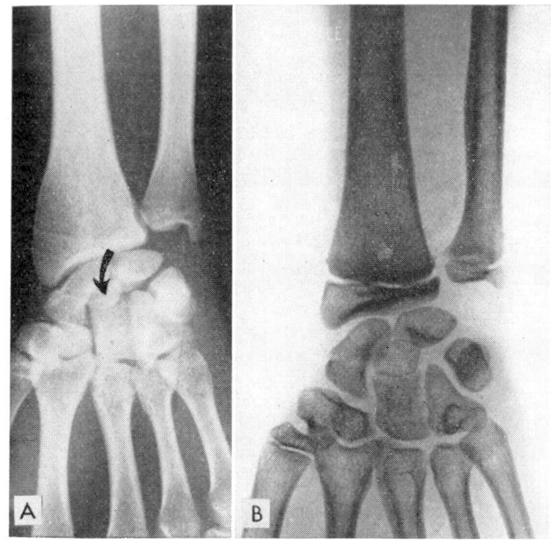

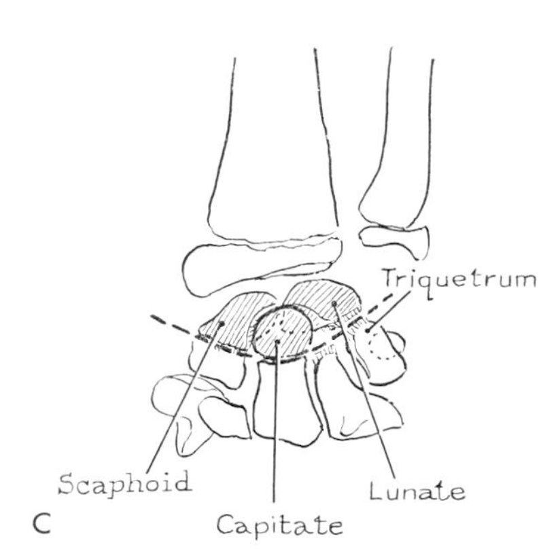

Figure 7–17. Fractures of the capitate bone.

A. Roentgenogram showing proximal fragment of broken capitate (arrow) rotated through 180 degrees. This must be the result of a self-reducing midcarpal dislocation. The proximal fragment was removed. Four weeks later the patient was doing his regular job as a laborer without complaints. (Courtesy Dr. Richard L. Fenton.)

B, C. The history suggested these carpals never were completely displaced. The fractures of scaphoid and capitate were stable. The scaphoid healed uneventfully. The capitate healed by fibrous union, as is suggested by beginning sclerosis at the fracture (B). It is apparent that the injuring force traversed the scaphoid, capitate, and the ligaments connecting the lunate and triquetrum (C). Completion of dislocation would have left the proximal fracture fragments (stippled) in normal relationship to the lunate.

hand dislocates the other carpal bones *on* the lunate (see Fig. 7–*13*, *F*, *G*). The brunt of such an injury is borne by the ligaments connecting the two carpal rows and, as these are disrupted, the capitate, accompanied by all or varying combinations of the other carpal bones, displaces dorsalward, while the lunate remains in normal position (Fig. 7–*15*).

Classification of the many combinations of fracture and dislocation peculiar to the injured carpus is of academic rather than therapeutic significance. Most of the carpals are firmly connected, directly or indirectly, to the keystone of the carpal mechanism, the capitate. All except the lunate tend to follow this bone into a displaced position. When the ligaments holding the lunate to the scaphoid and triquetrum are disrupted both these bones displace with the capitate, but if these intercarpal supports prove stronger than their bony anchorages a fragment of one or both bones may remain attached to the lunate, while the remainder displaces with the capitate. Occasionally the entire substance of one or both of these bones may remain with the lunate (Fig. 7–*16*). Similarly the dislocating scaphoid may fracture the radial styloid (Fig. 7–*12*) instead of disrupting the radial collateral ligaments. Occasionally, even, a fragment of the capitate may remain with the lunate (Fig. 7–*17*). To catalog all such injuries solely on a basis of roentgen findings is but a poor measure of what has happened to the elements of the complicated carpal mechanism. Often the most serious aspect of these injuries is ligament damage, which may remain unrecognizable in the early roentgenograms (Fig. 7–18).

Reduction by manipulation is easier and more certain than with dislocations of the lunate, because the wrist ligaments are widely disrupted and present no impediment to replacement of the dislocated carpus. Traction on the hand, accompanied by thumb pressure over the dorsum of the wrist, restores the carpal bones to a grossly normal position. However, the extensive ligament damage which facilitates reduction also may make maintenance of exact intercarpal relationships impossible. Small residual subluxations of one bone on another are common and rarely are controllable by external fixation. Reduction is maintained by splinting the flexed wrist for several weeks in the posture which maintains the best intercarpal relationship. Persistent subluxation of one or more carpals after three weeks of immobilization justifies continuance of splinting for several more weeks in the hope that undisturbed soft part healing will minimize the subsequent instability of the subluxed elements. Persistent severe pain and disability

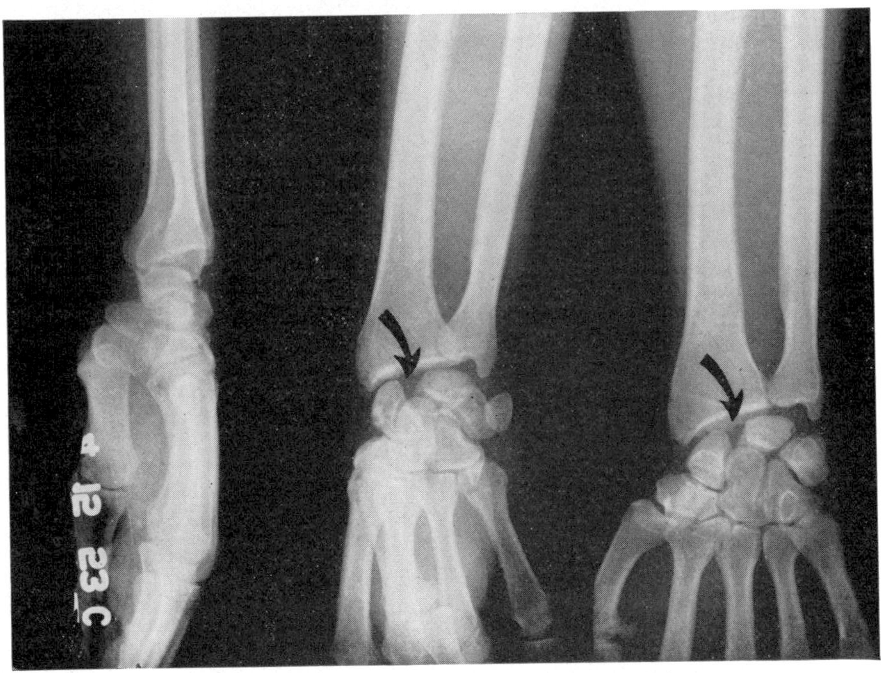

Figure 7–18. Carpal instability following perilunate dislocation.

A. A stiff, weak, and painful wrist many months after reduction of a perilunate dislocation. Note the rotatory displacement of the scaphoid in the lateral view. The proximal end of this bone projects dorsalward to impinge against the radius and impede wrist extension. There is abnormal motion between the scaphoid and lunate as demonstrated in the anteroposterior and oblique views (arrows). The significance of the damage to the scaphoid ligaments and their failure to heal soundly could not be recognized from the roentgenogram during the stage of active treatment. The scaphoid was excised with a good result.

from this complication necessitate excision of the offending carpals, or wrist fusion.

DISLOCATION OF OR ON THE LUNATE WITH SCAPHOID FRACTURE

This is the most common fracture-dislocation of the wrist (Fig. 7–19). The scaphoid is situated half in the proximal and half in the distal row of carpals. Figure 7–3 illustrates how an injury which drives the hyper-

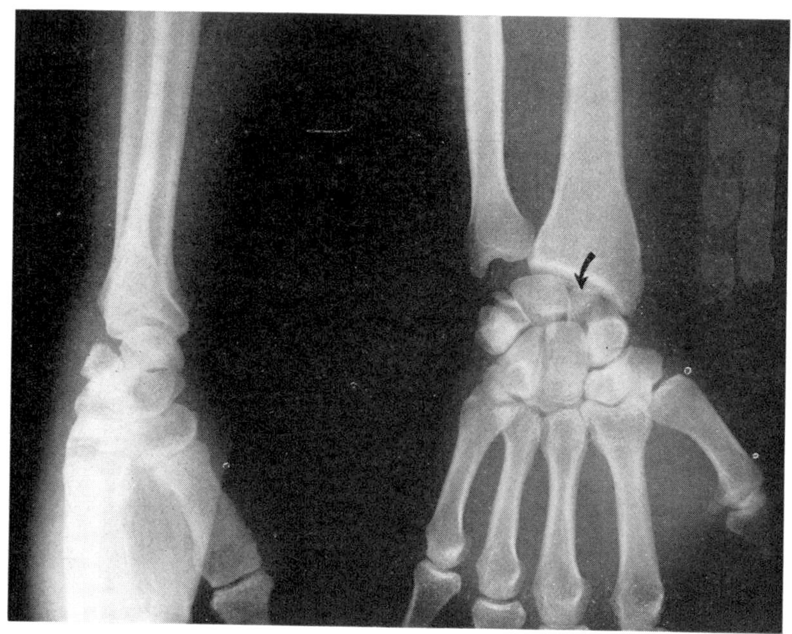

Figure 7–19. Perilunate dislocation with scaphoid fracture.
The proximal fragment of the fractured scaphoid (arrow) remains with the lunate in normal relation to the radius, and the distal scaphoid fragment is displaced with the capitate.

extended carpus dorsalward may well fracture the scaphoid and leave the proximal fragment behind with the lunate as the distal fragment displaces with the capitate. The counterpart of this lesion, a dislocation of the lunate accompanied by a fragment of scaphoid, is rare. In either instance the dislocation is reduced in the usual manner. It then becomes necessary to re-approximate accurately the fragments of the scaphoid. Due to the ligament damage attendant upon the dislocation these are always grossly unstable. A short period of immobilization with the wrist flexed no more than necessary to prevent redislocation is attended by soft part healing sufficient to prevent redisplacement of carpals on lunate. Treatment of the scaphoid fracture will be discussed, but in this instance the difficulties normally encountered with unstable lesions are magnified. Failure of union, avascular necrosis of the proximal fragment, and a painful weak wrist are to be expected. Late reconstructive procedures or wrist fusion often is necessary.

LATE UNREDUCED PERILUNATE DISLOCATION WITHOUT ARTHRITIS

Manipulative reduction is prevented by fibrosis. Open reduction is attended by a local tissue insult which vitiates the benefits obtained. Wrist fusion is a last resort. Resection of the proximal carpal row rapidly produces quite satisfactory results without precluding subsequent arthrodesis

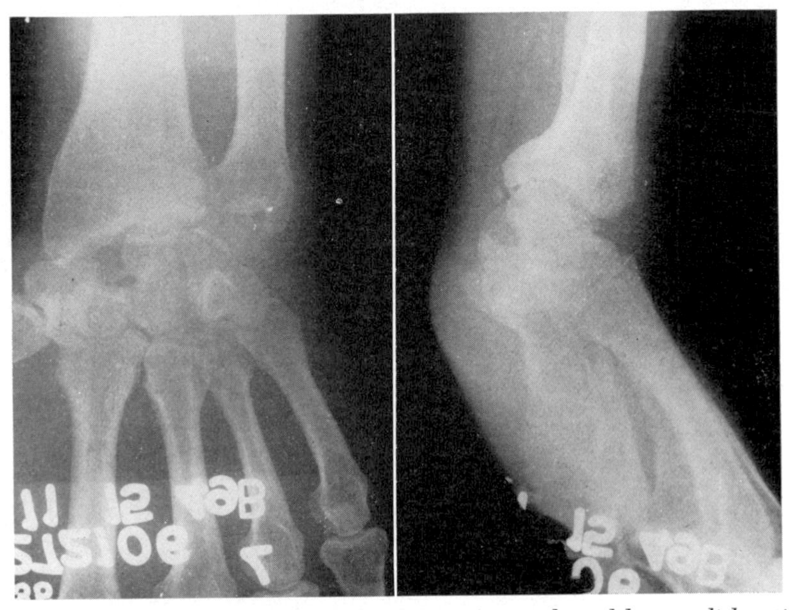

Figure 7–20. Proximal carpal row resection for neglected lunate dislocation. Roentgenograms show condition six years after operation, during which time the patient had performed all his duties as a farmer.

should the simpler procedure fail. If all components of the proximal row are removed (Fig. 7–*20*) a comfortable and useful wrist, marked by mild weakness and some limitation of motion, may be anticipated.

OLD UNREDUCED FRACTURE-DISLOCATION WITH ARTHRITIS

The use of a molded leather gauntlet, which prevents all except rotatory motions of the wrist, often produces adequate relief of pain. When palliative measures do not suffice, wrist fusion should be done. If symptoms of carpal tunnel compression are present in addition to wrist pain, division of the volar carpal ligament or removal of an extruded lunate should precede arthrodesis. Very old unreduced lesions (Fig. 7–*21*) are uncommon because persistent pain usually mandates operative measures long before the advent of arthritis.

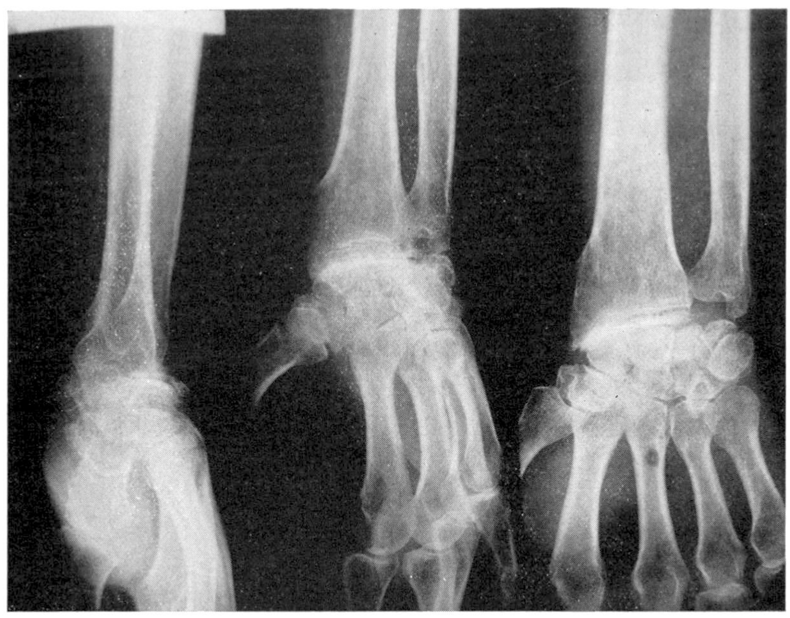

Figure 7–21. Unreduced fracture-dislocation of 62 years' duration.

This 86-year-old man had sustained a severe injury to his wrist while doing gymnastics at age 24 and had received no treatment. The wrist caused little trouble until three weeks prior to this examination, when he sustained a minor injury. This was followed by median nerve symptoms and severe wrist pain, both of which subsided gradually when the wrist was immobilized.

DISLOCATION OF CARPUS WITH MARGINAL FRACTURE OF RADIUS

The overhanging dorsal lip of the radius prevents backward dislocation of the lunate, but forward dislocation of the entire carpus may occur with an apparently insignificant marginal fracture of the radius (Fig. 7–22). The lesion is rare and difficult to manage. Reduction is easily accomplished by traction accompanied by thumb pressure over the flexion crease at the wrist, but is difficult or impossible to maintain except by skeletal traction. This is used in the manner described for certain Colles' fractures (see Fig. 7–8), and the wrist should be immobilized in a position of mild extension.

FRACTURES AND DISLOCATIONS INVOLVING THE CAPITATE

These are rare injuries. The essential lesion is a form of perilunate dislocation which may reduce spontaneously prior to examination, or may never displace completely. Undisplaced and stable fractures may heal with immobilization (Fig. 7–*17*), but it is questionable whether a strong fibrous union would prove serviceable enough to ensure a good result. Unstable (displaced) fractures (Fig. 7–*17*) require excision of the hypermobile proximal fragment. Following this the wrist should be immobilized for several weeks until soft part healing adequate to stabilize the remaining capitate fragment has been developed.

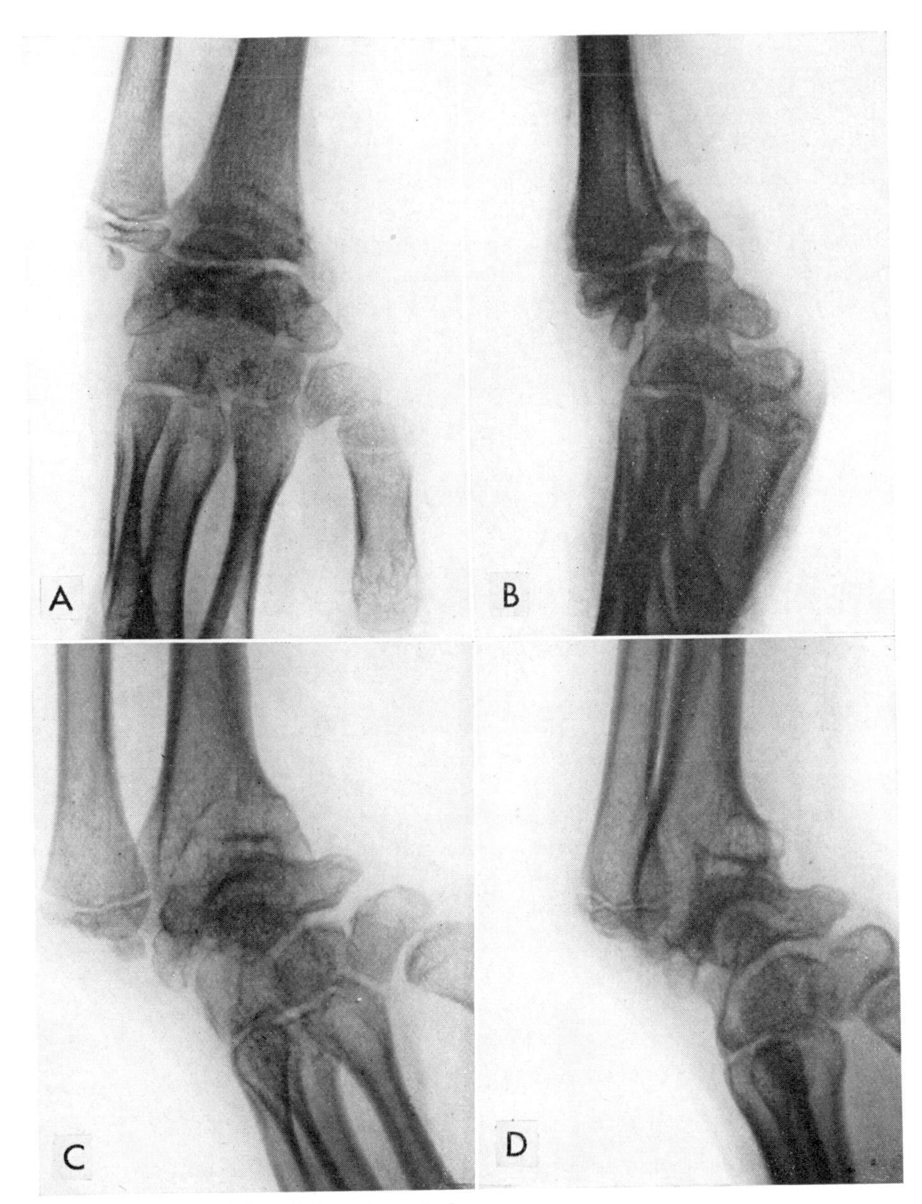

Figure 7–22. *Volar dislocation of the carpus.*

A, B. Roentgenograms of child seen some weeks after injury. Manipulative reduction was impossible, and it was considered that open reduction would do more harm than good. The median nerve and finger flexors were intact. A small marginal fracture through the volar lip of the lower radial epiphysis is apparent in the lateral view (B).

C, D. Roentgenograms four years later, no treatment having been given, show a grossly deformed and moderately disabled wrist due to carpal displacement and growth disturbance at the lower radial epiphysis. The median nerve remained functionally intact.

Adequate early treatment would have required skeletal pin traction, as illustrated in Figure 7–8, for certain maintenance of normal relationship between carpals and radius.

DISLOCATION OF THE SCAPHOID

This lesion may occur as the only demonstrable carpal disorder, but usually is accompanied by soft part damage which cannot be identified. The frequency with which rotatory subluxation of the scaphoid is observed following reduction of a perilunate dislocation suggests the occasional isolated scaphoid dislocation to be a residuum of a spontaneously reduced perilunate injury. When manipulative reduction proves successful, after-

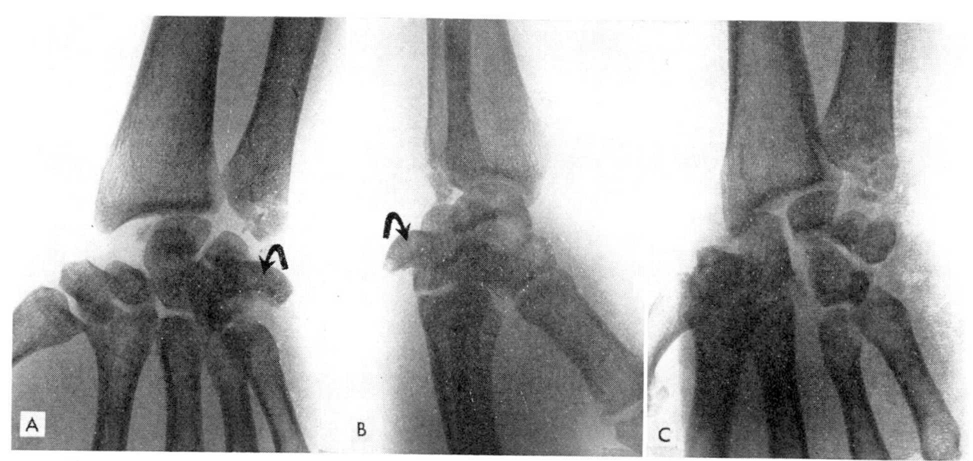

Figure 7–23. Dislocation of the scaphoid.

The primary lesion is a perilunate dislocation. The gross displacement of the extruded scaphoid (arrows in A and B) is indicative of very extensive soft part damage. Widespread intercarpal ligament disruption is confirmed by the spontaneous rearrangement of the remaining carpals following early excision of the scaphoid (C). The early result was fair; the late result is not known.

care should be the same as for a perilunate dislocation; otherwise, open reduction or excision of the scaphoid is necessary (Fig. 7–23).

INJURIES TO THE HAMATE BONE

A fall on the heel of the hand may fracture the hook of the hamate bone. This injury is painful, but not serious. As with fractures through many other bony appendages, fibrous union is likely. The early painful symptoms are palliated by rest, splints, and other local sedative measures. Occasionally persistent pain may require excision of the hook of the hamate. Dorsal dislocations of the hamate are quite rare. When manipulative reduction fails, operative replacement or excision should be done.

FRACTURE OF THE SCAPHOID

This is the wrist injury often accompanied by an apparently negative roentgenogram which, when examined casually and treated as a sprain, may never recover. As stated earlier, a wrist *sprain must be considered a fracture of the scaphoid until it is proved otherwise.* The true diagnosis is frequently missed. The penalty is often serious, but is by no means certain, since the incidence of spontaneous healing after scaphoid fracture is unknown. It is certain that in some cases union occurs without treatment, and it is well known that many untreated lesions eventuate with fibrous union and an essentially normal wrist until some subsequent trauma "shakes up" the pseudoarthrosis and initiates symptoms of pain, or perhaps merely necessitates a roentgenogram which discloses a long-standing but asymptomatic absence of bony union. It is reasonably certain, however, that failure to diagnose and treat an *unstable* scaphoid fracture will eventually result in painful arthritis of the radiocarpal joint.

DIAGNOSIS

Clinical Diagnosis

The history describes some injury which jammed the thenar eminence against the radius while the wrist was extended (see Fig. 7–3). One should not be led into a diagnosis of sprain by diffuse swelling, pain, and tenderness across the entire dorsum of the wrist. As the carpal scaphoid lies half in the proximal and half in the distal row of carpals, its fracture usually is accompanied by some diffuse damage to the intercarpal ligaments. Percussion of the tip of the stabilized thumb or index finger without wrist motion, when productive of a wincing pain just distal to the radial styloid, is strongly suggestive of scaphoid fracture, but there is no certain clinical method for differentiating sprain of the wrist from this fracture in the early stages after injury.

Roentgen Diagnosis

Roentgenography soon after injury may be as unreliable diagnostically as clinical examination. More often than not ordinary films are useless and misleading. The anteroposterior projection appears negative, because the tubercle of the scaphoid is superimposed over the fracture area; the lateral projection finds the scaphoid obscured by superimposition of the other carpals, and the temptation for a false negative interpretation is great. *An oblique view of the carpals throwing the scaphoid into true profile is mandatory. Even when all three projections appear negative, the examination should be repeated after two weeks.* During the interval decalcification occurs at a previously undiscernible fracture line to make it visible in the later films. Only when these later films remain negative can a fracture of the scaphoid be disproved with certainty.

TREATMENT DURING INTERVAL OF INDECISION

Following the dictum that a "sprained wrist" should be treated as a scaphoid fracture until subsequent films rule out bone injury, a snug plaster gauntlet is applied, to be removed in two weeks to permit roentgen re-evaluation. If the injury proves to be only a sprain this is excellent treatment; when a carpal fracture is present it may be essential.

PATHOLOGY OF SCAPHOID FRACTURE

The blood supply of the scaphoid enters through soft parts attached mainly to the distal half of the bone. The remainder of the bone is intra-articular, devoid of periosteum, and surfaced with articular cartilage. It has been customary to explain the high incidence of faulty healing and avascular necrosis of the proximal fragment of a fractured scaphoid on the basis of the level of the break and the consequent vascular privation of the proximal fragment. Operative exposure and inspection of early fractures reveal this thesis to be but a partial truth, and the intrinsic apposition and stability of the fracture fragments to be of equal importance.

Fracture Through Distal Third of Scaphoid

Both fragments are left with a good blood supply, but of equal importance, although much less appreciated, is the secure and perfect apposition of the fracture fragments guaranteed by intact common ligament attachments. Barring further injury and disruption of these soft-part splints, it appears probable that sound union might be expected, despite the type, presence, or absence of treatment. This is not to say that treatment is unnecessary, but rather to emphasize that optimum therapy must provide protection against re-injury, relief from pain, and not an indefinite abolition of function by prolonged immobilization.

Stable Fracture Through Waist of Scaphoid

The fragments are held securely in apposition by common soft-part attachments and relatively intact articular cartilage. When the articular cartilage is incompletely disrupted no more than a small hinge motion takes place at the fracture, even when the wrist is moved. Occasionally, despite a crack through the underlying bone, intact articular cartilage provides the fragments with ideal internal fixation. The wash of joint fluid in and out of the fracture gap is minimized or prevented, and neither rotatory nor shearing displacement of the fragments can take place. It would appear difficult to prevent the healing of such fractures.

Unstable Fracture Through Waist of Scaphoid

The fracture is complete in that the surrounding articular cartilage and soft parts are disrupted, as well as the bone. The fragments, lubricated by joint fluid, are greasy and slippery and skid about in all directions upon the slightest motion of thumb or wrist. Compression of the carpals against the radius, such as would result from muscle tension or finger function, creates shearing displacements of one fragment on the other, even when the wrist and thumb are held quite immobile. With each motion of the fragments, joint fluid washes through the fracture gap in a manner compatible with prevention of the first step in the bone-healing process, the formation of a clot. Free bleeding from the broken surface of the proximal fragment is uncommon. It is quite clear that complete immobility of the thumb and wrist does not provide complete immobilization of the bone fragments. In such unstable fractures healing is bound to be slow and likely to fail.

The stability or instability noted at operations on fresh scaphoid fractures has been variable, and it is likely that the prognosis depends to a large extent upon this factor. Roentgen evidence of any displacement is pathognomonic of instability. Unfortunately, an absence of displacement is not synonymous with stability. Often a fracture will appear stable and undisplaced by roentgenogram, only to prove quite unstable on fluoroscopic examination. Consequently, all fractures through or proximal to the waist of the bone must be considered as potentially unstable.

Fracture of Proximal Third of Scaphoid

A fracture of the proximal third of the scaphoid is unstable. It seldom occurs alone, and usually accompanies a lunate or perilunate dislocation, which may or may not reduce spontaneously prior to roentgen examination. The proximal scaphoid gives way, rather than its soft-part connections to the lunate. The proximal bone fragment is intracapsular, quite unstable, almost devoid of soft-part attachments, and therefore essentially avascular. The prognosis under any circumstances is poor. Healing, if it occurs at all, is certain to be slow, and avascular necrosis of the proximal fragment is common.

TREATMENT OF RECENT SCAPHOID FRACTURE

The forearm, wrist, and metacarpals should be dressed in a snug-fitting plaster gauntlet. In fractures of the distal third of the bone this usually may be discarded after about four weeks. In stable waist fractures evidences of union sufficient to permit removal of the gauntlet will be seen by roentgenogram after 8 to 10 weeks. Absence of any evidences of union in a waist fracture 12 weeks after injury is indicative of instability, and imperfect fixation sufficient to interfere with or prevent healing. Slow union is then to be *expected,* and nonunion to be *feared.* Any increase in the relative density of the proximal fragment indicates that inadequacy of the vascular supply is further complicating the healing process. In fractures through the proximal third of the bone both a failure or retardation of healing and a temporary or permanent avascular necrosis of the proximal fragment are common and unlikely to be controlled by external immobilization, regardless of its quality or duration.

Extent of Immobilization

Some surgeons contend that efficient treatment for a scaphoid fracture requires a plaster gauntlet which encloses the thumb, at least to the level of the interphalangeal joint. This efficiently obliterates function of the hand throughout the immobilization period. Others as staunchly advocate that the gauntlet should extend only to the metacarpophalangeal joint of the thumb. This allows fairly normal function of the hand, provided the thumb is opposed to the index finger. All report similar results. Observations at operation confirm that when the fracture is stable it makes no difference to its fixation whether or not the thumb is included in the gauntlet. Fixation and apposition are maintained securely in either case. When the fracture is unstable neither dressing produces complete fixation. Compression of carpals against radius, despite complete immobility of the entire wrist and thumb, results in a shearing motion of one fragment on the other. The advantages of immobilizing the thumb are theoretical and invalidated by operative findings; the penalties are practical and serious. *The thumb should be opposed to the index finger and allowed to move.*

The most perfect plaster gauntlet does not retain a snug fit and *should be re-applied every few weeks,* as atrophy makes it loose. The amount of motion sufficient to complicate the healing of an unstable fracture is certainly less than 1/8 inch, and such a range is possible after even a slight loosening of the plaster dressing. As in intracapsular fractures of the femoral neck, which are beset by problems similar to those of the fractured scaphoid, some form of internal fixation eventually may prove to be the optimum treatment for unstable lesions, but the exacting technique and specialized facilities necessary to the consistent success of such a procedure are not yet sufficiently developed and standardized to justify its general usage.

Slow Union and Duration of Immobilization

Should the surgeon sentence the man who earns a living with his hands to many months of immobilization (often amounting to disability and loss of wages) for a fracture of the scaphoid? Some authorities advocate immobilization for as long as a year or more in the presence of slow union. The patient cannot be reassured that, if immobilized well enough and long enough, all scaphoid fractures will eventually unite by bone, nor even that bony union is always synonymous with a strong and comfortable wrist.

When the fragments are well apposed and stable, uneventful bony union may be anticipated within 6 to 12 weeks. When no evidence of union exists after four months it becomes questionable whether it will ever be obtained, regardless of the duration of immobilization. When the ends of the bone fragments become sclerotic, further immobilization is futile and nonunion is established.

Cavitation of the scaphoid at the fracture site is a common index of some interference with the process of union. By roentgenogram the fracture gradually changes from a linear crack to assume the appearance of a decalcified cyst. Operative findings invalidate the concept that this process results from persisting hyperemia, but add little to a comprehension of its true cause. There are no soft tissues surrounding the fracture to become hyperemic. The proximal bone fragment is not hyperemic, but rather hypo-emic, yet cavitation of the proximal fragment develops coincidentally with that of the distal fragment. The phenomenon is not one of decalcification alone, but of actual cyst formation with loss of bone matrix as well as of mineral. Possibly the mineral migrates from the bone ends as in extra-articular fractures, but in increased amounts, since as it leaves the bone it is washed away into the surrounding lake of joint fluid. It is difficult to understand why the matrix of the bone ends should also disintegrate and disappear, but it has been seen that the process is not necessarily irreversible. Repair and obliteration of the cyst is by granulation tissue ingrowth from its walls, and the success or failure of this process is presumably dependent upon the intrinsic vascularity of the bone fragments. Granulations invading the fracture gap from both sides may eventually coalesce and calcify to produce a bony union, but clinical experiences indicate consummation of this reaction not only to be uncertain, but also to require many months to a year or more. It is upon a realization of these facts that the surgeon must predicate a treatment program for the scaphoid fracture which remains unhealed after several months of adequate immobilization.

Until four months after injury plaster immobilization should be discarded only when adequate roentgenograms show the presence of bony union. When no evidence of union is present after four months the plan of treatment should be re-examined. The patient should be told that his fracture has not healed, that it may be many months before healing occurs, and that bony union may never occur. He should also be advised that fibrous union may produce a very serviceable wrist, but that weakness and pain sometimes supervene at a later date. He should know that prolonged continuance of immobilization may eventuate in bony union, but that bony union in itself may not be synonymous with a good result. Above all, he should be reassured that measures are available for the relief of any pain or weakness which may occur. The implications of these measures, internal fixation, excision of one or both fragments of the fracture, bone graft, and arthrodesis of the wrist, should be discussed in detail. By a joint decision of both patient and surgeon, based on all the pertinent factors, a trial by use may then be elected, rather than the indefinite continuance of external immobilization.

TREATMENT OF ESTABLISHED NONUNION

Irreversible nonunion beyond the possibility of spontaneous repair exists when decalcification is replaced by sclerosis at the apposed margins of the fragments. This may occur with or without antecedent cavitation of the fractured ends. Roentgen evidences of sclerosis manifest the elaboration of a layer of compact bone at the broken surface of each fragment. The fragments are connected by fibrous tissue. The periphery of the resulting false joint is incompletely connected to the wrist joint capsule by fibrous adhesions, but a true fibrous union is rarely encountered, and wrist-joint fluid lubricates the pseudoarthrosis.

It is apparent that the absence or presence and severity of the symptoms depend upon the stability with which the ununited fragments are held together by these fibrous connections. Fluoroscopic examination of asymptomatic lesions reveals the fragments to be securely fixed so that little or no inter-fragment motion takes place. Exploration of symptomatic lesions reveals poor fixation, which allows hypermobile fragments (usually the distal) to jam against the dorsal lip of the radius on wrist motion. Four quite different procedures are available for relief of wrist pain and weakness resulting from nonunion of the scaphoid.

Excision of one or both fragments has been a topic of discussion and controversy for many years, chiefly because no surgeon has had the opportunity to observe a large enough number of cases to formulate an authoritative evaluation of the results. Such procedures present obvious advantages in that the operation is a minor affair requiring only a few

TABLE 7–*1*. RESULTS OF COMPLETE EXCISION OF SCAPHOID FOLLOWED FOR 5 TO 19 YEARS.

	Ratings *		
	Anatomy	*Function, Symptoms*	*Economic Recovery*
Case 1	4	4	4
Case 2	4	3	4 (slight pain on forced adduction; full work as a street cleaner)
Case 3	4	3	4 (mild pain on forced extension; 20° defect in extension)
Case 4	4	3	4 (5° defect in extension; 10° defect in flexion)
Case 5	3	3	4 (slight radial deviation of hand; 10° defect in extension; 33 per cent defect in strength of grip)
Case 6	4	3	3 (30° defect in flexion and extension —sufficient to interfere with work)

* Ratings are as follows:
4—100 per cent normal
3—99 to 75 per cent normal
2—74 to 50 per cent normal
1—less than 50 per cent normal

TABLE 7–2. RESULTS OF PROXIMAL FRAGMENT EXCISION FOLLOWED FOR 4 TO 13 YEARS.

	Ratings *		
	Anatomy	*Function, Symptoms*	*Economic Recovery*
Case 1	4	3	4 (30° extension and 10° flexion defect)
Case 2	4	3	4 (mild discomfort; full use)
Case 3	4	3	4 (mild discomfort on forced dorsiflexion)
Case 4	3	3	4 (ganglion present; mild discomfort on forcing motion; full use)

* See Table 7–*1* for explanation of ratings.

TABLE 7–3. RESULTS OF LUNATE AND PROXIMAL SCAPHOID FRAGMENT EXCISION FOLLOWED FOR 8 TO 11 YEARS.

	Ratings *		
	Anatomy	*Function, Symptoms*	*Economic Recovery*
Case 1	4	3	4 (40° flexion and 40° extension defect; good grip; no pain; full use)
Case 2	3	3	4 (15° extension defect; prominent ulnar head)
Case 3	3	3	3 (slight radial shift; extension 0; mild pain)

* See Table 7–*1* for explanation of ratings.

days' hospitalization and no postoperative immobilization. Immediate resumption of use and early restoration of a reasonably comfortable and strong wrist is the rule.

The accompanying tables show the results of the writer's experience in such cases employing complete excision of the scaphoid (Table 7–*1*), excision of the proximal fragment (Table 7–2), and excision of lunate and proximal fragment of the scaphoid (Table 7–3). One patient in whom the scaphoid was completely removed is omitted from Table 7–*1*. In this case treatment was rated a complete failure owing to faulty technique. The scaphoid was removed, but the associated dislocated lunate could not be found. Arthrodesis was subsequently carried out.

Drilling the fracture by multiple fine drill holes designed to break up its sclerotic margins and fashion avenues through which new tissues may unite the fragments has a disadvantage in that prolonged postoperative immobilization must be carried out. The results are uncertain.

Bone graft is often successful in promoting eventual union. Prolonged immobilization in plaster is required after surgery. The specialized operative technique and facilities necessary to success of this procedure contraindicate its use except by the skillful surgeon experienced in this type of work.

Intramedullary fixation by pin or screw rapidly relieves the painful wrist resulting from instability of the ununited fragments, but should not be used in the presence of arthritis or avascular necrosis. The morbidity is minimal and the early results are good, but bony union rarely occurs, and the enduring qualities of this procedure are not yet known.

Arthrodesis of the wrist is the operation of choice in the presence of arthritis. In other circumstances it may be done after failure of the other less radical measures.

Choice of treatment for nonunion of scaphoid. Several conditions influence the choice of treatment in established nonunion of the scaphoid.

(1) In the presence of radiocarpal joint arthritis wrist fusion should be done.

(2) In the absence of arthritis and the presence of avascular necrosis of the proximal fragment one or both fragments should be excised. If only

the proximal fragment is removed, the dorsal edge of the remaining fragment should be bevelled sufficiently to ensure that it does not impinge against the lip of the radius on dorsiflexion of the wrist. When the distal fragment is unstable and impinges grossly against the radius on dorsiflexion both fragments should be removed.

(3) In the absence of arthritis with two fragments of good vascularity bone graft should be done, provided postoperative immobilization is feasible. When a satisfactory result in a short time seems preferable to a somewhat better result requiring prolonged immobilization, ablation of one or both fragments is the method of choice.

(4) Internal fixation has produced gratifying early results in a small group, but the enduring qualities of this procedure (which has not been followed by bony union) are uncertain.

CHAPTER 8

INJURIES OF THE FOREARM

By HARRISON L. McLAUGHLIN, M.D.

FRACTURE OF FOREARM BONES IN CHILDREN

Reduction

MANIPULATION of forearm fractures in children requires anesthesia. There is often a temptation to try to correct a small angular deformity without anesthesia while the plaster splints are setting. If the fracture is greenstick in type, the angulation will recur in plaster (see Fig. 8–*4, A*); if it is complete, correction without anesthesia is not only uncertain but sadistic. In the average forearm fracture some combination of the following deformities necessitates reduction—shortening, rotation, displacement, and angulation.

Correction of length is not difficult, nor does it require great force. A child's muscles are small. Continued traction on the hand against countertraction at the elbow will restore normal length, except when all tissues are organized or the fracture partially healed. No other manipulation should be attempted until normal length has been restored.

Correction of rotation should coincide with traction. Not even a small child can overcome by growth the deformity produced by union of two fragments in a malrotated position. This is the worst deformity of all. It cannot always be identified in the x-ray films, except when the wrist and elbow are included in the same picture. Beware of the film which *shows a lateral view of the forearm bones at the elbow, and an anteroposterior or oblique view at the wrist* (see Fig. 8–*11*).

A fracture of the radius between the supinator and the pronator teres is immediately beset by two complicating factors: inaccessibility and uncontrollable rotation of the proximal fragment. This fragment is short, and buried under the mass of the forearm muscles. It cannot be grasped, let alone manipulated, and, despite all circumstances, assumes a position of flexion and supination due to unopposed biceps and supinator muscles (Fig. 8–*1, A*). The longer distal fragment, although pronated by unopposed teres and quadratus muscles, may be grasped, manipulated, and controlled by external forces. This controllable fragment, therefore, must be fitted to the uncontrollable proximal fragment, which means that re-

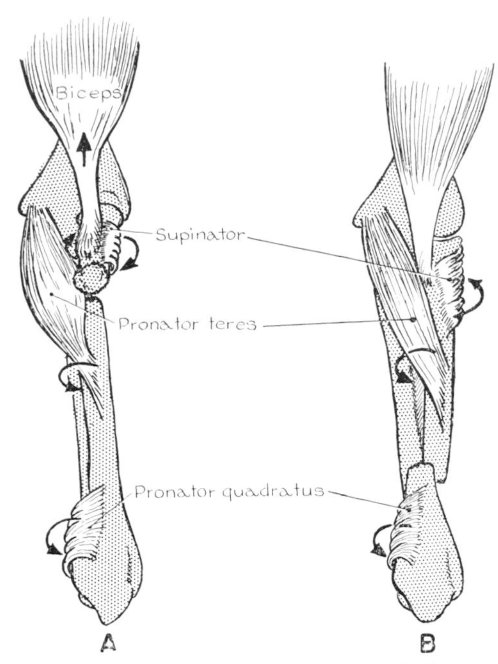

Figure 8–1. Rotatory muscle forces affecting radial shaft fractures.

A. In a fracture between the supinator and pronator teres insertions the proximal fragment is flexed and supinated by the biceps and supinator; the distal fragment is pronated by the pronator teres and quadratus.

B. In a fracture between the pronators the proximal fragment remains in balance; the distal fragment is pronated.

duction and fixation must both be done with the forearm flexed and supinated.

When the radius is fractured in its middle or distal portion, supinator action on the proximal fragment usually is balanced by the pronator teres (Fig. 8–*1, B*). The distal fragment remains controllable, even though the pronator quadratus is unopposed, and should be accommodated to the balanced position of the other by reducing and immobilizing the fracture with the forearm in neutral rotation.

Correction of displacement may be difficult, but perfection is not often necessary. Partial apposition of the fragments is better than a perfect fit obtained by force at the cost of much additional damage to the surrounding tissues. When the child is under eight years of age it is enough to lock the fragments sufficiently to make possible control of length and alignment by a plaster dressing. Residual displacement deformities are largely obliterated by growth. In older children, nature's power to correct residual bone deformity decreases, and the importance of obtaining a complete reduction increases progressively with the age of the patient. From adolescence on, perfection of reduction is desirable. However, at any age, residual displacement incurs the least penalty of all the deformities and by itself does not often produce a serious disability.

Many times the surgeon can reduce the radius or the ulna fracture, but not both. The first to be reduced persistently redisplaces during manipulation of the other. The radius must be reduced, even at the expense of leaving the ulnar fragments unapposed. The converse is never true. Reduction of the ulnar fracture without apposition of the radial fragments will be followed by recurrent deformity in plaster and a poor result.

Correction of angulation should be the final step in reduction. Generally, angulation with a volar apex requires the wrist to be immobilized in flexion; conversely, angulation with a dorsal apex requires immobilization in extension. While the plaster splints are setting they should be molded to conform with the normal volar curve of the radial shaft. A small residual increase in this curve has no ill effects, but reduction or reversal of the normal radial curve may interfere seriously with rotation. Young children have considerable ability to correct residual angular deformities, but this power decreases rapidly after ten years of age.

Factors Complicating Reduction

Interposition of tendon is not common, but should be excluded from among the causes of otherwise unexplainable inability to reduce fractures of the distal portions of the radius or ulna which have been grossly displaced. It is usually a fragment of the radius, which bore the brunt of the

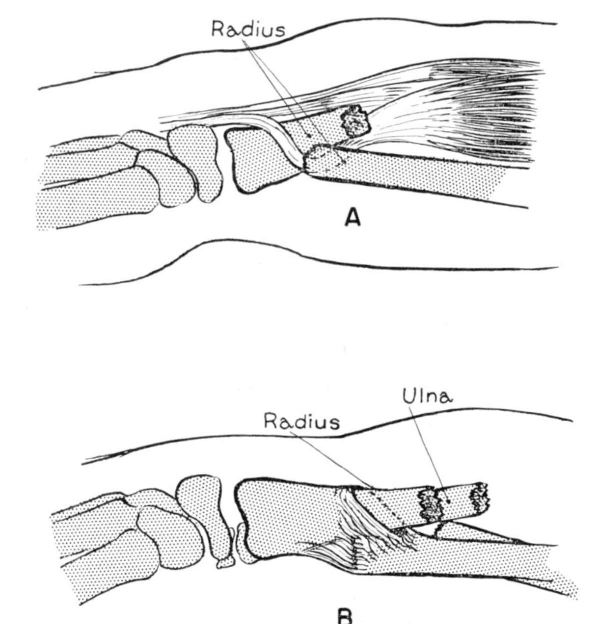

Figure 8–2. Complications of reduction.

A. Gross deformity in a fracture near the wrist may result in displacement of a flexor or extensor tendon to the wrong side of one of the fragments and prevent manipulative reduction.

B. The distal radial fragment has "buttonholed" its periosteum. Traction serves to tighten the grasp of the buttonhole on the projecting bone so that manipulative reduction cannot be accomplished.

injury and suffered the greater displacement, around which a flexor or extensor tendon becomes displaced to prevent reduction by any manipulative method (Fig. 8–2, *A*). Exploration and extrication of the interposed tendon must precede reduction.

Interposition of periosteum is not uncommon. When the bone snaps and the fragments displace, one fragment may pierce its periosteal sleeve through a veritable buttonhole (Fig. 8–2, *B*). Unless the adjacent periosteum is lacerated or widely stripped, this phenomenon can defy all attempts at manipulative reduction. Open reduction is required and the periosteal sleeve must be incised and released before the fragments can be reapproximated.

A toggle-joint fracture should be recognized in the first x-rays, approached with caution, and reduced by a special technique. Such a lesion

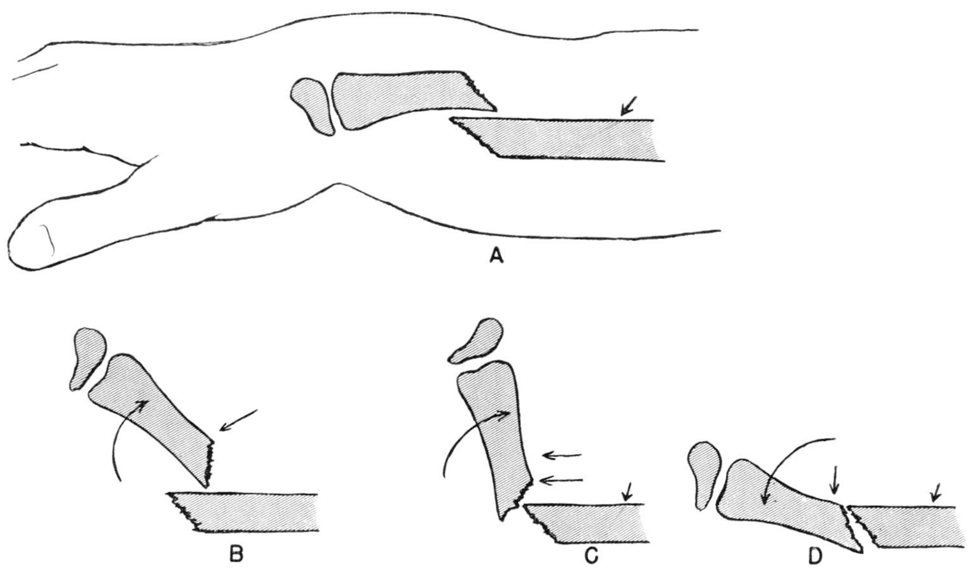

Figure 8–3. Reduction by toggle-joint maneuver.

Despite the optical illusion of shortening (A), the bone is of normal length. Reduction cannot be done by traction but requires (B) angulation and (C) pushing of the angulated fragment into end-on apposition to the other, followed by (D) correction of the angulation.

in one bone usually cannot be reduced by any manipulation when the other bone is intact. The fractured bone, despite an optical illusion of overriding, is actually about normal length (Fig. 8–3, *A*). Reduction by traction, which would require lengthening the bone the distance of the apparent overriding beyond its normal length, is impossible. Reduction by angulation is precluded by the intact other bone. Even when both bones are broken, reduction cannot be accomplished by traction. Successful reduction requires application of the carpenter's "toggle-joint" principle, as illustrated in Figure 8–3.

Greenstick fractures are common. One cortex breaks while the other remains essentially intact, only bent. The child's bone is resilient. The bend is easily straightened, but the bend recurs as soon as the corrective forces are removed. This recurrence of angulation is to be expected even within the best of plaster dressings (Fig. 8–4). When a greenstick fracture is sufficiently deformed to require reduction, *it should be made into a complete fracture* (Fig. 8–5). Until this is done, maintenance of correction remains an uncertainty. The intact cortex is cracked through by manual reversal of the angulation. This must be done carefully or the surgeon may produce a displaced, as well as a complete, fracture. Once the break is completed, correction of the angulation can be maintained by plaster dressings without fear of recurrence of the original deformity.

Many greenstick fractures need no reduction. An angular deformity

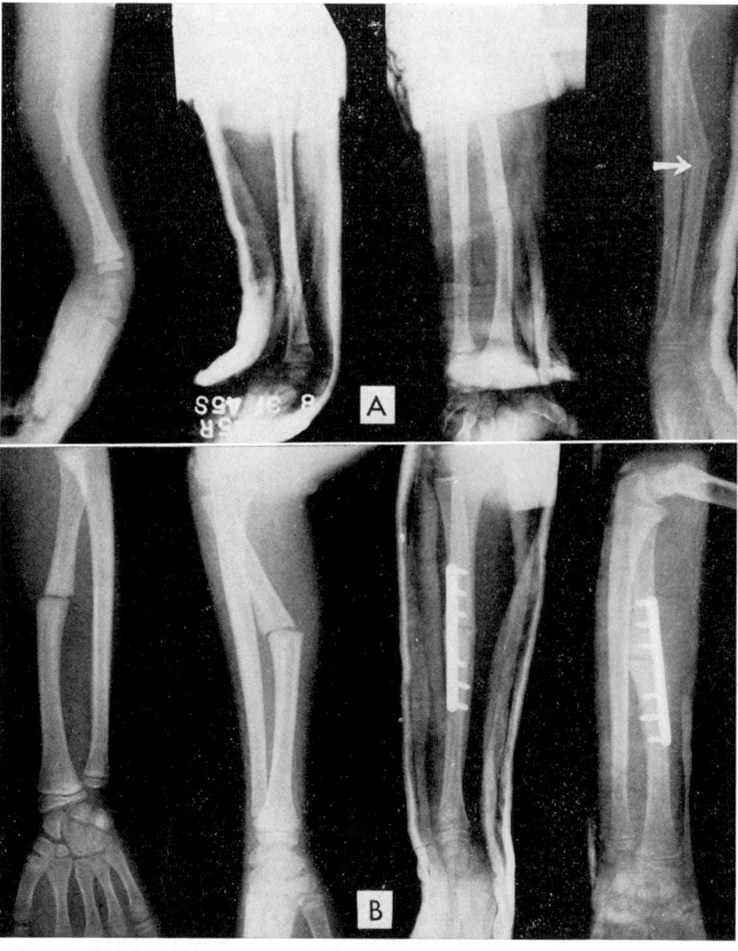

Figure 8–4. Greenstick fractures of radius and ulna.

A. The ulnar fracture was completed, the radius was merely straightened. The ulna healed perfectly; the radius healed with an angular deformity (arrow).

B. Three years later the angulated radius was accidentally refractured, which proved to be a fortunate circumstance. The angular deformity was corrected, and the eventual result was excellent.

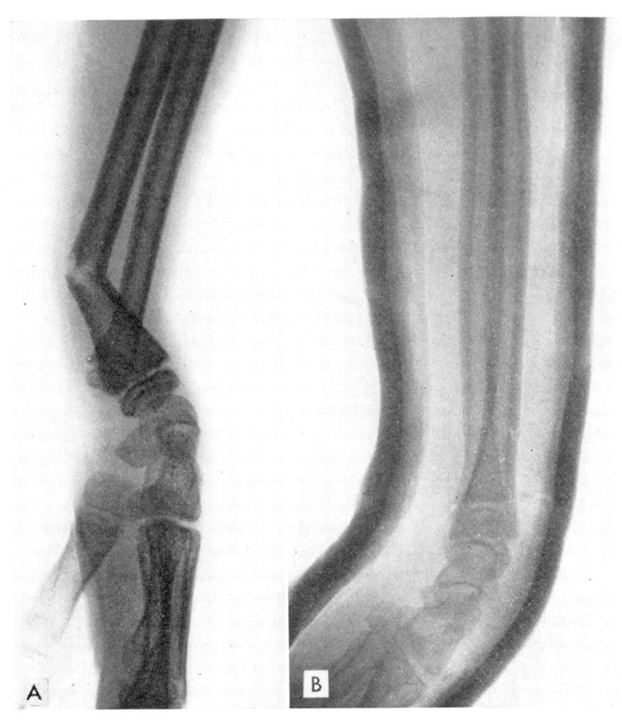

Figure 8–5. Greenstick fracture of the radius accompanied by a volar dislocation of the ulnar head—before (A) and after (B) manipulative completion and re-alignment of the fracture. The dislocated ulna reduced spontaneously and the ruptured inferior radio-ulnar ligaments healed soundly coincident with union of the fracture.

of 15 degrees or less, which accentuates the normal curve of the radius, produces no ill effects and needs no reduction, but the arm should be immobilized with the wrist in extension, lest the angulation increase. The opposite deformity, which flattens the radial curve, may interfere with rotation and should be corrected, except when the bone is angulated less than 10 degrees, or the injury is in a very young child. Under such circumstances the wrist should be immobilized in flexion.

Immobilization

It must be accepted that any immobilization applied to the extremity of a child will be subjected to continuously repeated insults throughout a period commencing a few days after application until it is removed. Splints must be designed to accept this abuse. The danger of late joint stiffness or of prolonged muscle atrophy and disability is absent. Plaster dressings more extensive than are required for management of the fracture alone are often advisable in the unruly child.

A circular plaster dressing has the advantages of strength and resistance to abuse and needs much less supervision than molded plaster splints which are bandaged in place. During the early stages following reduction, progressive swelling presents a real hazard if the limb is encased in a circular dressing. Frequent inspections to confirm a continuing intact circulation are mandatory. The parents must be warned against the cold white or blue hand, the loss of power to move the fingers, and the onset of unremitting pain; they should be instructed to examine for these signs of circulatory embarrassment every few hours throughout the first week. When swelling recedes a circular dressing becomes loose and presents a second danger, loss of reduction due to imperfect fixation. Proper utilization of circular plaster dressings, therefore, demands close and frequent inspection in the early stages after reduction, and removal and reapplication of new well-fitting dressings at appropriate intervals as swelling subsides or atrophy occurs. Care must be taken that the reduction is not lost at the time the plaster dressing is changed.

Molded plaster splints, which are bandaged to the limb, are weaker and less resistant to abuse than is circular plaster, but have the advantages that rebandaging permits reduction or increase of their compression of the limb without danger to the reduction, as the early swelling increases and later subsides. They must be inspected frequently throughout the entire period of use, or the bandages may loosen and the splints become ineffective.

The optimal immobilization program commences with the application of molded splints at the time of reduction. Appropriate tension is maintained by rebandaging throughout the period of increasing and subsiding swelling. When all swelling has subsided the final rebandaging is done with plaster instead of gauze bandages, making the dressing into a well-fitting circular encasement which usually will remain comfortable and efficient until union occurs. Only by some such program can integrity of the circulation be protected without risk of losing the reduction.

The extent of immobilization depends on the level of the fracture. In a small forearm containing a single fracture within 2 inches of the wrist, a secure grasp of both proximal and distal fragments is obtained by plaster dressings. Minor fractures in this region are adequately controlled by a "sugar tongs" splint (Fig. 8–6, *A, B*), which prevents rotation but merely reduces flexion and extension of the elbow. In all other forearm fractures, both the wrist and elbow should be securely immobilized by dressings which extend from the palmar flexion crease to the upper arm. Splints molded to the anterior and posterior surfaces of the limb are comfortable and efficient, and easily changed into a circular encasement by substitution of plaster for gauze bandages (Fig. 8–6, *C, D*).

The duration of immobilization is of special importance. Refracture through the region of the healed fracture is one of the more common late complications of forearm fractures in children. The responsibility for refracture within three months of the original injury rests squarely upon the surgeon, who should realize that, despite plentiful callus formation in the second month, considerable time must elapse before this new bone seasons

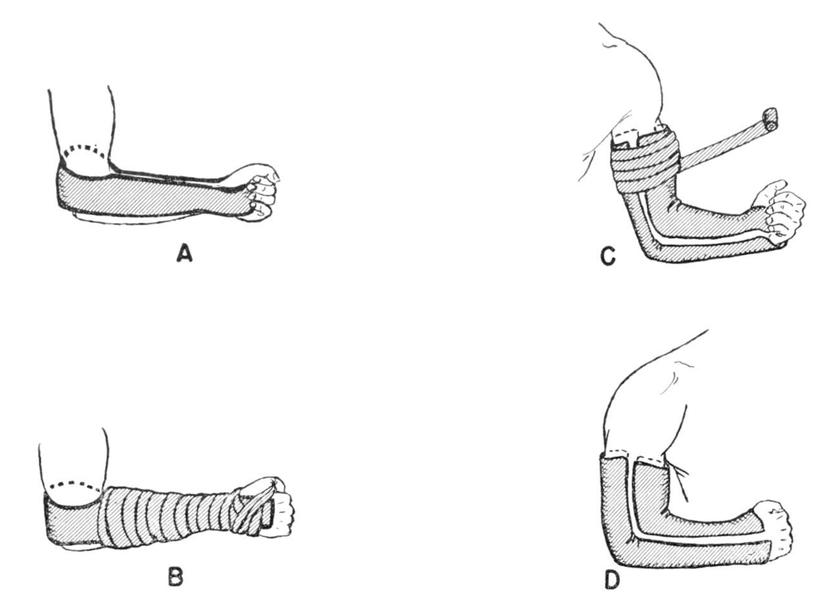

Figure 8–6.

A, B. Molded "sugar tongs" splint extending from the knuckles on the dorsum of the hand around the elbow, to end at the flexion crease in the palm: A, palmar view without bandages, and B, bandaged in place. The edges of the splint should be closely approximated on the radial aspect of the forearm.

C. Anterior and posterior molded splints—forearm supinated.

D. Anterior and posterior molded splints—forearm in neutral rotation.

and becomes strong and tough. He should also realize that, as soon as plaster splints are removed from a child, full strenuous activities and repeated traumas to the limb will follow very rapidly. Fractures through the shafts of both radius and ulna, therefore, should be immobilized at least two months and receive some protection for an additional month. Protection may take the form of supervision of activities, but this is often difficult to enforce. A useful device is a small molded splint which acts more as a constant reminder to the child than as a mechanical support to the healed but weak fracture site. It is appropriate to generalize that forearm fractures in the child require immobilization until united, and continued protection for about half as long again following union.

Refracture of Forearm Bones

Refracture through soft callus less than three months old has been discussed. Late refracture not uncommonly occurs, long after the original lesions are soundly healed (Fig. 8–7, *A;* see also Fig. 8–4, *B*). The child's bone is resilient, except at the site of a healed fracture. Here the shaft becomes thickened by callus, which roentgenographically appears to be the strongest segment but actually is brittle and inelastic by comparison with

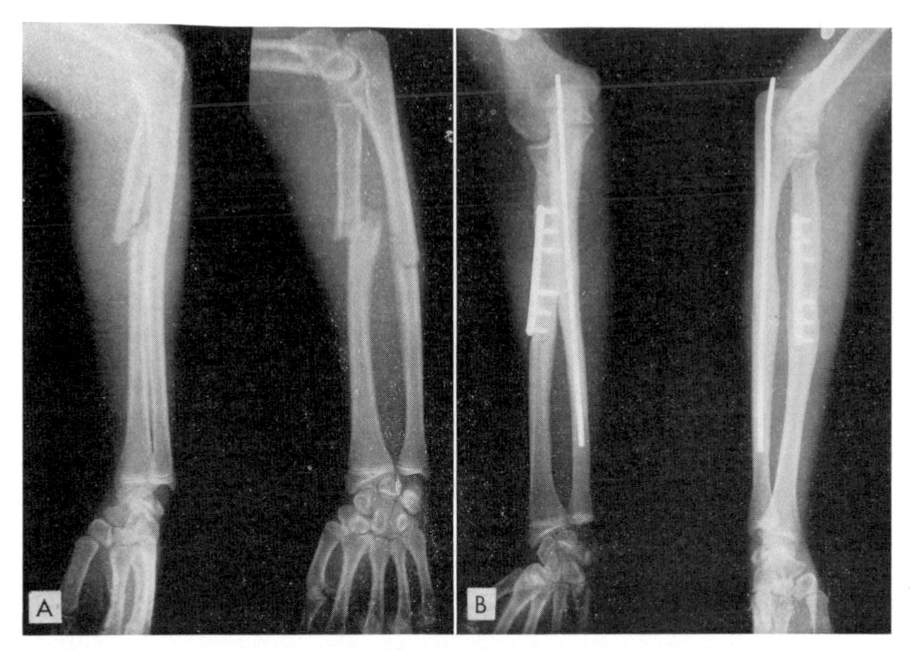

Figure 8–7. Fracture of shafts of radius and ulna.

A. Refracture three months after original injury. Note the bulbous mass of callus through which the radius fractured, and the small intermediate bone fragment which became wedged between the main fragments of radius to prevent successful manipulative reduction. Obliquity of the ulna fracture and loss of substance from the radial fracture created instability of the reduction, necessitating internal fixation. Complete epiphyseal fusion at the elbow allowed the use of an intramedullary rod for fixation of the ulna.

B. Roentgenograms showing results nine months later.

the rest of the bone. The remainder of the bone bends and the brittle segment snaps, in response to an adequate injury. As a general rule, refractures, both early and late, have a very much prolonged healing time in comparison with the original fracture.

Operative Treatment

Necessity, due to a failure to obtain or maintain adequate reduction, is the only justification of open reduction of a fractured forearm in a child. Comminution, loss of substance, and occasional obliquity of the fracture line are the only justifications for using internal fixation. These circumstances occur only rarely. The fracture line is usually fairly transverse and, when the fragments are reapproximated, maintenance of reduction by external dressings almost always proves secure. On the rare occasions when comminution, loss of substance, or an oblique fracture line prevents maintenance of reduction by external splints, the smallest amount of internal fixation compatible with maintenance of reduction should be inserted, and then supplemented by external immobilization. The presence of an epiphysis at either end of the child's bone contraindicates the use of intramedullary devices. If it proves necessary to use a plate as well as screws, the plate should be narrow and small and should be removed after the fracture is soundly united. To leave a plate in place is an invitation to refracture. The bone segment supported by the plate is stiffened and the remainder of the bone resilient. Late refracture at one end of this surgically stiffened segment is a constant potential danger.

FRACTURE OF SHAFTS OF RADIUS AND ULNA IN ADULTS

These are always complete and should be so treated even when they appear incomplete in the x-ray films. The problem they present is as difficult as that presented by their equivalents in the child is simple. Adult bones are no longer resilient and often shatter instead of breaking cleanly. Separate small intermediate fragments are frequently present. The resultant instability militates against the success of manipulative reduction and external immobilization. The fragments are subjected to the cross pull of strong rotator muscles, which often makes fixation difficult or impossible by any external immobilizing device. The time required for union must be measured in months instead of weeks. Delayed union is the rule, and fibrous union is common. The social and economic penalties attending prolonged disability in a productive adult are serious. Atrophy and joint stiffness are inevitable penalties of external immobilization and vary only in degree and duration. Some permanent defect is common.

Fracture of Lower Third of Shaft of Radius

This lesion is a pitfall for the unwary surgeon. It looks simple; the bone is broken cleanly, and usually in a short oblique line; and the deformity seems slight. The distal and often both fragment ends deviate toward the ulna. The temptation is to immobilize the limb after a mere gesture at reduction of this apparently insignificant deformity. The result is delayed union and eventual malunion, attended by serious permanent disability. Even when the significance of the deformity is appreciated, reduction accomplished, and immobilization carried out in strong ulnar deviation accompanied by continuous thumb traction in an attempt to maintain alignment of the radius, the results are uncertain. When the offending muscle forces are considered (Fig. 8–8, *A*), it is at once apparent that no form of external fixation can efficiently counteract them. In addition, the time often required for sound union (between 20 and 25 weeks in the last three patients treated with external immobilization by the writer) creates social and economic problems out of proportion to such a lesion, which responds so well to other methods of treatment. Open reduction and internal fixation is the treatment of choice. The internal fixation should eliminate or minimize the need for external immobilization,

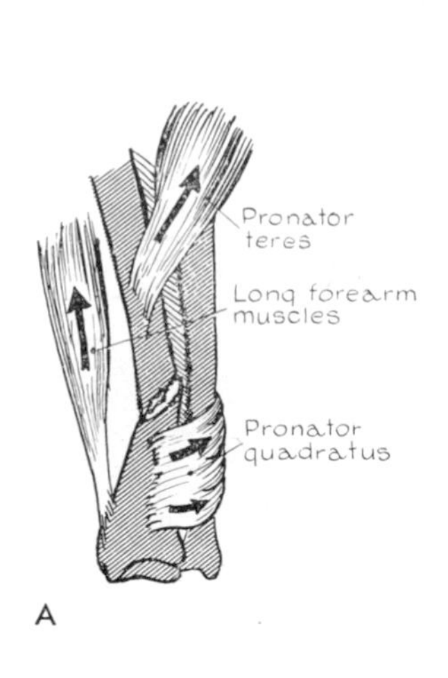

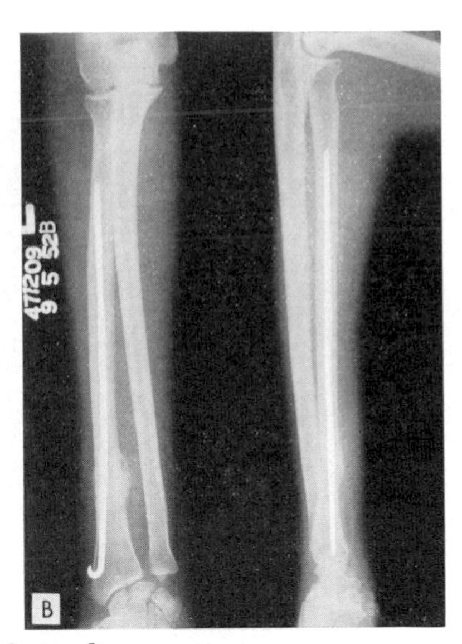

Figure 8–8. Fracture of lower third of radius.

A. Drawing showing muscle forces acting to displace segments after fracture of lower third of the shaft of the radius. These cannot be completely controlled by any form of external fixation.

B. Fracture of lower third of radius two months after open reduction and fixation by a Rush nail. Hospital stay 7 days. No external immobilization after operation. Patient returned to work as a laundress 3 weeks after operation. The result was excellent. The external callus represents consolidated "milled" bone grafts packed around the reduced fracture.

and use of bone grafts at the time of primary open reduction hastens sound union (Fig. 8–8, *B*).

Subluxation at the inferior radio-ulnar joint often accompanies a fracture through the lower half of the radial shaft, but actual dislocation occurs less frequently (see Fig. 8–5). Displacement results from stretching or disruption of the inferior radio-ulnar ligaments, replaces spontaneously with reduction of the radial fragments, and rarely requires any treatment in addition to that accorded the fracture.

Fracture of Upper Third of Shaft of Radius

This lesion is most frequently encountered in adolescents, but may also occur in adults. In young bones the fracture usually is somewhat of the greenstick type, angulated with apex volar and ulnarward, difficult to reduce, and more difficult to hold, and may require open reduction and internal fixation. Operative treatment is also commonly required in the adult for the same reasons. Here the fracture is always complete. The short proximal fragment buried under muscle bellies remains flexed and supinated and uncontrollable (see Fig. 8–*1*, *A*). When the distal fragment cannot be satisfactorily replaced, operative reduction and fixation should

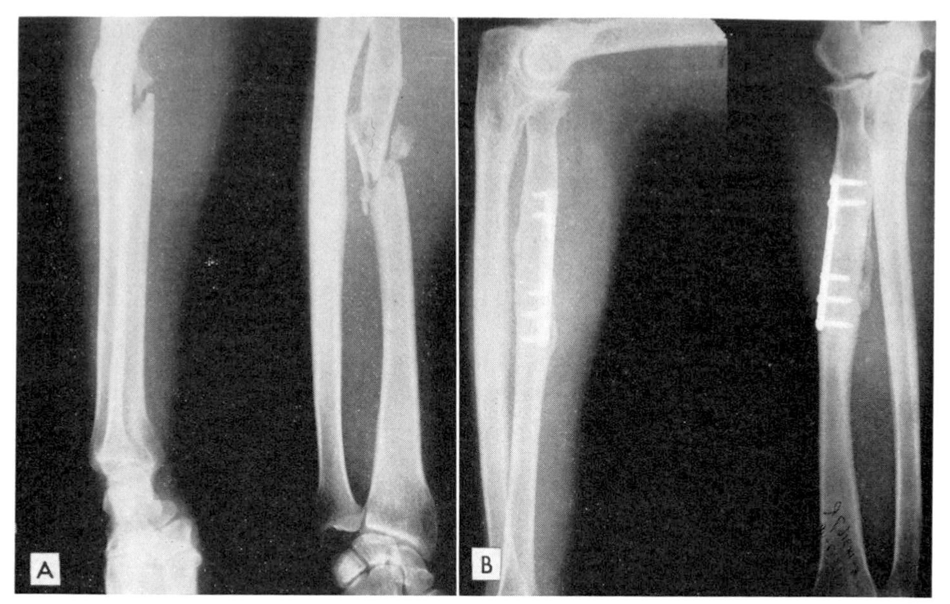

Figure 8–9. Fracture of upper third of radius.

A. Fracture of upper third of shaft of radius and avulsion of ulnar styloid. Open reduction in this type of lesion is mandatory to a good result. Comminution precluded rigid internal fixation.

B. A plate and screws were inserted to maintain length, axis, and rotation—supplemental external splints were needed.

be done. Care is required lest the dorsal interosseous nerve be injured in the course of exposing the fracture. Intramedullary fixation is contraindicated because it does not control rotation of the short proximal fragment. A small plate fastened by screws to the reassembled fragments provides optimal fixation (Fig. 8–*9;* see also Fig. 8–*4, B*).

Fracture of Shaft of Ulna

This fracture may occur without an associated dislocation of the head of the radius as a result of direct trauma. The deformity is consistent, and the presence of an intermediate small fragment is not uncommon. Muscle forces angulate the fragments toward the radius to produce displacement that may prove uncontrollable by any external dressing (Fig. 8–*10*). Bony union is apt to be delayed, and fibrous union may occur despite the extent or duration of immobilization. The treatment of choice for unstable lesions showing a tendency for recurrent angulation is open reduction and internal fixation by some intramedullary device.

Isolated fractures of the ulna in the middle or distal portions of the shaft remain more in balance than proximal lesions. Reduction usually can be maintained by a plaster dressing which immobilizes both wrist and elbow, but immobilization should be continued until strong union is present.

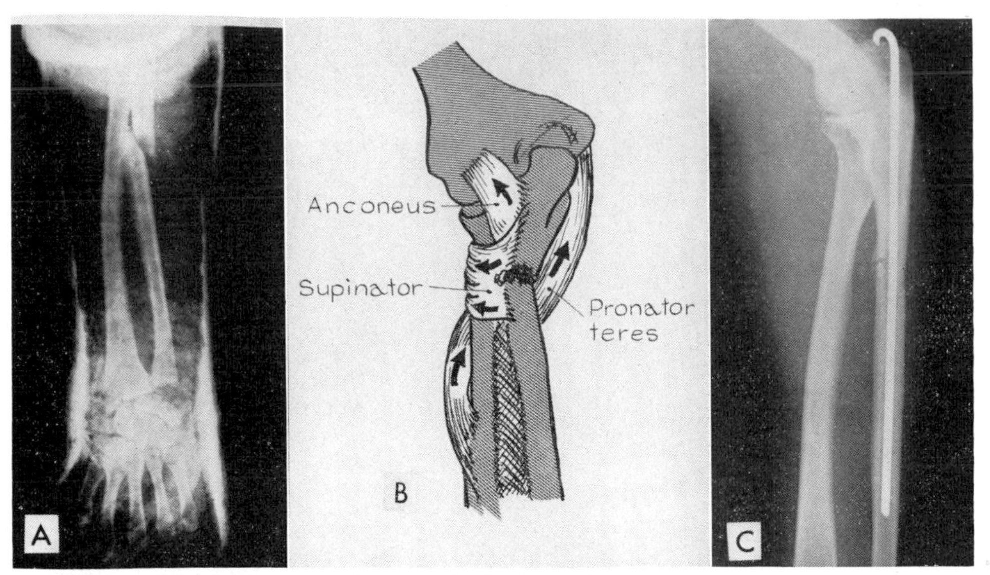

Figure 8–10. Fracture of upper third of the ulna.

A. Roentgenogram showing fracture, which could not be satisfactorily held in position by external immobilization.

B. Drawing showing muscle forces acting upon the fragments in such fractures and sometimes preventing maintenance of reduction.

C. Roentgenogram after open reduction. No supplemental external splints were used. Light use was resumed as soon as the operative incision healed.

Fracture of Shafts of Radius and Ulna

Treatment of fractures of the shafts of radius and ulna must be governed by the level of the fracture in the radius, and the stability of the reduction obtained. Unstable fractures at any level require open reduction and internal fixation, if consistently good results are to be obtained (Fig. 8–*11*). Intramedullary fixation is simple and efficient for maintaining ulnar alignment and apposition, but a plate is required for control of rotatory forces acting on the radial fragments (Fig. 8–7). Plates may be used for fixation of both bones, provided they are of appropriate narrow width (Figs. 8–*11*, 8–*12*). Fixation of only one bone invariably produces inferior results. Provision of fixation for both bones through separate incisions incurs no extra risk and has many advantages. The more rigid and secure the internal fixation, the less extensive and prolonged will be the supplemental external immobilization required. This is of considerable import to the wage earner, whose incapacity depends upon the period during which function of the limb is obliterated by plaster splints. The principle of "internal suture" by fixation with a single screw, etc., and dependence upon external splints to maintain reduction throughout the healing period, is wrong and accepts all the risks of operation without reaping its advantages, except when rigid internal fixation cannot be obtained.

Simple fractures of the forearm bones without undue displacement may do very well following manipulative reduction and immobilization, but

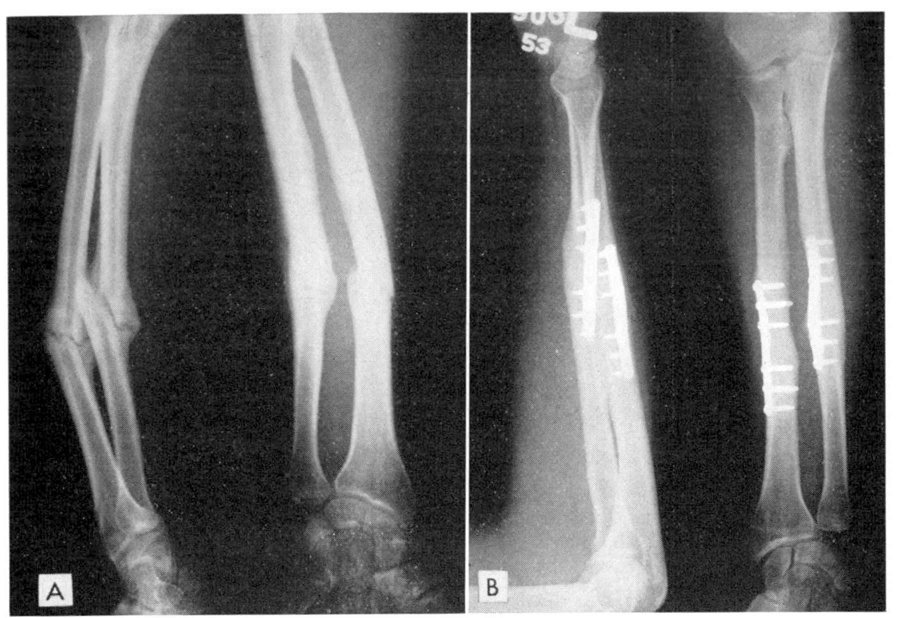

Figure 8–11. Fracture of shafts of radius and ulna.

A. A common end-result of attempting to control an unstable fracture of both forearm bones by external immobilization following manipulative reduction. In addition to the angulation, a gross rotation deformity is present.

B. Late osteotomy re-alignment and internal fixation of the fragments is required before the limb regains usefulness.

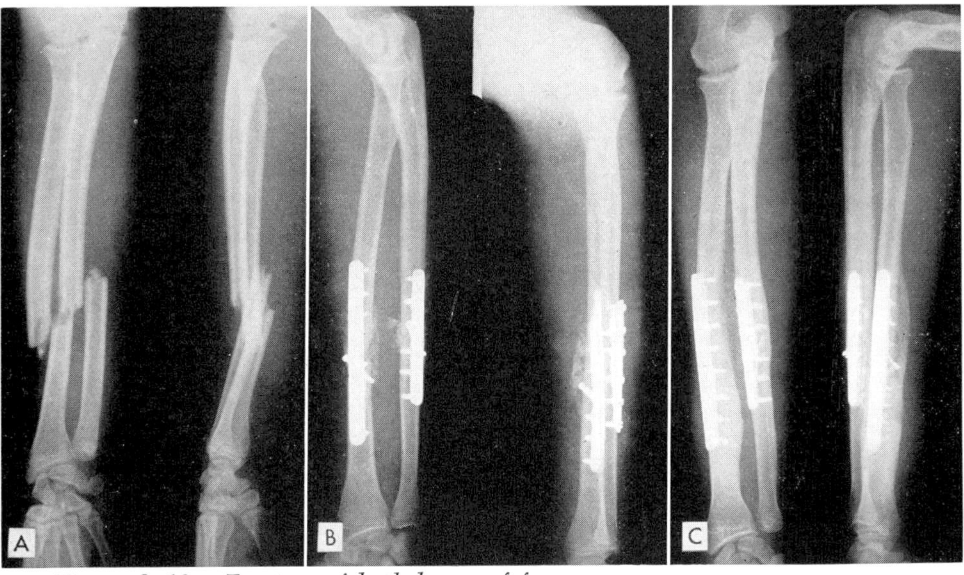

Figure 8–12. Fracture of both bones of forearm.

Both fractures are comminuted. The intermediate fragment of radius became wedged in the fracture site to prevent manipulative reduction. Open reduction, packing of milled bone grafts around each fracture, and rigid fixation by plates and transfixion screws. The result was good.

A. Original deformity.

B. Immediately after operation–note the milled bone around the fractures.

C. Results 2 months after operation.

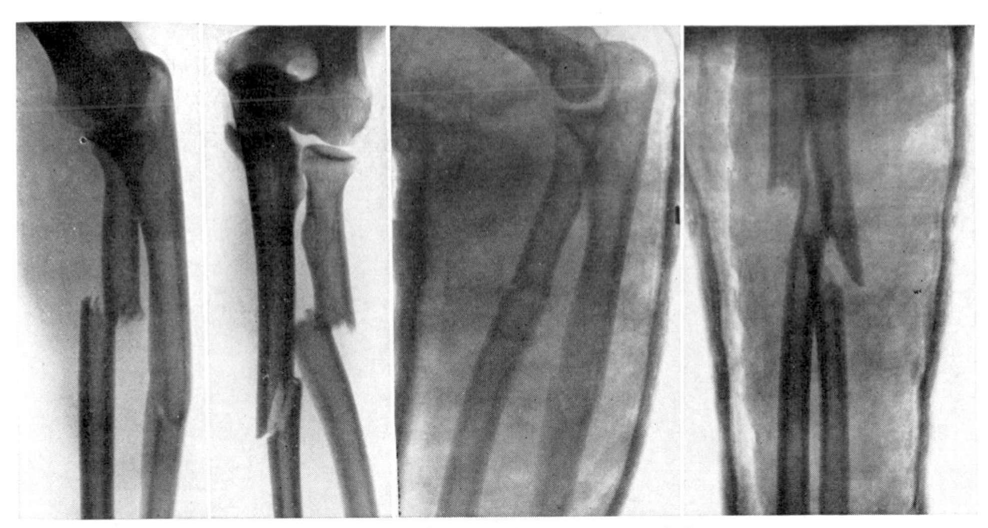

Figure 8–13. Fracture of both bones of forearm in adult.

An apparently perfect reduction was obtained in the lateral view. The anteroposterior film, however, reveals a totally unsatisfactory position of the fragments. The necessity for open reduction and internal fixation is obvious.

the great majority are unstable, defy adequate manipulative reduction, or redisplace within the best of plaster splints, due to the cross-pull of strong rotator muscles (Fig. 8–*13*). One attempt at manipulative reduction and immobilization from hand to upper arm with the forearm supinated or in midposition, depending upon the level of the fracture in the radius, is warranted. Comminution, obliquity of the fracture, inadequate reduction, or the first evidence of redisplacement in plaster constitutes an indication for open reduction and internal fixation.

FRACTURE OF SHAFT OF ULNA WITH DISLOCATION OF RADIAL HEAD

Monteggia in 1814 first described a fracture of the shaft of the ulna associated with an anterior dislocation of the head of the radius. This lesion is prone to many complications and is followed by a high percentage of poor results. Few of these are unavoidable. Almost all result from a failure to recognize the dislocation of the radial head or its implications. An *angulated* fracture of the shaft of the ulna is seldom an isolated lesion, for before gross angulation is possible the over-all length of the bone must decrease. Shortening cannot occur if the radius and radio-ulnar soft-part connections remain intact. All angulated fractures of the proximal half of the ulna should be considered to be accompanied by a dislocation of the radial head until it is proved otherwise.

Pathology of Orbicular Ligament

The radial head may dislocate forward or outward through a disrupted orbicular ligament, depending on the direction of ulnar angulation, but

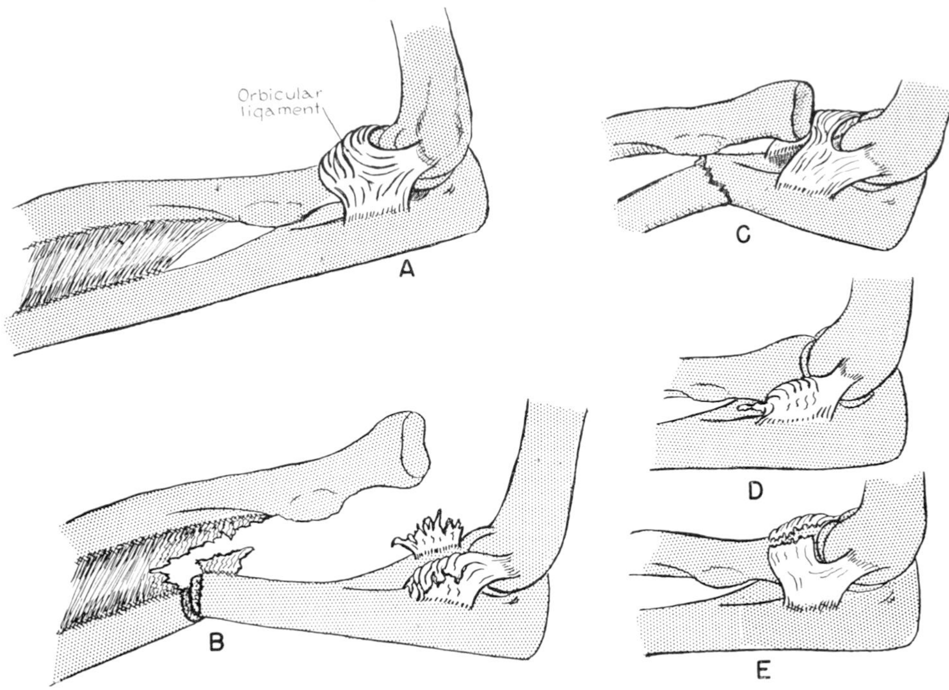

Figure 8–14. Variations in pathology of orbicular ligament in Monteggia fracture.
A. Normal appearance.
B. The radial head may disrupt, or
C. It may pull out from under the orbicular ligament.
D. The radial head may replace on top, or
E. It may replace within the orbicular ligament.

dislocation may also occur and the ligament be left essentially intact in continuity (Fig. 8–*14*). Under the latter circumstances, operative incision of the ligament, replacement of the radius, and ligament repair are mandatory to a good result. A disrupted ligament may remain open ready to receive the radial head when it is reduced, or it may collapse to become interposed between the ulna and the radius (Fig. 8–*14*). The former presages a good result, and the latter, a permanent disability.

Diagnosis

An angulated fracture of the ulnar shaft unaccompanied by a fracture of the radius justifies a presumptive diagnosis of Monteggia fracture, and some evidence of this is almost always present in the x-ray film. A line drawn through the long axis of an undislocated radius passes through the exact center of the capitellum or its epiphysis, regardless of the position of the elbow or the projection of the film. The least deviation from this alignment in the presence of an ulnar fracture is pathognomonic of orbicular ligament disruption. Pain, tenderness, swelling, and the frequent incidence of little or no clinical displacement of the radius make physical examination of little help in an early case. The status of the dorsal interos-

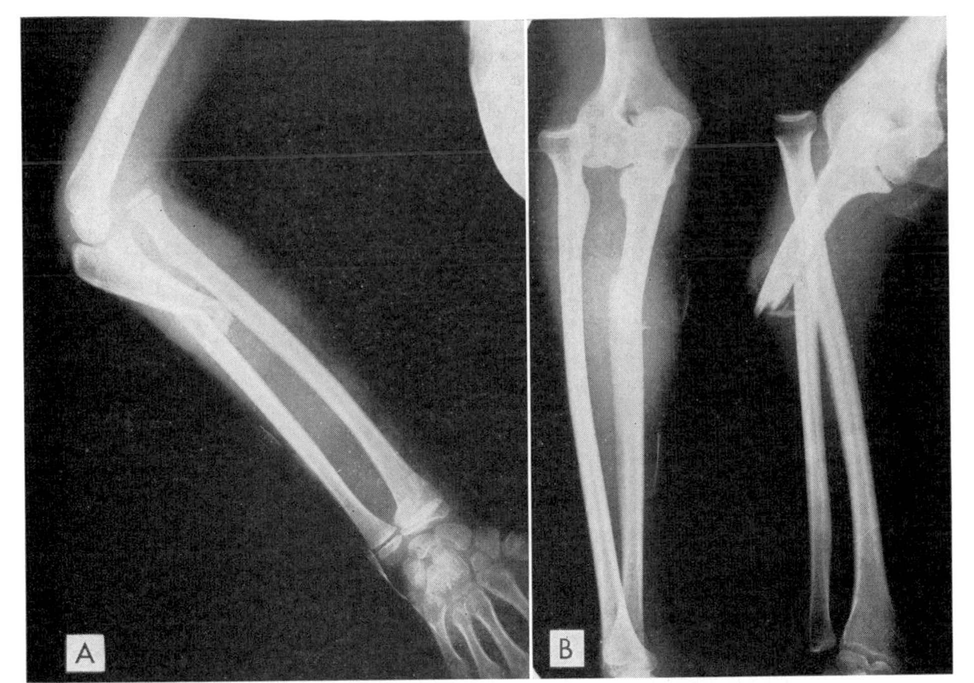

Figure 8–15. Displacement of the radius in Monteggia fractures. Consider the traction exerted upon the dorsal interosseous branch of the radial nerve which winds around the neck of the radius. A. Anterior displacement. B. Lateral displacement.

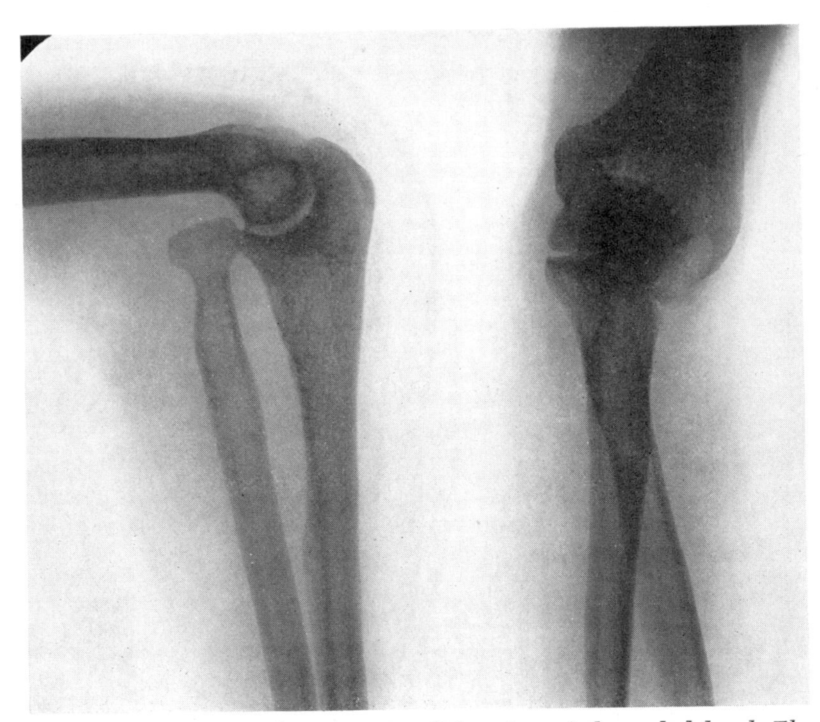

Figure 8–16. Long-standing anterior dislocation of the radial head. The anteroposterior film with the elbow in extension shows the head of the radius pulled medialward to lie in front of the ulna in the antecubital fossa.

seous nerve should always be checked, since it is carried into a displaced position with the radius and damaged by traction in more than 25 per cent of these lesions (Fig. 8–*15*). Clinical identification of a long-standing radial head dislocation is made by extending the elbow, upon which the radial head displaces forward to become palpable in the antecubital region (Fig. 8–*16*).

Treatment

Manipulative reduction and immobilization in plaster dressings is successful only in lesions with a stable fracture of the ulna and a ligament which is not interposed between the ulna and the reduced radial head. The elbow is extended, the length of the ulna is restored by steady traction, and the fragments are manipulated into apposition. Firm pressure is then made both on the apex of the ulnar angulation and on the radial head. When the latter has been pushed deeply into place against the ulna the elbow is flexed to 90 degrees and supinated. The ulnar reduction is maintained, and the elbow is then gently extended. If the orbicular ligament is interposed between the bones, redislocation of the radius occurs at once. If not, the radial head usually remains reduced, and immobilization extending from hand to upper arm with the elbow supinated and at right angles is justified. Only a perfect reduction will remain secure. X-rays should be taken at weekly intervals, and any recurrence of displacement of either the fractured ulna or the radial head is the forerunner of eventual failure of this method of treatment.

Operative treatment, when technically adequate and carried out early under appropriate auspices, produces consistently good and certain results. Exposure of both lesions through a single dorsolateral approach is contraindicated in recent injuries by the risk of excessive bone production in the interosseous space. Open reduction and internal fixation of the ulna through a dorsal approach and repair of the orbicular ligament over the replaced radius through an antecubital approach has proved to be a safe and efficient procedure. Internal fixation of the ulna should precede the ligament repair. Following operation the limb should be supported by plaster splints for six to eight weeks, until both fractured bone and ligament are well healed. The results are excellent. Complications which occur are the result of faulty technique. In 16 consecutive early lesions treated by this method the complications of myositis ossificans, radio-ulnar synostosis, nonunion, and infection have not occurred. In 9 of these cases operation followed failure of manipulative reduction or redisplacement following reduction. At operation in 10 cases an intact ligament with the radial head pulled out from beneath it or a torn ligament interposed between the radius and the lesser sigmoid notch of the ulna was found. During the same period only 9 patients progressed satisfactorily following manipulative reduction and plaster immobilization. These patients had a stable fracture of the ulna and a radial head that reduced completely and remained in place. The surgeon who elects to accept an imperfect reduction or a small recurrence of deformity following reduction should realize that he is accepting a permanent disability which can be prevented.

Old unreduced Monteggia fractures (Fig. 8–*16*) create disability by impingement of the radial head against the humerus. Excision of the head of the radius is the simplest and best treatment for this lesion in the adult, but should not be done in a child. To remove the radial head prior to epiphyseal closure almost invariably produces a subsequent derangement of the inferior radio-ulnar joint. In the child the procedure of choice is reconstruction by realignment of the malunited ulna, reduction of the displaced radial head, and repair or replacement of the orbicular ligament (Fig. 8–*17*). The results are good when this procedure is carried out before the shape of the dislocated radial head becomes distorted by growth.

"***Reverse Monteggia fracture,***" as fracture of the proximal ulna with posterior dislocation and fracture of the radial head is often called, is a separate entity which bears none of the stigmata of a Monteggia fracture. The orbicular ligament is rarely disrupted, and there is little or no risk of its interposition between radius and ulna. The radial head usually is frac-

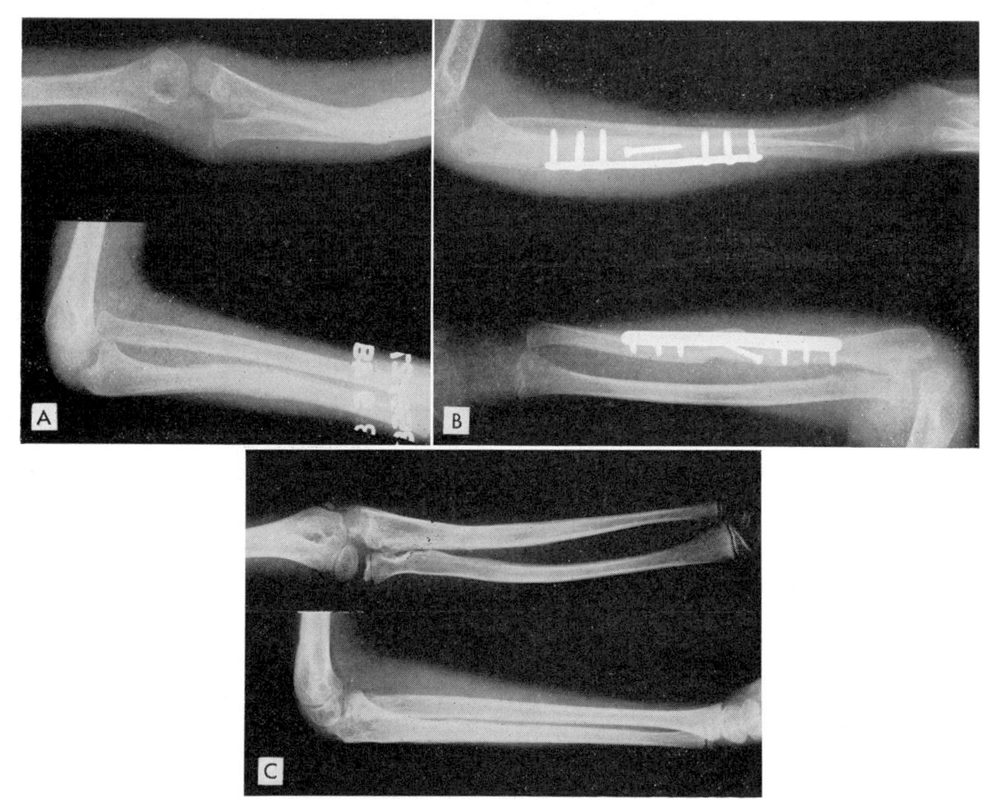

Figure 8–17. Unreduced Monteggia fracture (originally treated as a simple fracture of the ulna) in a child.

A. Six months after injury.

B. Three months after osteotomy and re-alignment of the ulna, replacement of the radial head, and repair of the orbicular ligament.

C. The result three years after operation. The limb is nearly normal.

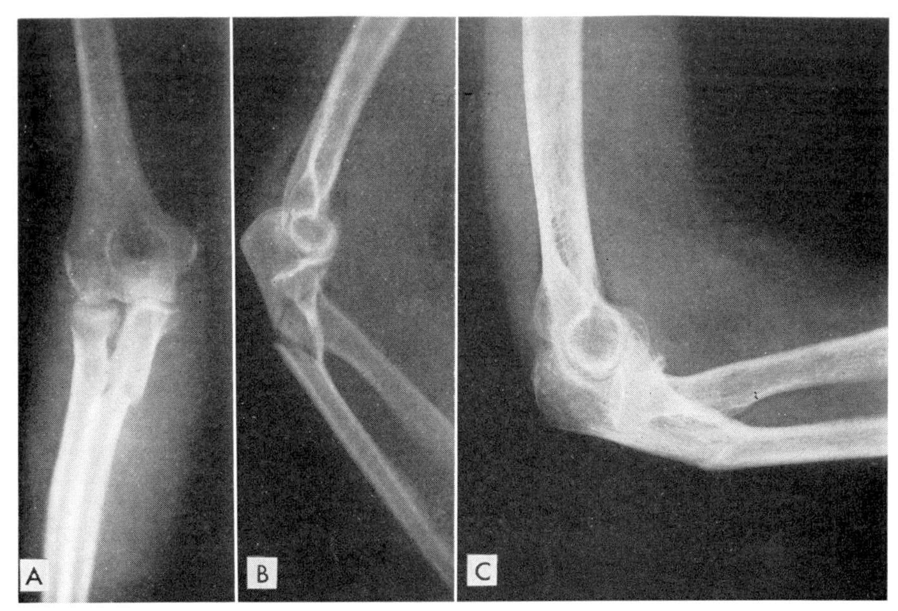

Figure 8–18. Fracture of proximal ulna with posterior dislocation and fracture of the radial head, which was reduced and immobilized with the elbow in flexion.

A, B. Films showing fracture.

C. The result after treatment. The deformity recurred and a permanent defect ensued.

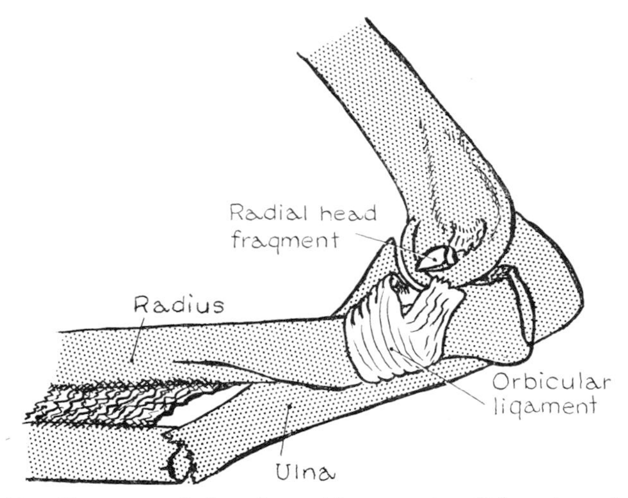

Figure 8–19. Fracture of the ulna with posterior dislocation of the radial head (a) *rarely disrupts the orbicular ligament;* (b) *usually fractures the radial head and lacerates the articular cartilage of the capitellum;* (c) *inflicts relatively little damage to the interosseous soft parts or the dorsal interosseous nerve.*

tured by impact against the capitellum (Figs. 8–*18*, 8–*19*). Correction of the angulation of the ulna, accompanied by traction with the elbow extended, results in spontaneous reduction of the dislocated radial head. Immobilization should be done with the elbow in full extension; flexion may result in early recurrence of the original deformity. An unstable frac-

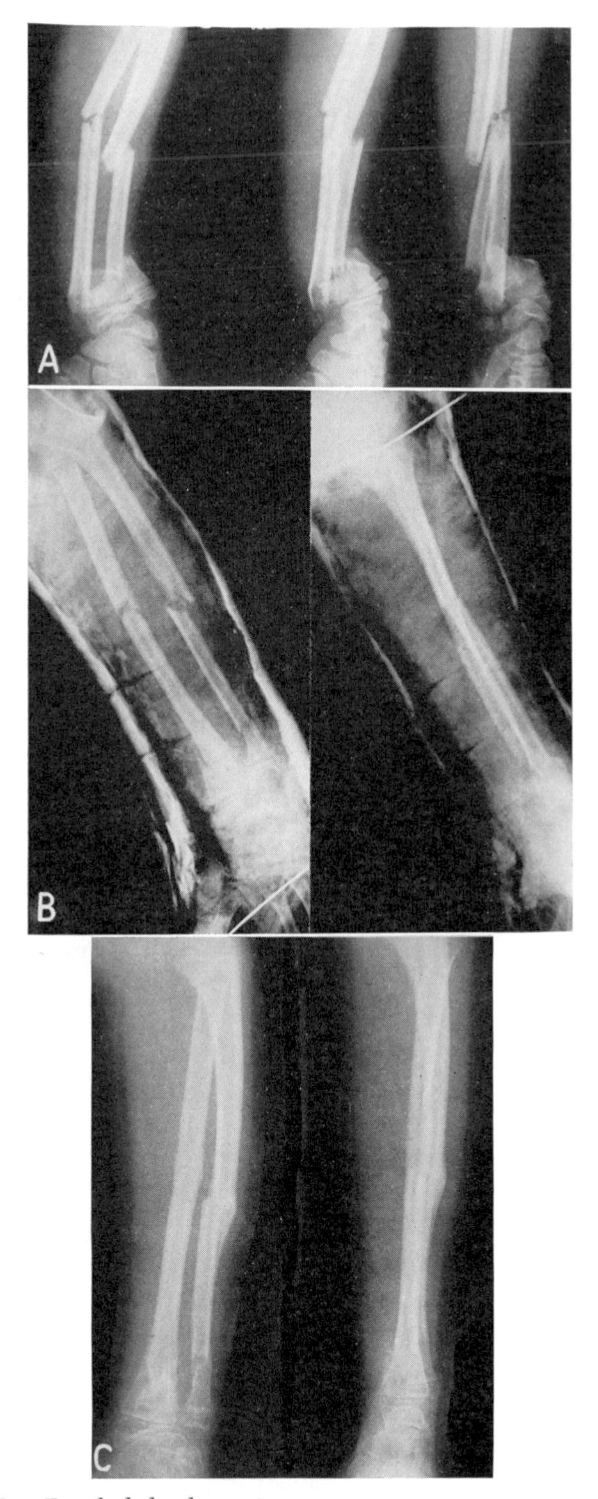

Figure 8–20. Fixed skeletal traction.

A. A severe open injury.

B. The wound was excised and reduction maintained by incorporation of traction pins in the immobilizing plaster dressing.

C. The result eight months after injury.

ture in the ulna or a large fracture of the radial head may require open reduction and internal fixation of the ulna and excision of the radial head. When this is done through a single approach use of an intramedullary device is the fixation method of choice, since the exposure necessary to the application of a plate to the upper ulna and the excision of the radial head carries some risk of excessive bone formation and radio-ulnar synostosis.

SUBLUXATION OF RADIAL HEAD

This fairly common lesion usually is incurred when an adult who is walking with a small child takes the infant's hand and attempts to lift him up to a step or over an obstacle. The child cries and refuses to move the limb. The parents are terrified. Sudden passive supination of the child's forearm invariably results in an astonishingly rapid and permanent relief of all symptoms. Use of the limb is resumed almost immediately, and no ill-effects of any kind are to be feared. The exact pathology is doubtful. The consistency of cause and cure indicates the most probable cause of symptoms to be a subluxation of the radial head from the sigmoid notch of the ulna.

MULTIPLE AND COMMINUTED FOREARM FRACTURES

Certain multiple or comminuted forearm fractures cannot be reduced satisfactorily by manipulation alone, nor can redisplacement and collapse be prevented by plaster dressings alone. When open reduction and internal fixation is contraindicated, these lesions can be managed efficiently by fixed skeletal traction pins applied through the olecranon and the bases (never the shafts or necks) of the metacarpals. After reduction, the pins are incorporated into a circular plaster dressing (Fig. 8–*20*). The pins should remain in place until healing is sufficient to prevent collapse when supported by plaster alone. Following their removal, the subsequent treatment until sound union is obtained is by plaster dressings alone.

CHAPTER 9

INJURIES OF THE ELBOW

By HARRISON L. McLAUGHLIN, M.D.
and BARBARA B. STIMSON, M.D.

ANATOMICAL CONSIDERATIONS

THE ELBOW JOINT is made up of three articulations contained within a single capsule. The ulnohumeral joint provides flexion and extension which is stabilized in all positions by the collateral ligaments whose humeral attachments correspond to the pivot of this hinge motion (Fig. 9–*1*). The radial head rests against the capitellum and the lesser sigmoid cavity of the ulna. The orbicular ligament, which holds the upper end of the radius in position, blends with the external collateral ligament, the elbow capsule, and the periosteal envelope enclosing the radial shaft (Fig. 9–*1*). Consequently the head of the radius may be removed without significant depreciation of total elbow function, provided the stump remains within the orbicular ligament.

The anterior capsule of the joint is supported by thin ligaments to

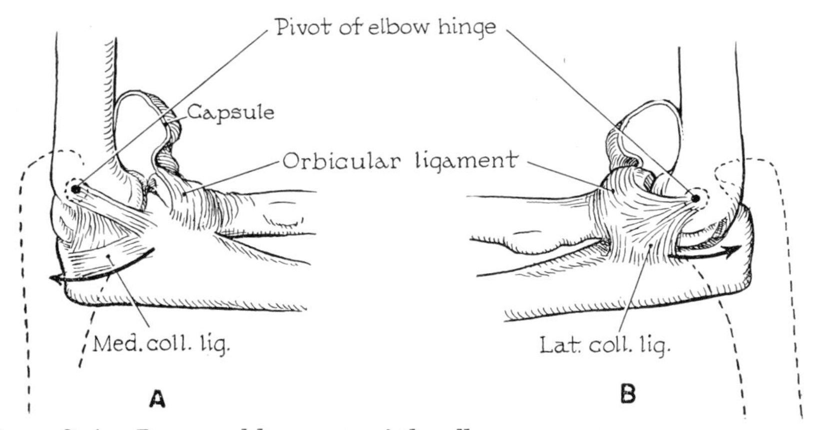

Figure 9–1. Bones and ligaments of the elbow.

Both the medial and lateral collateral ligaments attach to the humerus at the pivot of flexion and extension so that the joint is stabilized in all positions.

A. Mesial aspect of left elbow, showing medial collateral ligament.

B. Lateral aspect of left elbow, showing lateral collateral ligament.

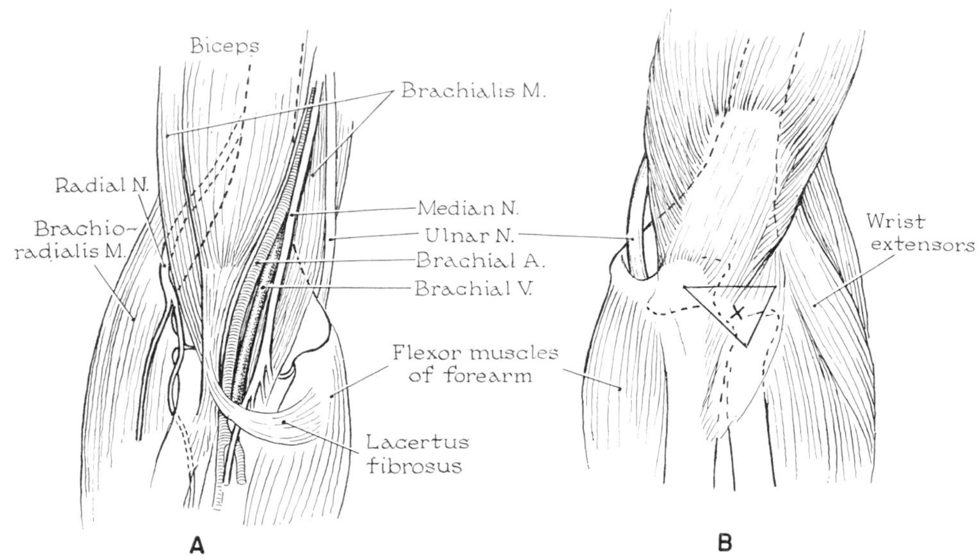

Figure 9–2. Soft parts of the elbow.
A. Normal structures of antecubital region.
B. Soft tissue structures covering back of the elbow. The center of a triangle (X) formed by the palpable prominences of the olecranon, radial head, and lateral epicondyle is the optimal point for insertion of a needle in aspiration of the elbow joint.

which the brachialis muscle is closely applied, but loosely attached. The tendon of the biceps muscle crosses the joint superficial to the brachialis and, at the level of the joint line, gives off the lacertus fibrosus which swings medialward to blend with the deep fascia of the forearm and form an arc under which pass the brachial artery and vein and the median nerve as they enter the forearm (Fig. 9–2). The radial nerve crosses the joint, buried deep in the interval between brachialis and brachioradialis muscles on the lateral aspect of the extremity.

The medial side of the elbow is covered by the mass of forearm muscles diverging from their common origin at the medial epicondyle. Crossing the joint just behind this bony point is the ulnar nerve (Fig. 9–2). The triceps tendon and aponeurosis attach to and enclose the olecranon region of the ulna. The palpable prominences of olecranon, lateral epicondyle, and radial head form a triangle, in the center of which is the optimal site for insertion of the needle in aspiration of the elbow joint (Fig. 9–2, *B*).

These bony landmarks (lateral epicondyle, radial head, and olecranon) remain palpable under almost all clinical circumstances. Normally they form a straight line in the extended and a triangle in the flexed elbow (Fig. 9–3). The radial head is palpable just distal to the lateral epicondyle. It is of some significance to the roentgen diagnosis of Monteggia fractures (p. 193) that the long axis of the radius goes through the center of the capitellum regardless of posture. The supinated forearm is abducted 15 degrees on the upper arm to form the "carrying angle," and the long axis of the extremity approaches a straight line only when the forearm is pronated (Fig. 9–3).

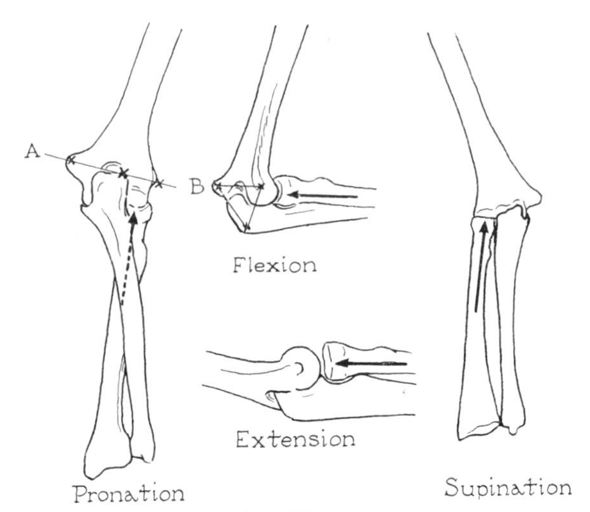

Figure 9–3. Bony landmarks of the elbow.

The olecranon and humeral epicondyles form a line (A) in the extended and a triangle (B) in the flexed elbow.

The long axis of the radius remains well centered in the capitellum in all positions (arrows).

The supinated forearm forms a 15-degree "carrying angle" with the humerus. The extremity approaches a straight line only when pronated and extended at the elbow.

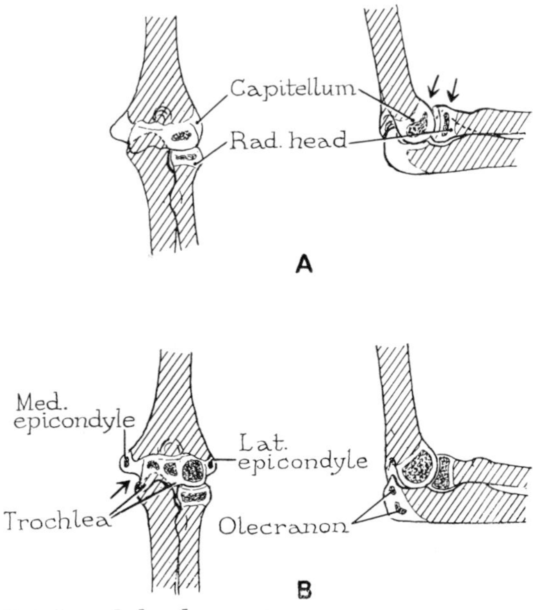

Figure 9–4. Epiphyseal development.

A. Until after age 5, epiphyseal centers for only the radial head and capitellum are visible in the x-ray film.

B. Between ages 10 and 13, additional centers for the trochlea, olecranon, and epicondyles appear in the roentgenogram.

The development of the epiphyses at the elbow is of some clinical importance. Normal ossification centers often are misinterpreted as fractures, and displaced epiphyses often pass unrecognized because they are not ossified. Normal elbows will show symmetrical stages of ossification on the two sides and roentgenograms should be obtained and compared in all equivocal cases. The approximate times of appearance of ossification in the epiphyses at the elbow (see Fig. 9–4) are as follows:

Capitellum	1 to 3 years
Radial head	5 to 6 years
Medial epicondyle	5 to 8 years
Lateral epicondyle	10 to 12 years
Olecranon	10 to 13 years
Trochlea	10 to 12 years

The lateral epicondyle, olecranon, and trochlea often show multiple ossification centers.

SOFT TISSUE INJURIES

"Tennis Elbow," Lateral Epicondylitis, Radiohumeral Bursitis

The etiology of these three clinically synonymous conditions is excessive wear and tear of the fibers of origin of the extensor communis muscle which are snapped across the epicondyle sharply by any activity which requires repeated pronation and flexion at the wrist.

The pathology consists essentially of attritional degeneration in the communis fibers exposed to such repeated minor traumas. Occasionally an amorphous deposit of calcium forms (Fig. 9–5) and produces an eventual

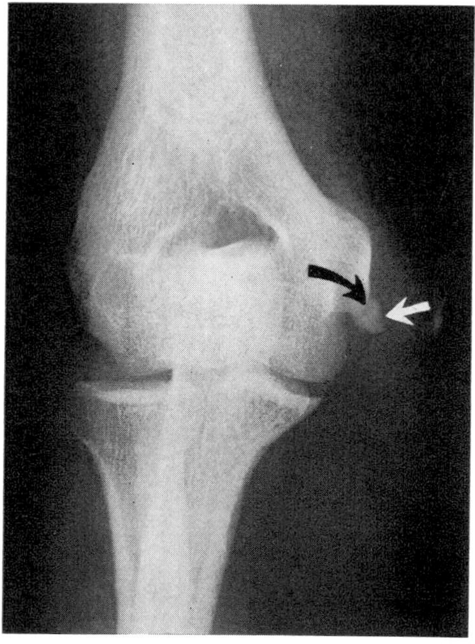

Figure 9–5. Tennis elbow, lateral epicondylitis, or extensor communis tendonitis, with a visible calcium deposit (arrows).

inflammatory response similar to that more commonly encountered in the shoulder tendons. Small cavities simulating bursae, but histologically of degenerative origin, may be encountered at operation.

The clinical picture is constant. There is a dull boring pain in the outer side of the elbow, which is accentuated by use of the extensor muscles. This pain often radiates down the dorsal aspect of the forearm to, but not past, the wrist. There is a trigger point of tenderness at the lateral epicondyle. Resisted extension of the fingers and forced passive flexion and pronation of the hand (with the elbow extended) increase the pain at the region of the lateral epicondyle.

Duration. The condition is self-limiting, but spontaneous recovery often does not occur until after symptoms have persisted for six months or more. A "cock-up" splint for relaxation of the extensor apparatus is of some palliative benefit. "Needling" of the trigger point, using 1 per cent procaine hydrochloride, produces temporary, and at times permanent, relief. Physiotherapeutic measures produce nothing but temporary palliation.

Treatment. Because the etiology is so often occupational this minor condition may produce a major disability worthy of curative therapy. A 3-cm. incision is made over the lateral epicondyle and deepened to the origin of the extensor communis, which is then stripped from the epicondyle and allowed to retract distalward. This removes most of the tension from the painful fibers and usually results in rapid and permanent relief of pain.

Medial Epicondylitis

This is pathologically identical and etiologically the reverse of lateral epicondylitis. It results from an occupation entailing repeated forceful flexion and supination of the wrist. A common example is the baseball pitcher who snaps his wrist into flexion and supination in the act of throwing a ball which curves. After a full game, acute medial epicondylitis requiring several days of rest and palliation is commonplace.

Olecranon Bursitis

The subcutaneous olecranon bursa over the point of the elbow is quite vulnerable to direct contusion and chronic mechanical irritation. There is no difficulty in making a diagnosis of the egg-shaped soft swelling at the point of the elbow. Often a tender, somewhat mobile nubbin of tissue is palpated in the center of the swollen area, but more often than not very little pain or tenderness is present. Many such lesions, especially when they result from a direct contusion, subside spontaneously. Early aspiration, followed by rest of the elbow and support by a pressure dressing, may effect a cure. The inflamed bursa exposed to or resulting from repeated mechanical irritation rapidly becomes thick walled and fibrotic and is no longer amenable to conservative measures. Excision through a transverse incision, with precautions against damage to the ulnar nerve, is the only certain curative therapy for such a chronic enlarged and fibrotic bursa. *Incision for release of bursal fluid is to be condemned* as a common precursor of chronic bursal infection eventuating in osteomyelitis of the olecranon.

Rupture of Distal Biceps Tendon

The predisposition to this uncommon injury is attritional degeneration of the fibers of the biceps tendon at or near its insertion on the tuberosity of the radius. The immediate cause of rupture is a sudden forceful flexion of the elbow against resistance. The lacertus fibrosus which transmits biceps contractions to the forearm via the deep fascia almost invariably remains intact. Consequently, although a measurable weakness of supination power follows avulsion of the biceps tendon from the radius, the total flexion power of the elbow is not often seriously decreased. A comfortable and useful but somewhat weakened extremity will result spontaneously. Operative repair of the rupture, therefore, is a matter of election and becomes mandatory only on those rare occasions when the lacertus fibrosus is also disrupted.

FRACTURES AT LOWER END OF HUMERUS

SUPRACONDYLAR FRACTURES IN CHILDREN

These common childhood injuries result from a fall on the outstretched hand and may present simple treatment problems attended by excellent prognoses or vexing therapeutic riddles calling for the utmost in surgical judgment in order to forestall catastrophe. The fracture line is generally transverse and situated at the junction of the cancellous condyles with the cortical portion of the humerus where this bone is virtually hourglass-shape in cross section (Fig. 9–6, *A*). The displacement pattern is constant, consisting of some combination of posterior tilt, displacement, rotation, and overriding of the small distal fragment from the shaft of the bone (Fig. 9–6). The absence or presence and degree of these four displacements determine the extent of concomitant damage to the adjacent soft tissue structures and, *ipso facto*, govern the urgency and technique of treatment and the prognosis. A therapeutic classification would segregate almost all supracondylar fractures into three broad categories.

Type I—Greenstick or Undisplaced Supracondylar Fracture

The deformity amounts to nothing more than a reduction of the forward inclination of the condyles from the shaft of the humerus. This deformity rarely requires correction, but should be prevented from increasing. This is accomplished by dressing the extremity in a posterior molded plaster splint with the elbow flexed about 60 degrees for three weeks (Fig. 9–6, *C*). Complete recovery is to be expected.

Type II—Displaced Supracondylar Fracture

Despite displacement of the fracture fragments, the posterior humeral periosteum is intact. Anything more than a small amount of displacement

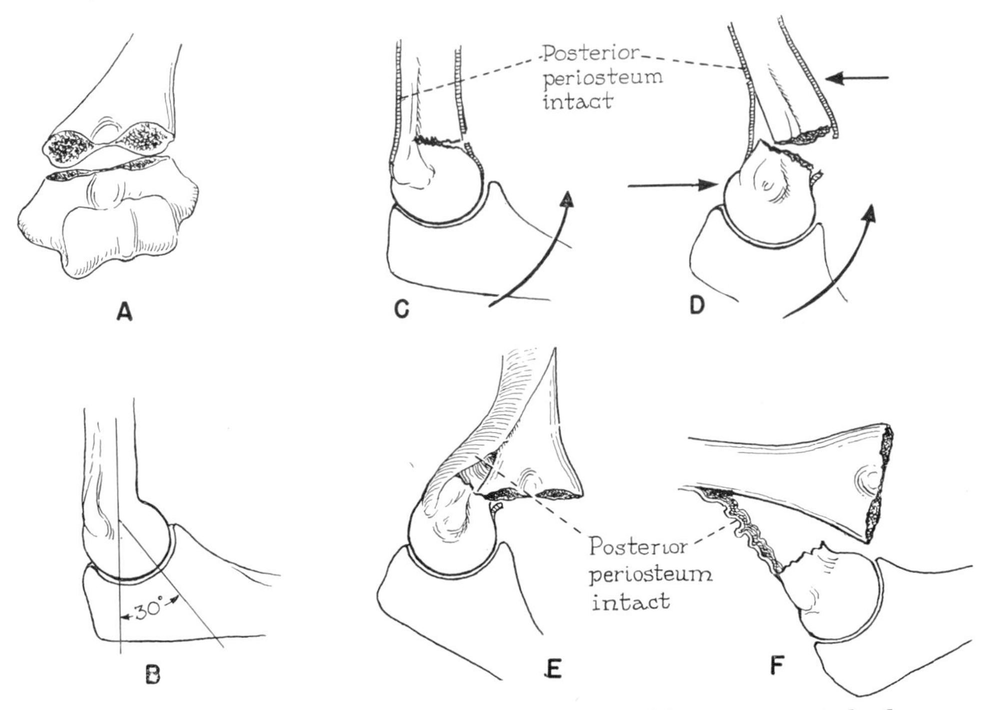

Figure 9–6. The four displacements in supracondylar fracture of the humerus.

A. The level of the fracture is such that the fragment ends are hourglass shape in cross section.

B. The lower end of the humerus normally inclines forward to form an angle of 30 degrees with the axis of the shaft.

C. A "greenstick" fracture requires only flexion (arrow) for restoration of the normal angle.

D. The lower fragment of a displaced fracture must be replaced (arrows) before the elbow is flexed.

E. Rotational displacement is common and must be corrected (see Figure 9–7, D).

F. Overriding is the precursor of vascular embarrassment (see Fig. 9–7, A) and nerve damage (see Fig. 9–7, B).

In all displacements a tongue of posterior periosteum and soft parts remains intact and is the most important agent in maintenance of reduction (see Fig. 9–7, E).

should be corrected. The status of the nerves and circulation distal to the fracture must be checked before and after reduction, which, in a child, should be carried out under general anesthesia.

Reduction is not accomplished by merely supinating the forearm and flexing the elbow. This does little except to increase existing compression of the brachial artery and all other soft parts in the antecubital space (Fig. 9–7, *A*). The first step in reduction is to extend the elbow gently to 180 degrees coincident with steady traction and countertraction along its axis (Fig. 9–7, *C*). Traction is maintained until humeral length has been restored. Not until this has been accomplished is it possible to carry out the second step, i.e., digital replacement of the small distal fragment under the shaft of the bone (Fig. 9–7, *D*). When the fragments have been reapproximated the third step, correction of rotatory displacement, should

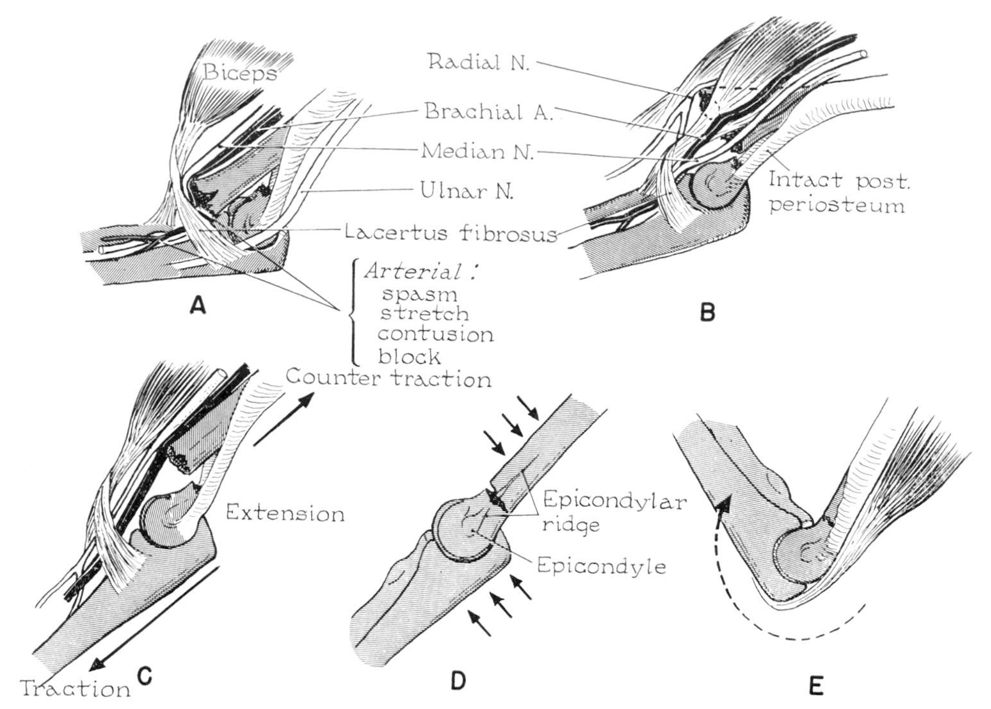

Figure 9–7. Concomitant soft part damage and technique for reduction of supracondylar fracture.

A. The lacertus fibrosus is displaced with the distal fragment and the forearm. The neurovascular structures in the antecubital compartment are stretched, contused, and constricted between the lacertus fibrosus and the overriding humeral shaft.

B. If the distal fragment is displaced inward, the median nerve and brachial artery may escape damage, but the radial nerve then lies directly in the path of the humeral shaft.

C. The folly of primary elbow flexion is obvious in A. The first maneuver in reduction is extension and restoration of length by traction (arrows). This also relieves the constriction of soft part structures in the antecubital space.

D. Following restoration of length the distal fragment is pushed into place under the shaft. Rotation is then corrected by lining up the palpable epicondylar ridges.

E. Flexion then tightens the intact posterior periosteum and triceps and makes the reduction stable.

be done. The distal fragment is derotated until its easily palpable epicondyles are realigned with the equally palpable epicondylar ridges of the proximal fragment. Traction should be maintained throughout the entire procedure until the next and final step, flexion of the elbow, stabilizes the reapproximated fragments (Fig. 9–7, *E*) by tension of the intact posterior periosteal sleeve. Elbow flexion is carried out with a finger on the radial pulse, for not only the stability of the reduced fracture but also the risk of cutting off the arterial supply to the forearm and hand increase in direct proportion to the amount of elbow flexion. The optimal amount of flexion for immobilization is the least amount necessary for stabilization of the fracture without jeopardizing the distal circulation.

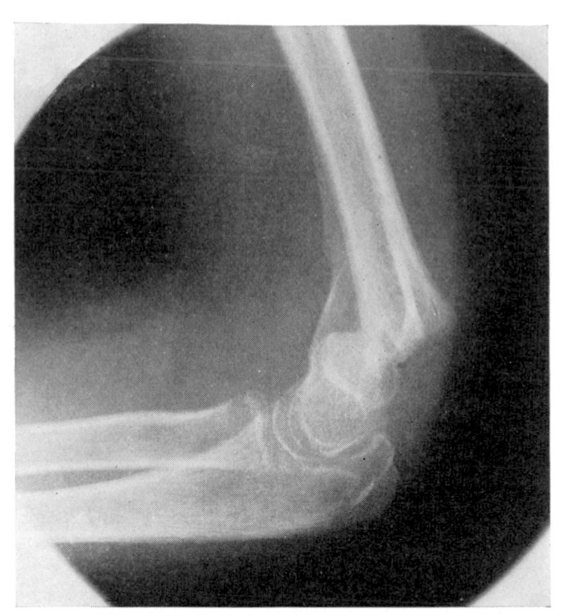

Figure 9–8. Supracondylar fracture with anterior displacement which was incorrectly fixed in flexion. The reduction was unstable because the intact anterior periosteal sleeve, which can be seen to have filled in with new bone formation, was allowed to remain slack. The original deformity recurred. This lesion must be dressed in extension.

Fixation requires maintenance of posterior periosteal tension by immobilization of the extremity with a molded plaster splint extending from the metacarpophalangeal joints to the upper humerus. The forearm is in full supination to prevent recurrence of internal rotation displacement of the small distal fragment on the humeral shaft. The elbow is flexed in the position elected at the time of manipulation. The child should be hospitalized or kept under constant surveillance, and the circulatory status of the hand checked hourly until it is normal. The splint is discarded in three to four weeks, after which physical therapy is not only unnecessary but often harmful. Forcible stretching and the carrying of weights in an attempt to hasten recovery of extension at the elbow are to be condemned as procedures which do great harm. *The normal activities of childhood consistently produce maximal rehabilitation in the shortest possible time.*

Supracondylar fractures with anterior displacement. These uncommon injuries result from a fall on the back of the flexed elbow. Mechanically and from the viewpoint of reduction and fixation, they are the direct opposites of ordinary supracondylar fractures. The intact periosteal sleeve is on the anterior surface of the fracture, necessitating immobilization in *extension* rather than flexion in order to provide stable fixation of the reduced fragments (Fig. 9–8). Damage to the antecubital nerve and vessel is not common, but the ulnar nerve may often be seriously injured.

Type III—Supracondylar Fracture with Cold White Hand

This is an emergency to be measured in minutes. The elbow is grossly deformed and swollen. Early antecubital ecchymosis may testify to laceration of the deep fascia and brachialis muscle by the widely displaced bone fragments. The circulation distal to the elbow is deranged by stretch, compression, and distortion of the arterial supply (Fig. 9–7, *A*, *B*), and impediment to the venous return. As a result the hand is cool and pale, little or no finger motion can be obtained, the slightly cyanotic nail beds blanch poorly, and the radial pulse is weak or absent.

Volkmann's ischemic paralysis is imminent. Once established, even for an hour or two, this dreaded crippling lesion often proves irreversible. The basic etiology is of vascular origin, including spasm and mechanical blockage of the brachial artery at the fracture and an impeded venous return. Poorly understood neurological phenomena contribute to the end-result, but the most important single etiological factor is anoxia of the tissues distal to the elbow. The primary cause of anoxia is displacement of the fracture fragments and the only efficient single corrective measure is prompt reduction of this displacement. Until this has been accomplished, procaine hydrochloride block of the stellate ganglion or the use of vaso-relaxing drugs will be of little help; elevation of the extremity may do more harm than good if, as is usually the case, arterial deficiency is the important culprit; and decompression of the antecubital space by incision of the deep fascia or the instillation of hyaluronidase will prove of little avail. When these ancillary measures are carried out as the primary therapy, time passes, and often also the point of no return from tissue anoxia. *The urgent primary measure for relief of impending or early Volkmann's ischemia is reduction of the fracture.*

THE SUPRACONDYLAR DILEMMA

The grossly displaced fracture has been reduced. When the elbow is flexed sufficiently to stabilize the reduction the radial pulse cannot be obtained. When flexion is released the pulse returns, but the fracture redisplaces. In short, the amount of elbow flexion necessary to maintain reduction obliterates the distal circulation. This dilemma is encountered in about 10 per cent of supracondylar fractures, and attempts to meet both aspects of the problem by plaster fixation of the reduced fracture are almost always predestined to failure.

TREATMENT

Fixation by Skeletal Traction

Maintenance of reduction by skeletal traction obviates the necessity for elbow flexion, decompresses the antecubital compartment, assists drainage of the injured area by gravity, and leaves the entire extremity accessible for the frequent assessments of circulation that should be done (Fig. 9–9). The skin of the elbow region is prepared as for operation. A Kirschner wire is passed transversely through the upper end of the ulna

(1) ***distal to the radial head,*** since a more proximal position may transfix and produce a subsequent growth derangement of the olecranon epiphysis;

(2) ***from the medial to the lateral surface of the bone,*** so that the ulnar nerve may be pushed out of danger at the point of wire insertion;

(3) ***with the forearm in supination,*** since, if the wire is inserted in the pronated position, subsequent supination may compress the motor branch of the radial nerve between it and the neck of the radius to produce "drop wrist."

The child is placed in bed and the fracture is reduced by manipulation. The extremity is then suspended with the humerus vertical and the forearm horizontal (Fig. 9–9). Sufficient traction is applied via the Kirschner wire to raise the shoulder from the bed. The forearm is suspended in a hammock. Five to 8 pounds of traction suffices to maintain length and axis of the broken humerus and general approximation of the fracture surfaces even in the absence of acute flexion. Rotatory displacement is corrected by adjusting the position of the forearm hammock so that the hand is suspended above the child's face or umbilicus as the deformity may dictate. Plaster splints are not used.

This method of treatment has been required in about 10 per cent of the cases of supracondylar fracture in the writer's experience (Fig. 9–*10*). No Volkmann lesions have ensued, and a group of patients with early or

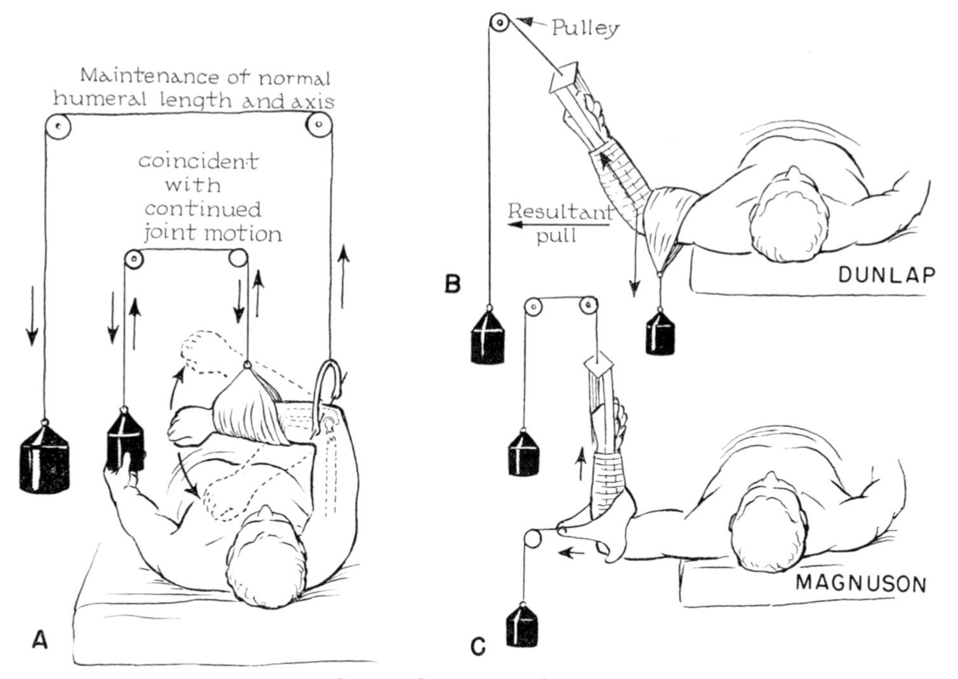

Figure 9–9. Fixation of humeral fractures by traction suspension.

A. Skeletal traction by a pin through the olecranon permits maintenance of humeral length and axis coincident with continued joint motion, and the abolition of all encircling dressings or splints.

B, C. Skin traction maintains humeral length and axis, but permits little or no motion of the joints and superimposes some added circulatory embarrassment to the extremity.

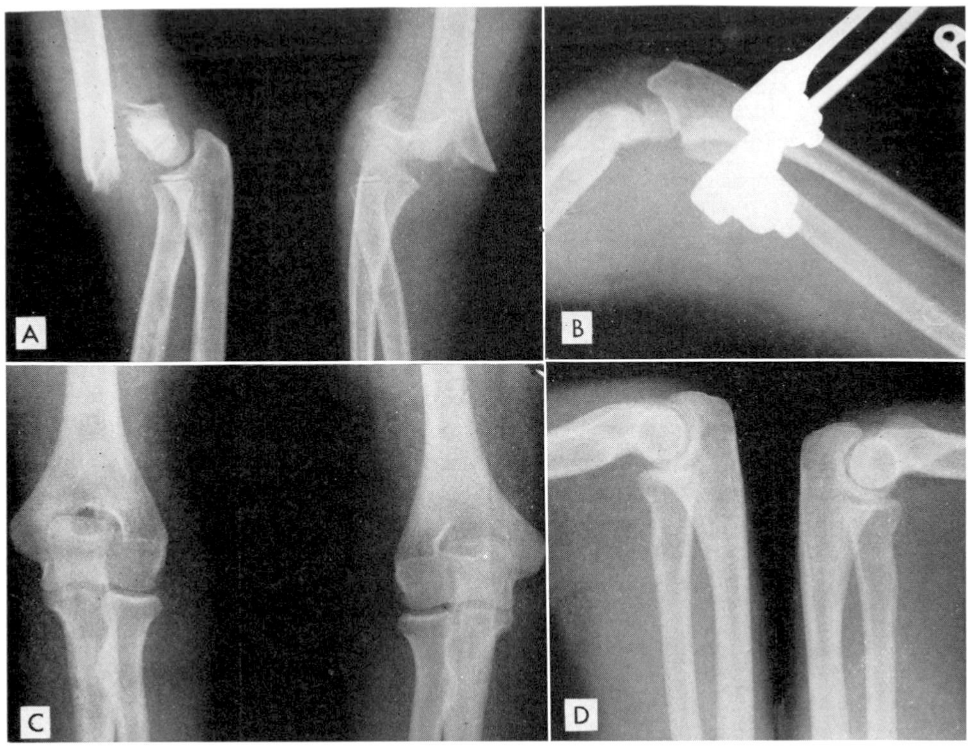

Figure 9–10.

A. A supracondylar fracture of 6 hours' duration with a cold, white hand, imperceptible pulse, and great pain on the slightest finger motion.

B. Following reduction and fixation by skeletal traction as in Figure 9–9, A. The impending Volkmann ischemia subsided slowly over 24 hours.

C, D. The result and the normal elbow 6 years later.

impending ischemia recovered completely. Open reduction has proved unnecessary and unwise. Incision of the lacertus fibrosus alone has proved of very questionable benefit. Auxiliary measures, e.g., stellate ganglion block, vasorelaxing drugs, and subfascial hyaluronidase instillation, rarely have been required. After 7 to 14 days the traction is replaced by a molded plaster splint, and the child may be treated as an outpatient.

FRACTURES OF DISTAL HUMERAL EPIPHYSES

A sprained elbow in a child is unusual. What appears to be a sprain is almost always an injury to the upper radial or distal humeral epiphysis. The diagnosis cannot be made by x-ray, but clinical examination discloses the focus of pain and tenderness to be located at one of the elbow epiphyses, and not at its ligaments. Protective dressings should be used until pain and tenderness are no longer present. The parents should be warned concerning the possibility of later growth disturbance.

Displacement of Capitellar and Trochlear Epiphyses

This uncommon injury is the anatomical equivalent of a supracondylar fracture, but the fracture line traverses epiphyseal cartilage and is not seen in the roentgenogram. Consequently the diagnosis is often missed or misinterpreted as a dislocation of the elbow or fracture of the lateral condyle. Only the ossification center for the capitellum may appear displaced, but close scrutiny will disclose that the ulna also is in abnormal relationship to the humerus (Fig. 9–*11*). The problem is recognition of the lesion.

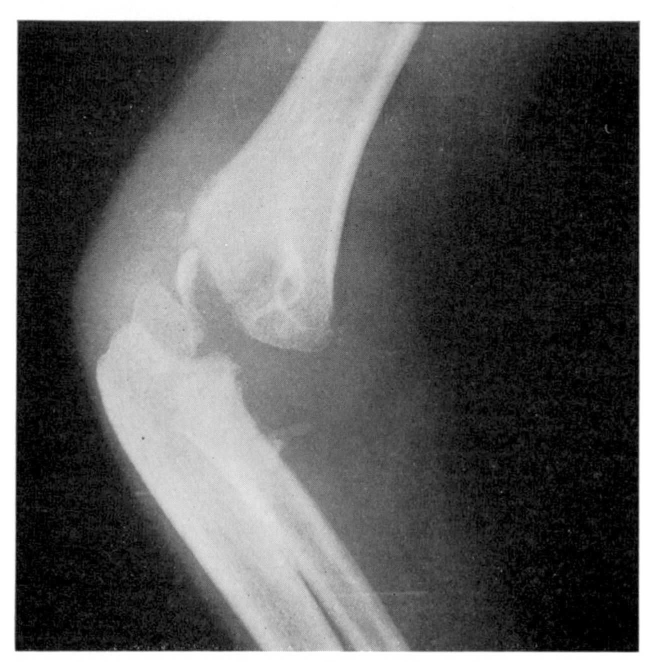

Figure 9–11. Displacement of entire humeral epiphysis.

At first glance this appears to be a fracture of the lateral condyle (capitellum), but the ulna is also displaced in relation to the humerus. The unossified trochlear epiphysis is displaced along with the capitellum. The diagnosis was missed until several weeks after injury. The child has a permanent disability at the elbow.

Reduction and aftercare are identical to those for a displaced supracondylar fracture. The prognosis must be guarded as gross deformities may result from the extensive epiphyseal damage associated with displacement of the entire lower humeral epiphysis.

Fracture of Capitellar Epiphysis (Lateral Condyle)

Forced abduction of the forearm may produce a shearing fracture of the external condyle if the medial collateral ligament remains intact. The fracture line splits apart the trochlear and capitellar epiphyses and traverses both the capitellar epiphyseal plate and the diaphysis of the lower humerus (Fig. 9–*12*). The intracapsular cartilaginous portion of the broken fragment is devoid of blood supply save for that from the meager soft

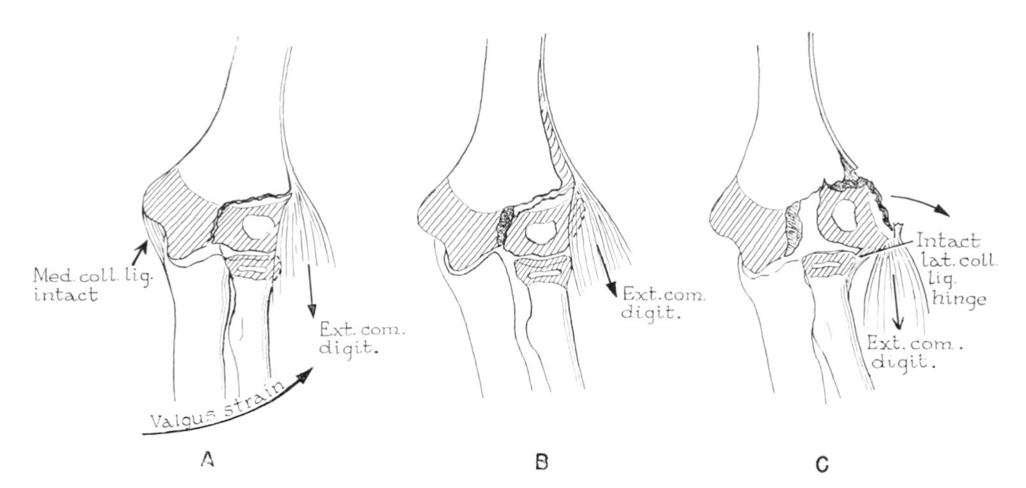

Figure 9–12. Fracture of capitellar epiphysis (lateral condyle).

A. The injury splits apart the capitellar and trochlear epiphyses and shears off a shell of lateral condyle metaphysis.

B. If the soft-part envelope of the lower humerus remains intact, little displacement occurs.

C. If the soft parts are disrupted, the fragment is tilted out of the joint on a hinge formed by the external collateral ligament. The elastic displacing factor of the extensor communis usually prevents manipulative reduction.

parts attached to the epicondyle and the diaphyseal shell. Accurate reduction is necessary to bony union. Incomplete reduction is followed by fibrous union, increased lateral displacement of the condylar fragment, an increased carrying angle predisposing to late ulnar palsy, and an altogether unsatisfactory result. It is, therefore, of great importance to obtain and maintain complete reduction of any existing displacement.

Treatment. When the fragment remains in the joint the surrounding soft parts are essentially intact (Fig. 9–*12*, *B*). Reduction is accomplished by manual compression of the elbow and is usually quite stable when the elbow is flexed. Immobilization in flexion for three or four weeks is followed by bony union and a relatively low incidence of subsequent growth deformities. When the soft parts enclosing the lower humerus are extensively torn (Fig. 9–*12*, *C*), the extensor digitorum communis rotates the condylar fragment out of the joint on a pivot of the lateral collateral ligament. The empty lateral joint cavity must then be opened by adducting the extended forearm on the humerus before the fragment can be replaced in the joint. One early attempt to manipulate even the most grossly displaced fragments should be made. If it is unsuccessful, open reduction is strongly indicated, but exposure of the fragment requires very precise dissection lest the circulation carried by its few remaining soft-part attachments be destroyed. Adequate internal fixation can usually be obtained by suture of the surrounding soft tissues. When this is not possible the diaphyseal rather than the epiphyseal portion of the fragment should be transfixed if pins or screws are used for fixation.

FRACTURE OF MEDIAL EPICONDYLE EPIPHYSIS

Epicondyle Avulsion with Intact Elbow Ligaments

Until it fuses to the humerus in late adolescence the epiphysis of the medial epicondyle is vulnerable to avulsion by the flexor muscles, arising from a common origin. So long as the elbow ligaments remain intact this is a minor injury, essentially equivalent to a small tear of the site of common flexor origin. The epicondyle may be separated but undisplaced from the humerus, or retracted as much as 2 cm. toward the wrist, depending upon the amount of tearing of the adjacent soft tissues (Fig. 9–*13*). Reduction of such displacement cannot be obtained or maintained except by operative replacement and fixation, which is neither necessary nor advisable except when there is evidence of concomitant damage to the ulnar nerve. Otherwise this injury should be treated for what it is, incomplete avulsion of a muscle attachment. The elbow is flexed to 90 degrees and dressed in a molded splint, but only for 7 to 10 days while the acutely painful symptoms subside. Active motion and use are then resumed progressively, and function will return steadily if no attempts are made to stretch the elbow forcibly. If immobilization is prolonged for several weeks, many months must pass before extension is regained.

Healing is usually by fibrous rather than bony union, and the bone fragment remains in its original displaced position (Fig. 9–*14*). Late overgrowth or deformity of the epicondyle fragment is not uncommon. The former may produce a visible deformity simulating cubitus valgus, but this

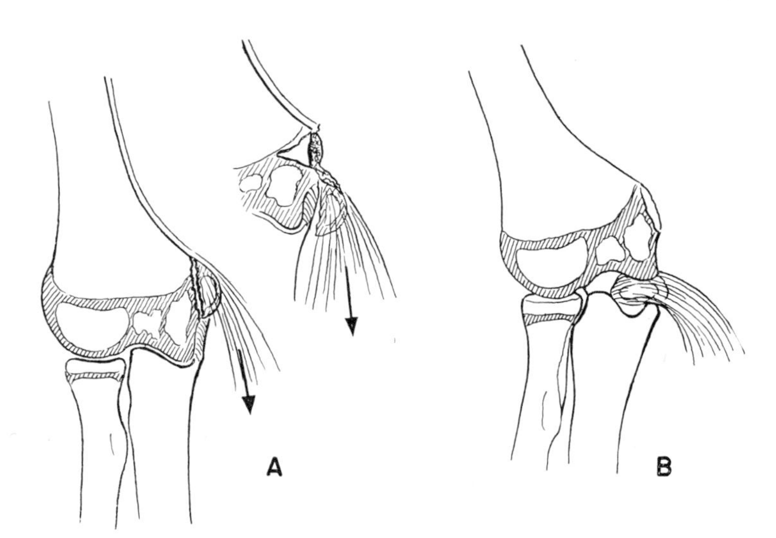

Figure 9–13. Avulsion of medial epicondyle.

A. The epicondyle is avulsed by the flexor muscles of the forearm (arrow) arising from a common origin. Displacement is proportional to the amount of laceration of the soft parts enveloping the epicondyle.

B. If the medial ligaments of the elbow are ruptured and the joint opens (as in dislocation), the epicondyle may become caught between trochlea and ulna. When this occurs the fractured (flat) surface of the epicondylar fragment rotates 90 degrees and faces distalward in the x-ray film.

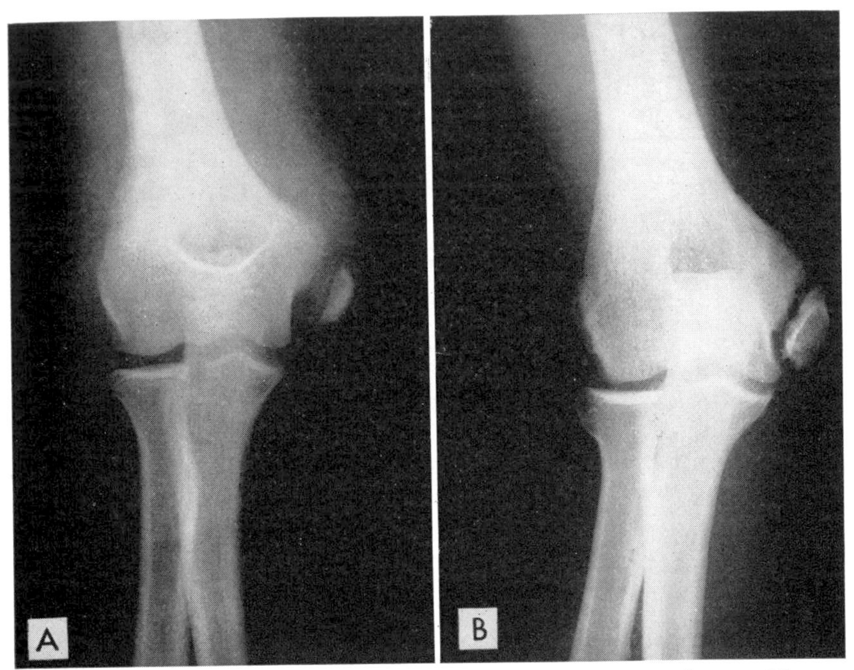

Figure 9–14. Avulsion of medial epicondyle by common flexors. The partially avulsed site of origin of the muscle contains the medial epicondyle.

A. The lesion after reduction of the concomitant dislocation of the elbow.

B. Fourteen months later, showing fibrous union and calcification in the injured external ligaments.

is nothing more than an illusion caused by undue prominence of the epicondyle. Despite all such imperfections, there is no deficit in elbow motion or flexor muscle strength.

The ulnar nerve may be damaged from contusion by the displaced fragment at the time of injury, or from compression by scar many months later. Careful assessment of ulnar nerve function is therefore necessary at every visit, and at suitable intervals after recovery. Early nerve deficits in the presence of gross displacement warrant operative replacement and suture of the epicondyle (or excision of the fragment and repair of the soft part defect), followed by neurolysis and transposition of the nerve to the anterior aspect of the epicondyle. Late development of ulnar palsy, which is relatively uncommon, also constitutes a strong indication for anterior transposition of this nerve.

Epicondyle Avulsion with Ruptured Elbow Ligaments

Avulsion of the epicondyle coincident with a valgus strain sufficient to rupture the medial collateral ligament, or with a posterior dislocation of the elbow, creates a potentially complicated and hazardous situation. As the ligaments rupture the elbow joint opens so that the epicondyle fragment becomes caught between trochlea and ulna (Fig. 9–*13*, *B*). The joint is locked and, even under anesthesia, motion is limited. On casual examination the gross anatomy seems normal. The multiplicity of ossification centers in the child's elbow makes radiographic diagnosis difficult. Certain catastrophe will follow unless it is recognized that the epicondyle has been displaced into the elbow joint.

The diagnosis of inclusion of the epicondyle into the elbow joint is not difficult. Whether or not a dislocation has recently been reduced, the inner aspect of the elbow is swollen and ecchymotic. Palpation of the bony landmarks reveals absence of the medial epicondyle. Elbow motion is blocked

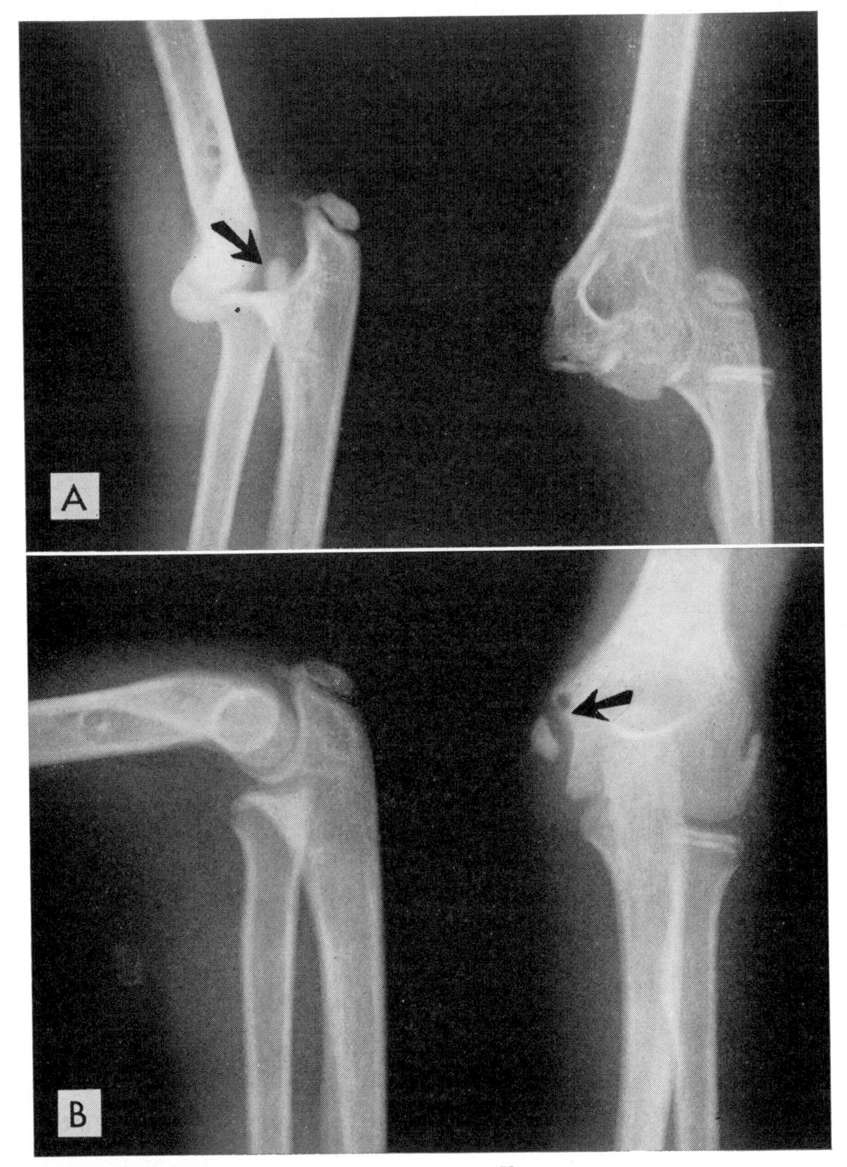

Figure 9–15. Epicondyle inclusion in the elbow joint.

A. The original dislocation with the avulsed epicondyle interposed between the bones.

B. After extrication and suture through drill hole in the humerus. Fibrous union.

even under anesthesia. Evidence of damage to the ulnar nerve is commonly present. Comparison of x-ray films of the two elbows will clinch the diagnosis (Fig. 9–*15*). The epicondyle will be found to be absent from its normal position and located in a displaced position, despite the confusion of overlapping ossification centers, if the films are carefully compared. Rotation of the displaced bone fragment so that its flat (broken) surface faces distalward is almost pathognomonic of inclusion into the joint.

Treatment. It is occasionally possible to milk the bone fragment out of the elbow joint by manipulation, but this is an uncertain procedure at best and apt to create considerable additional damage to the articulating surfaces of ulna and trochlea. The elbow should be exposed through a medial incision. The epicondyle and site of common flexor origin will be found tucked between the humerus and ulna and may be extricated gently with small hooks. The avulsed fragment should be restored to position and its surrounding soft parts repaired by suture. When indicated, the ulnar nerve should be transposed to an anterior location. The results are good if the lesion is recognized and repaired early. The prospects for complete recovery diminish in proportion to the duration of uncorrected inclusion in the joint. Unrecognized, neglected lesions justify a poor prognosis for recovery of function following late extirpation of the fragment from the elbow.

Epicondyle Avulsion Prior to Ossification

Young children in whom no ossification centers are visible may suffer injuries to the internal epicondyle identical to those discussed here. Roentgenography not only fails to assist in diagnosis, but contributes to a false sense of security on the part of the surgeon. There remains little excuse for not making the diagnosis, however, for *the clinical evidence can always be elicited if the lesion is suspected.*

FRACTURE OF LOWER EXTREMITY OF ADULT HUMERUS

This injury occasionally occurs in young adults, but is encountered chiefly in persons past middle age. The elbow is flexed, as in carrying a bundle, so that when a fall occurs its impact is received at the olecranon or over the back of the lower end of the humerus. The relatively brittle condylar segments shatter and the olecranon is driven upward like a wedge to split apart and displace the fragments. The elbow "feels like a bag of beans," with absence or gross distortion of the landmarks. Early ecchymosis and massive swelling are present. Nerve injuries are common, but recovery is usually spontaneous. There is often an open wound at the point of impact on the dorsal aspect of the elbow. Fracture lines enter the joint to distort the articular surface of the humerus. All periarticular soft tissues are lacerated or infiltrated with hemorrhage so that massive periarticular fibrosis is the usual consequence of healing. *Prolonged immobilization, therefore, is usually followed by fibrous ankylosis of the elbow. Mobility is essential to the usefulness of the elbow and should be maintained at all costs, including, when necessary, the acceptance of malunion with gross bone deformity.*

Comminuted Fractures—Dicondylar, Intercondylar, Transcondylar, T and Y Fractures

The appellation given this injury is unimportant. The humeral condyles are shattered, split apart by the olecranon wedge, and rotated into grotesque positions by their epicondylar muscle attachments. Comminution precludes a *stable* reduction by any method. Healing sufficient to protect against loss of reduction is not present for four to six weeks after injury. Plaster immobilization of this duration almost certainly ensures permanent stiffness. Internal fixation is useless, and open reduction should not be done. Arthroplasty (excision of the elbow joint) should not be considered until the acute reaction has subsided and the periarticular tissues have "jelled" sufficiently to serve as a hinge for motion. Only two therapeutic alternatives warrant consideration—to ignore anatomy and concentrate on maintenance of function alone, or to maintain normal length and axis of the shattered humerus by a form of traction which allows continued mobility of the elbow throughout the healing period of the fracture.

Treatment by early mobilization. Manual traction is made on the semi-extended elbow and the condyles are compressed. A molded plaster splint is applied from wrist to shoulder with the elbow extended at least 135 degrees. These injuries are flexion fractures, and maximal collapse and displacement will occur if the arm is dressed with the elbow in flexion. The function of this splint *is not maintenance of reduction,* but provision of comfort, rest, and protection to the injured area. Although the weight of the *dependent* extremity is helpful in stabilizing the position of the fracture fragments, it is more important that the extremity is *elevated* for the next few days so that the fluid products of the injury may be drained by gravity. As soon as the acute reactions to trauma subside (within 7 to 12 days) the splint should be removed periodically and all motions of the elbow resumed gradually but progressively. From this time on the splint should be reapplied only when its use is dictated by comfort, fatigue, or protection against external forces. It should be discarded as soon as this can be tolerated. The result will be marked by roentgenographic evidence of gross malunion and an elbow which is visibly deformed anatomically, but which is reasonably strong and mobile and usually quite comfortable and useful. This is far superior to the elbow which, although normal by roentgen and anatomical criteria, is permanently stiffened by the immobilization used to maintain reduction.

Treatment by traction. The essential objective of treatment by traction is to maintain normal humeral length and axis coincident with continued elbow joint motion. Normal humeral length and axis can be well maintained by various forms of skin traction (Fig. 9–9), but only at the expense of motion. Both objectives can be attained by skeletal traction. The olecranon is transfixed with a traction pin proximal to the radial head in the axis of the humerus. The extremity is suspended by sufficient traction

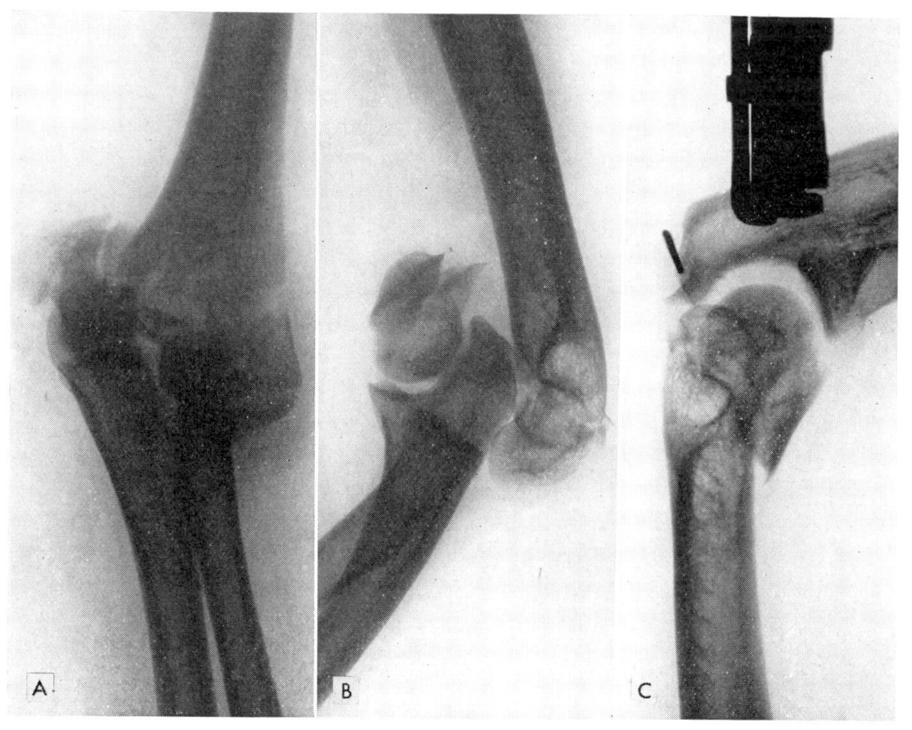

Figure 9–16. Comminuted fracture of lower end of humerus.
A, B. Roentgenograms before treatment.
C. After overhead suspension by a Kirschner wire through the intact olecranon. Motion in balanced suspension gradually molded the humeral fragments into a shape congruous with the radial and ulnar articulating surfaces.

to lift the shoulder from the bed (5 to 8 pounds). The fracture is then reduced as well as possible by manual compression. The forearm is suspended in a hammock so that it can be passively flexed and extended by the uninjured hand (Fig. 9–9). The patient is taught to flex and extend the injured joint in this way at frequent intervals and in gradually increasing amounts. Within a week a total arc of 30 to 40 degrees is usually possible within the limits of pain. It is this *early* motion of the intact articulating ends of the radius and ulna which tends to remold the shattered humeral fragments into a congruous shape before they become fixed in granulations (Fig. 9–*16*). After four or five weeks, traction may be discontinued in favor of a protective posterior splint which, over the next several weeks, is removed at progressively increasing intervals for exercises and resumption of normal use.

Treatment by open reduction. Open reduction and internal fixation is not justifiable unless the lesion is early, uncomminuted, and amenable to internal fixation compatible with continued elbow motion throughout its healing period. Such a combination of circumstances is uncommon, and open reduction should never be considered except by the most experienced surgeon.

FRACTURE OF THE HEAD OF THE RADIUS

Radial head fracture is produced by impact against the capitellum. The usual injury is a fall on the outstretched hand or a posterior dislocation of the elbow. These fractures are divisible into four categories, each of which calls for specific treatment.

Type I—Radial Head Fracture with No or Minimal Displacement

Sprain of the elbow almost never occurs. What appears to be a sprain usually is a mere fissure fracture of the radial head, unrecognized because

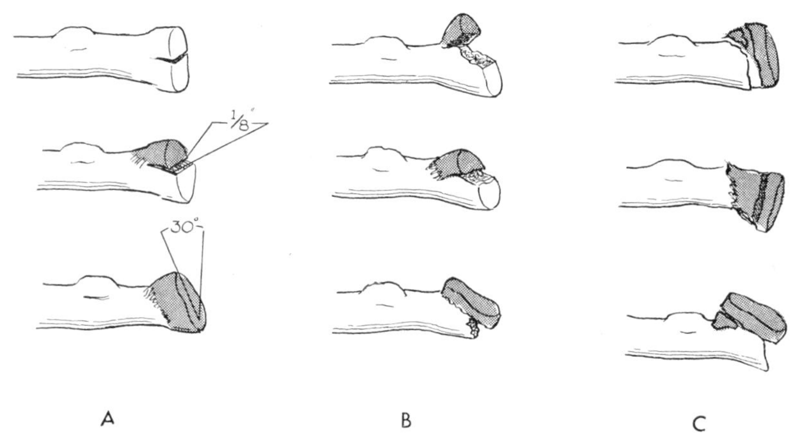

Figure 9–17. Common categories of radial head fracture.

A. An undisplaced crack, displacement less than ⅛-inch or angulation less than 30 degrees, should be treated by aspiration of the hemarthrosis, when needed, and early motion.

B. Gross displacement, with the head fragment remaining within the joint, should be treated by radial head excision.

C. In the child, a mild epiphyseal displacement or angular radial neck fracture should be treated by rest in a plaster splint. If the epiphysis is grossly out of place, open reduction, if the patient is below age 13, and radial head excision, if above age 13, should be done.

x-ray films fail to show it in profile, and productive of symptoms by virtue of a sequential hemarthrosis. Type I fractures with small displacement are recognizable by x-ray. A segment of radial head is depressed ⅛ inch or less, or the radial articular surface is tilted 30 degrees or less (Fig. 9–*17*, *A*). Within these limits the deformity is compatible with good function and should not be corrected. *Immobilization is unnecessary and harmful.* Treatment should be designed to relieve pain and preserve function. Pain and limitation of elbow motion result not from the fracture, but from joint distention by a tense hemarthrosis. Aspiration consistently produces a comfortable movable elbow.

Aspiration of the elbow joint for decompression of hemarthrosis, diagnosis, suppuration, or instillation of medication is done by insertion of the needle in the center of the triangle formed by three palpable bony landmarks—the radial head, olecranon, and lateral humeral epicondyle (Fig. 9–2). At this point there is little between skin and joint capsule except anconeus muscle. A tense, tender, elastic or fluctuant swelling in the same area constitutes the clinical evidence that a joint effusion is present.

After aspiration the elbow should be rested by sling or splint for 24 hours until the danger of recurrent hemarthrosis subsides. Motion and use of the extremity then should be encouraged up to the point of pain or fatigue. Patients having sedentary occupations usually can return to their jobs within a few days, and manual workers within two or three weeks. The most common error is to treat this lesion by immobilization because it is a fracture. Bone union takes place swiftly and surely, and is quite independent of therapy. Motion within pain limits from the start incurs no risk of increased displacement of the fragments. *Immobilization for more than 48 hours does no good and much harm.*

Type II—Displaced Fracture of the Radial Head

Deformity in excess of that which delineates Type I fractures is rarely correctible and never acceptable (Fig. 9–*17, B*). Attempts at reduction and fixation are not indicated. The radial head should be removed. Provided this is carried out without damaging the radial nerve as it winds around the neck of the radius, and in such a way that the radial stump remains stabilized by the orbicular ligament, recovery will be rapid and unmarked by any significant depreciation of elbow function. The entire radial head, *not the displaced fragment alone,* should be removed. Following operation, except when the elbow has become stiffened by unnecessary immobilization, a return to all but manual laboring jobs may be expected in three or four weeks. The end-results are very satisfactory.

Borderline lesions. In a large group of radial head fractures the deformity is neither minimal nor gross. Treatment by aspiration and early mobilization produces satisfactory results in about 80 per cent of these cases, but the average time of return to work is delayed for six to eight weeks. The remainder of these patients suffer from persisting painful symptoms and many eventually require radial head excision. Since early ablation of the radial head returns most workers to their jobs in a matter of several weeks, the importance of the primary decision on treatment is obvious. In doubtful cases conservative treatment risks nothing but an increased disability period, and does not preclude late radial head excision when the choice proves to have been wrong.

Type III—Injuries to Radial Head Epiphysis

The radial head in a child is not subject to the fissured or segmental depressed fractures so common to the adult. Rather, its articular face is tilted from the axis of the shaft by a greenstick fracture of the radial neck, or a displacement of the entire epiphysis accompanied by a triangular fragment of metaphysis (Fig. 9–*17, C*). In general, 30 degrees of articular tilt represents the borderline below which the deformity may be accepted and beyond which it should be corrected. Unlike similar lesions in the adult, however, *the radial head should not be removed.* Excision of the radial head in a child under 13 years of age results in overgrowth of the capitellum and loss of radial length, with subsequent deformity and derangement of the inferior radio-ulnar joint.

Unacceptable epiphyseal displacement should be corrected by manipulation. Under general anesthesia the elbow is fully extended and the forearm adducted. The wrist is then rotated until the displaced radial head epiphysis presents laterally in a position where strong digital pressure can push it back into alignment with the shaft of the bone. The elbow is immobilized in flexion for four to six weeks. As a rule, even when an excellent reduction has been obtained, subsequent partial recurrence of the original deformity occurs. The result is eccentric rotation of the radial head in relation to the axis of the shaft (Fig. 9–*18*). Temporary acceptance of this defect until the wrist and elbow epiphyses have matured, followed by late excision of the deformed radial head, when necessary, is good treatment. When manipulative reduction fails, operative replacement of the displaced radial head should always be done in children under 13 years. In older children it should be done whenever possible, but the radial head may be removed in this age group with relatively little risk of subsequent growth disturbance.

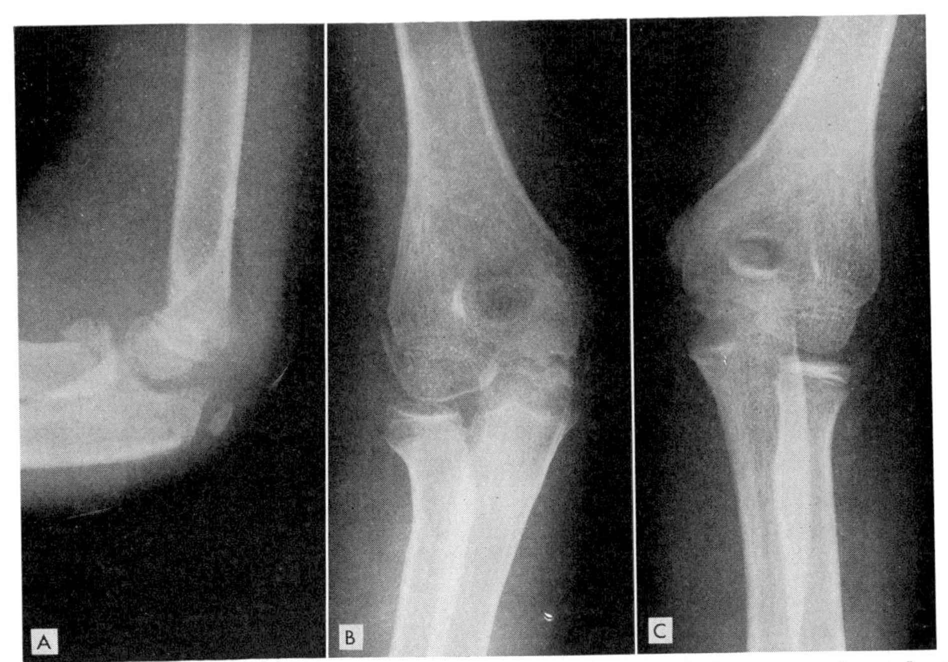

Figure 9–18. Eccentric malunion after displacement of the proximal epiphysis of the radius.

A. Incomplete reduction.

B. The radial head epiphysis is closing early and has healed so that it rotates eccentrically.

C. The normal elbow.

Type IV—Radial Head Fracture with Gross Anterior Displacement

This injury is a concomitant of posterior dislocation of the elbow but, if the dislocation has been reduced, the apparently isolated radial head fracture is a surgical trap. The dire potentialities of the lesion often pass unrecognized, along with the fact that its local pathology constitutes an emergency to be measured in hours. The anterior elbow joint capsule is ruptured and the brachialis muscle lacerated (Fig. 9–*19*, *B*) by the dislocation. The urgency for specific treatment depends not upon the dislocation or the radial head fracture, but upon the small fragment of radial head which, even after reduction of the dislocation, remains displaced in a

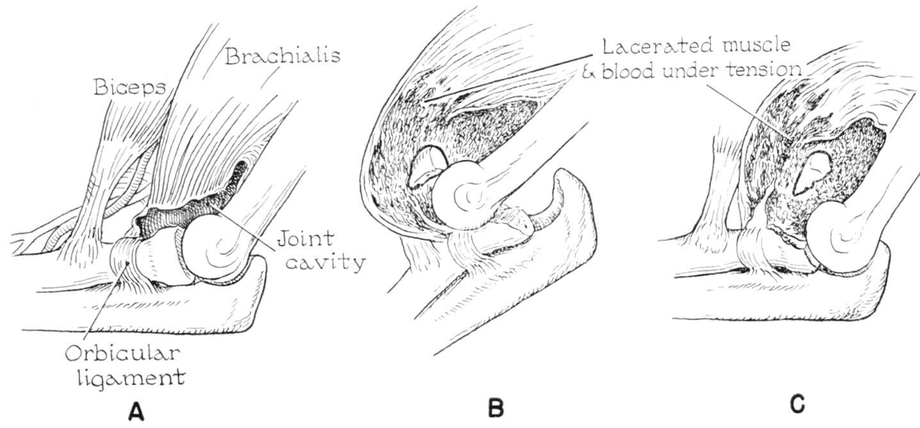

Figure 9–19. Etiology of myositis ossificans at the elbow.

A. Normal relations of elbow.

B. Posterior dislocation, radial head fracture with gross anterior displacement of the fragment, and rupture of the elbow capsule and overlying brachialis.

C. The dislocation is reduced but the radial head fragment remains in a puddle of hemorrhage and damaged muscle to form a nidus for ossification in the hematoma.

puddle of hemorrhage and damaged brachialis muscle (Fig. 9–*19*, *C*). *Myositis ossificans,* producing permanent stiffness of the elbow joint, is to be expected unless appropriate preventive measures are taken *at the earliest possible moment, and not later than 24 hours after the injury* (Fig. 9–*20*).

The writer's experience prior to 1938 was marked by the development of myositis ossificans and some degree of elbow stiffness in 50 per cent of such lesions. Assessment of these unsatisfactory results disclosed certain contributing therapeutic errors, many of which remain common practice, for example:

(1) Removal of the radial head, or fragment, later than 24 hours after injury. Operations done from a few days to a few weeks after injury fail to affect the incidence of myositis ossificans.

(2) Incomplete removal (removal of displaced fragment only) of the radial head.

(3) Operative exposure through a posterior or lateral approach, which failed to decompress the antecubital compartment.

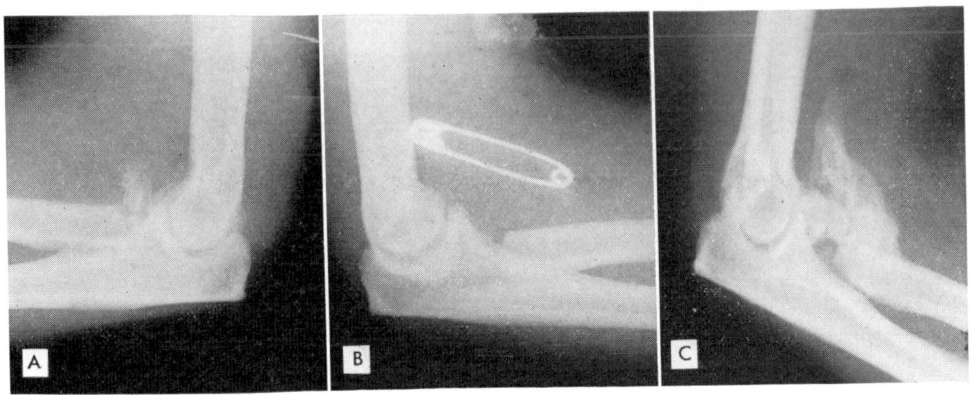

Figure 9–20. Conditions conducive to myositis ossificans.

A. Anterior displacement of radial head fragment following reduction of the concomitant dislocation.

B. Radial head removed late, *through a* lateral approach, *with a* Gigli saw, *and the wound* closed tightly.

C. End-result—a permanently stiff elbow.

(4) Removal of the radial head by a Gigli saw, leaving considerable bone dust in situ.

(5) Incomplete hemostasis, not only of the lacerated soft tissues, but also of the radius stump.

(6) Tight layer-by-layer closure of the operative wound, which serves to perpetuate deep tissue tension.

(7) Energetic aftercare, e.g., heat, massage, forceful exercises, or passive stretching.

Subsequent to 1938, in the writer's experience, myositis ossificans has not developed in any patient with such a lesion, provided therapy embraced the following:

(1) Operation within 24 hours after injury. When this cannot be done, all thoughts of operative treatment should be deferred for several months.

(2) Complete removal of the radial head as well as of all separated fragments.

(3) Removal of the radial head by a sharp instrument (osteotome or rongeur).

(4) Complete hemostasis, including cauterization of the radial stump.

(5) An anterior operative approach which permits decompression of the subfascial antecubital compartment.

(6) Loose closure of the skin and no closure of the deeper fascial layers.

(7) Prohibition of all physiotherapeutic measures during the postoperative period. Gradually increased active motion and use within the limits of pain and fatigue should be encouraged.

DISLOCATION OF THE ELBOW

Posterior dislocation of the radius and ulna from the humerus (Fig. 9–*21, A*) is a common injury resulting from disruption of the elbow liga-

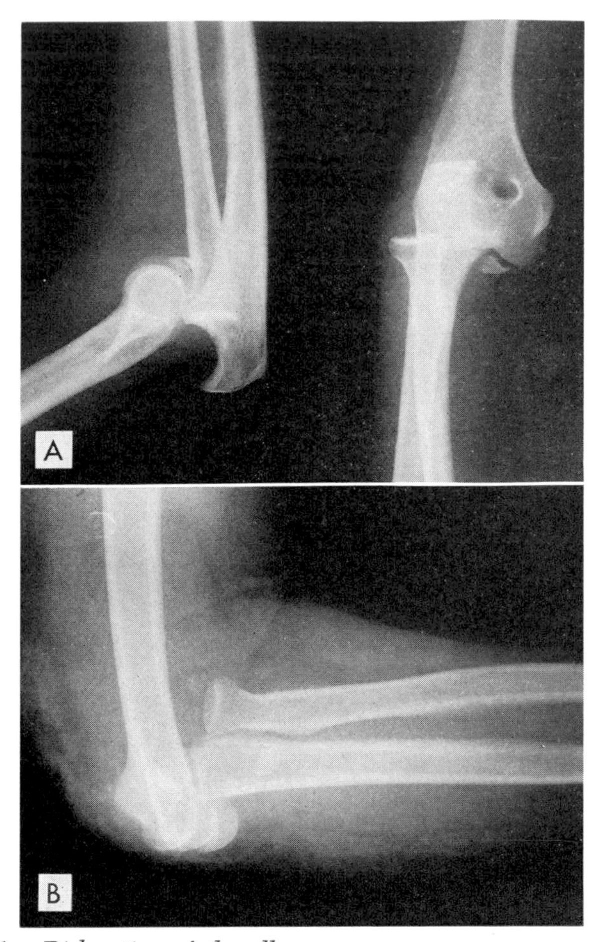

Figure 9–21. Dislocation of the elbow.

A. Posterior dislocation of the elbow with fracture of the coronoid.

B. A pure lateral dislocation of the elbow. Note the marked pathology of the soft parts.

ments by a force applied to the forearm lever. Depending upon the direction of the offending leverage, the disengaged forearm bones may also be displaced in a medial or lateral direction. Pure lateral dislocations (Fig. 9–*21, B*) are less common, and medial displacements are extremely rare. In any event the elbow is greatly deformed, immobile, tender, and painful, and soon becomes markedly swollen. Differentiation from a displaced supracondylar fracture is established by gross distortion of the epicondyle-olecranon relationships. Anatomical distortion also predisposes to frequent concomitant injuries to the nerves and vessels crossing the joint. *The circulatory and neurologic status of the hand must be assessed before and after reduction.*

Reduction by Manipulation

Reduction by force increases soft part damage. Atraumatic reduction depends primarily upon elimination of the massive spasm which locks the forearm bones in their displaced position. Anesthesia is essential. Posterior displacement is corrected by steady gentle traction with the elbow extended. Occasionally preliminary hyperextension for disengagement of the ulnar coronoid process from the olecranon fossa is advisable. A lateral dislocation requires only that the lower end of the humerus be grasped between the surgeon's hands from behind and the forearm bones shifted into proper position by thumb pressure.

Aftercare

The reduction must be confirmed, and concomitant small fractures excluded, by x-ray. The functional integrity of the circulation and nerves distal to the elbow must be certified. Elbow extension must be prevented until the disrupted collateral ligaments and other damaged periarticular soft tissues heal firmly enough to prevent redislocation. This is done by a posterior molded plaster splint with the elbow flexed to a right angle. After three or four weeks, gradually progressive resumption of motion and use within the limits of pain and fatigue should be encouraged. Extension is always the last motion to be regained, and *should never be forced by passive stretching.* Such action is an invitation to catastrophe, and the most common cause of a stiff elbow due to myositis ossificans.

FRACTURE-DISLOCATION OF THE ELBOW

Fracture of Coronoid of Ulna

Chip fracture of the coronoid is a common but clinically insignificant concomitant of elbow dislocation (Fig. 9–*21, A*). The chip displaces and replaces with its parent ulna, to which it remains firmly attached by soft tissues. Eventual bony union is the rule. This lesion is of no therapeutic or prognostic import, except on rare occasions when a major portion of the coronoid is separated from the ulna to jeopardize stability of reduction by mechanical deficiency of the trochlear notch. Under such circumstances open reduction and internal fixation of the displaced coronoid may be required.

Fracture of Radial Head

Radial head fracture by impact against the capitellum during the act of dislocation is not uncommon. The most common and dangerous form of this complication requires urgent and specific treatment. See discussion of Fracture of the Head of the Radius (p. 221).

Avulsion of Medial Epicondyle

It is probable that many avulsed epicondyles included in the elbow joint following reduction were extra-articular prior to manipulation. Extension of the elbow as a preliminary step in the reduction of a pure lateral dislocation may facilitate inclusion of an otherwise extra-articular epicondyle into the joint, and undue opening of the joint by hyperextension of a posterior dislocation also invites this complication. See discussion of Epicondyle Avulsion with Ruptured Elbow Ligaments (p. 215).

Anterior Fracture-Dislocation of Elbow

Occasional anterior dislocations unaccompanied by a fracture of the olecranon or medial humeral condyle are primarily lateral dislocations with secondary forward displacement of the forearm by an appropriate continuing force. The first step in reduction is reproduction of the lateral dislocated position, following which complete correction of the deformity becomes a simple problem. Direct anterior dislocation does not occur, except as a sequel to fracture of either the olecranon or the lower humerus caused by an impact from behind. The point of the elbow is poorly protected by soft parts so that an associated open wound is common. These injuries are severe, anatomical distortion is great, and serious damage to the nerves and vessels crossing the elbow joint is frequent.

Anterior Dislocation with Fracture of Olecranon

A comminuted fracture of the olecranon, which destroys the stabilizing function of the trochlear notch, is the most common concomitant of anterior dislocation. Manipulative reduction and immobilization is rarely successful, but should be attempted in children prior to operative manipulation of injured epiphyses (Fig. 9–22). Stability of reduction depends

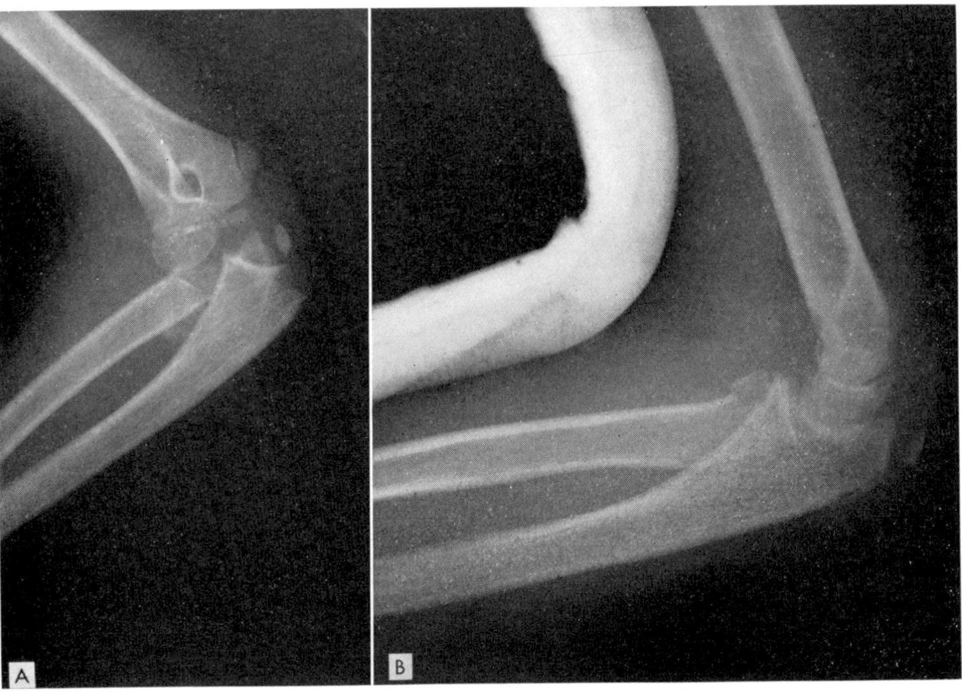

Figure 9–22. Comminuted fracture-dislocation in a child.
A. Before treatment.
B. After manipulative reduction and immobilization in a molded splint. Figure 9–18 shows the late result.

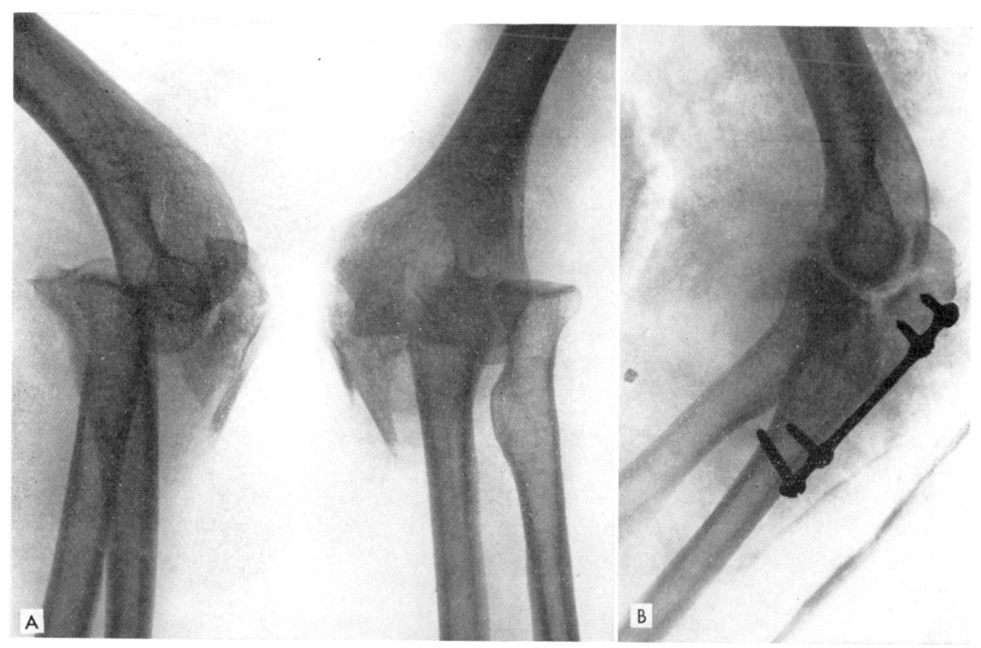

Figure 9–23. Fracture-dislocation with comminuted olecranon and demolition of trochlear notch.

A. Before treatment.

B. After open reduction with reconstruction and internal fixation of the olecranon.

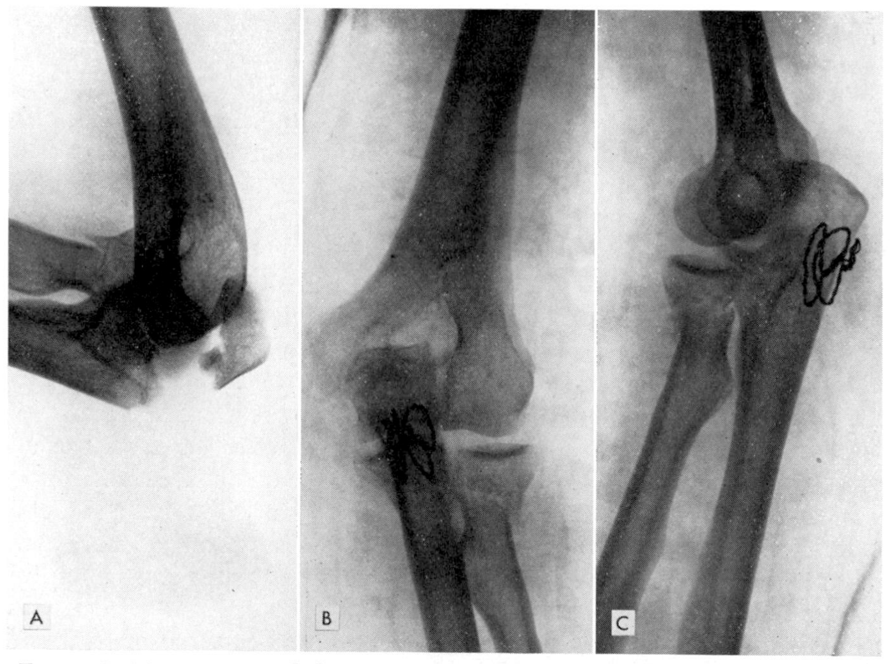

Figure 9–24. Fracture-dislocation with fracture of both olecranon and radial neck.

A. Before treatment.

B, C. After treatment. The olecranon is sufficiently uncomminuted to make suture feasible and the position of the radial fragments is stable.

upon reconstruction of the trochlear notch of the ulna. Open reduction and internal fixation of the olecranon fracture is almost always necessary (Fig. 9–*22;* see also Fig. 9–*23*). When secure fixation can be obtained, aftercare is the same as that for uncomplicated dislocations.

Fracture of the radial head or capitellum may also occur as the forearm bones are driven forward (Fig. 9–*24*). Removal of the radial head or fragment of capitellum, often the procedure of choice in the absence of an associated dislocation, greatly increases the instability of the reduced elbow joint. Such fragments should be replaced whenever their retention contributes to stability. Their excision later, when necessary, is a minor and much safer procedure.

Anterior Dislocation with Fracture of Humerus

This is a most unstable lesion due to comminution and great soft part damage. It is usually impervious to fixation by external immobilization and difficult or impossible to stabilize by internal fixation. Skeletal traction (see Figs. 9–*16*, 9–*9*, and 9–*10*), made possible by an intact olecranon, is the procedure of choice until healing is sufficient to permit continued support by external immobilization.

FRACTURE OF OLECRANON

Olecranon Fracture by Indirect Trauma

Indirect trauma produces an avulsion of the olecranon by violent contraction of the triceps in opposition to forcible elbow flexion. Retraction of the avulsed fragment is proportional to the amount of associated damage suffered by its soft-tissue attachments. When the triceps aponeurosis remains intact the fracture is undisplaced, and the ability to extend the elbow against gravity is preserved. When the triceps aponeurosis is disrupted the avulsed fragment is retracted, but seldom past the upper limit of the olecranon fossa, and active elbow extension is lost. Under any circumstances the objectives of treatment should be maintenance or restoration of triceps function, a smooth trochlear notch, and normal mobility of the joint.

Olecranon avulsion with intact triceps function. The olecranon is fractured, but the fragments are undisplaced, and extension against gravity is preserved (Fig. 9–*25*). The patient requires relief of pain; the elbow requires maintenance of function; and the fracture requires nothing other than protection against external forces which might disrupt the intact soft-part fixation of its fragments. Immobilization is therefore unnecessary. Comfort and protection are provided by a molded splint from shoulder to knuckles, but this should be removed early and often for gradually progressive exercises and use. It should be reapplied for three or four weeks, whenever the patient is exposed to forces beyond his control, and then discarded.

Olecranon avulsion with absent triceps function. The avulsed olecranon is retracted and elbow extension against gravity cannot be maintained (Fig. 9–25). Operative fixation of the fracture and suture of the torn triceps aponeurosis should be carried out without delay. This is a necessary rather than an elective procedure. It is technically adequate only when the status of the local repair becomes comparable to that of an undisplaced fracture with an intact triceps aponeurosis. Once the operative wound has healed, aftercare then requires not immobilization but a program of protection and early mobilization similar to that for undisplaced fractures.

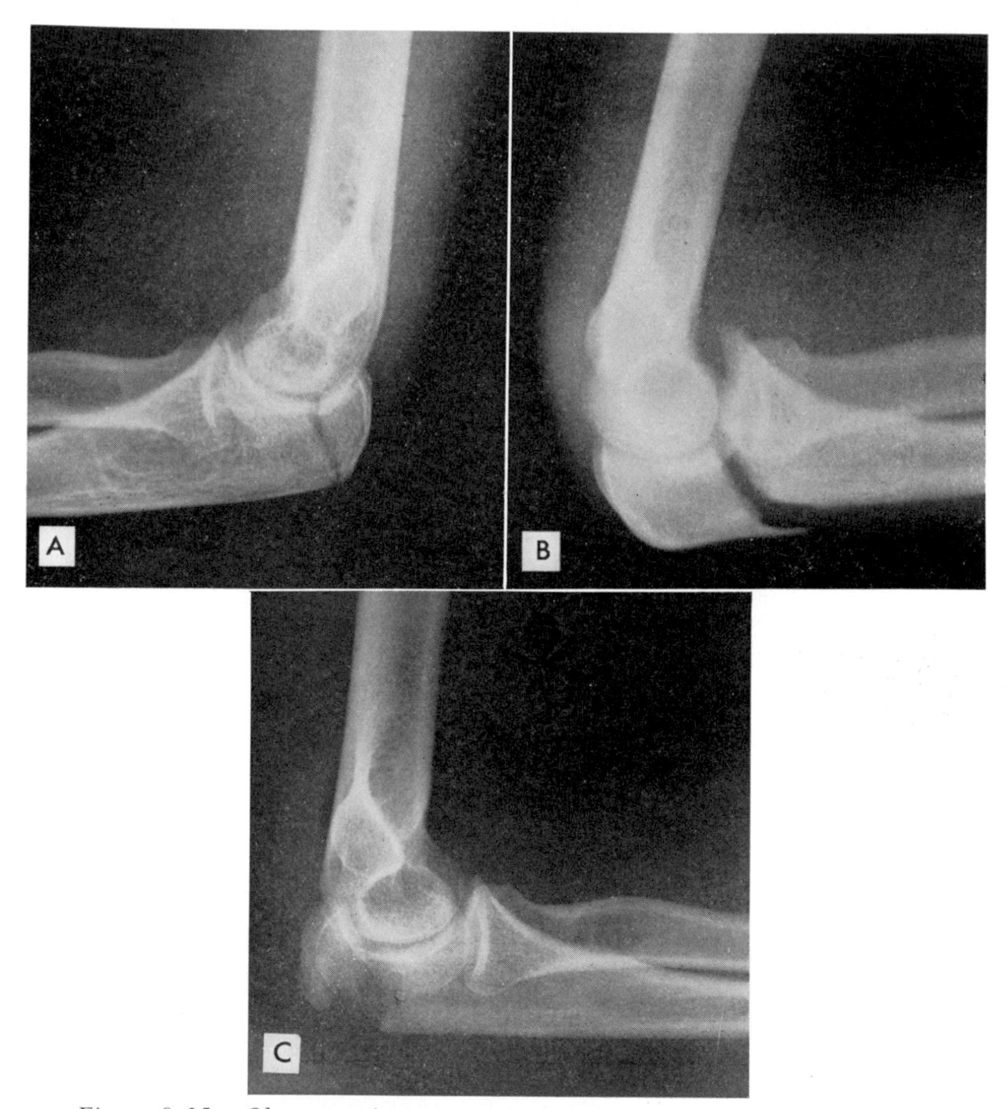

Figure 9–25. Olecranon fracture.

A. With intact triceps function, needing nothing but comfort, protection, and maintenance of motion.

B. With an intact triceps, but a jeopardized trochlear notch. Operative fixation is desirable but, if it is not feasible, the arm must be dressed in full extension.

C. With absent triceps function, requiring operative repair.

Occasionally operative repair cannot be done. If the fragments are separated, early mobilization of the elbow will result in a fibrous union and an elongated triceps. The former may or may not prove to be a significant complication, but the latter inevitably produces weakness of extension power. The elbow should be immobilized by an anterior molded splint *in full extension.* The avulsed fragment is replaced in proper position by digital manipulation, and may be bound firmly into place by snug bandages or adhesive strapping. Immobilization in extension must be continued for four to six weeks, following which attempts to recover motion should be limited to active exercises and use. Convalescence is prolonged over many months, and some permanent motion defect is the rule.

Olecranon Fracture by Direct Impact

These lesions which result from a fall or blow on the point of the elbow may allow anterior dislocation of the forearm bones if more than half of the trochlear notch is involved (p. 228). In lesser injuries the olecranon is comminuted, but remains relatively undisplaced and enclosed within an intact soft-part envelope. Triceps function is preserved. As a rule, some roughening of the articular surface of the trochlear notch is present but, in view of existing comminution, correction by manipulation is impossible, and operative reduction is unsuitable.

The elbow is splinted in 90 degrees flexion for three to five weeks, after which motion is allowed within pain limits. Recovery of function is slow and imperfect; no good and much harm will be caused by attempts to hasten or improve the result by forcible passive stretchings.

In the presence of an open wound or displacement in excess of 1 cm. operative treatment may become mandatory, and small displaced fragments may be removed or replaced, as circumstances dictate. When necessary, as much as the proximal half of the olecranon may be removed without serious effect, so long as the triceps is firmly reattached to the remaining stump of bone.

CHAPTER 10

INJURIES OF THE SHOULDER AND ARM

By HARRISON L. McLAUGHLIN, M.D.

ANATOMICAL FEATURES OF THE SHOULDER

THE SKELETON of the shoulder girdle is composed of the clavicle, scapula, and humerus. The clavicle and scapula are suspended from the vertebral column by the trapezius, rhomboid, and levator scapulae muscles (see Fig. 10–2). The scapula is held out from the thorax by the clavicle, which, by bridging the gap between sternum and acromion, constitutes the only rigid connection between the upper extremity and the remainder of the skeleton (Fig. 10–*1*). The inner end of the clavicular strut is provided with stable mobility by the costoclavicular ligament, which maintains it in close relationship to the first rib, and by ligaments circumferentially incorporated into the capsule of the sternoclavicular joint (Fig. 10–*1*). This is a universal joint which moves only through a small range, but which participates in almost every motion of the shoulder girdle mechanism. The scapula is suspended from the clavicle by the coracoclavicular ligaments

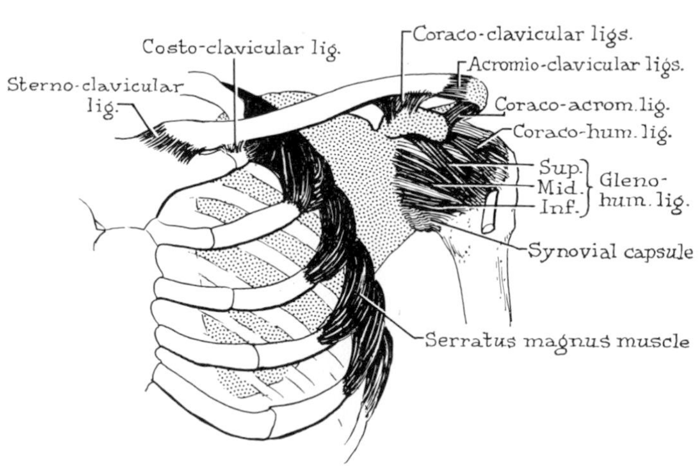

Figure 10–1. Ligaments of shoulder girdle and serratus magnus muscle.

The serratus magnus muscle arises from the vertebral edge of the anterior surface of the scapula and inserts into the anterior wall of the thoracic cage. It holds the scapula against the chest wall and is the main motor for moving the entire shoulder girdle forward.

(Fig. 10–*1*), and the acromioclavicular articulation is supported by ligaments incorporated into its joint capsule. The clavicular strut prevents the scapula from sliding too far forward on the thoracic cage, and the tone of the serratus magnus muscle prevents its sliding backward. The inferior angle of the scapula is stabilized by a small slip of the latissimus dorsi muscle (see Fig. 10–*4*), and by the actions of the teres major and minor muscles (Fig. 10–*2*).

The glenohumeral joint is a modified type of ball-and-socket joint, but not in a mechanical sense. The hemispherical humeral head rests against, rather than within, the only slightly concave glenoid. The synovial capsule is weak and loose, has a capacity 50 per cent greater than that of the humeral head which it encloses, and is but sparsely supported by ligaments. A tripartite sling of glenohumeral ligaments supports the anterior aspect of the joint capsule and defends against anterior dislocation of the humerus (Fig. 10–*1;* see also Fig. 10–*16*), but tendons are substituted for ligaments to support the remainder of this joint. The coracohumeral ligament (Fig. 10–*1*) extends downward and forward from the lateral aspect of the coracoid and blends with the fibers of the supraspinatus tendon as they insert into the humerus.

The coraco-acromial ligament (Fig. 10–*1*) is a purely scapular structure that forms an arch under which the tuberosities of the humerus must pass when the arm is elevated.

The movements of the shoulder are a product of many complex muscle motors acting upon four joints. The glenohumeral and both clavicular joints are universal joints, and the scapula is extremely mobile. Every muscle has multiple actions which change, and sometimes are reversed, depending upon the positions of the three bones involved when action commences. Consequently, the number of combinations are almost unlimited. A complete comprehension of the muscle dynamics of the shoulder is virtually impossible, but a working knowledge of the muscles responsible for gross motion patterns is essential to the surgeon.

Internal rotation results from synchronized actions of the subscapularis, pectoralis major, teres major, and latissimus dorsi muscles (Fig. 10–*2*). The total force is formidable and greatly in excess of that available for external rotation, which is produced mainly by the supraspinatus, infraspinatus, and teres minor (Fig. 10–*2*). The posterior fibers of the deltoid are potential external rotators; the anterior fibers, internal rotators.

Adduction is the total product of the action of the pectoralis major, teres major, and latissimus dorsi (Fig. 10–*2*), as well as of all of the intrinsic muscles below the level of the pivot point of humeral elevation (see Fig. 10–*26*). This also is a formidable force and greatly in excess of that available for abduction, which depends mainly upon the intrinsic muscle forces superior to the humeral head and the deltoid, with contributions by the serratus magnus and the trapezius.

Mechanics of abduction. It would be impossible for one man to raise a long ladder to a standing position if it was lying upon a smooth surface. As soon as he picked up one end, the other would slide. However, if a

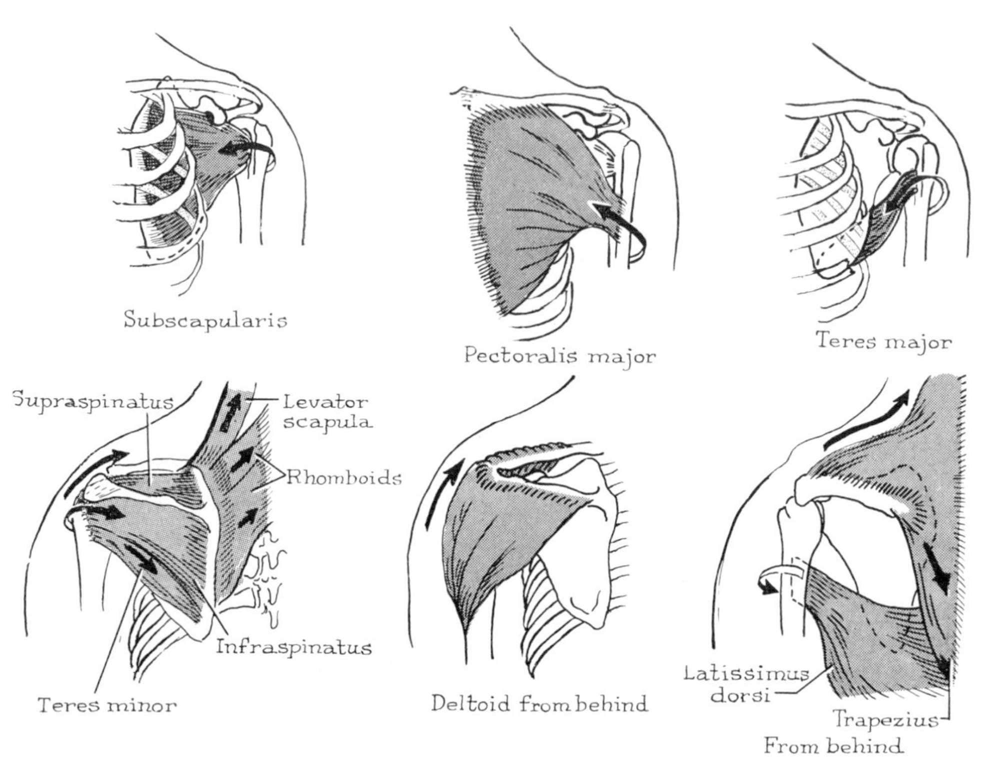

Figure 10–2. Muscles of shoulder girdle (except serratus magnus).

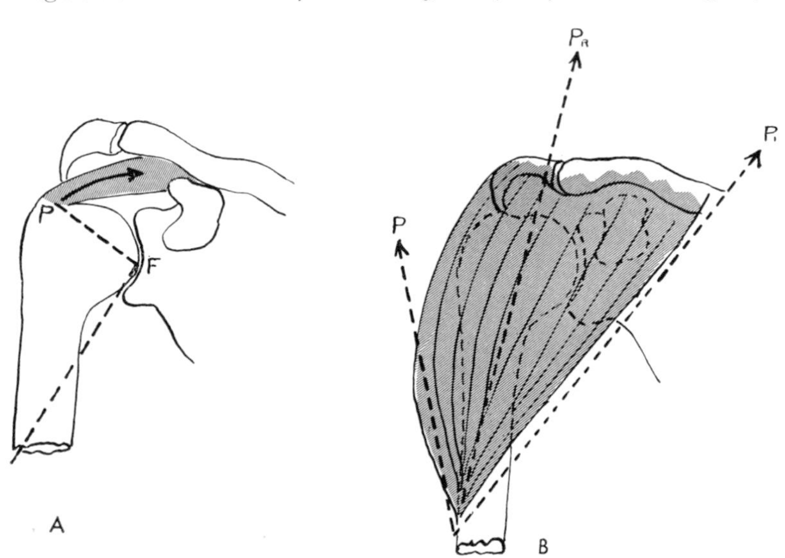

Figure 10–3. Mechanics of abduction.

A. That portion of the intrinsic muscle cuff superior to the humeral head applies power to the short arm of the lever PF and provides a sliding fulcrum on the glenoid.

B. Force of the outer fibers of the deltoid P would produce a fulcrum on the acromion. Force of the inner fibers, P_I, could provide a fulcrum on the glenoid only in adduction. The resultant force of all deltoid fibers, P_R, merely lifts the humerus toward the acromion.

Only when the glenohumeral joint is stabilized by the intrinsic muscles has the powerful deltoid a fulcrum over which it can abduct the limb.

second man merely put his foot against the far end of the ladder, the first man could raise it to a standing position with ease. It is equally impossible for the deltoid alone to elevate the limb, or to do more than slide the humeral head toward the acromion, until the intrinsic muscles simultaneously stabilize the glenohumeral fulcrum (Fig. 10–3).

THE SCAPULA

The scapula has three main functions: (1) to connect the upper limb to the remainder of the skeleton via the clavicle; (2) to articulate with the humerus, and (3) to provide attachment for many muscles with widely divergent forces. All or any part of it may be ablated subperiosteally or along with the associated muscles at a surprisingly small cost to total shoulder function. Total subperiosteal removal occasionally is required for the control of osteomyelitis and leaves a comfortable, useful limb, which is difficult to raise above the horizontal. Neoplasm may require removal of all associated musculature, as well as the bone. The result is a flail shoulder and a limb that is comfortable and useful only when it is dependent. Partial scapulectomy, except when the glenoid is removed, is followed by little or no functional defect.

INJURIES OF THE SCAPULA

Fractures of Body of Scapula

These uncommon lesions result from a combination of direct violence and the sudden contractions of divergent muscles. The strong fasciae enclosing the intrinsic muscles limit displacement of the fragments, but great tension and pain may be produced because they also enclose hemorrhage and other products of tissue damage. Manipulative reduction approaches the impossible, and even when the position can be improved fixation is prevented by the many muscle forces involved. Fortunately, the penalty of malunion is consistently negligible, except when a large fragment or mass of callus encroaches upon the interscapulothoracic space to produce pressure symptoms. Removal of the offending fragment or callus may be expected to produce relief.

Treatment. Reduction and fixation are unattainable, and normal bony anatomy is not necessary to good function. The essentials of treatment, therefore, are directed to control of pain and maintenance of function. Early infiltration of the tense subfascial spaces with a mixture of procaine hydrochloride and hyaluronidase accelerates decompression and relief of pain. The weight of the arm should be removed from the scapula by use of a sling, or by bed rest with the limb in balanced suspension. Rest of the part for a short time is justifiable, but *immobilization may produce a stiff shoulder*. Gravity-free motion should commence within a few days, and gradually progressive resumption of use should be encouraged from the start. Comfort and usefulness may be anticipated within a few weeks, but maximal recovery will not be present until after several months.

Complications. These fractures result from great violence. The dorsal spine and thoracic cage or its contents are prone to coincident damage, which may remain masked by the more superficial injury, or may be so severe that the fractured scapula becomes a matter of minor import in the over-all picture.

Fractures of Neck of Scapula

These fractures are usually comminuted and often impacted. Disimpaction and correction are difficult to accomplish and maintain by any means. Bed rest with the limb in balanced suspension is continued until the stage of severe pain is over, and then a progressive program of exercises and gradually increasing resumption of use should be prescribed. A slow but satisfactory recovery is to be expected.

Fractures of Coracoid Process

The coracoid process is most commonly fractured by impact of the dislocating humeral head, but may also be avulsed by violent muscle contraction. When the coracoclavicular and coraco-acromial ligaments remain intact, gross displacement is prevented. Fibrous union of the fracture is not uncommon. No treatment, other than that for dislocation, is needed and no residual defect follows upon the fibrous union.

Avulsion of Glenoid Rim (by Triceps)

This injury is peculiar to athletes and is usually caused by a violent throwing motion. The avulsed fragment varies between 0.5 and 1 cm. in diameter. It may be devoid of a sharp profile in the roentgenogram and is easily mistaken for a calcium deposit. Displacement seldom exceeds 0.5 cm., and it would appear that the majority of such lesions remain asymptomatic. Fibrous union is common. Occasionally a wincing pain is produced by jamming of the fragment of bone between humeral head and glenoid as the arm is drawn back, as for throwing or batting in baseball. Ablation of the fragments is followed by complete relief of symptoms.

Fractures of Acromion

These are uncommon. External trauma to the acromion usually disrupts the acromioclavicular joint rather than the bone. Occasionally the acromion may be fractured by a humeral impact (see Fig. 10–23). Usually the displacement is mild. Bony union is the rule, despite the presence or absence of immobilization, provided the fragments are in apposition. Fibrous union occasionally follows failure to recognize that soft tissues are interposed between the fragments. Symptomatic nonunion or malunion can be relieved by subperiosteal removal of enough acromion to include the offending lesion.

Fracture of Inferior Angle

Avulsion of the inferior angle by the teres major may occur. The size of the bone fragment and the amount of displacement are variable, but in any event reduction and fixation are impossible, except by operative measures. Symptoms should be controlled and function maintained. Gross displacement of a large fragment may warrant early operative replacement and suture, or the displaced fragment may be removed, but the majority of such lesions respond well to expectant therapy. Persistent late pain is relieved by removal of the fragment.

Violent lifting strains often produce a partial rupture of the fasciculus of the latissimus dorsi attaching at the inferior angle of the scapula (Fig. 10–4). The diagnosis is made on a history of sudden lifting strain accompanied by a sharp pain which persists at the inferior scapular angle. The area is tender, and pain is accentuated by passive stretch or active contraction against resistance of the latissimus. X-ray films are negative, and other local causes for pain are excluded. Little except symptomatic therapy is possible or necessary. Spontaneous recovery is the rule, but a protracted period of pain is to be expected if heavy labor is continued.

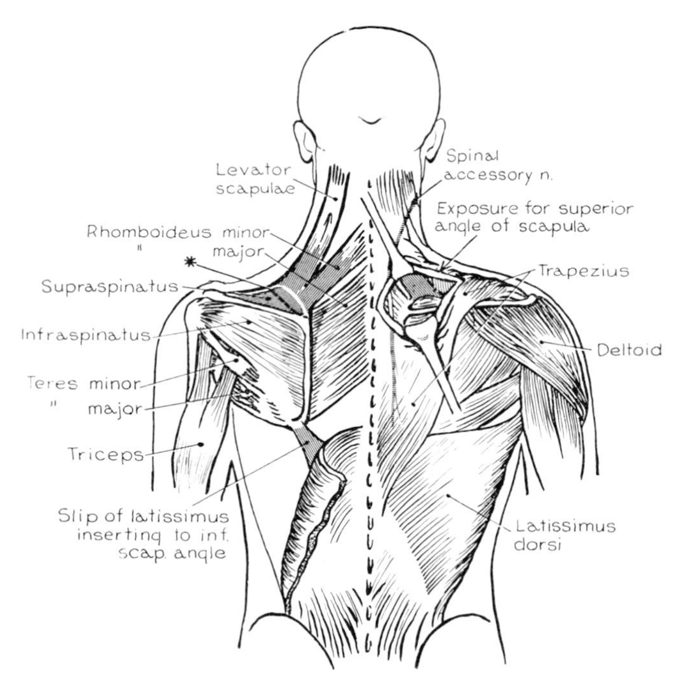

Figure 10–4. Muscles of scapular region.

Note the location of the small slip of latissimus dorsi which inserts into the inferior angle of the scapula and may be damaged by lifting strains.

Chronic spasm may produce pain and tenderness at the insertion of the levator scapulae. Palliation may require subperiosteal removal of the superomedial angle of the scapula as outlined on the left (*) through the operative approach indicated on the right. The spinal accessory nerve must be protected from operative damage.

Injuries of Superior Angle—Grating Scapula, Scapulothoracic Syndrome, etc.

The superomedial angle may be cracked by direct violence to the "winged" scapula, but this lesion is rare and there is usually no displacement. Involvement by callus or scar, partial rupture, or chronic irritation of the inserting fibers of the levator scapulae muscle is much more common. The resultant "scapulothoracic" syndrome may be no more than a nuisance but often amounts to a real disability. The basic pathology is similar to that of the more widely recognized tennis elbow or lateral epicondylitis.

The clinical picture is pain in the back of the shoulder, aggravated by use of the limb and not always relieved by rest. It is unaffected by motion of the cervical spine, and the painful area, unlike the somewhat similar situation resulting from a cervical disc lesion, is the seat of localized tenderness. The onset of symptoms is preceded by some sudden lifting strain, or by long-continued occupation requiring constant use of the limb in a position of forward flexion. It is a common complaint of the infantry soldier who constantly hunches the shoulders to adjust his pack. Obliteration of symptoms by infiltration of the tender area with procaine hydrochloride clinches the diagnosis. The crepitus which led to the term "grating scapula" is not always present.

Palliative measures will fail until the patient ceases the activities which irritate the levator mechanism. A change of job usually is followed by relief. Persistently painful lesions are consistently relieved by subperiosteal excision of the angle of the scapula (Fig. 10–*4*).

NERVE INJURIES

Brachial Plexus Traction Injuries

The brachial plexus is derived from the roots of the fifth cervical to the first thoracic nerves (Fig. 10–5). Each is snubbed to its transverse process by fasciculi of prevertebral fascia. This stabilization of the roots, which is relatively weak at birth, is a safeguard against the transmission of traction to the spinal cord. Consequently, traction injuries produce a preponderance of root damage in the newborn, but cause more distally placed nerve trunk damage in the adult. As the cords of the plexus approach the coracoid after passing between the clavicle and the first rib, they are fixed to both of these bones, along with the axillary artery, by the clavipectoral fascia. Just distal to this point all cords pass under the coracoid. These anatomical features account for the mechanics of traction injuries to the brachial plexus (Fig. 10–5). Any force which tends to increase the distance between the two points of fascial fixation stretches the nerves. Abduction of the arm stretches the nerves under the pulley of the coracoid, and addition of external rotation accentuates this stretch. Contralateral deviation of the head or depression of the shoulder stretches the nerves over the pulley of the first rib, and,

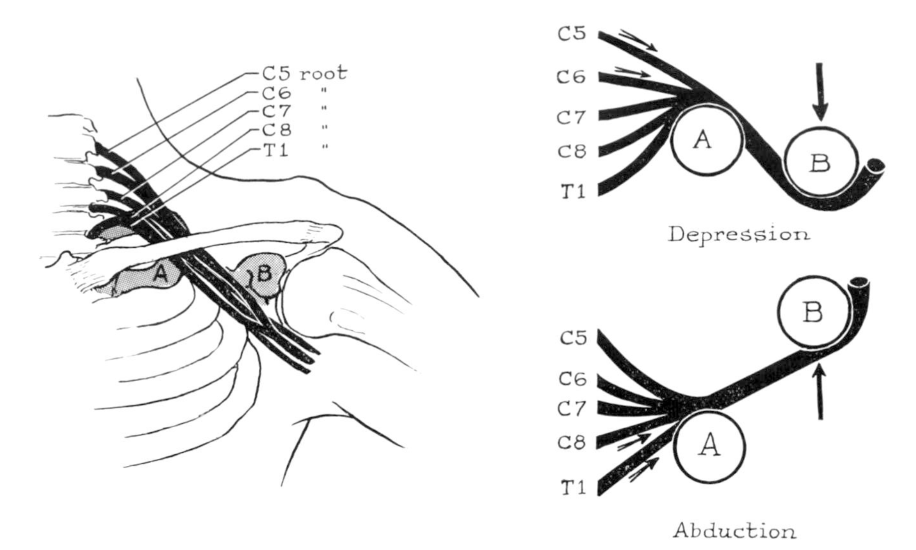

Figure 10–5. Stretch injury to brachial plexus.

The nerve roots, C5 to T1, of the brachial plexus are snubbed to the transverse processes of the respective vertebrae, and are fixed by the clavipectoral fascia between the clavicle and the first rib. The first rib (A) and the coracoid (B) act as pulleys over which traction injuries to the nerves are produced. When the shoulder is depressed violently the upper elements of the brachial plexus receive the brunt of the stretching impact; conversely, when the arm is forcibly hyperabducted the nerves are pulled taut under the pulley of the coracoid and the lower elements are more likely to be injured. Most traction injuries produce a mixed upper and lower type of brachial plexus lesion.

if the shoulder is forced backward, the nerves not only are stretched but may also be compressed between clavicle and rib. Treatment of a stretch injury to the brachial plexus is usually fruitless.

Erb-Duchenne or "Upper Type" Birth Palsy

This rather loosely used term implies birth damage to the fifth and sixth cervical roots. There is paralysis of the spinati, deltoid, biceps, brachialis, and brachioradialis muscles. The levator scapulae, rhomboids, and serratus are less commonly involved, depending upon the level of the damage. The shoulder sags, the arm hangs limp in internal rotation, and the wrist is pronated. If the deformity is allowed to persist, posterior subluxation of the humeral head from the glenoid is to be expected.

Treatment requires that the deformity be overcome, and the weight of the limb removed from the shoulder. A brace which maintains the limb in abduction and external rotation accomplishes both purposes. The mother is instructed in a program of passive motion of the paralyzed joints and gentle massage. The speed and completeness of recovery are surprising in many infants.

Klumpke-Déjerine or "Lower Type" Birth Palsy

This syndrome involves the eighth cervical and first dorsal roots. Sensory changes are much more marked than in upper type lesions, and vasomotor phenomena may occur. The flexors and extensors of the forearm and the intrinsic muscles of the hand are paralyzed. The triceps is involved, but the wrist extensors and supinator and pronator teres remain intact. Operative redistribution of the remaining intact muscle motors to compensate for those which are without function is the only available treatment.

Traction Injuries in Older Children and Adults

These injuries follow no consistent pattern, are of a mixed upper and lower type lesion, and rarely if ever conform to the classic syndromes encountered in the newborn. Violent traumas may produce an actual rupture of nerves, or may stretch and tear fibers of both the nerve trunks and their fascial investments. The result is hemorrhage and eventual scarring and adhesion formation. Therefore, when the trauma is one of violence, early exploration should be contemplated with the idea of nerve suture or fascial sheath decompression and of obtaining hemostasis designed to minimize eventual fibrous tissue formation.

Many such injuries result not from violence but from continued traction. Hyperabduction of the limb for blood pressure readings or intravenous medication during anesthesia is the classical and too frequent example. Spontaneous eventual recovery of such lesions may be expected after a period more often measured in months than in weeks. During the paralytic period the involved muscles should be supported by appropriate splints and may be kept somewhat in tone by electrical stimulation.

Pressure Injuries of Brachial Plexus and Its Branches

The nerves involved and muscles paralyzed depend upon the area of pressure. *Crutch paralysis* is usually the fault of the surgeon. Every patient given crutches must be warned against the consequences of carrying his weight on his arm pits, and be taught to carry his weight on his hands. He should be checked frequently for evidences of axillary pressure on the nerves. Crutch walking should cease immediately with the first sign of a neurological deficit and should not be recommenced until complete recovery occurs. *Shoulder braces during anesthesia* in a high Trendelenburg position may produce nerve damage by pressure in the posterior cervical triangle. *Saturday night paralysis* results from sleeping with the limb hanging over the arm of a chair in a position appropriate for nerve pressure. *A displaced fragment* of a fractured clavicle may contuse or even lacerate the brachial plexus cords, and most commonly involves the ulnar tract. *Tumors* in the neck and occasionally an *aneurysm of the subclavian artery* are infrequent offenders. *Fracture and/or dislocation of a cervical vertebra* and *protrusion of a cervical intervertebral disc* may involve the nerve roots by pressure.

Dislocation of the shoulder is commonly complicated by signs of traction or pressure upon the axillary nerve.

INJURIES TO INDIVIDUAL NERVES

Spinal Accessory (Trapezius)

This nerve is superficially placed and quite vulnerable to incisional injury as it traverses the superior apex of the posterior cervical triangle. It is not infrequently divided by a careless surgeon in the course of some minor procedure for incision and drainage of suppuration, or the removal of enlarged nodes from the side of the neck. The trapezius is paralyzed to produce a consistent deformity marked by shrinkage at the base of the neck, sagging of the shoulder, and a rotation of the scapula toward the humerus. There is weakness in hunching the shoulder and elevating the limb. An attempt should be made to repair the nerve by direct suture and, if this proves impossible, the descending hypoglossal nerve may be anastomosed to the distal segment of the spinal accessory with expectations of some improvement.

Long Thoracic Nerve of Bell (Serratus)

An isolated lesion of this nerve may be caused by pressure in the neck, but most frequently it is seen in association with occupations which require repeated heavy lifting with the arms elevated, or the carrying of heavy weights on the shoulder. The characteristic deformity is a "winging" of the scapula, which is most marked when the patient pushes against a wall with the arms horizontal. There is a weakness in lifting and considerable difficulty in elevation of the arm owing to impaired fixation of the scapula. Spontaneous recovery is to be expected, if the primary offending activity is discontinued. During the period of paralysis, however, the weight of the limb should be removed from the scapula by use of some form of brace or sling.

Axillary or Circumflex Nerve (Deltoid, Teres Minor)

Strangely enough, the axillary nerve is rarely injured by fractures at the surgical neck of the humerus around which it winds, but it is frequently injured by one type of anterior dislocation of the shoulder (p. 252). Absence of motor power cannot be demonstrated in a dislocated shoulder, but examination will disclose some sensory deficit in about 25 per cent of all cases of anterior dislocation. Usually this deficit disappears almost immediately following reduction of the dislocation. When evidence of axillary nerve damage persists, it usually proves to be but one manifestation of a brachial plexus traction injury involving the upper cords, mainly the fifth cervical. Deltoid paralysis resulting from axillary damage is occasionally compensated for by hypertrophy of the spinati so that very little disability exists, but most patients have great difficulty in abduction and few can move the hand to their hip pocket until nerve function returns.

Pseudoparalysis of the deltoid is a consistent manifestation of complete avulsion of the rotator cuff tendons from the humerus in the aged patient. Some 20 such lesions have been encountered by the writer, and most of them had been diagnosed as an axillary nerve lesion. It is worthy of note that in the absence of rotator cuff action the deltoid is powerless to abduct the arm due to instability of the glenohumeral fulcrum. The differential diagnosis depends upon the demonstration of intact sensory function of the axillary nerve, and often a mild inferior subluxation of the humerus. In doubtful lesions this may be confirmed by electrical tests. If the humerus remains subluxated for more than a short time, signs of brachial plexus damage due to traction usually supervene to confuse the picture.

Conservative treatment of paralyzed deltoid. For many years support of the arm in an abduction brace has been the accepted and unquestioned procedure. The validity of this is questionable. The position of abduction relaxes only the central segment of the deltoid, but the anterior and posterior segments, as well as the teres minor and the axillary nerve, are maintained at a relative stretch. Removal of the weight of the limb from the deltoid by a sling in the dependent position is more compatible with the anatomical features involved, and certainly is much more comfortable for the patient.

DISLOCATION OF THE SHOULDER

The glenohumeral joint is an unstable mechanism. The relatively oversized humeral head is held against, rather than within, the small and shallow glenoid cavity by muscular control. Ligamentous support is absent, except for that provided by the glenohumeral ligaments. The acromion prevents upward and gross backward displacement of the humerus. The only inelastic protection against forward displacement is the glenohumeral ligament sling. The inferior aspect of the joint is virtually unprotected, except by muscles. Under normal circumstances, before the humerus can displace enough to place a strain on the acromion or glenohumeral ligaments, the first line of defense against dislocation must falter. This is the synchronized stabilizing action of all the muscles crossing the joint (Fig. 10–*6*). Consequently, dislocation may result from a major trauma, which overpowers the muscles, or from a lesser injury, which catches them off guard.

The soft, large, and redundant joint capsule is little protection against dislocation, except in its anterior and antero-inferior parts, where it is reinforced by the glenohumeral ligaments. In order to allow the great range of motion of the shoulder the actual capacity of the capsule is much greater than the enclosed humeral head (Fig. 10–7; see also Fig. 10–*1*). On the superior and posterior aspects of the joint the capsule blends with the inserting fibers of the rotator cuff tendons, and anteriorly both capsule and glenohumeral ligaments fuse with the deep surface of the subscapularis tendon at its insertion. Their anatomic location makes the external rotators

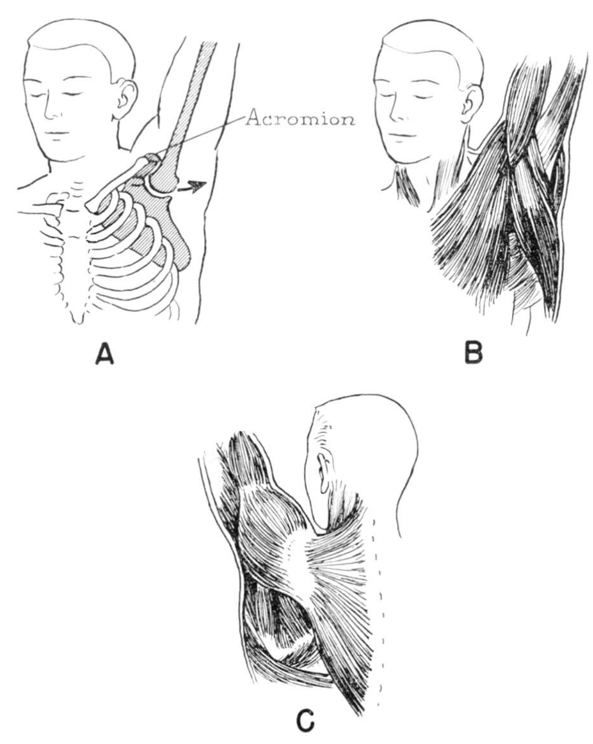

Figure 10–6.

A. Elevation of the arm tends to lever the humeral head out of the glenoid fossa over the fulcrum of the acromion.

B, C. Displacement of the humerus is counteracted by the support of all the muscles crossing the shoulder joint.

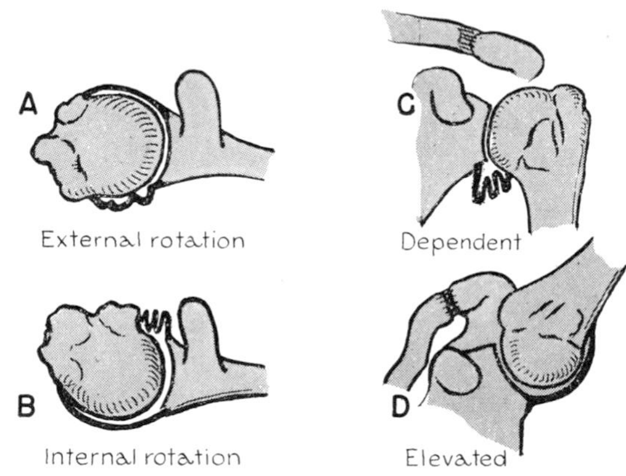

Figure 10–7. Redundancy of the shoulder capsule is a prerequisite to the great range of motion available in this joint. The capacity of the joint capsule is much greater than the humeral head which it contains. Consequently, few dislocations of the humerus are extracapsular. External rotation (A) and elevation (D) place the anterior and inferior (least protected) portions of the capsular structures on stretch.

a defense against anterior, and the subscapularis a defense against posterior dislocation.

PRIMARY ANTERIOR DISLOCATION OF THE SHOULDER

Forward dislocation of the humerus from the glenoid requires disruption of the structures supporting either the front (glenohumeral ligaments) or the back (external rotator tendons) of the joint. When the weaker of the two gives way the other is usually spared (Fig. 10–8). There is good evidence that during youth, and regardless of the mechanics of the injury, the anterior joint supports are disrupted and the dislocating humerus drags the intact external rotator tendons across the face of the glenoid cavity. During the third and fourth decades the incidence of disruption is about equally divided between the anterior and posterior joint supports. After age 40 the average humeral head has become relatively brittle, and the intrinsic tendons are weakened by attritional changes. The anterior supports then give way in only about 10 per cent of dislocations, and the usual disruption takes place in the external rotator tendons or, even more commonly, in the tuberosity into which they insert. In these circumstances the intact anterior supports of the joint act as a hinge upon which the humeral head swings into the dislocated position. It is of interest that the great majority of neurological complications accompany this type of dislocation. Possibly the intact anterior capsular hinge may pull the displacing humerus down

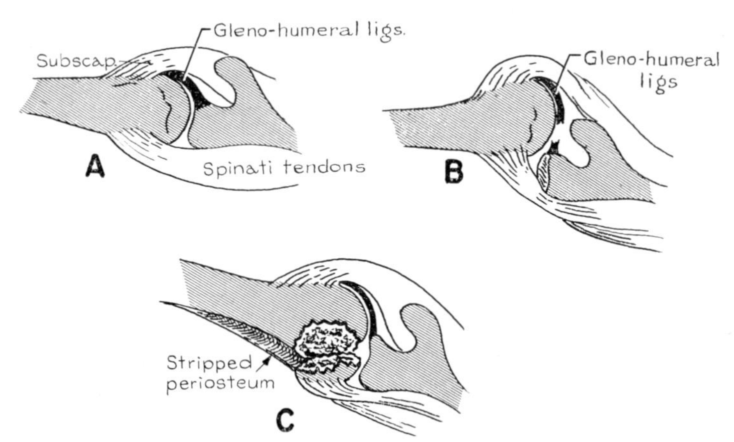

Figure 10–8. Section of left shoulder viewed from above with arm abducted.

A. Anterior displacement of the humerus is defended by the glenohumeral ligaments supporting the front of the joint and the pull of the spinati tendons from behind. When one of these supports gives way to allow anterior dislocation the other is usually spared.

B. Glenohumeral ligaments ruptured—the dislocating humerus drags the spinati tendons behind it across the glenoid.

C. Posterior supports disrupted—the humerus dislocated forward and the intact but redundant anterior supports act as a hinge to guide the direction and final location of the humerus. It is in this type of dislocation that the great majority of nerve injuries are encountered.

into close proximity with the nerve trunks, whereas when the anterior capsule gives way it might more easily stay above them.

Diagnosis

The acromion is unduly prominent and there is an absence of the subacromial fullness normally produced by the humeral head (Fig. 10–9).

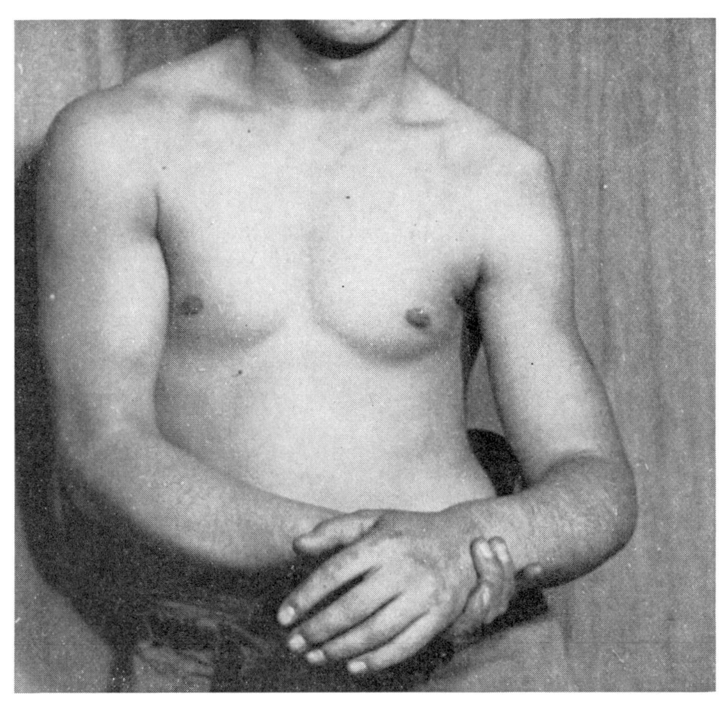

Figure 10–9. Dislocation of the left shoulder, of 30 minutes' duration. Compare the visible abnormality of the left shoulder with the clinical signs of dislocation.

The long axis of the arm points to the base of the neck when it is viewed from in front, and points anteriorly to the acromion when it is viewed from the side. Little movement is possible, and pain is severe. The displaced humeral head may be palpated deep to the pectoral mass. The elbow cannot be made to touch the side. A straight edge can be made to touch the acromion and lateral epicondyle simultaneously. The palpable absence of the humerus from its usual position below the acromion is obvious. Measurement from acromion to lateral epicondyle is equal to or greater than that in the other arm. *If this measurement is definitely shortened,* beware of fracture-dislocation, and consequent greater danger of brachial plexus damage from manipulations of any type. No diagnosis is complete until the neurologic and the vascular status of the limb have been assessed.

Reduction

Coincident with dislocation, all muscles in and around the shoulder joint go into strong protective spasm, thereby locking the humeral head in its displaced position. Obliteration of this spasm is by far the most important feature of any reduction procedure, for in the absence of muscle forces to maintain malposition the humerus slips back into the glenoid with the greatest of ease, *unless prevented by some interposed structure*. The essence of any reduction, therefore, is (1) reduction of pain and, *ipso facto*, reduction of spasm by anesthesia or opiates; and (2) traction to stretch the contracted but relaxing muscles. These alone will reduce all uncomplicated early lesions. When steady traction under anesthesia for 30 seconds fails to effect reduction, it usually means that a small irregularity of humeral head is hooked on the lip of the glenoid, and gentle rotatory motions will clear such an obstruction in short order. Countertraction is rarely needed in a heavy person and, when it is required, is most safely supplied by an axillary swathe, rather than by the operator's foot in the axilla.

The Hippocratic method of reduction, consisting of manual traction on the wrist against countertraction of the operator's foot in the axilla, is an inheritance from the era antedating anesthesia. It is efficient in generating sufficient power to overcome existing spasm by brute force alone. With spasm controlled by anesthesia or opiates the maneuver is unnecessary. When used skillfully by a surgeon well versed in the anatomy of the region it is safe. Under other circumstances it incurs a real risk of catastrophe.

Kocher's method of reduction was designed as a manipulation to guide the humeral head back into normal position. With adequate relaxation by opiates or anesthesia this maneuver is no longer necessary, except in lesions of 36 or more hours' duration, after which muscle spasm is augmented by edema and tissue organization. The patient is supine and under general anesthesia. The elbow is flexed to a right angle. Steady traction is then made in the line of the humeral shaft. As the muscles commence to give, the wrist is grasped and slowly the arm is brought into full external rotation. At this point reduction often occurs. If it does not, the elbow is then carried slowly across the front of the chest, using the thorax as a fulcrum to lever the humeral head in the direction of the glenoid. Once reduced, the arm is brought back into internal rotation. All movements must be slow and steady and, *above all,* gentle. Forceful or snapping maneuvers can do nothing but harm.

Reduction without anesthesia or opiates can be accomplished in most uncomplicated early lesions. Place the patient prone on a table so that the involved limb is hanging over the edge and clear of the floor. Make him as comfortable as possible and leave him there. The dislocation will reduce spontaneously when the weight of the arm tires and relaxes the spastic musculature.

Regardless of the technique employed, it is safe to postulate that, following adequate reduction of muscle spasm, the early dislocation which fails to reduce after steady gentle traction in the line of the humerus, coupled with slight rotatory motions, contains an unrecognized complicating feature which may prevent reduction by any form of manipulation. It is folly to try for reduction through force, and worse to do many repeated unsuccessful manipulations, each of which is less likely to succeed than the preceding. When a dislocation refuses to reduce, the surgeon should stop and find out the reason.

Complications Militating against Reduction

Biceps tendon interposition. Fracture of the greater tuberosity accompanying dislocation may involve the bicipital groove to such an extent as

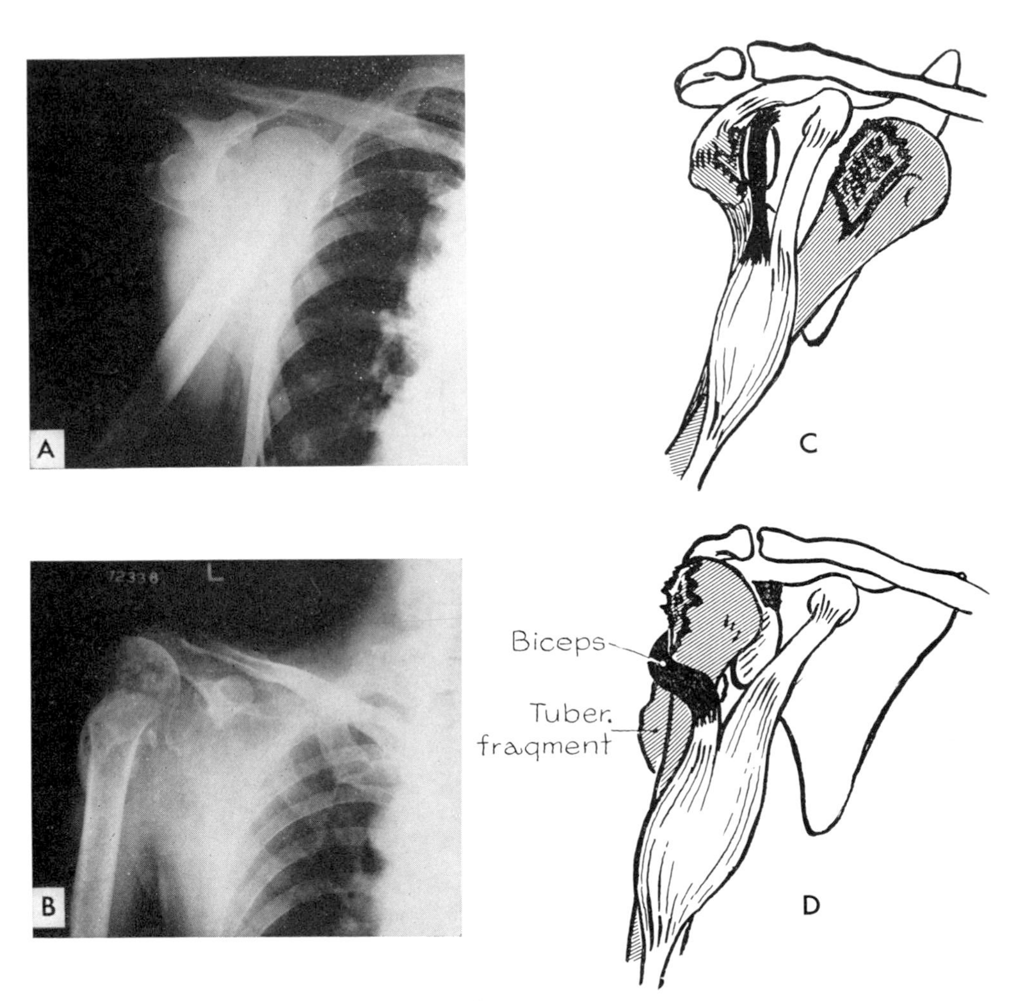

Figure 10–10. Dislocation of shoulder.

A. Roentgenogram showing original dislocation (note the humeral head is displaced medial to the coracoid).

B. Roentgenogram made one year later, after five unsuccessful attempts at manipulative reduction and a long period in a plaster spica.

C. Dislocation with humeral displacement to the medial side of the coracoid ruptures the biceps tendon or, more often, avulses it from the bicipital groove. This tendon remains stretched across the glenoid to prevent reduction.

D. The operative findings. The tuberosity fragment was firmly healed to the posterior aspect of the humerus and the interposed biceps tendon fixed so securely in place by fibrous adhesions that reconstruction proved impossible. Arthrodesis was required.

to release the biceps tendon from its normal channel. As the humeral head dislocates forward the tendon remains behind (Fig. 10–*10*). Reduction can be accomplished by force, but subluxation immediately recurs since the tendon remains behind the humerus. Such a complication should be anticipated whenever the humeral head is displaced medial to the coracoid (Fig. 10–*10*, *C*). When such gross displacement exists it must be assumed that the biceps tendon is fractured or stretched across the joint behind the humerus. Rupture is excluded by the absence of a retracted biceps muscle belly. One gentle attempt at manipulative reduction is justifiable. The necessity for open reduction is almost inevitable.

Engagement of humeral head crater with glenoid. The glenoid lip occasionally becomes engaged in the humeral head defect created by a tuberosity fracture and is held there firmly by the relatively intact anterior and inferior capsule (Fig. 10–*11*). The dislocation may be irreducible by manipulation. Even at open reduction it is sometimes necessary to divide the anterior capsule before the two bones can be disengaged and the dislocation reduced. Repeated attempts to manipulate such a lesion accomplish only a marked increase in the existing damage. Open reduction should be decided upon as soon as it becomes apparent that the bones are so jammed together that manipulative disengagement is impossible.

Rotator cuff interposition. Dislocation in the elderly sometimes is accompanied by massive avulsion of all three external rotators from the humerus. The detached tendon cuff may fall across the glenoid and cover

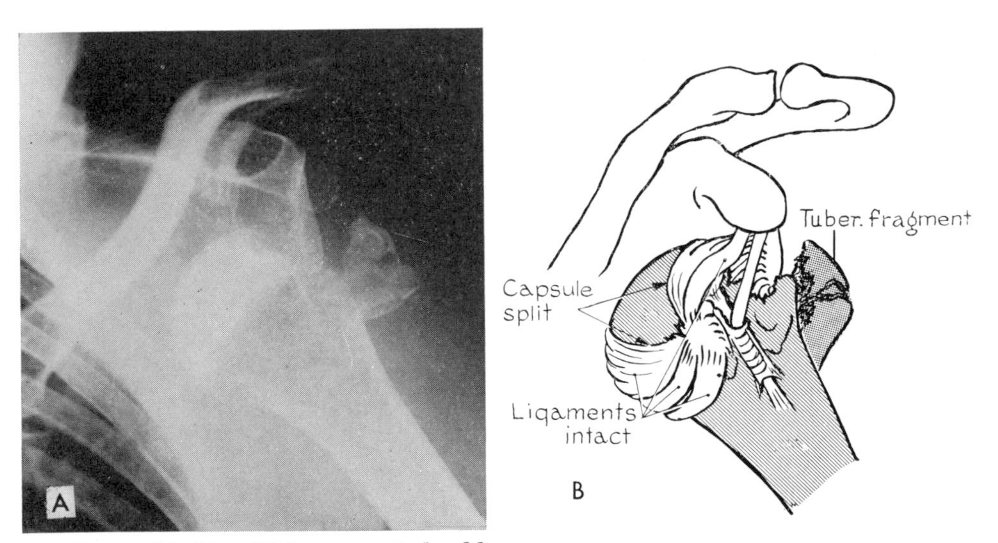

Figure 10–11. Dislocation of shoulder.

A. Roentgenogram showing dislocation which could not be reduced by manipulation.

B. Operative findings. The anterior lip of the glenoid was engaged in the donor cavity of the tuberosity fragment and held there securely by the anterior capsule which, although split horizontally, was intact in continuity. Even with these structures in full view, the humerus could not be manipulated or levered into the glenoid until the tight intact anterior capsule was released.

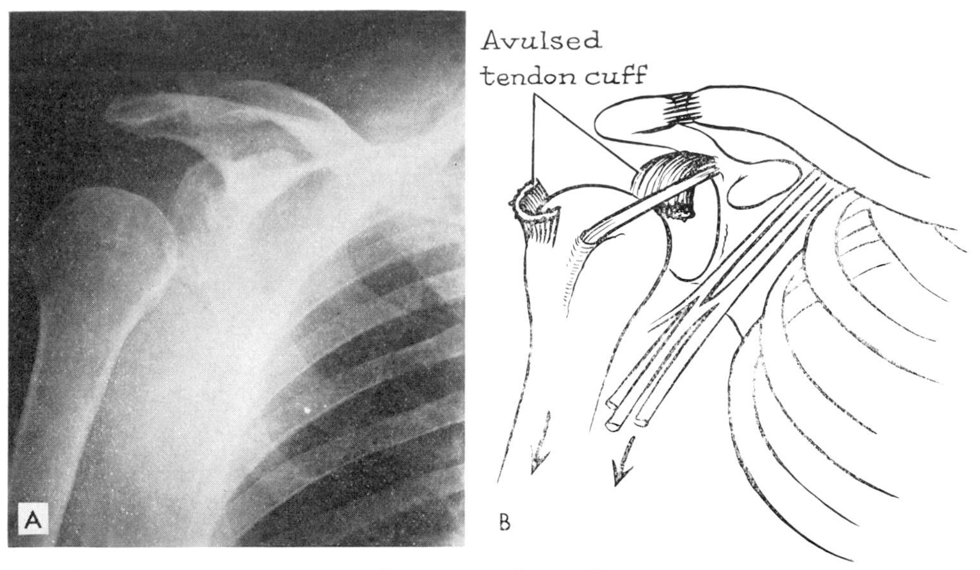

Figure 10–12. Massive avulsion of tendon cuff.

A. Persistent inferior subluxation of the humerus following reduction of anterior dislocation, in the presence of intact suprascapular and axillary nerves, indicates a complete tendon cuff avulsion.

B. Without the suspensory action of the intrinsic muscles, the weight of the limb produces traction on the cords of the brachial plexus. The avulsed cuff may drop across the face of the glenoid cavity like a curtain to block replacement of the humerus by manipulation.

its surface like a veil (Fig. 10–*12, A*). Accurate reduction may be impossible, despite a very mobile humeral head. No "click" into place will occur. Whether or not the cuff is between the bones, the dislocation may seem to reduce, but as soon as the patient stands a palpable sulcus forms between acromion and humeral head. Inferior subluxation will persist (Fig. 10–*12, A*). Complete inability to abduct will suggest deltoid paralysis, but the sensory function of the axillary nerve remains intact. Within a short time the weight of the limb produces progressive neurological signs of traction on the brachial plexus. All patients with late lesions of this type encountered by the writer have been referred from the Neurological Department, where they had been sent with a diagnosis of either deltoid palsy or brachial plexus injury. Exploration and reattachment of the rotator cuff should be done as soon as possible. The results are fair to good, and vary in proportion to the duration of the lesion. Without operative repair the result is eventually an irreversible and crippling neurological deficit in a limb which cannot be raised from the side.

Old unreduced dislocations. These are the most difficult of all. Occasionally manipulative reduction will occur with surprising ease. Therefore, one attempt to reduce by manipulation is worthy of trial. Force should never be used, especially the leverages implicit in a Kocher maneuver. After several weeks the humerus becomes soft, weak, and decalcified, and will fracture far more easily than the surrounding organized tissues will stretch. Often the lesion produces surprisingly little in the way of symptoms or disability and should be left alone, especially in elderly patients. Open reduction (without doing more harm than good) is one of the most difficult problems with which a surgeon can be faced. It is not so much that the replacement of the humeral head in the glenoid is difficult, but many essential soft-part structures may have to be destroyed before this can be done. In addition, all the great vessels and nerves of the region are immobilized in malposition as firmly and by the same fibrous adhesions as the humerus. Excision is sometimes wiser than reduction of the humeral head.

Complications Following Reduction

Tuberosity fracture. A fracture of the greater tuberosity of the humerus often accompanies anterior dislocation of the shoulder, but it is not always a complication. The avulsed tuberosity remains imbedded in posterior capsular structures suspended between the rotator tendons and the sleeve of periosteum pulled away from the humerus (Fig. 10–*13*). The intact anterior joint capsule is the hinge upon which the humerus swings into the dislocated position. Reduction of the dislocation replaces the tuberosity fragment in normal position; indeed, it cannot be elsewhere so long as its soft tissue attachments remain intact. Bony union between humeral head and tuberosity fragment is the rule, following which both anterior and posterior joint supports are strong and sound. These dislocations rarely occur

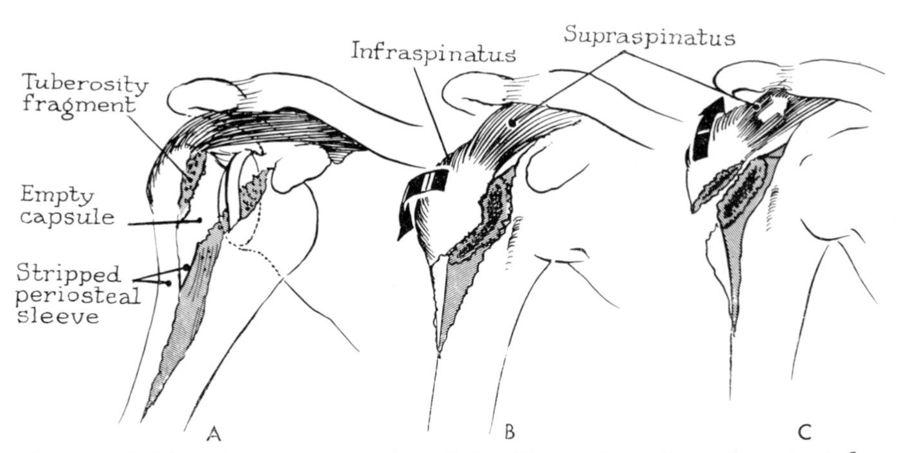

Figure 10–13. Anterior dislocation of shoulder with fracture of greater tuberosity.

A. The tendon cuff, the empty posterior capsule, and the stripped periosteal sleeve remain intact; reduction of the dislocation is accompanied by perfect reduction of the tuberosity fragment.

B. Extensive splitting of cuff and periosteum allows the infraspinatus to create an external rotation displacement of the tuberosity fragment on the humerus following reduction of the dislocation (see Figure 10–15).

C. Transverse laceration of the periosteal sleeve allows the supraspinatus to retract or tilt the tuberosity fragment toward the acromion following reduction of the dislocation (see Figure 10–14).

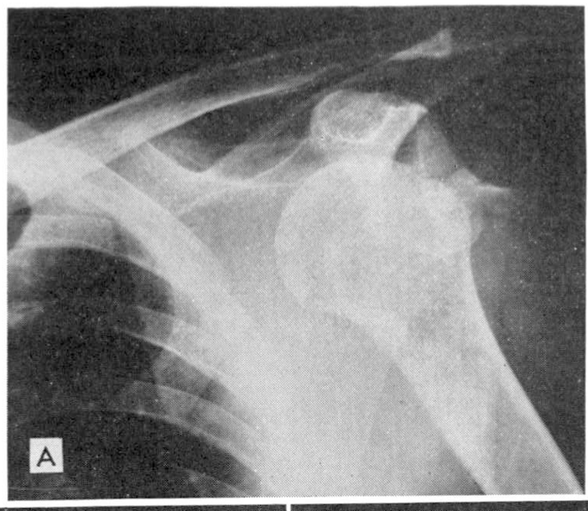

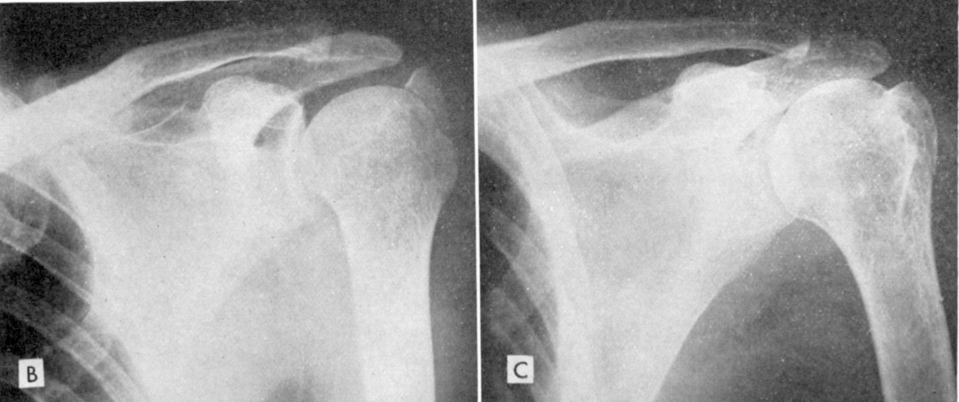

Figure 10–14. Residual displacement of tuberosity fragment.
A. Original dislocation.
B. Following reduction by simple traction.
C. Following cuff repair and re-attachment of the tuberosity fragment. The result was excellent.

in young people and rarely, if ever, become recurrent. This was confirmed by analysis of 573 primary anterior dislocations reviewed by the writer. In about 33 per cent of this group there was fracture of the tuberosity and none became recurrent, regardless of variations in treatment. In about 75 per cent of these lesions reduction of the dislocation was accompanied by spontaneous anatomical reduction of the tuberosity fragment, which was maintained despite early active motion of the limb. Nevertheless, all such patients have a prolonged disability period, which is due to internal derangement of the subacromial mechanism by the healing process. Maximal recovery does not occur for three months or more, and some of the patients never quite regain full elevation.

Nerve damage. Some nerve damage occurs in about 30 per cent of all dislocations accompanied by a tuberosity fracture. Similar neurological complications occur in only 5 per cent of all other anterior dislocations, and usually in those in which the dislocation is made possible by disruption of the soft-part supports of the back of the joint. It seems probable that in dislocations allowed by disruption of the posterior joint support by either the tuberosity or rotator tendons, the intact anterior joint supports maintain the humeral head in close proximity to the nerve trunks, even when dislocated, whereas when the anterior joint supports are ruptured the humeral head may more easily slip by the nerve trunks.

Residual displacement of tuberosity fragment. In 25 per cent of dislocations accompanied by a tuberosity fracture roentgenograms following reduction disclose some residual displacement of the fragment (Figs. 10–*14*, 10–*15*). Reduction and maintenance of position, or residual displacement of the tuberosity fragment, depend upon the status of its soft-part attachments. When these are damaged, secure operative repair is essential to a good result. The fragment itself is of relatively little import and often is better excised, unless large and hard enough to be useful in the repair. Residual tuberosity displacement of 1 cm. or more is indicative of extensive soft part laceration, and will produce a major permanent disability unless it is repaired as soon as possible. Displacement of 0.5 to 1 cm. produces some permanent disability, which in 20 per cent of cases is serious enough to require a late operation. This will not be followed by as rapid or satisfactory a result as would have resulted from early repair. Displacement of less than 0.5 cm., although usually attended by delayed recovery, occasionally produces late symptoms or disability sufficient to warrant operation. Such residual displacements are easy to identify and measure when the

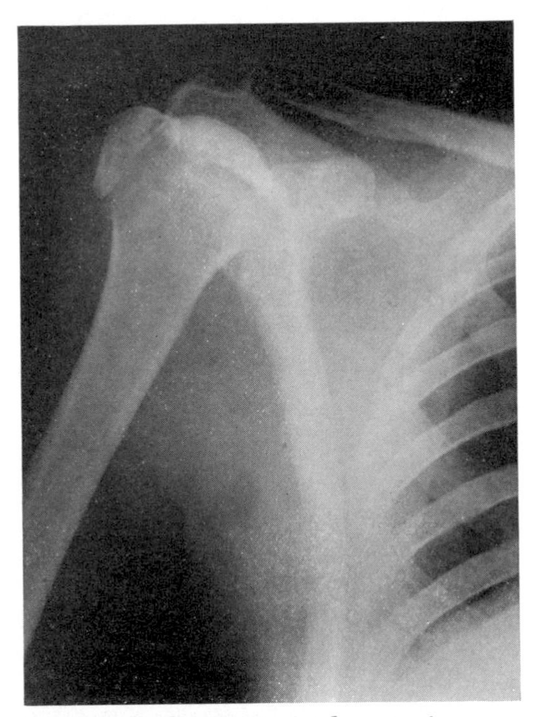

Figure 10–15. Residual displacement of tuberosity fragment.

Persistent external rotation of tuberosity fragment following reduction of anterior dislocation. This displacement became obvious only when an anterior posterior film was taken with the arm internally rotated.

tuberosity fragment is retracted toward the acromion (Fig. 10–*14*). On the other hand, the displacement may be difficult to demonstrate by x-ray until the fragment is brought into true profile, especially when the deformity is an external rotation tilt of the tuberosity (Fig. 10–*15*). Films taken in multiple positions of rotation may be necessary for accurate evaluation of such a lesion. Occasionally the fragment will be found to be in excellent position when the arm is externally rotated, but tilted grossly out of place in internal rotation. The alternative to operative repair for residual displacement of the tuberosity fragment is support of the abducted and externally rotated limb by brace or plaster spica until healing occurs. This treatment is inferior to repair. Gross displacement only occasionally can be well reduced by posture. True mobilization is impossible. The attempt to immobilize incurs a great risk of subsequent shoulder stiffness, and the general results of this type of treatment are inconsistent and unreliable.

Cuff tear. A large percentage of anterior dislocations without tuberosity fracture in patients over age 40 are followed by persistent pain and disability. The clinical picture is almost always that of damage to the intrinsic tendon cuff. Some permanent defect is the rule, and in about 20 per cent of patients this is sufficiently disabling to justify late exploration and repair. The incidence of mechanical subacromial derangement complicating dislocation in patients over 40 is equal to that of recurrent dislocations in younger patients, and by comparison the resultant symptoms and disability are more severe. The predisposition to cuff tear increases with age of the patient, and complete avulsion of all external rotator tendons is not uncommon in the elderly patient (Fig. 10–*12*).

Aftercare of Primary Dislocation

The main complications to be feared following reduction of a primary dislocation are recurrent episodes in the young, and subacromial derangement in the middle-aged and older groups. The converse is also true. There is little danger of subacromial derangement in the young, and less than 10 per cent risk of recurrence in the older group. Up to age 30 aftercare should be designed to minimize the likelihood of recurrence. Immobilization of the dependent arm by a sling and a swathe, which binds it to the thorax for four to eight weeks, is amply justified in order that the disrupted anterior joint supports have a maximum opportunity to heal. The prognosis should always be guarded. Despite adequate immobilization maintained for as long as eight weeks, many such lesions recur sometimes within the following three years. As the age of the patient increases, the danger of late stiffness, pain, and disability due to subacromial derangement replaces that of recurrent dislocation. The duration of immobilization should be decreased progressively with the advance in years. In primary dislocations occurring after the age of 40, protection against re-injury by sling and swathe is justified only when the convalescing patient is exposed to external forces beyond his control and when he sleeps. At all other times he should be encouraged to maintain shoulder function by a regulated program of gradually progressive resumption of use. During the first few weeks after reduction gravity-free exercises should be insisted upon. Elevation of the limb against gravity may progress as the symptoms subside. A similar program is appropriate for all dislocations accompanied by a tuberosity fracture which reduces spontaneously and which shows no or less than 0.5 cm. residual displacement. Early motion does not jeopardize the position of the fragment. Under any circumstances, with or without a tuberosity fracture, if dislocation first occurs after age 40 maximal rehabilitation will require three or more months. Immobilization will result in prolongation of this period and increase the likelihood of a serious permanent defect.

RECURRENT ANTERIOR DISLOCATION OF SHOULDER

This condition is peculiar to young people. There is evidence that the great majority of dislocations recur when the primary episode precedes age 20; that about 60 per cent recur when the onset is between the ages of 20 and 30; and that after age 30 the incidence of recurrence drops sharply. When the primary dislocation occurs after age 40 recurrence is uncommon. It is reasonably certain that these data remain constant, not because of etiologic or therapeutic factors, but because, in the young, the dislocating humeral head tends to disrupt the anterior supports of the joint, and, in the older group, the posterior supports. It is also clear that no data pertaining to recurrences are valid unless the patients involved are followed for a long period. Only 50 per cent of first recurrences take place within 18 months; the remainder occur between 18 months and 5 years after the primary dislocation.

Primary Pathology of Recurrent Anterior Dislocation

The glenohumeral ligaments (Fig. 10–*16*) are the only inelastic protection against anterior dislocation of the humerus. Some disruption or functional derangement of these structures constitutes the primary cause of recurrent dislocations. They originate from almost the entire anterior and inferior rim of the glenoid and converge into a common insertion, which fuses with the deep surface of the subscapularis tendon at its humeral attachment. Often they are seen as poorly defined thickenings of the joint capsule, but the superior and middle ligaments may be well defined separate structures within the capsule. Not only is this sling of ligaments stretched by abduction and external rotation, especially when carried to a point where the humeral head is levered forward on the fulcrum of the acromion (Fig. 10–*17*), but also the pressure of the spherical humeral head has a tendency to split the ligaments apart. The same effect follows hyperextension or any force which drives the humeral head directly forward. Rupture, avulsion from either humerus or scapula, or a horizontal laceration which splits these ligaments is not likely to heal. Indeed, it is difficult to see how any such tear could ever heal when the raw surfaces are bathed in anticoagulant joint fluid and every slight movement, even respiration, causes some move-

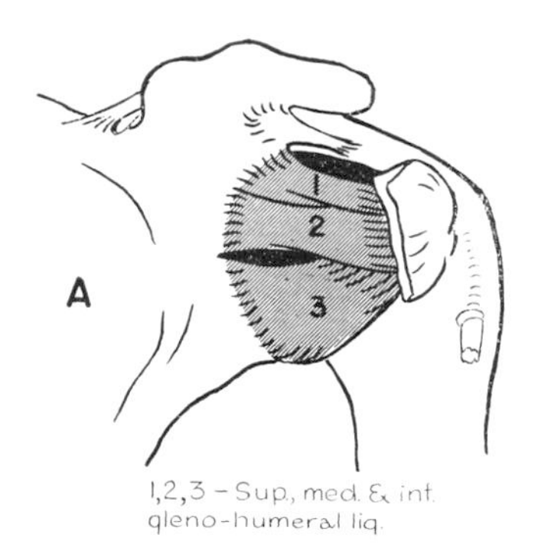

Figure 10–16. Glenohumeral ligaments, the only inelastic defense against anterior displacement of the humeral head.

A. Left shoulder viewed from in front. The three ligaments form a triangular sling supporting the humeral head in front and inferiorly.

B. Left shoulder joint cavity viewed from the side with the humerus removed.

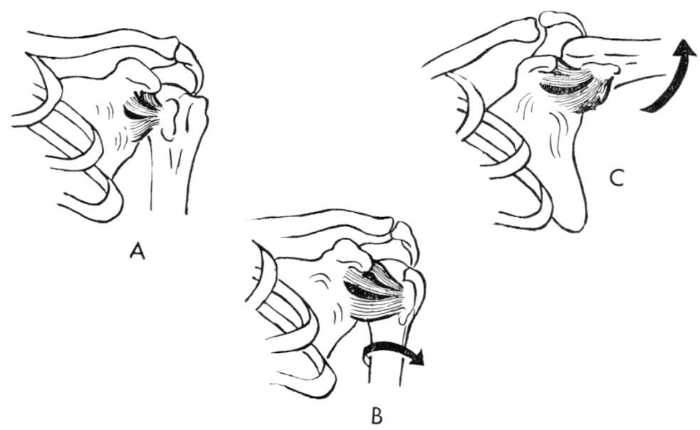

Figure 10–17. The tripartite glenohumeral ligament sling.

A. The sling is loose when the arm is dependent.

B, C. External rotation (B) and elevation (C) tighten the ligaments over the anterior and inferior aspects of the humeral head.

ment of one fragment on the other. Consequently, all such injuries predispose to recurrence, which may happen when the arm assumes a posture creating some functional demand upon the unhealed ligaments and the shoulder musculature is caught off guard.

Depending on the amount and location of ligament damage, recurrent

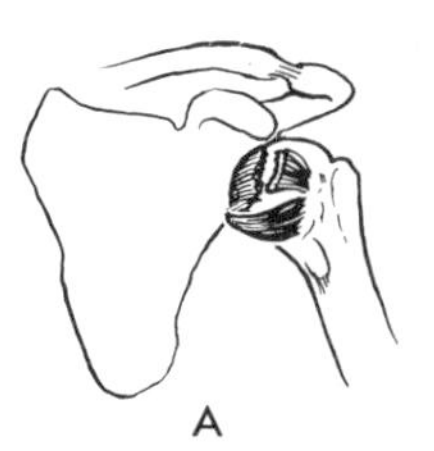

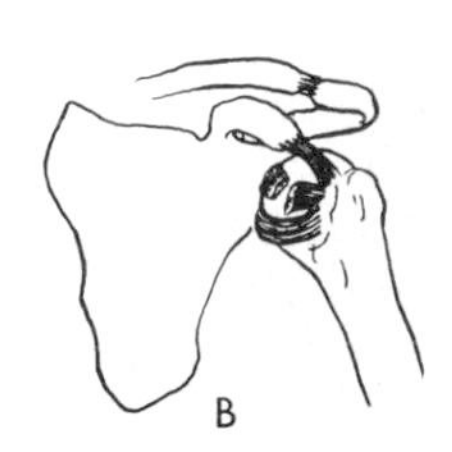

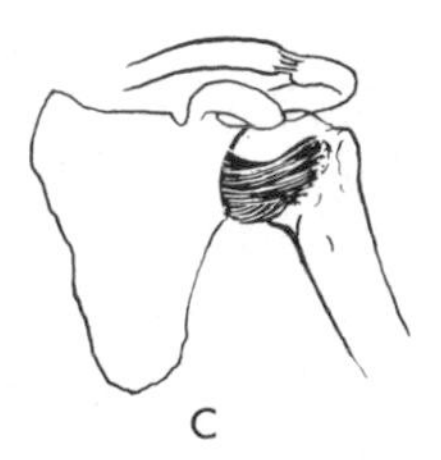

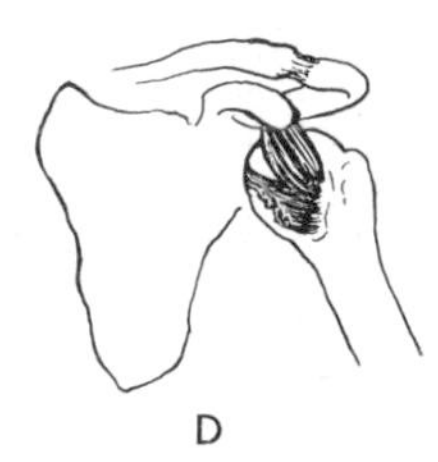

Figure 10–18. Injuries to the glenohumeral ligaments.

A. Rupture through the substance of the ligaments removes the only inelastic *defense against anterior dislocation of the humerus.*

B. Rupture or avulsion of the middle ligament, or a horizontal rent, divides the ligament sling into two halves, between which the humeral head may dislocate.

C. Avulsion of the superior ligament allows the entire sling to slip under *the dislocating humeral head.*

D. Avulsion of the inferior ligament from the scapula makes the entire sling hypermobile so that it slips over *the dislocating humeral head.*

episodes will be subluxations which the patient can reduce, or dislocations requiring manipulative reduction. Generally a little extra damage accumulates with each episode, so that recurrent subluxations eventually become dislocations. The mechanisms by which recurrent episodes are allowed by disruption in continuity of the ligament sling are obvious. A horizontal split permits humeral head displacement due to hypermobility of the split halves of the ligament sling, that above the split sliding over, and that below sliding under the presenting humeral head (Fig. 10–*18*, *B*). This phenomenon accounts for the majority of recurrent dislocations which at exploration are found to have but minor evidences of damage at the rim of the glenoid. Avulsion, even though small in extent, of the superior scapular attachments of these ligaments allows the entire sling to slide under the dislocating humeral head (Fig. 10–*18*, *C*). Conversely, a small avulsion of the inferior ligament from the scapula may produce enough hypermobility to allow the ligament sling to slide over the dislocating humeral head (Fig. 10–*18*, *D*).

The glenoid labrum (Fig. 10–*16*) is a mere appendage to the medial attachment of the glenohumeral ligaments whose main anchorage is to the scapula. It may be avulsed with the scapular attachment of the ligaments or may remain in normal position. Under any circumstances it sustains some injury as the dislocating humeral head passes over the rim of the glenoid. Consequently, in many instances laceration of the glenoid labrum is the result and not the cause of recurrent dislocations, and in the remainder its avulsion from the glenoid is nothing more than an indication of the location and extent of glenohumeral ligament avulsion from the scapula. After repeated injury by many dislocations this meniscus may become extremely lacerated or even disintegrate and disappear.

Secondary Pathology of Recurrent Anterior Dislocation

The anterior segment of the glenoid labrum may be injured in conjunction with avulsion of the scapular attachment of the glenohumeral ligaments or, as has been mentioned, by passage of the humeral head over the glenoid rim. After the cushioning effect of this meniscus is destroyed the anterior rim of the glenoid receives the full impact of the dislocating humerus. There are two common results of this phenomenon. The sharp rim of the glenoid progressively becomes bevelled and smooth, and at times a veritable slide is formed to facilitate excursions of the humerus. In the dislocated position the posterior aspect of the anatomical neck of the humerus is jammed against the glenoid rim, and the progressive development of a vertical groove at this pressure point is common. All these entities have been advanced as causes of recurrent dislocations. Although it is true that, once established, each makes it easier for the humeral head to displace forward, these lesions are the results and not the causes of recurrent dislocations.

Treatment of Recurrent Anterior Dislocation

Nonoperative prevention of recurrent dislocations is possible by the use of a harness which limits elevation of the arm to 60 degrees. Any such program, which must be carried out indefinitely, is harsh treatment for the young person usually afflicted with this condition. Most patients learn instinctively to guard against elevation and do so most of the time. This prevents participation in athletics and many of the other physical activities enjoyed by young persons. Innumerable operations have been devised for the correction of recurrent dislocations. The majority fall into three main categories: humeral suspension operations, creation of a checkrein to limit external rotation, and implantation of a bone block to obstruct forward displacement of the humerus. Most of these operations are successful in many instances. All are attended by a significant incidence of failures, since none attack the primary cause. The operation of Gallie recognizes the importance of glenohumeral ligament injury by reinforcing the ligaments with fascial implants. Bankhart's operation concentrates upon the glenoid labrum injury, and consequently is unsuccessful in cases in which this lesion is the result and not the cause of recurrences. The best procedure, and the only one with a chance to succeed in every case, may be epitomized as follows: Obtain adequate exposure and explore the joint mechanism thoroughly. Identify and repair whatever lesion is found to be the primary cause of the recurrent dislocations. If the lesion proves irreparable, as is sometimes the case when disruption occurs through the substance of the ligaments, reinforcement by fascia or the implantation of a bone block should be done.

Aftercare of Recurring Dislocation

Many recurrent dislocating lesions require manipulative reduction. Symptomatic and functional recovery is very rapid, often a matter of only several days. The lesion is beyond the stage where healing can be expected. Little or nothing in the way of additional tissue damage is normally produced by an individual recurrence. The symptoms should be treated and the patient allowed to return to his usual activities as soon as he can tolerate them.

POSTERIOR DISLOCATION OF THE SHOULDER

Posterior dislocations are uncommon, seldom enter the mind of the surgeon examining a shoulder, and consequently often remain undiagnosed for long periods. About 30 per cent of such lesions result from convulsive seizures due to epilepsy and therapeutic or occupational shocks. The remainder consistently result from trauma to the adducted and internally rotated arm. An accurate description of the injury is the best evidence to differentiate between a posterior and an anterior dislocation when reduction was accomplished or occurred spontaneously prior to examination.

Diagnosis

The clinical picture is constant, but the signs often escape notice. The coracoid is unduly prominent to palpation. The anterior aspect of the humeral head is less prominent than the normal. There is a palpable prominence of the humeral head below the posterior edge of the acromion. Usually these abnormalities are barely visible and the long axis of the humerus appears grossly normal. The limb is fixed in internal rotation and abduction is markedly limited. Motion in the very small range available is attended by severe pain. Roentgen diagnosis by films taken in the ordinary projections is difficult and at times impossible (Fig. 10–*19*, *A*). Good axillary views are precluded by the absence of abduction. Transthoracic films are often unsatisfactory. A film should be taken with the patient standing and facing the cassette obliquely so that the central ray corresponds to the long axis of the scapular spine (Fig. 10–*19*, *B*).

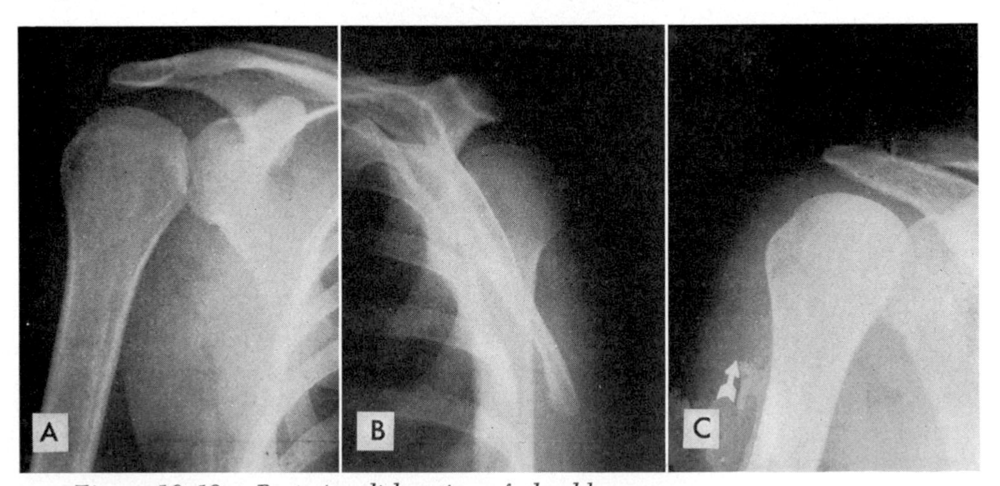

Figure 10–19. Posterior dislocation of shoulder.

Roentgen diagnosis may be difficult or impossible by ordinary films.

A. Primary posterior dislocation, of 30 minutes' duration, ordinary anteroposterior view.

B. Tangential view prior to reduction leaves no doubt about the diagnosis.

C. The same shoulder, immediately following reduction.

Treatment

Primary posterior dislocation. These lesions are easy to reduce by anesthesia and traction in the axis of the humerus, coincident with gentle external rotation and, when necessary, a push against the humeral head from behind. Once reduced there is little tendency to redislocate. Temporary rest and protection of the limb by sling and swathe for only a few days to a week are all that is required. Complete symptomatic and functional recovery occurs within two or three weeks. The results are good. Occasionally a late complication occurs in the form of transient "locking" symptoms, presumably caused by spontaneously reduced subluxations. These may occur for several years, but mild symptoms of this type may be expected to subside eventually.

Recurrent posterior subluxation. These lesions are usually reduced immediately by some motion of the shoulder and are seldom available to examination. The patient presents himself in the surgeon's office with little except a history that his shoulder "goes out of joint." Under these circumstances it is usual that some operation designed to correct recurrent anterior dislocation is advised. If carried out, the procedure is a complete failure. The risk of making this mistake can be minimized by ascertaining the position of the arm (adduction and internal rotation, or abduction and external rotation) which predisposes to the "locking" or "popping out of joint" episodes described. Operative repair offers the only hope for relief of persisting symptoms.

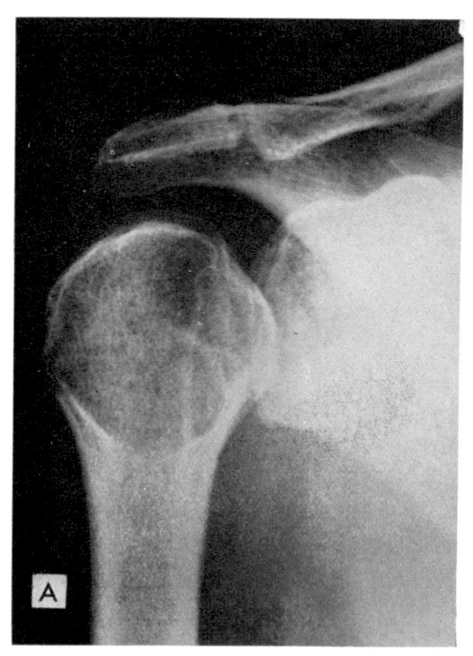

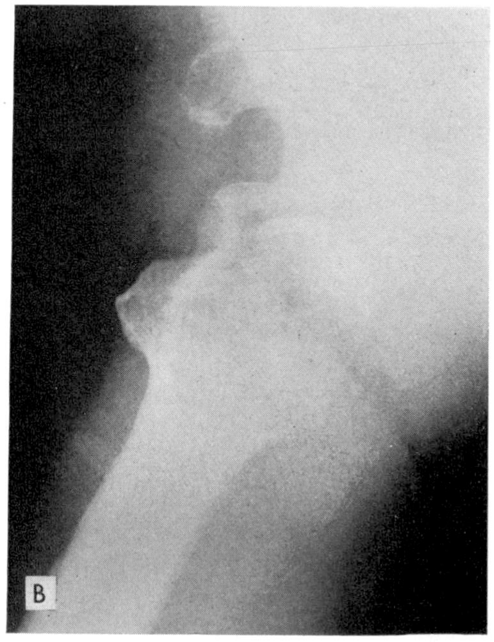

Figure 10–20. Posterior dislocation of the shoulder.

A. Old unreduced posterior dislocation. Overlapping of glenoid and internal rotation of humeral head is apparent. Humeral head defect is suggested.

B. Same patient following repair and restoration of elevation of the arm, illustrating the size and location of the humeral head defect.

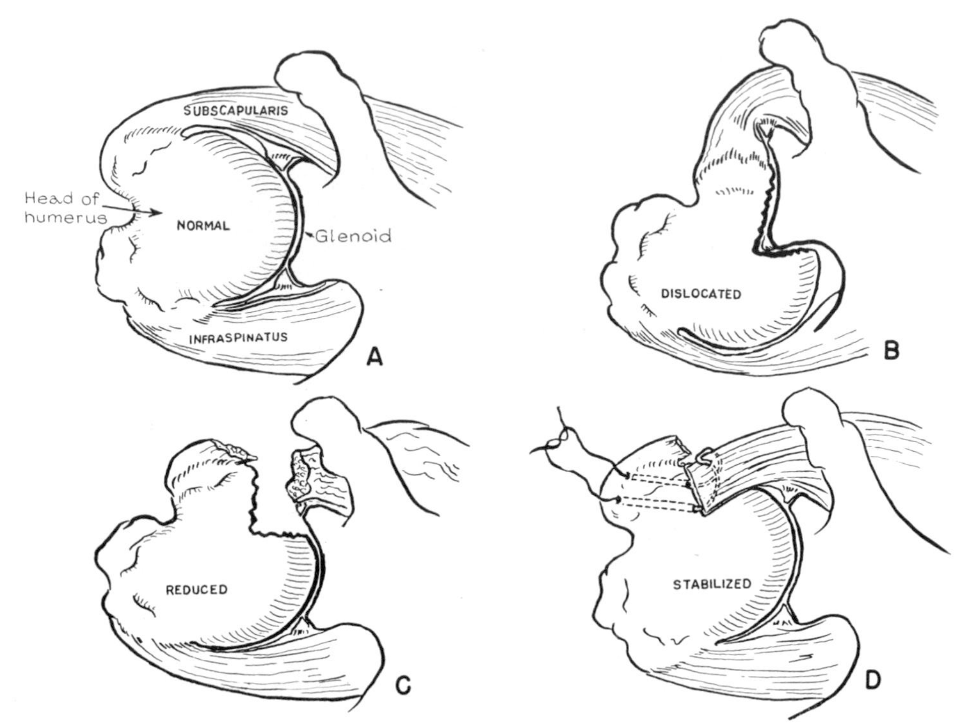

Figure 10–21. Operative stabilization of old unreduced posterior dislocation of the shoulder.

In some instances, with fracture of the posterior glenoid rim, supplemental stabilization by a posterior bone block is advisable.

A. The left shoulder viewed from above.

B. The deformity of posterior dislocation with engagement of the posterior glenoid rim in an anterior humeral head defect.

C. Reduced, but still very unstable; redislocation occurs with internal rotation, flexion, or adduction. Subscapularis divided.

D. Technique for stabilization by medial transposition of the subscapularis insertion into the humeral defect.

Old unreduced posterior dislocation. Longstanding fixed posterior dislocations result from a failure of diagnosis and consequent neglect. The majority of patients travel from doctor to doctor receiving treatments for what is called a "frozen shoulder." The anterior aspect of the humeral head remains jammed against the posterior rim of the glenoid. A deep vertical groove (Fig. 10–*20*) forms in the soft bone of the humeral head and engages the glenoid rim. Once this engagement becomes secure, manipulative reduction cannot be accomplished. Open reduction should be carried out (Fig. 10–*21*).

UNUSUAL DISLOCATIONS OF THE SHOULDER

Luxatio Erecta

This uncommon lesion results from violent force in the plane of true abduction. The acromial fulcrum levers the humerus away from the glenoid

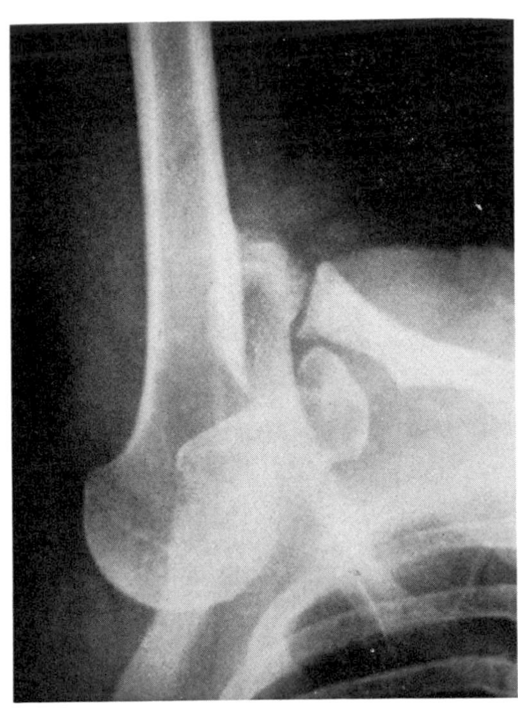

Figure 10–22. Luxatio erecta.

The humeral head is extracapsular. All soft tissue attachments to the upper end of the humerus have been peeled from the bone or ruptured. The acromial edge is fractured by humeral impact. The amount of soft part disruption militates for easy reduction by simple traction in the long axis of the humerus.

and the inferior capsule is widely disrupted. The head of the humerus enters the axilla and the axis of the arm points overhead. This is almost the only form of dislocation in which the humeral head is extracapsular (Fig. 10–22). All of the intrinsic muscle attachments are peeled or torn from the humerus. The biceps tendon is dislocated from its groove. Unless the latter slips behind the humeral head, reduction is easily accomplished by traction in the axis of the humerus until it is reapproximated to the glenoid, following which the limb may be brought to the side. These lesions should be immobilized for two to three weeks so that the peeled-off sleeve of periosteum and musculotendinous cuff attachments may adhere firmly to the humerus.

Superior Dislocation

This lesion cannot occur unless permitted by a coincident fracture of the acromion (Fig. 10–23). Gravity tends to reduce the deformity, and it is impossible to estimate the actual amount of displacement which existed at the time of the injury. The musculotendinous cuff may split in the coronal plane, allowing the humerus to displace upward through the aperture. Under such circumstances the anterior and posterior parts of the split tendon cuff may grasp the surgical neck of the humerus firmly. Down-

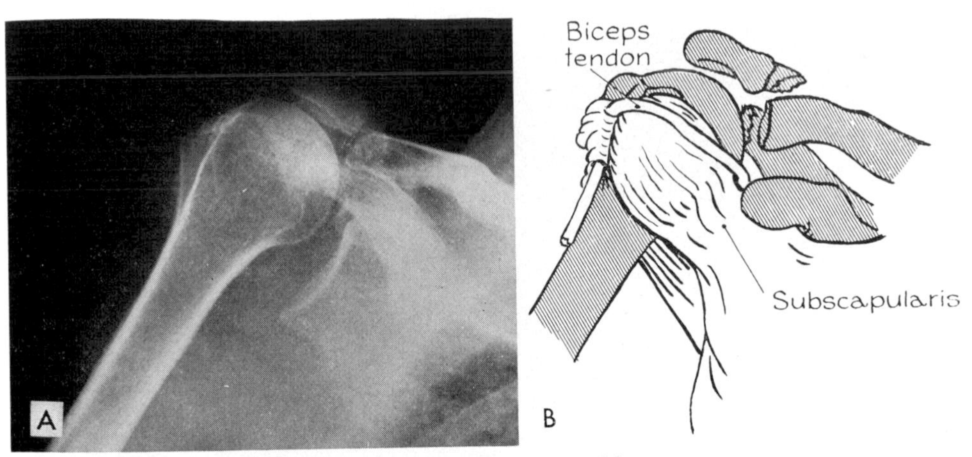

Figure 10–23. *Superior dislocation of the shoulder.*

Superior dislocation of the humerus requires fracture of the overlying acromion. Persistent upward subluxation indicates distal displacement of the longitudinally split tendon cuff, both halves of which tightly embrace the surgical neck. The displaced biceps tendon may also contribute to persistent subluxation. Attempts to reduce by traction serve but to tighten the grasp of these misplaced soft structures around the neck of the bone. This dislocation proved irreducible by manipulation. Open reduction, replacement, and repair of the cuff tendons, and excision of the outer fragment of acromion was carried out.

ward traction simply tightens this embrace on the humeral neck so that manipulative reduction proves impossible. Open reduction, replacement and repair of the cuff, and excision or fixation of the acromion fragment should be done.

FRACTURE-DISLOCATION OF THE SHOULDER

This injury, which rarely occurs in the young, results from the same traumas which produce fractures of the upper humerus without dislocation, and dislocations without humeral neck fractures, but is produced in only 1.1 per cent of the cases of such trauma (see Table 10–*1*). Variations in concept of what constitutes a fracture-dislocation have made the literature

TABLE 10–*1*. TYPES OF SHOULDER INJURY ENCOUNTERED IN 1796 CASES.

Type of Injury	*No. of Cases*		*Incidence*
Fracture neck of humerus		921	51.2%
Dislocation			
Anterior (without fracture)	759		
Anterior (with tuberosity fracture)	71		
Posterior	25	855	47.7%
Fracture humeral neck with dislocation			
Anterior	17		
Posterior	3	20	1.1%

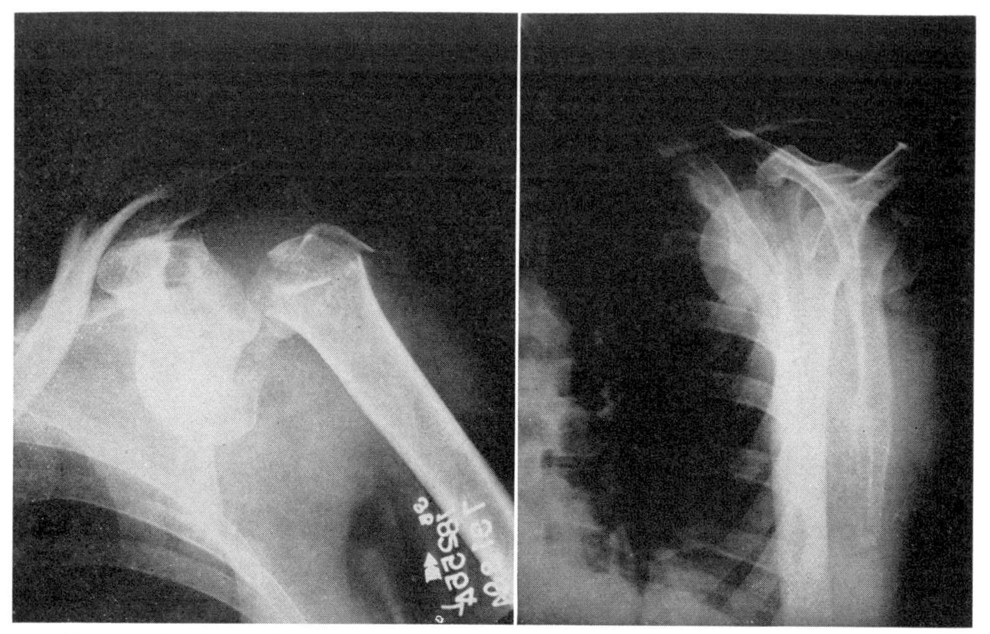

Figure 10–24. A true fracture-dislocation.
The naked head fragment is extracapsular, the greater tuberosity fragments are pulled backward, the lesser tuberosity fragment is pulled forward and the shaft upward into the interval between the tuberosities.

pertaining to treatment and results very confusing. The true lesion (Fig. 10–*24*) has a consistent pattern of four fracture fragments—the humeral head, the shaft, and the greater and lesser tuberosities. The head fragment is extruded from the capsular cavity. In only 2 of 20 cases encountered by the writer did it remain impacted on the shaft. In the others it was free, extracapsular, often rotated 180 degrees, and essentially devoid of soft-part attachments. Usually it rested against the cords of the brachial plexus, but in three instances it had been driven backward and rested in the sub-spinous position. The lesser tuberosity is pulled forward by the subscapularis, the greater tuberosity backward by the external rotators, and the shaft upward by the long muscles of the arm.

Treatment

Treatment is difficult. The dislocation can be reduced by very gentle traction on the abducted or elevated arm when the humeral head and shaft fragments remain impacted. Attempts to reduce by manipulation are almost always unsuccessful when the head fragment is free. Open reduction may be done. However, the end-results of both open and closed reductions are poor. The incidence of late aseptic necrosis of the head fragment is very high, regardless of the method of reduction. Progressive pain and stiffness are to be anticipated, but may not become severe until several years have passed, and the necrosis has become well established.

Simple excision of the free head fragment produces better results than any reconstruction procedure. These are not good surgical results, but the patients are happy and satisfied, with shoulders that are comfortable and useful, although limited in motion and subject to early fatigue. The early results of humeral head replacement by prosthesis are astonishingly good, but this procedure has not as yet withstood the test of time.

FRACTURES AT UPPER END OF HUMERUS

FRACTURES CAUSED BY DIRECT IMPACT

The cancellous humeral head responds to a direct blow like shatterproof glass; it cracks, and fissures radiate from the point of impact, but the bone does not shatter nor do the fragments displace. The prominent greater tuberosity bears the brunt of the blow and may be the only part of the bone to suffer damage, but fissures may extend across the humeral head or neck in any direction. Rapid bone healing cannot be prevented and need not be assisted. Soft-tissue attachments hold the bone fragments in place more efficiently than any device available to the surgeon. Immobilization is unnecessary and is in fact harmful since the main complication to be avoided is a stiff shoulder. The essentials of treatment are limited to relief of pain and maintenance of function. Simple palliative measures—temporary and intermittent rest in a sling and progressive early motion and use, regulated according to the subsidence of pain—will be followed by rapid and complete recovery.

FRACTURES CAUSED BY MUSCULAR VIOLENCE

Avulsion of Lesser Tuberosity (by Subscapularis)

Isolated lesions are quite rare. Their significance is proportional to the size and displacement of the avulsed bone fragment. When a major portion of the tuberosity is displaced medial to the glenoid (in anteroposterior roentgenograms), it is likely to jam between humeral head and coracoid when the arm is adducted or rotated internally. A serious permanent defect is to be anticipated unless the fragment is sutured back in place without delay. However, when the avulsed fragment is but a small shell of tuberosity this injury is equivalent to an isolated rupture of the subscapularis tendon. Treatment of the symptoms and early resumption of motion and use will be followed by a good result. Maximal recovery without any serious permanent defect occurs within several months. Deficient subscapularis function is amply compensated by the remaining intact adductors and internal rotators.

The lesser tuberosity may be avulsed in conjunction with a posterior dislocation of the humerus. This lesion, which is a counterpart of the greater tuberosity avulsion so commonly associated with anterior glenohumeral dislocation, is especially prone to accompany posterior dislocations which result from convulsive episodes. Early operation and suture of the avulsed tuberosity in place is indicated as the most simple and best preventive against redislocation.

Avulsion of Greater Tuberosity (by Spinati)

This fracture often accompanies anterior dislocation of the humerus. Reduction of the dislocation may result in spontaneous reduction of the fractured tuberosity fragment. The penalties and problems attending a residual displacement of the tuberosity are discussed on page 253. When avulsion of the greater tuberosity appears to be an isolated lesion, the probable cause and abnormality are those of an incomplete or spontaneously reduced anterior dislocation and should be treated as such.

FRACTURES CAUSED BY INDIRECT IMPACT

The force of a fall on the elbow or outstretched hand is transmitted through the shaft of the humerus to impact its head against the glenoid and acromion. Leverage and torque may alter the mechanical forces and the result of this secondary impaction. The neck of the humerus and one or both tuberosities usually are fractured. Displacement of the tuberosity fragments follows a consistent pattern dictated by the pull of the subscapularis and spinati muscles. The angle of incidence between the humeral head and shaft fragments usually is altered to produce an apparent varus (adduction fracture) or valgus (abduction fracture) deformity. This deformity is determined by the position of the humerus at the moment of impact, the head fragment assuming whatever position into which it may be pushed by the shaft of the bone. Treatment based purely upon deformity

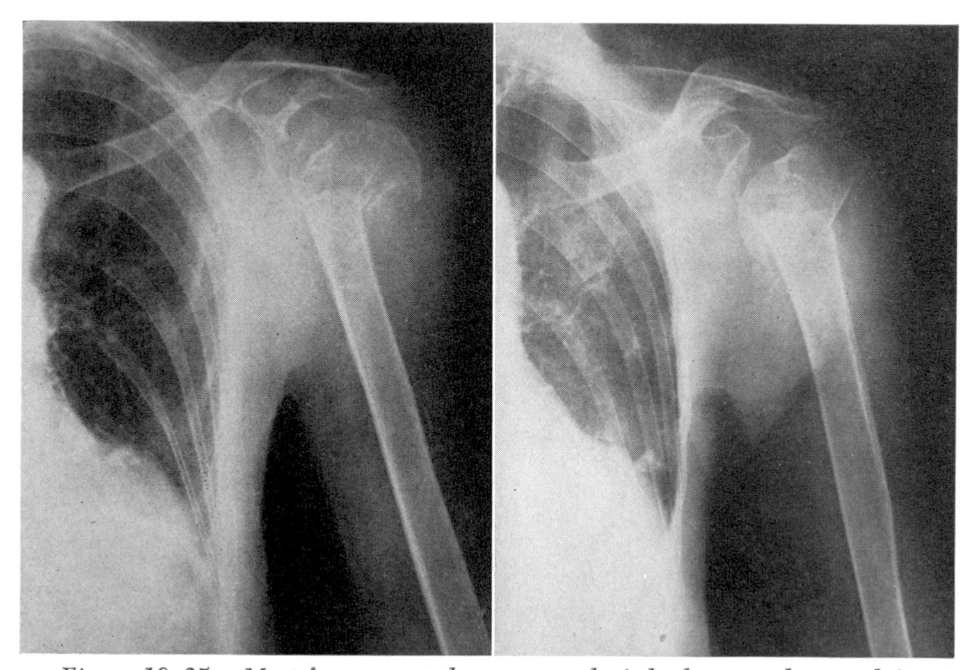

Figure 10–25. Most fractures at the upper end of the humerus have a deformity marked by anterior angulation due to action of the pectoralis major. If the roentgenogram is taken with the arm in a sling (internal rotation–left) it will disclose an "abduction" fracture; however, if the limb is lying by the side in external rotation (right), the appearance will be that of an "adduction" fracture.

or anatomical location of the fracture is precarious and uncertain. Almost all humeral neck fractures have some angular deformity, apex forward. Films taken with the arm in a sling (internal rotation) disclose an abduction fracture, but if the arm is externally rotated another film will show the same lesion to be what is commonly termed an adduction fracture (Fig. 10–25). Good treatment depends primarily upon a correct choice between the following alternatives: (1) *reduction of the fracture,* or (2) *acceptance of the existing deformity.*

Indications for and against Reduction

Penalties of immobilization. These are serious. The great majority of these fractures occur in persons past middle age. Reduction requires fixation. The inexorable penalty of immobilization is prolonged and often permanent stiffness of the shoulder. The surgeon must have good and logical reasons for correcting anatomical deformity at such a cost.

Functional unimportance of humeral head anatomy. Few surgeons have failed to be astonished at the excellent function following malunion with gross deformity of a fracture at the upper end of the humerus. Many have rued the excellent roentgen result which followed reduction and immobilization but was attended by persistent stiffness and pain. The explanation of such an apparent paradox seems reasonably clarified by the following:

(1) Between the fractured bone and the skin are several tissue layers containing many muscles. Not only each layer, but each muscle, must move freely on the others before glenohumeral motion can take place. Following the fracture the deep muscles are lacerated and the tissue planes infiltrated with hemorrhage. Whether or not the fracture is reduced, it is normal for these moving parts to adhere to each other by fibrous union if motion is obliterated throughout the healing period. In an elderly person even a normal shoulder will become stiff, contracted, and painful after a short period of immobilization.

(2) The glenohumeral articulation is not a ball-and-socket. It resembles one-half of a billiard ball which rests against, but not within, a slightly concave 1-inch coin. As long as any portion of the humeral ball remains in apposition to the glenoid coin a potentially adequate articulation is preserved. Total shoulder motion is the sum of four joints: scapulohumeral, sterno- and acromioclavicular, and glenohumeral. Motion of a normal shoulder utilizes only a portion of the range available in each. Reduction of available glenohumeral motion produces a compensatory increase in the contributions of the other three joints to total motion of the shoulder.

(3) The individual muscles of the shoulder are complicated in their function but, when considered as a unit, are extremely versatile and adaptable. Malunion alters but does not obliterate the functions of the intrinsic muscles. Normally these functions include suspension of the humerus, rotation of the humerus, and stabilization of the glenohumeral fulcrum. Malunion does not seriously hamper any of these functions. *Normal anatomy of the humeral head is not necessary to normal function of the shoulder.*

Healing potential of the fracture. The fracture involves cancellous bone. With two exceptions, (1) gross retraction of a tuberosity fragment into the shoulder joint, and (2) interposition of a complete barrier of soft parts between the fragments, healing of the fracture is swift, sound, certain, and independent of therapy.

Stability of the fracture. Existing displacement results from laceration of the soft tissues enclosing and attaching to the fracture fragments. An increase in displacement requires additional laceration of the remaining intact soft parts. The main fragments are held to the biceps tendon like beads on a string. Manipulative reduction adds to soft part damage and decreases the intrinsic stability of the fragments. Gentle, progressive, gravity-free motion creates no risk of additional tissue damage so long as the limits of pain are not passed.

The considerations for or against reduction of fractures of the upper humerus in patients past middle age may be summarized as follows:

(1) Perfect reduction is unnecessary to satisfactory function.

(2) Any but gross displacement is compatible with a useful, comfortable shoulder.

(3) Immobilization is unnecessary to maintenance of the existing position of the fragments.

(4) Appropriate early exercises do not jeopardize maintenance of existing position.

(5) Early motion is necessary to the prevention of stiffness.

Reduction is indicated by the following local factors:

(1) Loss of contact between humeral head and shaft.

(2) Gross angular displacement (approaching 90 degrees) of an unimpacted humeral head fragment.

(3) Displacement of an avulsed tuberosity fragment into the shoulder joint.

(4) Gross soft tissue interposition between head and shaft fragments.

Reduction

The fallacies of abduction are obvious, but often unrecognized. It is not only instinctive, but sometimes advocated, that the extremity be abducted in order to facilitate manipulation of the shoulder. It is widely accepted that the supraspinatus produces a fixed abduction deformity of the relatively uncontrollable head fragment. This is not true, for depressor muscle forces more than compensate for supraspinatus action (Fig. 10–*26*). The head fragment will be found to rest in a position where it was pushed by the shaft. Persistent abduction of this fragment in relation to the shaft results from impaction or engagement of the fragments. When impaction is broken up or the fragments disengaged, the head fragment will rest in neutral position, for its muscle attachments remain relatively intact, in continuity and in balance. The only place for abduction in the manipulation of an angulated fracture is for purposes of disimpaction prior to reduction.

Abduction is even more illogical and potentially harmful in the reduction of a completely displaced fracture of the humeral neck. The deformity is constant (Fig. 10–*27*). The head fragment rests in about neutral posi-

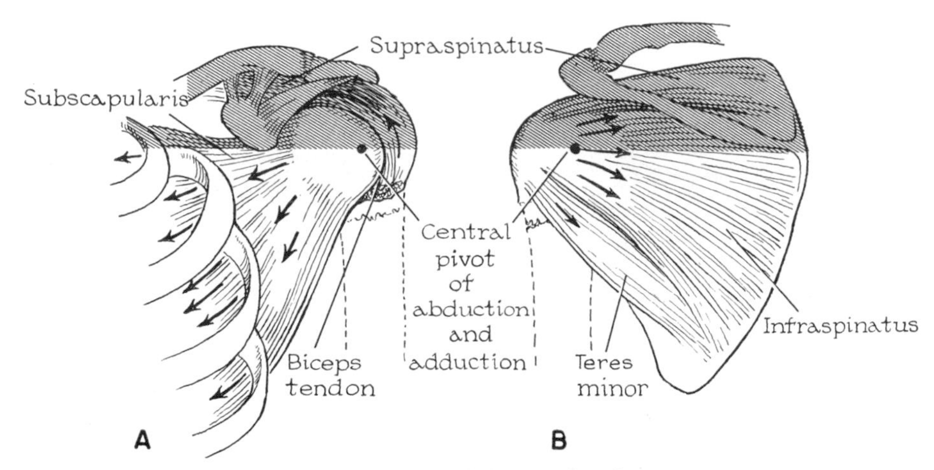

Figure 10–26. The fallacy of fixed abduction by the supraspinatus.

When the humeral neck is fractured the pivot of humeral head rotation remains unchanged. The intrinsic muscles above this pivotal point exert an abduction force, but this is balanced by equal or greater depressor forces. The head fragment remains in muscle balance and displaces in whatever direction it is pushed by the shaft fragment.

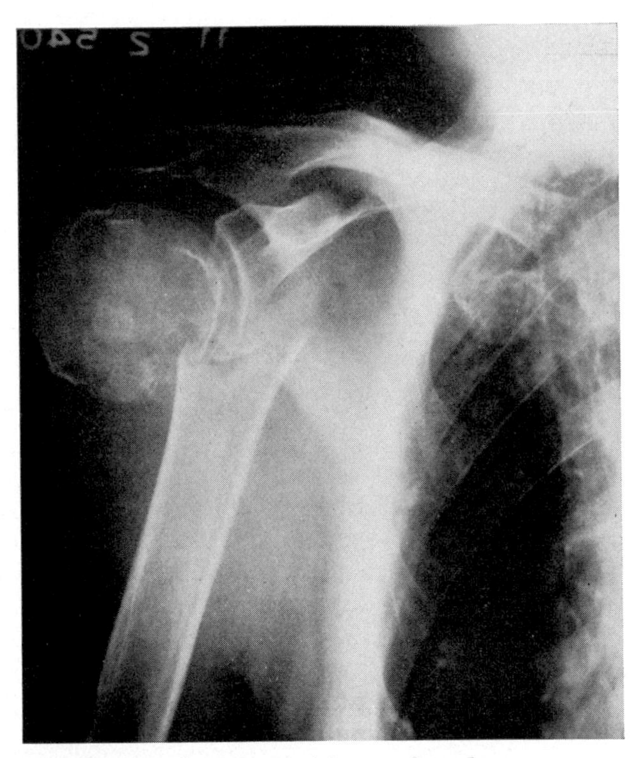

Figure 10–27. Displaced fracture of humeral neck.

Completely displaced fractures of the humeral neck show a consistent deformity pattern: The long muscles of the arm produce shortening; the adductors pull the shaft fragment toward the thorax.

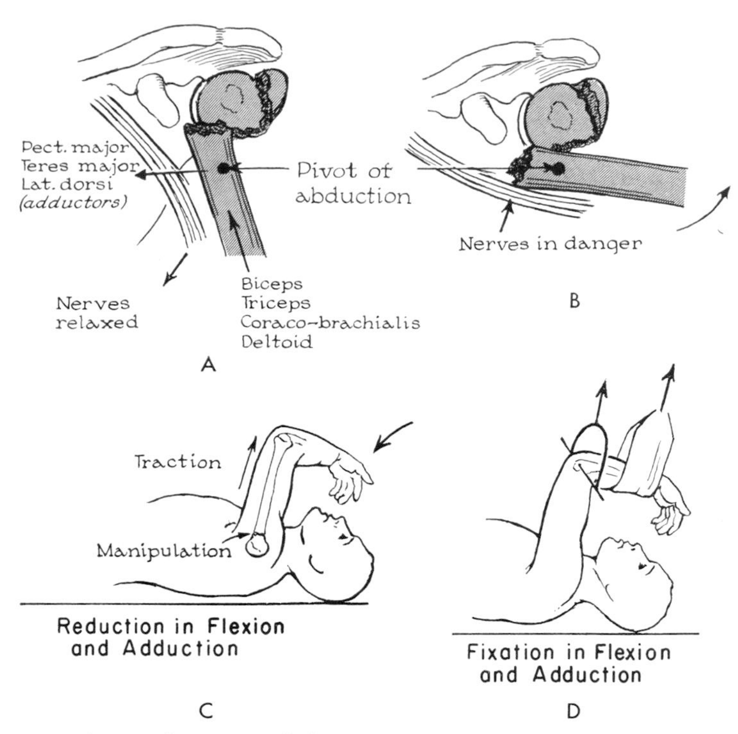

Figure 10–28. Reduction and fixation of fracture at neck of humerus.

A. The shaft fragment is pulled medialward by the adductor muscles. Shortening is produced by the long muscles of the arm. The pivot of shaft abduction is lowered from the humeral head to the level of the pectoral insertion.

B. Abduction tightens pectoral muscle, hinders reduction, and tilts the proximal end of the shaft fragment further into the axilla.

C. Reduction by overcoming shortening and manipulative correction of displacement should be done with the arm flexed and adducted for relaxation of the displacing muscles.

D. Fixation requires continued pectoral relaxation by continued flexion and adduction; humeral length is maintained by skeletal traction.

tion. The shaft fragment is displaced into the axilla by the adductors, forward by the pectoralis major, and cephalad by the long muscles of the arm. The sharp end rests in close proximity to the great nerves and vessels of the axilla. Abduction invites laceration of these structures, increases the displacing forces of the offending musculature (Fig. 10–28), and impedes rather than facilitates reduction.

The essentials of reduction by manipulation include:

(1) Muscle relaxation by adequate anesthesia.

(2) Restoration of humeral length by traction—along the axis of the flexed and adducted humerus.

(3) Reapposition of shaft to head by manipulation. It is a simple matter to replace the shaft under the head of the bone once length has been restored and the displacing effect of the pectoralis major neutralized by flexion and adduction of the arm.

Fixation

Perils of immobilization. The penalties of immobilization are temporary and acceptable in the young patient, but permanent and serious in the patient past middle age. Moreover, immobilization by a plaster dressing is not necessary to maintenance of reduction. A plaster spica is used in the treatment of shoulder lesions in persons past middle age under two ordinary situations, namely joint suppuration and arthrodesis. This statement is made with appreciation of the continued popularity of immobilization in the abducted position for treatment of humeral neck fractures, with a strong conviction born of logic and experience that such treatment usually does more harm than good, and with the realization that this choice of an elevated position for the immobilized arm is not unrelated to the fact that this is the optimal position for a stiff shoulder. Reduction can be maintained without jeopardizing function, by manipulative impaction of the reduced fragments or a short period of skeletal traction.

Fixation by surgical impaction. Return of the arm to the side after reduction of the fracture is commonly attended by recurrence of the original deformity. More often than not this can be prevented or an acceptable degree of reduction maintained by manual impaction of the cortical shaft fragment into the cancellous bone of the humeral head. This impaction must be done without undue force lest the shattered head and tuberosities are spread apart, their remaining soft-part connections disrupted, and the deformity increased. Engagement of the fracture surfaces sufficient to ensure that both fragments move as a unit is optimal, and permits simplified aftercare by early mobilization.

Fixation by skeletal traction. Failure to engage or impact reduced fragments so that they move in unison calls for additional fixation. The displacing muscle forces are unchanged. Reduction requires these to be neutralized by traction in flexion and adduction. Maintenance of reduction requires their continued neutralization. This is simple and efficient when implemented by Kirschner wire olecranon traction with the arm flexed and adducted and the elbow at a right angle so that the supine patient looks at the palm of the hand (Fig. 10–28).

The traction pull should be at least 5 and not in excess of 10 pounds, or sufficient to keep the shoulder off the mattress. *This is not immobilization.* Some motion of all the joints of the extremity coincident with continuous neutralization of the displacing muscle forces can and should be practiced from the start. For the first few days palpation reveals the shaft to move independently of the head fragment. Usually the fragments will be felt to move in unison after 10 to 14 days. This results from early soft part healing in and around the fracture. The traction may then be removed, the patient allowed out of bed, and the injury treated as if movement in unison had existed from the start.

Treatment by Early Mobilization

This method of treatment obtains for fractures of the humeral neck which have been reduced and impacted, or held by skeletal traction until

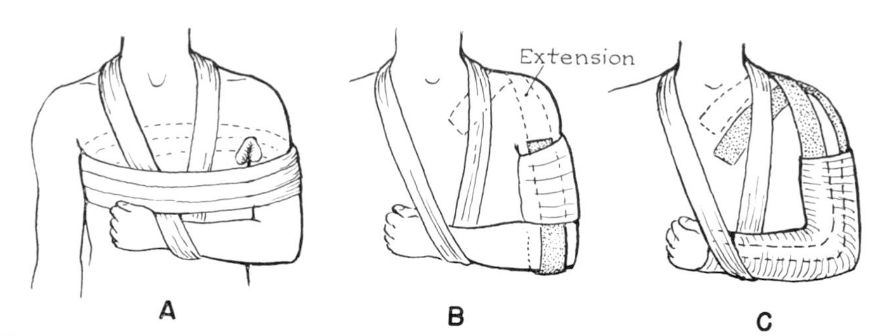

Figure 10–29. Dressings for fractures of shoulder and arm.

A. Dressing for fracture of humeral neck region. The limb is suspended from the wrist so that its weight provides traction, and is bound comfortably to the chest by an elastic bandage.

B. Molded "sugar tongs" splint, which may be extended over the shoulder (dotted line) for stabilization of humeral shaft fractures.

C. More extensive molded splints for humeral shaft fractures in children and unreliable adults.

the fragments move in unison, and for all others, impacted or not, in which some apposition of shaft and head is preserved. Its essentials consist of (1) relief from pain, (2) protection against further tissue damage, and (3) maintenance of function. The extremity is dressed in a sling and bound to the chest by a swathe. The sling should suspend the extremity at the wrist rather than the elbow, so that the weight of the arm hangs from the shoulder (Fig. 10–29, *A*). This is sufficient traction. *A hanging plaster should not be used* for it is unnecessary, will produce some elbow stiffness, and will predispose to inferior subluxation of the humerus from the glenoid. The swathe should be discarded as soon as symptoms permit, except when the patient is sleeping or is exposed to forces beyond his control. Any simple palliative measures available should be used as needed until pain and spasm subside spontaneously. Above all, the patient must be persuaded that the sling and swathe is for comfort and protection and not for immobilization, and that the resultant restriction of motion is a necessary disadvantage of early treatment which must be compensated for by added efforts on his part a little later.

Active gravity-free pendulum motions of the extremity should be started within a few days, or as soon as pain permits. The sling is removed and the patient stoops forward with the arm hanging limply from the shoulder. He is then taught to swing the extremity in a gradually increasing arc. This is done at home at frequent intervals and the scope of the exercises is increased as pain subsides. Within about two weeks gently progressive aided active exercises against gravity are permissible and safe (Fig. 10–*30*). All tolerable light use of the extremity is encouraged from the start. *Normal use is the best exercise.*

The limits of pain and fatigue constitute the yardstick of early mobilization. Within these limits all motion and use of the arm are safe and beneficial, but beyond them there is risk of further tissue damage until the fracture has healed. A single daily exercise period at the surgeon's

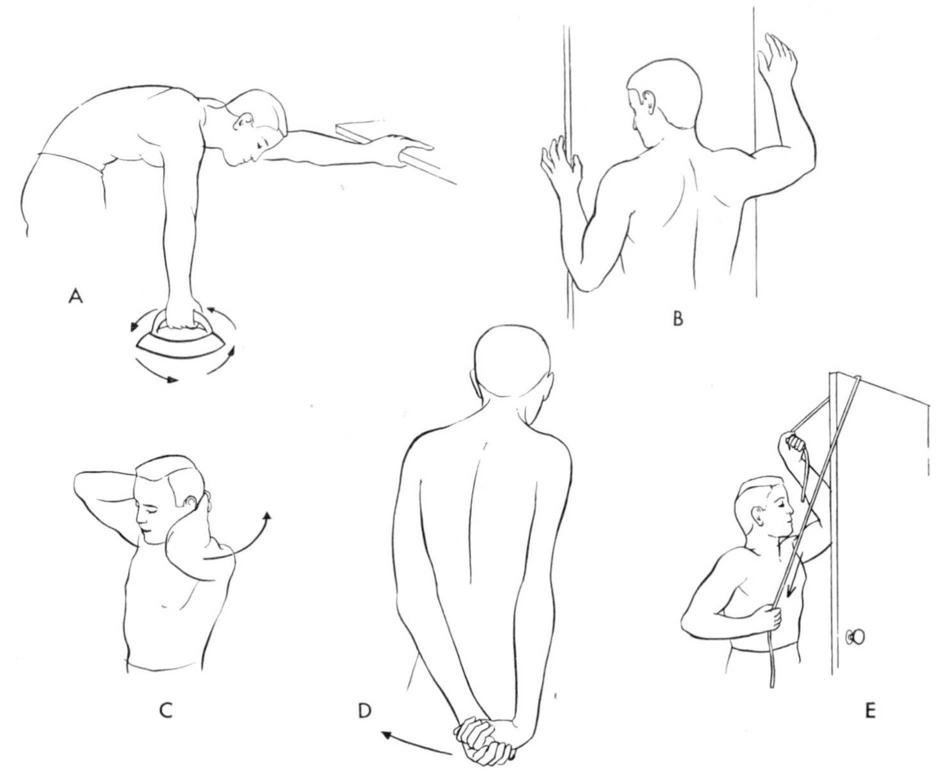

Figure 10–30. Mobilization of injured and painful shoulder.

A. Gravity-free pendulum exercises are more comfortable and efficient with a weight in the hand.

B. Crawling up the wall, assisted elevation; a strip of adhesive is placed on the wall to be marked in pencil as a record of the elevation attained each day.

C. Exercise for restoration of external rotation.

D. Exercise for restoration of internal rotation.

E. The normal extremity assists in elevation of the injured member.

office or a rehabilitation center is almost useless. Exercises should be done *hourly*, but not for more than *a few minutes at a time*. A longer exercise period is apt to induce sufficient pain, spasm, and fatigue to vitiate its otherwise beneficial effects. Physiotherapeutic modalities alone are harmful. Their proper functions are limited to the palliation of discomfort prior to and resulting from exercises. Subsidence of pain and recovery of function are the indications for resumption of ordinary activities. The x-ray films should be ignored in making this decision.

Inferior Subluxation of Humerus

This common complication of fractures at the neck of the humerus is seldom recognized at once since the first x-ray films are usually taken with the patient recumbent, or with the weight of the arm supported by a sling. The cause is not entirely clear, except that the suspensory action of the

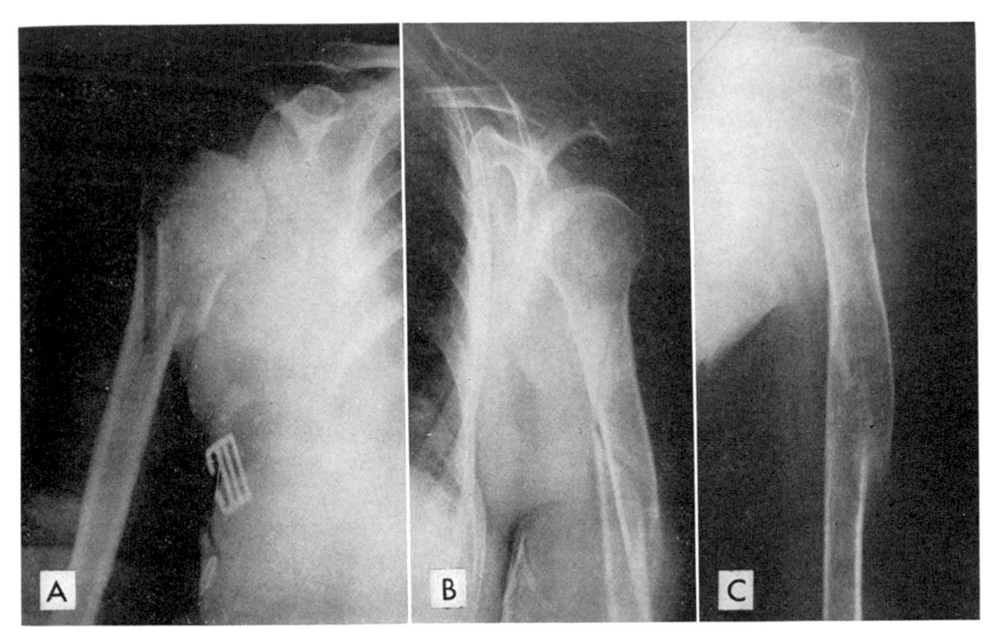

Figure 10–31. Fractures of upper end of humerus.

A. Comminution of upper shaft, humeral neck, and tuberosities with undisplaced fissures of the shaft distal to the main injury. Hanging plaster–inferior subluxation of the humerus.

B, C. Comminuted fractures of the upper half of the humeral shaft held in satisfactory position by intact soft part connections, (B) before and (C) after healing.

Note the inferior subluxation of the humerus which was produced by application and relieved by removal of a hanging plaster in both cases.

intrinsic muscles is temporarily defective. Consistent spontaneous recovery after weeks or months suggests that contusion or stretch of the motor (transverse scapular nerve) supply to the spinati may be the primary lesion. Nevertheless, while the subluxation persists it is attended by serious disability. It is important, therefore, to recognize this phenomenon at an early date by taking the first roentgenograms with the patient erect and the extremity dependent. When subluxation is present it may be assumed that its duration will be directly proportional to the length of time the dysfunctional intrinsic muscles are allowed to remain "on the stretch." Use of a hanging plaster under such circumstances (Fig. 10–*31*) is apt to delay recovery for many months, and sling support of such a lesion should be at the elbow and not at the wrist. Otherwise, the injury may be treated by an early mobilization program, but the weight of the arm may well be supported by sling, at least intermittently, until all risk of "stretch paralysis" of the temporarily defective intrinsic muscles has passed.

FRACTURES OF PROXIMAL HUMERAL EPIPHYSIS

Epiphyseal injuries result from violent trauma often producing gross displacement. Either fragment may impale the surrounding soft tissues and large masses of muscle may become interposed between the fragments to make manipulative reduction difficult or impossible. The misconception that all these lesions are adduction fractures creates a dangerous tendency toward uniformity of treatment. They may, in fact, result from a force from any direction, and there is no consistent deformity. Treatment must be tailored to fit the individual problems of each lesion. Skeletal traction through the olecranon is frequently necessary to restoration and maintenance of humeral length. The use of an abduction frame which greatly limits the choice of arm position is only occasionally an adequate method of treatment. When the original deformity is enough to necessitate reduction and fixation the child should be hospitalized. On rare occasions, reduction can be maintained by plaster splints. Usually it is necessary to apply sufficient continuous skeletal traction to maintain humeral length with the extremity in balanced suspension in whatever axial and rotatory posture proves to neutralize the displacing muscle forces. Such a regimen should be maintained for about four weeks, after which ambulation with the arm in protective splints should be continued until healing is secure.

Growth disturbance is the complication to be feared. Nature consistently corrects or compensates for even gross deformity (Figs. 10–32, 10–33), and union is to be expected even in the face of considerable soft part interposition (Fig. 10–32). However, the major portion of humeral length depends upon this epiphysis, and cessation of its growth in a small child is a real catastrophe. Repeated attempts at manipulative reduction, each of which damages the epiphyseal plate, should not be made. Open reduction in children under the age of 10 years is justified only by a complete failure to achieve any approximation of the fragments. Adequate humeral length and axis can be obtained without undue surgical insult of the epiphyseal

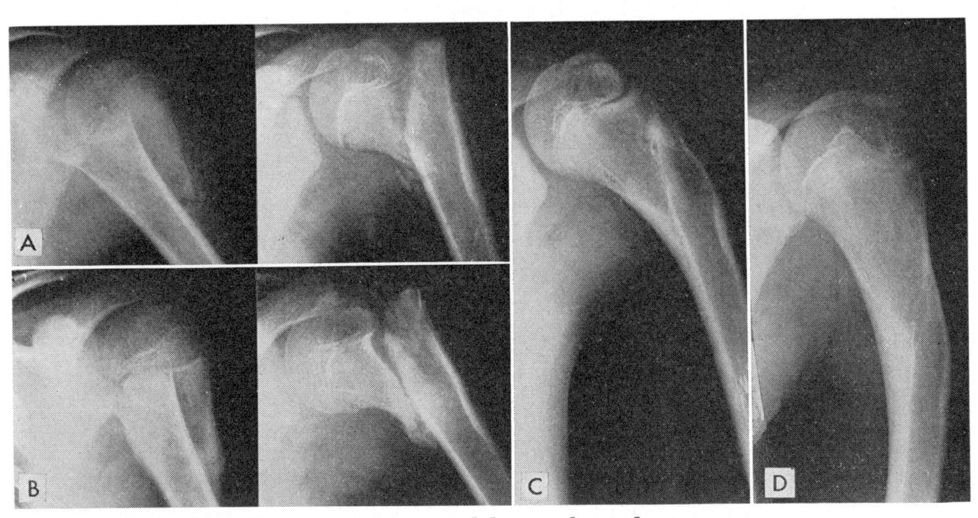

Figure 10–32. Fracture at proximal humeral epiphysis.

A, B. Films taken in September and November, 1943, showing unreduced fracture with gross tissue interposition between the fragments and marked original deformity.

C, D. Films taken in September, 1944, and September, 1946, respectively. Note that union and correction of the deformity eventuated spontaneously.

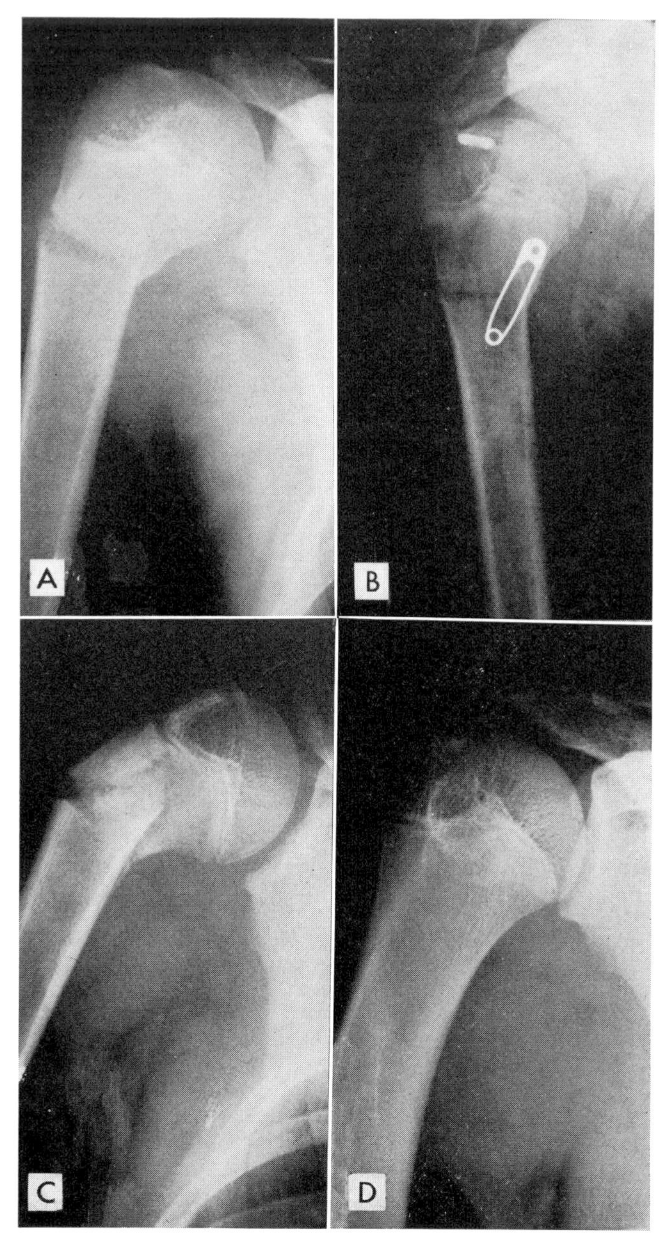

Figure 10–33. Fracture of neck of humerus in a child.
A, B. Before and after reduction and fixation.
C. The result of removing the fixation prematurely.
D. Spontaneous correction of deformity after 2½ years.

plate by continuous traction suspension and, although good apposition of the fragments is desirable, it is not essential. Continuance of epiphyseal growth, even in the presence of deformity, is better than a humerus with a perfect reduction and an irrevocably damaged growth potential.

FRACTURES OF HUMERAL NECK IN CHILDREN

Greenstick fracture through the neck of the humerus is not uncommon in children. The fracture should be completed and the angulation corrected only on those rare occasions when gross angulation is present. Under such circumstances reduction proves difficult to maintain, except by a regimen of continuous traction suspension. Up to 30 degrees of angular deformity may be accepted so long as the greenstick lesion is firm and there is no tendency for the deformity to increase. The arm is dressed in protective splints (Fig. 10–*29*) until union is sound.

FRACTURES OF SHAFT OF HUMERUS

Humeral shaft fractures result from torque, leverage, direct impact, or some combination of these forces. It is popular to predict consistent deformity patterns according to the level of the fracture and its theoretical effect upon the displacing potential of the muscles involved. Such theories are predicated upon cadaver anatomy and are not commonly of any clinical significance. Of real importance are the following facts:

(1) Intermuscular septa which are intact in continuity and attached to each fragment constitute excellent internal splints which minimize all except angular displacements.

(2) The weight of the dependent limb is almost always enough to preclude angulation and neutralize the theoretical displacing forces of the muscles, including shortening. In short, the weight of the dependent limb will preserve normal humeral length and axis.

(3) A fracture through the middle segment of the humerus opens up broken surfaces comprised almost entirely of hard cortical bone with but a tiny central medullary opening, but in the proximal or distal segment opens up vascular cancellous bone which heals rapidly and well.

(4) Excessive motion or other harmful factors are diffused throughout the extensive healing area of a spiral or oblique fracture and are unlikely to have any localized deleterious effect upon union of the fracture, but the brunt of similar strains is concentrated at the one localized spot where callus must bridge the fragments of a transverse fracture, hence delayed union is not uncommon and nonunion may occur.

Fractures of Proximal Humerus

These lesions are usually spiral and oblique, as well as comminuted (Fig. 10–*31*). Undisplaced fissures radiating from the main fracture and militating against stable internal fixation often pass unrecognized in the early films. Concomitant humeral neck and tuberosity fractures are not uncommon. Large areas of vascular cancellous bone surfaces are opened so that union takes place rapidly. The limb is suspended by a collar and wrist cuff (Fig. 10–*29*) and bound lightly to the chest by an elastic bandage. The weight of the limb is almost always sufficient to maintain adequate humeral length and axis and satisfactory position of the shattered fragments. A hanging plaster is a dangerous device in the treatment of these injuries. More often than not it will produce an inferior subluxation of the humerus which may delay recovery of function long after the fracture is healed (Fig. 10–*31*). Gravity-free pendulum exercises should be started early. A program of early mobilization and progressive resumption of use, graduated according to the limits of pain and fatigue, will eventuate in a reconditioned limb by the time union occurs. Immobilization throughout the same healing period will produce a stiff shoulder. Open reduction and internal fixation is only occasionally required, usually for the extrication of soft tissues from between grossly displaced fragments.

Fractures of Middle Third of Humerus

An uncomminuted spiral fracture is a simple lesion. Humeral length and axis can be preserved by the weight of the dependent extremity, and apposition of the fragments can be maintained by molded plaster splints (Fig. 10–*29*). These measures provide support and stabilization, but not immobilization of the fracture. Many such lesions are treated by a "hanging plaster," but the added traction provided by this elbow-stiffening device is not often really necessary, except when unusually strong muscles create persisting displacement despite the weight of the extremity. Clinical union compatible with beginning gentle shoulder and elbow motions is usually present in less than two months. The fingers and wrist are moved from the start. Nonunion is uncommon, except when soft tissue interposition between the fragments has passed unrecognized.

A transverse fracture looks simple, but the prognosis in such cases should be guarded. The fragment ends are small, circular, and composed mainly of dense cortical bone with but a tiny central medullary opening. The horizontal fracture line provides little or no defense against torque, leverage, or displacing strains. The effect of motion of the fragments is concentrated at the one small fulcrum which must be bridged by healing. The mass of reparative tissue is small and may be repeatedly disrupted in its formative stages by fragment mobility which would have little or no effect if it were diffused throughout a more extensive area of healing. The fact that many such fractures heal uneventfully despite inadequate or minimal stabilization does not detract from the logic which dictates a necessity for secure and continued fixation until bony union occurs.

A comminuted fracture is often spiral in type with a third triangular fragment. Whether or not gravity traction by the weight of the dependent extremity, combined with external splint fixation, will prove adequate depends upon the amount of laceration of the soft tissues surrounding the lesion and can be determined only by trial. If soft part damage is small, this lesion may successfully be treated as if it were a simple spiral fracture.

If the soft parts, and especially the intermuscular septa, are extensively torn, persistent displacement of the unstable fragments may call for open reduction and internal fixation.

Concomitant radial nerve injury. Radial nerve paralysis is the most common complication of fracture through the middle third of the humerus. This is almost always the result of contusion or stretch, but occasionally the nerve is lacerated or severed, or interposed between the bone fragments. Statistically the prognosis for spontaneous recovery of nerve function is good, but far from certain. Whenever appropriate facilities are available the fracture should be explored, reduced, securely stabilized by internal fixation, and the nerve repaired or insulated from the fracture site by transposition of a triceps pedicle flap. Under any circumstances stretching of the paralyzed muscles must be prevented by splinting the wrist and metacarpophalangeal joints in a position of extension until nerve function is regained.

Soft part interposition. A barrier of soft tissues interposed between the fragments is the most frequent cause for nonunion of a humeral shaft fracture. This bone is completely surrounded by muscles and some soft tissues become caught between the fragments of bone in all fractures in which the displacement is significant. Bony union occurs despite small amounts of interposed muscle, but is effectively prevented by larger amounts. The presence or absence of interposed soft parts must be ascertained by attempting to educe *bone crepitus* at the first examination. This must be done gently, lest the movement of the fracture fragments damage the adjacent radial nerve. Failure to obtain bone crepitus is an indication for early operative treatment of the fracture.

Segmental Fractures of Humeral Shaft

Segmental fractures have two common denominators: (1) the fracture at one end of the intermediate segments heals slowly or fails to unite, and (2) stable fixation by external immobilization is impossible. A good result requires anatomical reduction and secure and prolonged fixation. Usually these prerequisites are possible only by open reduction and internal fixation (Fig. 10–*34*). This is a task for the most experienced and technically adept surgeon available, and is an invitation to catastrophe in less competent hands. The arm must be opened widely, yet in such a way that the blood supply of the intermediate fragment is not jeopardized. The problem of fixation, which must be tailored to fit the needs of the individual lesion, is always complicated. Nevertheless, consistently good results are to be expected in these complex lesions if accurate reduction and secure fixation can be provided.

Fractures of Distal Humeral Shaft

Fractures of the distal humerus above the supracondylar level involve vascular bone once again becoming cancellous as the elbow joint is approached. Usually they are oblique or spiral (Fig. 10–35). Perfect reduc-

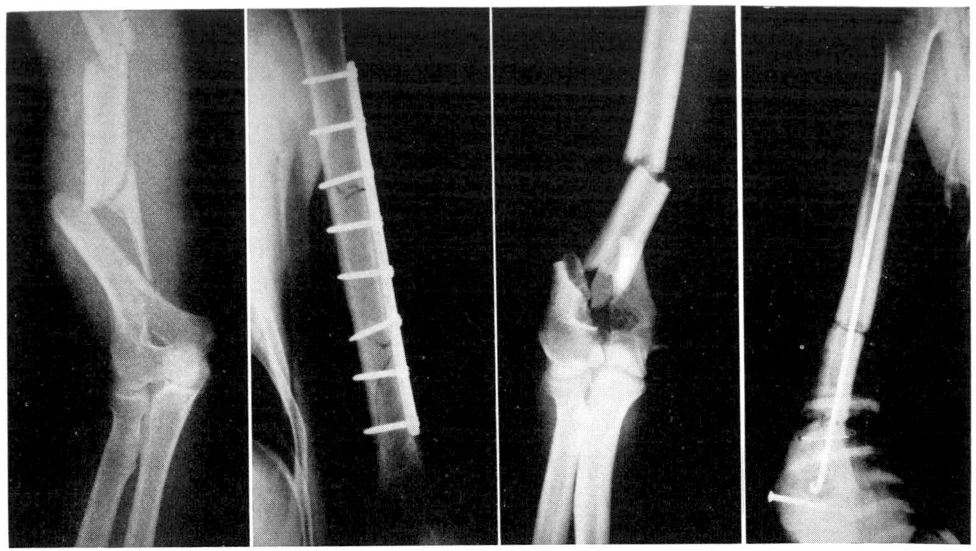

Figure 10–34. Segmental fractures of humerus.

These are always unstable and unsuitable for treatment by external immobilization. Operative exposure must not destroy the blood supply of the loose segment. Internal fixation must be tailored to fit the characteristics of the fracture. Recovery in each of these injuries was rapid and complete.

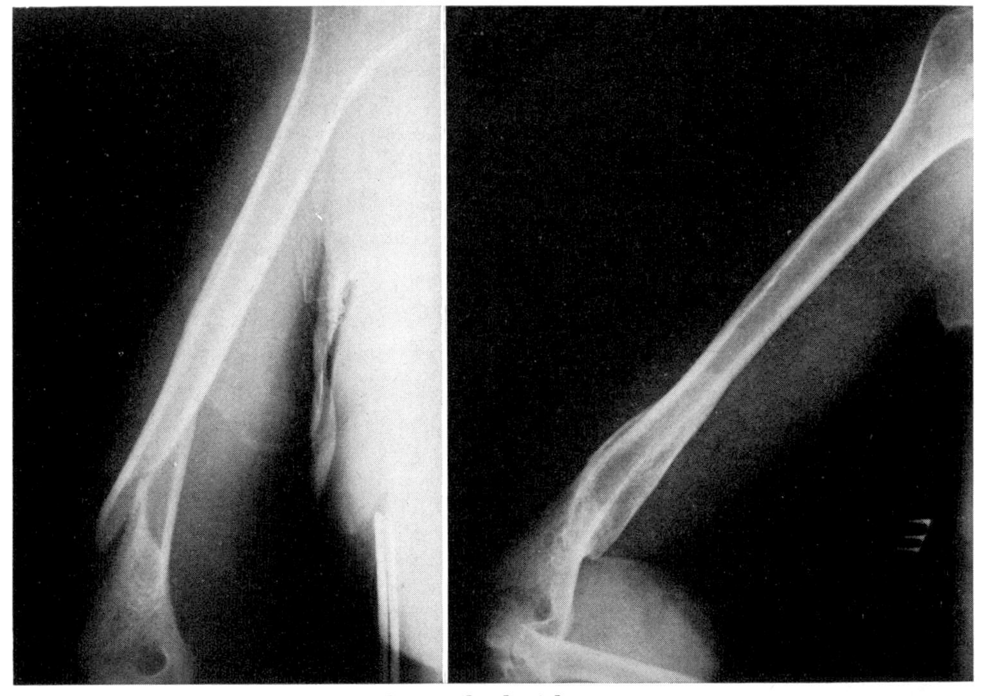

Figure 10–35. Fracture of lower third of humerus.

Before and after treatment by molded splints. A perfect reduction is unnecessary to full recovery.

tion is unnecessary. Apposition of the fragments can be maintained by molded splints. The elbow is immobilized in 90 degrees flexion, since extension is likely to create displacement of the short distal fragment by tension of the muscles crossing the joint. Union occurs within three months and the results are good.

INTERNAL DERANGEMENT OF THE SHOULDER

CALCIUM DEPOSITS

These lesions are not of traumatic origin, but the onset of associated symptoms commonly follows a minor injury or unaccustomed exertion. They are not peculiar to the shoulder, but may be encountered in any tendon. Symptoms are most common in the shoulder because this is the only location in which tendons pass between two bones (the acromion and the humerus) on every motion. The resultant syndrome is often termed "calcified bursitis." Codman amply demonstrated in 1931 that the offending deposit is neither calcified nor is it in the subdeltoid bursa.

Pathogenesis

A deposit begins as localized hyaline degeneration in the collagen of the tendon fibers. Soon the nuclei disappear, and the tendon fibers become fibrillated. Meanwhile motion continues to grind them into a mass of necrotic debris enclosed within the tendon substance. Inorganic salts of calcium are deposited and eventually identification and location of the mass is possible by x-ray.

Such a lesion is self-limiting. In the middle-aged approximately 10 per cent of asymptomatic shoulders contain such deposits. So long as the deposit remains within a necrotic walled tendon cavity there are no symptoms. However, the enclosed material is a foreign protein. Eventually it escapes to the tendon surface and comes into contact with the vascular coverings of the tendon (the synovial floor of the subdeltoid bursa). A foreign protein reaction then occurs, and within hours the symptoms of inflammation supervene. A large quantity of the material reaching the surface produces an acute reaction. Repeated release of only a few particles at a time produces chronic intermittent symptoms. An acute episode is essentially the manifestation of a chemical furuncle presenting in the floor of the subdeltoid bursa. By comparison the chronic lesion resembles an acne. Eventually, either by an acute reaction or by chronic repeated episodes, the irritant material is phagocytosed and eliminated. The cavity granulates and is replaced by fibrous tissue.

Treatment

Because the lesion is self-limited, therapy has been confused with empiricism. Spontaneous recovery eventually occurs, regardless of the type, presence, or absence of treatment. All therapy is palliative, except that designed to remove the material causing the symptoms. Acute lesions

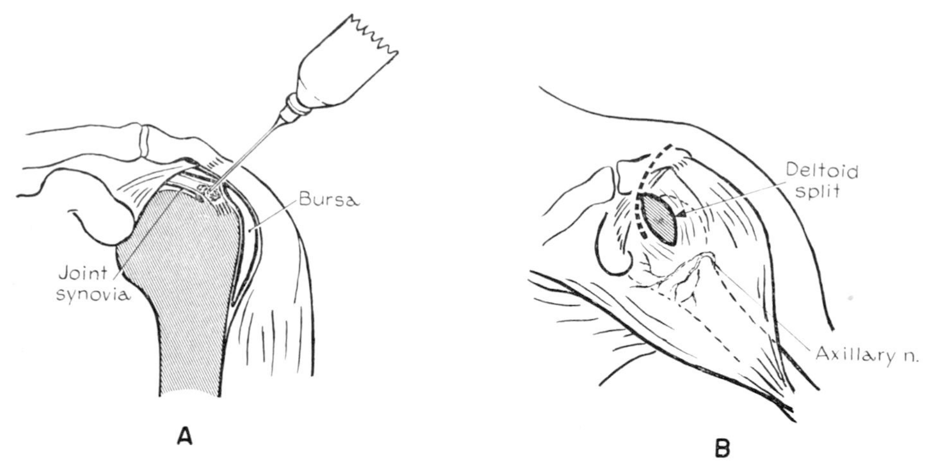

Figure 10–36. Surgical treatment of painful calcium deposits in rotator tendons.

A. The deposit is in the tendon. The inflammatory reaction is occasionally in the synovial lining of the joint, but is usually in the synovial floor of the bursa. Severe pain indicates an acute chemical furuncle. Needling procedures to be successful must result in decompression of this furuncle.

B. The operative approach for removal of a calcium deposit (dotted line) should be curved for a good cosmetic result, and should not exceed 3 cm. in length. The deltoid fibers should be spread apart close to the acromion. Otherwise branches of the axillary nerve may be damaged. The deposit is delivered into the operative field by manipulation of the humerus.

(furuncles) may be decompressed by needle puncture, which is the equivalent of incision (Fig. 10–36). Drainage is unnecessary since the material is absorbed rapidly once it gains access to the subdeltoid bursa. Chronic deposits are dry and under no tension; they will rarely be helped by any needling procedure, and are not benefited by radiotherapy. They must be treated by palliative measures or removed.

The indications for treatment are simple. The patient with chronic pain should be told that he has a condition which is not dangerous, and from which he will eventually recover; that the only significance is the painful symptoms; that there are many palliative measures; that the only quickly curative treatment is removal of the offending deposit; that the longer he can tolerate the symptoms, the nearer he will be to the point of spontaneous recovery; and that, on a basis of the duration and severity of the symptoms, he should decide between expectant and curative therapy. The patient disabled by an acute episode should be reassured that the acute symptoms will probably subside within 5 to 10 days under any circumstances; that subsidence of pain usually coincides with spontaneous rupture of the furuncle and elimination of the deposit; and that once this occurs no future attacks are to be feared. Decompression by needle hastens recovery. Operative incision of the furuncle produces the most certain early relief. Radiotherapy (not exceeding a total of 600 roentgen units) is a logical treatment for the acutely inflamed lesion, but the results, however spectacular they sometimes appear, are similar to those obtained by the simpler palliative measures in control cases. The patient with a history of acute pain, which reached a peak and then commenced to subside prior to examination, has ruptured the furuncle and may confidently be assured of spontaneous relief within a few days. In the writer's experience operative intervention has been justified in less than 5 per cent of persons afflicted with a painful deposit.

RUPTURES OF MUSCULOTENDINOUS CUFF

The tendons of the intrinsic muscles of the shoulder fuse together to form an aponeurotic cuff before inserting into the tuberosities of the humerus (Fig. 10–37, *A*). The tendon fibers are peculiarly prone to attrition

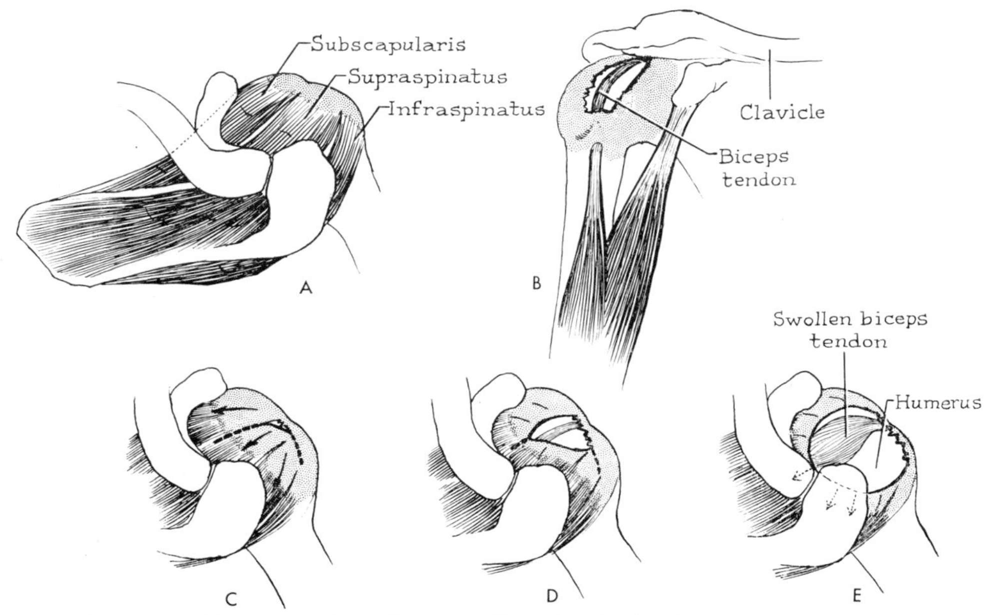

Figure 10–37. Musculotendinous cuff (right shoulder).

A. Viewed from above, the intrinsic muscles fuse to insert into the humerus by a common aponeurotic tendon cuff.

B. Disruption of the tendon cuff often lays bare the biceps tendon which becomes irritated and swollen, due to mechanical irritation of motion.

C. A tear begins and may extend across the inserting tendon fibers, or the divergent muscle forces (arrows) may split the tendon longitudinally to enlarge the primary defect.

D. Extension of the tear produces a triangular defect.

E. A crescentic hiatus is the final result.

at their insertion. Once they are worn and weakened, transverse rupture or a splitting apart of the fibers may occur from minor traumas. The tear tends to enlarge even in the absence of additional injuries, due to the divergent muscle forces (Fig. 10–37, *C*). Usually the biceps tendon is uncovered and becomes greatly enlarged and inflamed due to friction against the acromion and coraco-acromial ligament (Fig. 10–37, *E*). Eventually the hiatus in the tendon cuff becomes crescentic (Fig. 10–37, *E*).

Diagnosis

There are two pathognomonic signs of a cuff tear:

Roentgen demonstration of the escape of gas or opaque material through the ruptured cuff into the subdeltoid bursa, after its injection into the shoulder joint.

Displacement of a fractured tuberosity from the humeral head, which cannot occur with an intact cuff.

Two signs of value to the differential diagnosis are constantly present:

The absence of contracture. In a series of several hundred proven cuff tears, none was associated with a stiff shoulder. In a large series of stiff shoulders explored, none had a cuff tear. The shoulder containing a torn cuff often seems stiff when moved against gravity, but the defect in motion results from pain and there is little or no defect in passive or gravity-free motion.

Selective myopathy. Within two weeks after cuff rupture there is visible atrophy and palpable atony of the spinati muscle bellies. The deltoid, if abnormal, eventually hypertrophies. This is in contradistinction to the deltoid atrophy and spinati integrity common to most other painful conditions in the shoulder.

Four dependable signs of cuff tear are usually present and demonstrable:

The absence of a deposit. In several hundreds of calcium deposits removed and an equal number of ruptured cuffs repaired, the two lesions coexisted only twice. The presence of a deposit, therefore, is strong evidence against a cuff tear.

Palpability of lesion. Palpation of the rupture is almost always possible. Through a relaxed deltoid the tear can be felt as a hiatus or irregularity just proximal to the greater tuberosity.

Crepitus. Cuff rupture produces a characteristic soft palpable crepitus on motion of the arm. This must be differentiated from that produced by a redundant thickened bursa, and at times by the biceps tendon.

Absent or reduced function of the intrinsic muscles. Painless or only mildly uncomfortable inability or weakness in maintaining the abducted arm against gravity or resistance, in the presence of intact axillary and suprascapular nerves, is supportive evidence of a cuff tear.

TABLE 10–2. ANALYSIS OF 100 CONSECUTIVE CASES OF PROVED RUPTURE OF MUSCULOTENDINOUS CUFF

Type of rupture	Massive	Full-thickness	Incomplete-thickness
Number of patients	18	66	16
Average age	57	51	41
(*age spread*)	(41 to 74)	(19 to 72)	(16 to 63)
Sex			
Male	16	42	9
Female	2	24	7
Occupation			
Laborers	12	28	5
Sedentary	6	38	11

The adage that a ruptured cuff is peculiar to males past middle age who do manual labor is unreliable, as is shown in the analysis of 100 consecutive cases presented in Table 10–2.

Indications for Operative Repair

Despite the fact that ruptured tendons elsewhere in the body generally warrant repair, many cuff ruptures need no repair, and few need repair immediately. This is amply substantiated by many facts, among which are the following: A torn cuff is found in 20 to 30 per cent of unselected cadavers (age at death over 60). Many patients, in whom the clinical signs of rupture are clear, recover spontaneously if given a chance. Almost all ruptures occur through degenerated tendon tissue, so that the tear is the equivalent of an old chronic lesion as soon as it occurs. Hence there is little advantage to be gained by early operative intervention. In addition, pain often precludes an accurate diagnosis during the early stages following injury. Finally, the results of early and late repair are about identical.

Early operative repair, therefore, is contraindicated in all except massive lesions which are certain to produce serious defects. A minimum of two weeks' observation is wise, following which, if symptoms fail to abate and the diagnosis remains definite, repair should be carried out. So long as subjective improvement continues, conservative therapy should be maintained. When symptoms become stationary, the decision for or against operative repair should be governed by their severity and the resultant disability.

Conservative Treatment

Immobilization of the limb in abduction accomplishes more harm than good and often incurs a penalty more severe than that of the untreated cuff tear. Pain should be controlled and the mobility of the shoulder maintained. A sling may be used to support the arm during the early painful phase, but this should be discarded as soon as its absence can be tolerated. Gradually progressive exercises and resumption of use at frequent intervals, up to but not past the limits of pain, should be insisted upon. Under such a program almost half of the patients in whom the evidence of rupture is definite will recover a comfortable, useful extremity. When this does not take place, operative repair deserves consideration and is attended by a good prognosis, provided the surgeon ignores the anatomical features of the rupture and accomplishes (1) snug apposition of healthy to healthy tissue without tension, (2) restoration of continuity between the spinati muscles and the humerus, and (3) a smooth tendon surface for articulation with the acromion (or removal of the acromion).

RUPTURE OF LONG TENDON OF BICEPS

In cadaver studies the long head of the biceps is often found to be ruptured, and the distal fragment reattached to the bicipital groove. This and clinical observations indicate the intra-articular portion of the tendon to be functionally insignificant. It may be ablated with impunity. Frequently, following traumatic rupture, the distal fragment retracts, owing to contraction of the muscle belly. The result is an unsightly lump of muscle at midarm, unaccompanied by much functional disturbance, provided the biceps rupture occurs as an isolated lesion. In other cases the tendon wears away and finally ruptures because it has been uncovered by a cuff tear (Fig. 10–37). When this occurs, some pain and disability are common, but result from rupture of the cuff rather than of the biceps. Consequently, since a biceps rupture alone produces neither permanent symptoms nor disability and rarely warrants operative repair except for cosmetic purposes, the same lesion accompanied by persistent pain and disability in the shoulder should arouse suspicion of a cuff rupture. Total strength is only a little weakened by rupture of the long head, since the short head of the muscle is amply able to compensate for the lost power.

SNAPPING SHOULDER

Several conditions can cause a painful "catch" on certain motions of the shoulder. Few of these are amenable to conservative therapy, and the symptoms may warrant exploration.

Chronic Recurrent Subluxation of Biceps Tendon

This condition may result from stretch or rupture of the cuff expansions holding the proximal end of the tendon in the bicipital groove. The mechanical irritation resulting from hypermobility causes inflammation of its synovial investment so that shoulder motion is impeded by a painful jog as it slips in and out of the groove. There is no conservative treatment. Operative stabilization of the tendon or ablation of the intra-articular portion, and reattachment of the distal fragment in or about the bicipital groove, is the treatment of choice.

Tear of Glenoid Meniscus

This injury may occur without dislocation. The nature of the tear is as variable as it may be in tears of the menisci of the knee. Painful locking symptoms, similar to those encountered in the deranged knee, may occur. Excision of the torn portion of labrum is the only measure available for relief when symptoms are serious.

Thickened Subdeltoid Bursa

Subdeltoid bursitis from any cause which results in a thickening of the bursal roof may produce painful snapping episodes on motion as the thickened walls of the bursa heap up into folds which snap rather than slide under the edge of the acromion and the sharp anterior edge of the coraco-acromial ligament. The most efficient treatment is excision of the bursa and division of the ligament.

Tendon Cuff Irregularity

A small tear in the cuff may produce little in the way of symptoms, except when the irregularity it creates in the surface of the tendon cuff catches against the edge of acromion or coraco-acromial ligament as the arm is elevated or lowered. Repair, accompanied by division of the coraco-acromial ligament, is indicated.

Incomplete Glenohumeral Dislocation

Recurrent subluxation of the shoulder should always be considered in the differential diagnosis of any disability characterized by snapping or locking episodes.

FROZEN SHOULDER

The shoulder, in common with all other joints, stiffens when it is not used. The position of disuse is dependency and internal rotation. In the adult any condition in or distant from the shoulder which predisposes to prolonged dependency of the arm is a potential primary cause of a stiff shoulder. Causes outside the shoulder include all lesions productive of pain on elevation of the arm, for example, cervical arthritis and disc lesions, apical lung tumors, pulmonary tuberculosis or chronic pleurisy, cardiac disease, and even some inflammatory conditions in the abdomen. A common cause is the prolonged use of a sling for treatment of some lesion in the hand or wrist. Intrinsic causes include low-grade infections in the shoulder or clavicular joints, painful mechanical derangements of the acromioclavicular joint, neglected painful deposits in the shoulder tendons, and post-traumatic immobilization of the injured shoulder. In about 10 per cent of the cases there is no demonstrable cause for the stiffened shoulder. It is common to such lesions that the patients are past middle age and under some emotional stress.

Secondary Effects

The side effects of a frozen shoulder confuse the diagnosis. Chronic protective muscle spasm produces pain, which radiates from the shoulder like the spokes of a wheel, to the deltoid tubercle and at times into the forearm, and up the trapezius to produce occipital tension headaches, across the pectorals to produce mediastinal symptoms, and down the back along the scapular muscles. These symptoms may simulate radicular pains, but a careful examination demonstrates them to follow muscle bundles, rather than nerve tracts, and to stop short of the hand, in contradistinction to true nerve-root symptoms which follow the nerves and usually involve the fingers. In addition, constant protective spasm and, *ipso facto*, chronic sympathetic stimulation produce some vasomotor change in the limb. Secondary sensory symptoms from hypoxia, and reflex changes due to muscle spasm, may then further confuse the picture. Hence, many so-called "shoulder-hand" syndromes may result from some primary cause unconnected with either shoulder or hand.

Pathology

The condition in most stiff shoulders is self-limited, but often lasts 6 to 18 months, if allowed to become well established. The findings are variable. When the lesion results from some primary cause of prolonged dependency of the arm there are contracture and loss of elasticity of all periarticular tissues, but no significant microscopic evidences of pathology. Most idiopathic lesions show, in addition, an obliteration of the redundant capsular folds by a proliferative inflammatory synovitis. This process often interferes with mobility of the biceps tendon by inflammatory fixation of its synovial investment, and has led to use of the term "bicipital tenosynovitis." Contrary to widespread belief, the subdeltoid bursa rarely shows adhesions or becomes obliterated, but is merely anemic and atrophied by disuse.

Treatment

Forceful manipulation of the frozen shoulder is to be condemned. Operative observations show that manipulation not only does not break adhesions but does rupture and tear the biceps and subscapularis tendons, the glenohumeral ligaments and contracted joint capsule, and many other normal anatomical structures. It is little wonder that such procedures are often followed by an increase, rather than a decrease, in pain and stiffness. Gentle passive stretching of the joint within pain limits may be beneficial, but in the last analysis the contracted structures must be stretched gradually by active exercises, made possible by palliative therapy. Progress is always slow and most patients will become so disheartened as to need all the reassurance and encouragement at the surgeon's command before success is achieved. Such a program is facilitated by preliminary removal of whatever organic or emotional primary cause predisposed to prolonged dependency of the arm. When the primary cause is irreversible, the prognosis is poor.

Summary of Cause and Management of Frozen Shoulder

1. The shoulder, in common with all joints, and to a degree affected by the age of the patient and the presence of some undue mental tension, tends to stiffen with disuse.
2. No shoulder which moves through a normal range as many as a few times each day will become frozen.
3. The immediate cause of all frozen shoulders is prolonged dependency of the limb.
4. The primary factors causing prolonged dependency may be intrinsic or far removed from the shoulder.
5. The best treatment is prophylactic—the shoulder should not be allowed to become stiff.

6. Once the condition is established, the most efficient and safest plan for management is elimination of primary causes of dependency and active gradual mobilization of the joint by the patient.

7. Forceful manipulation is to be condemned in all but exceptional circumstances, and operative mobilization of the joint should be reserved as a last resort.

FRACTURE OF THE CLAVICLE

The clavicle is the only rigid connection between the upper limb and the remainder of the skeleton. Fracture usually results from a fall on the outstretched hand, as the force of the impact is transmitted from the extremity to the torso through this small bone. The deformity may be negligible in greenstick fractures, but is constant and characteristic when the fracture is complete. The inner fragment appears elevated, but is actually balanced between sternocleidomastoid muscle and costoclavicular ligament in about normal position. The shoulder girdle, bereft of its single bony strut, falls downward and medially and rolls forward on the thorax, carrying with it the outer clavicular fragment.

Treatment

Reduction requires the shoulder girdle as a whole to be pulled upward and backward until it is symmetrical with the normal side. This maneuver realigns the fracture fragments, and residual displacement may be corrected by digital manipulation at the fracture site.

Fixation requires the whole shoulder girdle to be maintained in normal position, since the clavicle cannot be stabilized directly by any external splint. This is most simply accomplished by a figure-of-8 or T splint dressing (Fig. 10–38), but no form of external fixation provides true immobilization of the fragments. As a result, continued mobility predisposes to exuberant callus formation. When the best possible cosmetic result is mandatory, the patient should be put to bed with a pillow between the scapulae and light traction on the arm, which is suspended so that its long axis corresponds to that of the clavicle.

Open reduction is not indicated in children, but may be of great benefit in comminuted fractures in the adult, especially when a displaced fragment presses upon the underlying brachial plexus or subclavian vessels. Open reduction and intramedullary fixation (Fig. 10–39) is simple, sure, and attended by little morbidity when carried out with certain pitfalls and safeguards in mind. The intramedullary device should always be inserted from the inner to the outer fragment and never in the opposite direction. The procedure should never be done "blind," but only with the lesion well exposed. The end of the fixation device, which is left protruding from the bone for easy removal, should be crimped to forestall its migration into undesirable locations. The patient may resume all but heavy activities as soon as the skin is healed, but must look forward to removal of the fixation device after union of the fracture. Congenital pseudarthrosis and fibrous

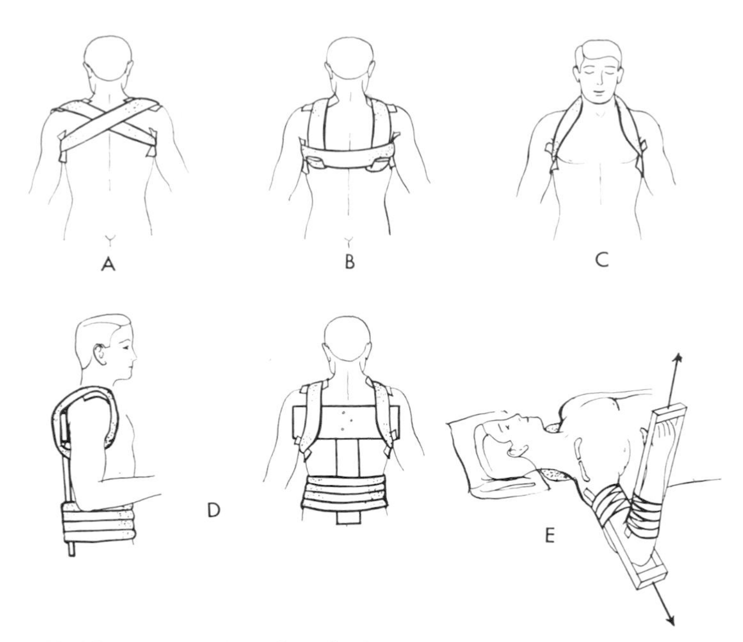

Figure 10–38. *Fixation of clavicle fractures.*

A. Figure-of-8 supportive bandage or molded splint (appropriate for small children, but inefficient in larger children and adults).

B. A more efficient dressing than that shown in A, in that the shoulders are held back more efficiently (rear view).

C. Front view of A and B; axillae and bony prominences on the superior surface of the shoulders must be padded.

D. A T *splint, as shown here, is relatively inefficient and uncomfortable, but is a simple expedient when plaster of paris is not available.*

E. Treatment by traction and bed rest. A pillow between the scapulae throws the shoulders back. Humeral traction should be parallel to the long axis of the fractured clavicle. Forearm lift should be just enough to counterbalance the weight of the suspended limb.

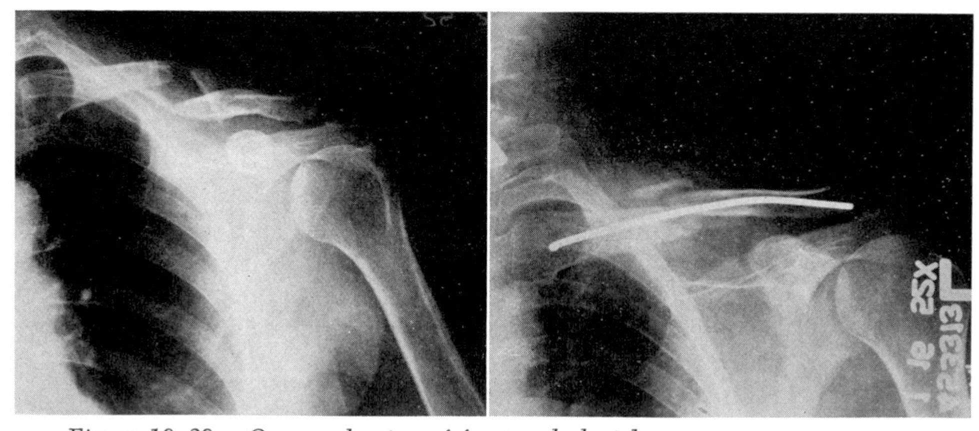

Figure 10–39. *Open reduction of fractured clavicle.*

A comminuted unstable fracture in an adult. Signs of ulnar nerve irritation, which subsided subsequent to open reduction and fixation by an intramedullary device. The latter is crimped at its medial end to prevent migration.

union of the clavicle, formerly difficult problems, have been greatly facilitated by intramedullary fixation with or without a bone graft.

Fracture of the Clavicle in Infants

Fracture of the clavicle in small infants is not uncommon. No dependable history is available. The infant screams on examination of any part of the limb. Demonstrable local signs may not be present and, since most such lesions are greenstick or mildly buckled fractures, the x-ray film may require close examination before the diagnosis becomes certain. The lesion, per se, is of little significance, but the mother's fears are great. A definite diagnosis, a flannel figure-of-8 dressing, and reassurance that recovery without permanent defect will occur in a week or two, will allay both.

Complications of Clavicle Fracture

The late complications of clavicle fracture are uncommon and almost entirely restricted to adults. Occasionally a branch of the supraclavicular nerves may be compressed by callus to produce paresthesias and pain. Nonunion is to be feared, and early operative fixation should be considered when the fracture occurs in a large muscular male, for most forms of external fixation will fail to control the weight of his shoulder and the powerful muscles involved. Dressings such as that described by Sayre and Velpeau, which obliterate function and motion of the entire limb, have properly fallen into discard, since their use is commonly productive of prolonged and serious stiffness and disability throughout the entire extremity. Above all it must be realized that no external dressing really immobilizes a fractured clavicle, and that the optimum effect of conservative treatment is to maintain alignment of the fragments coincident with continued motion and some use of the extremity. Bony union is the rule within three to four weeks in adolescents, but may be delayed for six to ten weeks in adults.

DISLOCATION AT THE STERNOCLAVICULAR JOINT

A trauma which forces the shoulder backward and downward levers the clavicle over the first rib and may disrupt the sternoclavicular ligaments and displace the inner end of the clavicle forward and upward (Fig. 10–*40, A*). The costoclavicular ligament remains intact, and the weight of the limb maintains the clavicular displacement. Conversely, violence which forces the shoulder upward and forward may drive the inner end of the clavicle downward and medially behind the sternum. The much more common anterior dislocation is marked by hypermobility and a prominent projection of the inner end of the clavicle, and eventually some mild discomfort on motion of the arm. Posterior dislocation (Fig. 10–*40, B*) causes pressure first on the trachea to produce dyspnea, and at times dysphagia, and then on the great vessels to produce cyanosis from the neck up. This

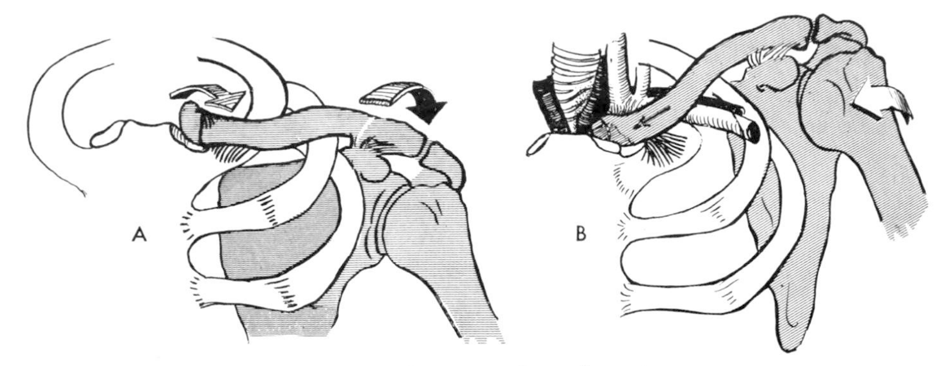

Figure 10–40. Dislocation at the sternoclavicular joint.

A. The first rib is the fulcrum; downward and backward depression of the shoulder levers the inner end of the clavicle forward from the sternoclavicular joint.

B. Forward and medial compression of the shoulder drives the inner end of the clavicle downward behind the sternum to press upon the trachea and great vessels.

is an alarming syndrome accompanied by little in the way of visible deformity.

Treatment

Reduction of either type follows immediately upon traction on the shoulder in a line parallel to the long axis of the clavicle. Many anterior dislocations require nothing more than to push the displaced end of the clavicle into place.

Fixation is difficult. The weight of the limb must be supported or the displacement recurs immediately. Respiratory motions preclude true immobilization. The mechanical problems involved and the dressings which most efficiently answer the problem are similar to those described for fracture of the clavicle.

Open reduction is sometimes required in chronic lesions for cosmetic reasons, or as a result of symptoms produced by instability of the end of the clavicle. Reconstruction procedures which attempt to replace and maintain the clavicle in position seldom are completely successful, and are followed by a risk of late painful arthritis in the joint. The most simple and efficient procedure is subperiosteal excision of the medial 2 cm. of the clavicle, taking care that the stump remains stabilized by the costoclavicular ligament, and that the internal mammary artery, which lies immediately behind the segment to be resected, is not injured. The morbidity is minimal, and the usefulness of the limb returns as soon as skin healing occurs. The results are very satisfactory.

INJURIES AT THE ACROMIOCLAVICULAR JOINT

The acromioclavicular mechanism is stabilized by ligaments reinforcing the joint capsule and by the coracoclavicular ligaments, which are the only inelastic structures suspending the scapula (and the weight of the limb) from the clavicle (see Fig. 10–*41*). A circular fibrocartilaginous meniscus, subject to lacerations, improves the efficiency of this universal joint. The great majority of acromioclavicular injuries result from a direct impact which drives the acromion downward from the clavicle. Displacement may stop short at, or continue and rupture the coracoclavicular ligaments.

INCOMPLETE DISLOCATION

Incomplete acromioclavicular disruption leaves the coracoclavicular ligaments intact, but ruptures the acromioclavicular ligaments. Gravity rotates the scapula toward the arm. On clinical examination the end of the clavicle appears elevated—actually the acromion is depressed (Fig. 10–*41*). The intra-articular meniscus is torn and the joint severely disrupted. Eventual traumatic arthritis is to be expected after some years free from symptoms or disability.

Treatment

Reduction is simply accomplished by lifting the arm and pressing the outer end of the clavicle into place.

Fixation is difficult. The weight of the limb must be removed from the shoulder by a sling, and the end of the clavicle held in place by a dressing which maintains a fixed distance between acromion and elbow. The almost invariable result is some persistent subluxation and hypermobility which in time leads to post-traumatic arthritis and painful symptoms.

COMPLETE DISLOCATION

Complete acromioclavicular dislocation disrupts both the acromioclavicular and coracoclavicular ligaments. The scapula drops away from the

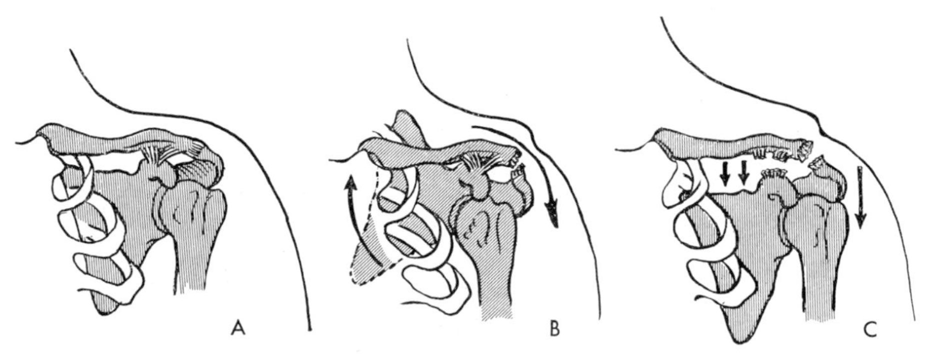

Figure 10–41. Injury to acromioclavicular and coracoclavicular joints.

A. The acromioclavicular and coracoclavicular ligaments (uninjured).

B. The acromioclavicular ligaments alone are ruptured. Gravity rotates the scapula clockwise.

C. Both sets of ligaments are ruptured. The entire limb drops away from the clavicle.

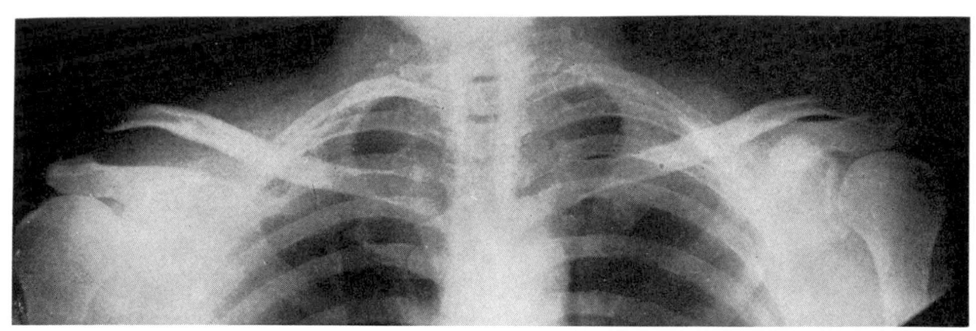

Figure 10–42. Roentgen diagnosis of complete acromioclavicular dislocation.

The film includes both shoulders. The patient is erect, holding small weights in each hand. The discrepancy in measurements from clavicles to coracoids is certain evidence of conoid and trapezoid ligament rupture on the right side.

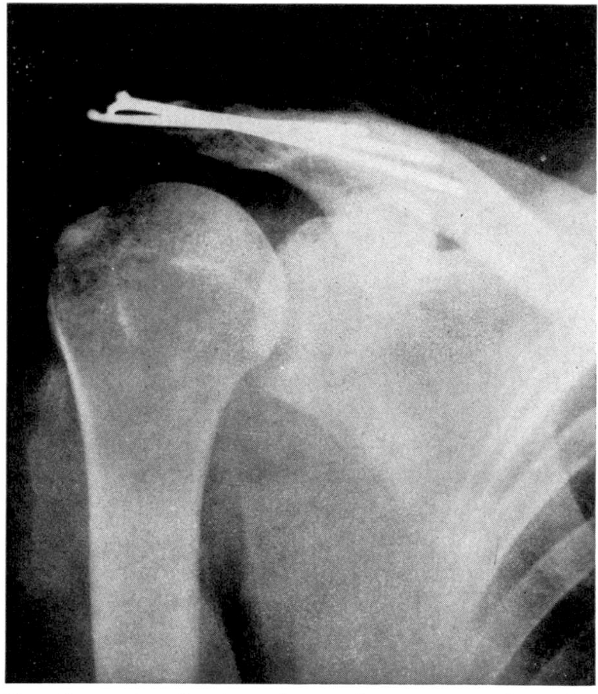

Figure 10–43. Operative fixation of complete acromioclavicular dislocation.

Three stiff wires transfix the acromion and clavicle. The lateral ends of the wires are crimped to prevent migration medialward. The coracoid is held at a normal distance from the clavicle despite gravity. The wires must be removed about six weeks after operation, at which time fibrous union is secure.

clavicle (Fig. 10–*41*). In contradistinction to incomplete lesions attended by no permanent defect, except pain at the deranged joint, this lesion often disables the manual worker by weakness in the limb. Conservative treatment by strapping is not often followed by a good result. Operative fixation is a matter of election for the sedentary patient, but is strongly indicated for the manual worker.

Differential Diagnosis

The differential diagnosis between complete and incomplete lesions cannot be made by clinical evidence, nor can it always be made from routine roentgenograms. The only certain evidence of a conoid and trapezoid ligament rupture is found in an anteroposterior film showing both shoulders and taken with the patient standing erect and, if possible, holding a small weight in each hand. An increase in the distance between clavicle and coracoid (Fig. 10–*42*) is certain evidence of ligament disruption.

Operative Treatment

Many operations have been advocated for the management of an early complete dislocation. The simplest and most efficient of these is open reduction and transfixion of the repositioned bones by two or three stiff wires (Fig. 10–*43*). The arm is carried in a sling for several weeks, but all joints of the limb should be moved frequently. The wires are removed after six weeks, otherwise they will work out through the skin of their own accord. The results are good, and no weakness ensues, since the scapula is held in proper relationship to the clavicle during the period of formation of a mass of fibrous tissue which replaces the broken ligaments.

OLD UNREDUCED DISLOCATIONS OR PAINFUL PERSISTENT SUBLUXATIONS

Repair in such cases is difficult and followed by only fair results. Subperiosteal excision of at least 2 and not more than 3 cm. of the outer end of the clavicle is the procedure of choice. The stump of the bone must be left long enough to retain a connection with the coracoid, by scar tissue, if not by ligaments, and short enough so that it does not impinge against the acromion when the arm is abducted. The resected segment of bone is replaced by a fibrous cord and a comfortable and serviceable shoulder may be expected.

INTERNAL DERANGEMENT OF ACROMIOCLAVICULAR JOINT

Wrenching injuries, as well as direct traumas, to the acromion may stop short of producing actual subluxation of the joint but injure the intra-articular meniscus. The resultant syndrome is marked by pain and tenderness in the joint without x-ray signs until many years later, when arthritic changes supervene. Occasionally such lesions are painful enough to be quite disabling. The diagnosis is strengthened when symptoms are relieved temporarily by injection of a few milliliters of procaine hydrochloride into the joint cavity. Meniscectomy alone relieves the symptoms when the lesion is early and unattended by articular cartilage damage or degeneration. The most certain results follow excision of the outer end of the clavicle.

Fracture of the outer end of the clavicle is the equivalent of an acromioclavicular injury, except that the disruption takes place through bone rather than the adjacent ligaments. So long as the coracoclavicular ligaments are intact, displacement cannot occur. Bony union is to be expected and little except symptomatic therapy is required. Displacement makes the lesion the equivalent of a complete acromioclavicular dislocation, and warrants treatment as such.

Part III

THE LOWER EXTREMITY

CHAPTER 11

INJURIES OF THE FOOT

By FREDERICK S. CRAIG, M.D., and

HARRISON L. McLAUGHLIN, M.D.

ANATOMICAL FEATURES OF THE FOOT

TWELVE OF THE 26 bones making up the skeleton of the foot, or all excepting those in the toes, are arranged in the form of an arch which parallels the long axis of the foot. The arch is not symmetrical, but has an architecture defying detailed mechanical analysis, being considerably higher on the medial than on the lateral aspect of the foot (Fig. 11–*1*, *A*), and having a shorter posterior segment and a longer anterior curve.

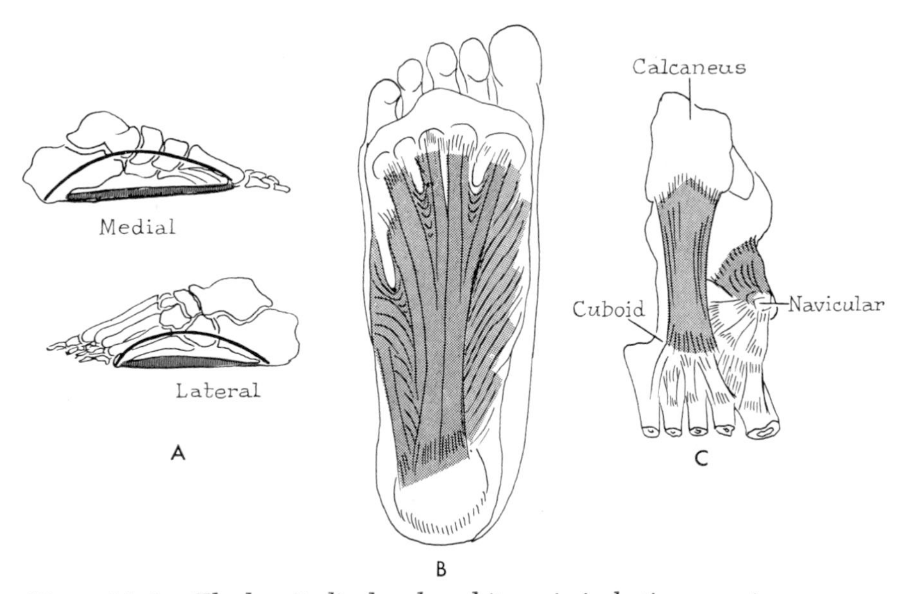

Figure 11–1. The longitudinal arch and its main inelastic supports.

A. The bony arch of the foot is longer and higher on the medial than on the lateral surface, and is supported in the manner of a bowstring by the subcutaneous plantar fascia.

B. The plantar fascia, viewed from below.

C. The calcaneocuboid and calcaneonavicular ligaments, viewed from below. These and many other smaller ligaments support the plantar concavity of the longitudinal arch and augment the bowstring function of the plantar fascia.

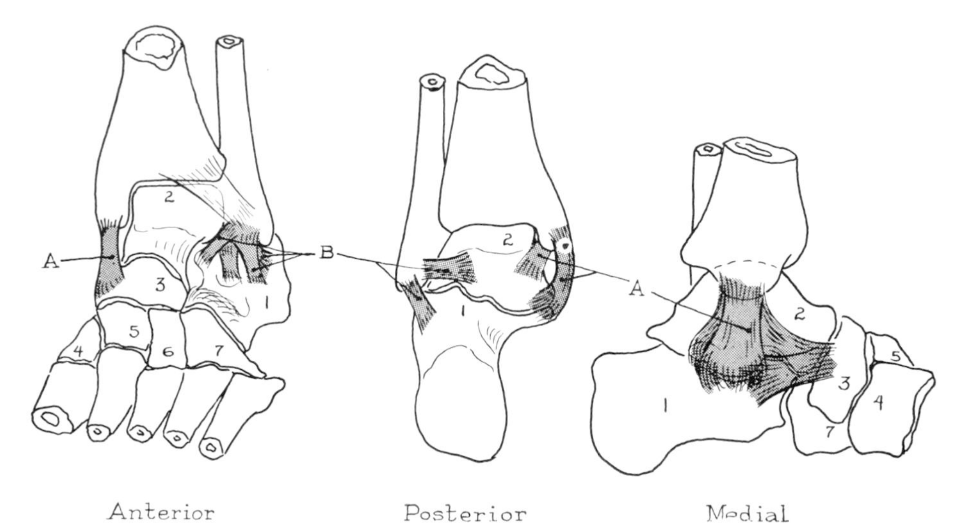

Figure 11–2. The principal bones of the foot and their ligamentous attachments to the leg, in anterior, posterior, and medial views.

1. *Calcaneus (os calcis).*
2. *Talus (astragalus).*
3. *Navicular.*
4. *Medial cuneiform bone.*
5. *Intermediate cuneiform bone.*
6. *Lateral cuneiform bone*
7. *Cuboid bone.*

A. *Medial collateral (deltoid) ligament of ankle.*
B. *Lateral collateral ligament of ankle.*

The tibiotalar joint moves only in flexion and extension; the talocalcaneal joint moves only in inversion and eversion.

Body weight is transmitted from the tibia through the talus (astragalus), which is at the apex of this arch. Below the talus, and forming the short posterior segment of the arch, is the calcaneus. The remainder of the bones of the foot comprise the longer anterior segment of the arch. Both talus and calcaneus are connected to the leg bones by strong collateral ligaments (Fig. 11–2), and the talus is grasped firmly, like a tenon, in the mortise formed by the malleoli, so that no motions except flexion and extension can take place at the talotibial articulation. Inversion and eversion of the foot occur in the talocalcaneal articulations.

In the standing position weight is borne by the calcaneus and the metatarsal heads. There is no significant transverse arch. The metatarsal heads all bear equal portions of weight, except the first metatarsal, which accepts double the load of each of the other four. Weight bearing on these points without collapse and flattening of the longitudinal arch of the foot is made possible by strong inelastic and elastic arch supports. The superficially placed plantar fascia (Fig. 11–*1*, *B*), as well as multiple more deeply situated ligaments, are stretched across the concavity of the bony arch in the manner of bowstrings (Fig. 11–*1*, *A*, *C*). Supporting and defending

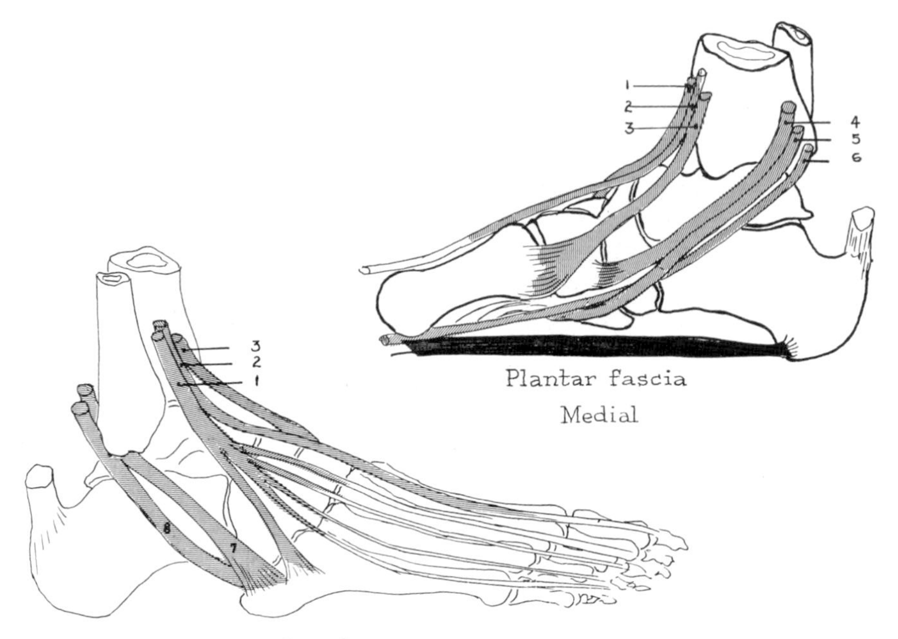

Figure 11–3. The tendons supporting and motivating the foot, in lateral and medial views.

1. *Extensor digitorum longus.*
2. *Extensor hallucis longus.*
3. *Tibialis anticus.*
4. *Tibialis posticus.*
5. *Flexor digitorum longus.*
6. *Flexor hallucis longus.*
7. *Peroneus brevis.*
8. *Peroneus longus.*

against any sudden overloading of these inelastic struts is the motor power of a group of strong muscles, arising in the leg but inserted into the foot with mechanical advantages designed to suspend the arch of the foot from above (Fig. 11–3).

PROBLEMS COMMON TO INJURIES OF THE FOOT

EDEMA

Edema is common to all foot injuries. The prevention of swelling is much easier than its eradication. Once a foot has become grossly swollen, which may occur with great rapidity, adequate treatment of the injury may be precluded until edema has been eradicated. Prolonged edema is followed by fibrosis, stiffness, and pain. The resultant disuse perpetuates and predisposes to increased edema. A vicious cycle invalidating treatment and preventing recovery, despite all forms of treatment, may be established.

Prevention of Edema

Prevention of edema requires some combination of elevation, compression, and rest. The foot should be higher than the knee, and the knee higher than the hip. A snug compression dressing should be fashioned with many layers of sheet wadding, cotton, or mechanic's waste, and secured circumferentially around the entire foot with an elastic bandage. Usually an adequate compression dressing also provides immobilization sufficient to place the injured tissues at rest. In the presence of gross fractures additional splints may be required.

Treatment of Established Edema

Delay in treatment may permit the formation of tense swelling of all the tissues, and blistering of the skin. These products of neglected tissue damage often must be controlled before the actual injury can be treated. Large blisters may be aspirated with aseptic technique. At times a tense localized hematoma may require aspiration or incision. Gentle motions of all joints within the limits of pain and safety help to restore an efficient circulation to and from the foot. Elevation should be maintained. Lumbar sympathetic block by procaine hydrochloride has a palliative effect, but does not often increase circulatory efficiency to a measurable degree.

IMMOBILIZATION

Immobilization by plaster of paris dressings is useful or necessary in the management of many injuries of the foot, but immobilization begets stiffness, and should be used only when its benefits will outweigh the disadvantages inherent in what may prove to be a long period of post-immobilization stiffness and pain.

Molded plaster splints have advantages over circular plaster dressings. Circular dressings fit only when applied, after which they progressively become loose or unduly tight with variations in the degree of swelling. Molded splints can be rebandaged in place with appropriate tension as often as the need arises.

Except on rare occasions, the foot should be immobilized in a position of neither plantar flexion nor extension, but at right angles to the leg, and neither inverted nor everted. Prolonged plantar flexion predisposes to calf contracture and a fixed equinus deformity (Fig. 11–4). Overuse of the toe extensors in an attempt to extend the foot against such a contracture may produce clawing of the toes, followed by painful and unsightly corns. Prolonged immobilization in a position of inversion may stiffen the foot in this position so that its outer border is overloaded by weight bearing and becomes painful. Attention to these small details during the application of immobilizing dressings may prevent a long and unnecessary period of painful disability after the dressings are removed. Except when rare and specific indications are present, the injured foot should be immobilized in the position of use.

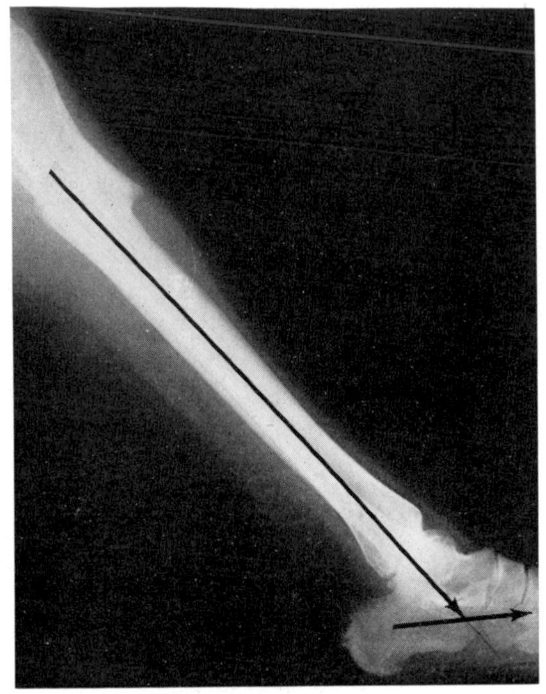

Figure 11–4. Equinus deformity following prolonged plaster immobilization for a fracture of the tibia with the foot in plantar flexion. The maximum dorsiflexion is demonstrated.

MOBILIZATION

It is beneficial to maintain motion of an injured foot within the limits of pain, fatigue, and safety. Even when the foot itself requires immobilization, toe motion must continue. Passive motion is of little or no value, and may be harmful. Active motion, on the other hand, is produced by the muscles whose contractions implement the venous and lymphatic pump to reduce edema, increases the local metabolic demand to augment the blood supply, and minimizes both stiffness and vascular stagnation at the injured area. The convalescent period consistently is decreased in proportion to the degree of normal foot or toe motions which are permitted by the circumstances of the injury and the treatment employed.

SOFT TISSUE INJURIES OF THE FOOT

RUPTURE OF THE ANTERIOR TIBIAL TENDON

Diagnosis

This injury, which results from a misstep usually causing sudden forcible flexion or eversion of the foot, and which almost always occurs at a weak point of degeneration in the tendon, is quite rare. Normally, the tense tibialis anticus tendon is easily palpable and visible, 1 inch in front of the medial malleolus, when the foot is inverted or extended. Weakness or absence of these motions, absence of the tense tendon to sight and touch, and the usual stigmata of a local injury establish a clear-cut diagnosis.

Treatment

Operative repair or reinsertion of the tendon should be done as soon as possible. A severely painful everted foot consequent to unopposed peroneal muscle action is likely to result from failure to restore continuity and function of the tibialis anticus. Secure repair permits ambulation in a plaster of paris boot during convalescence. Removal of the boot and progressive resumption of unsupported function may be allowed after two months.

TENDON DEPOSITS

Amorphous deposits with pathogenesis and life cycles identical to those described in Chapter 10, on Injuries of the Shoulder and Arm, may be encountered in any of the tendons of the foot. By far the most frequent location is in the peroneus longus tendon at its point of entrance into the groove on the plantar surface of the cuboid bone (Fig. 11–5).

Diagnosis

The clinical picture, as with similar lesions elsewhere in the body, is one of a very acute local reaction often marked by a sterile cellulitis, but productive of little or no systemic response. Roentgenographic evidence

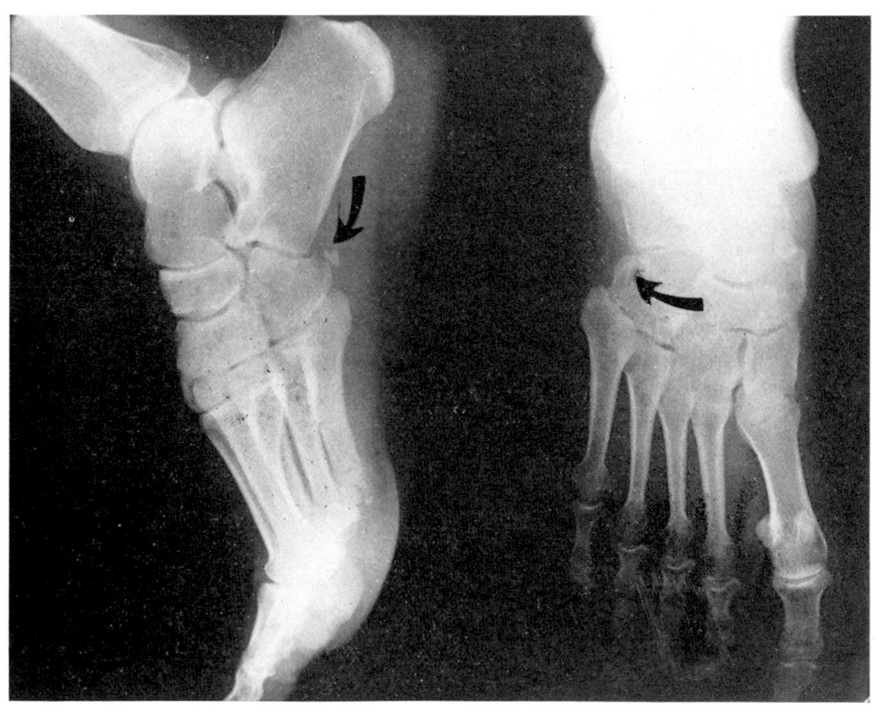

Figure 11–5. A painful deposit in the peroneus longus tendon; not to be confused with a sesamoid bone common to the same area.

of the deposit, which should not be confused with the somewhat similar appearing sesamoids common to certain tendons of the foot, and especially to the peroneus longus tendon, confirms the diagnosis.

Treatment

Since all such conditions are self-limited, treatment should be designed primarily to control the pain until spontaneous recovery takes place. The foot should be placed at rest in a plaster splint. Warm soaks and other gentle palliative measures may be required. When an acutely inflamed deposit is large and accessible, decompression of the chemical furuncle by needle hastens relief of pain. Decompression by incision is rarely necessary, because recovery within a few days may be expected under any circumstances.

TENOSYNOVITIS

Tenosynovitis may occur at a point of friction of any tendon. The rubbing of a new shoe or a minor local injury may be the primary offending agent. Prolonged use of a foot with an unduly high arch, such as in hiking or dancing, not uncommonly results in a synovitis of the anterior tibial tendon sheath. Molded arch supports may be required to reduce the strain on this tendon and prevent recurrence following excessive use of the foot.

Diagnosis

Acute synovitis is characterized by local pain, tenderness, swelling, and redness in the local area, and spasm of the muscle belly motivating the involved tendon. In subacute and chronic conditions, similar but less marked signs and symptoms often are accompanied by crepitus on motion, as though there were sand in the tendon sheath. In chronic synovitis pain is usually limited to the extremes of motion of the tendon, or to manipulations which place the tendon under maximum stress, such as passive stretch by the examiner or strong contraction of the involved muscle against resistance. At rest or with weight bearing, the foot will be held in an abnormal position which reduces tension upon the painful tendon–tendon sheath entity, but which also creates imbalance of the foot, as a whole, and results in additional painful symptoms from overloading of other uninflamed structures. Temporary abolition of pain by injection of the suspected tendon sheath with procaine hydrochloride may be useful for identification of the specific tendon sheath involved.

Treatment

Acute synovitis requires rest in a splint, elevation, and the application of gentle heat. Symptoms subside rapidly when the inflammation is of mechanical origin, after which gradual resumption of motion and use is permissible and safe. Full activity should not be permitted until all symptoms have subsided completely. Otherwise, the synovitis may recur and become chronic.

Chronic synovitis often is resistant to therapy. When the painful and tender area is well localized, abolition of pain by procaine hydrochloride infiltration may permit sufficient temporary active motion to restore a more normal gliding motion in the tendon–tendon sheath structure. Occasionally the benefits of the injection are permanent. Whether this is the result of rupturing small adhesions by the motion temporarily made possible by the local anesthetic is unknown. Reduction or removal of the load ordinarily accepted by the inflamed tendon–tendon sheath structure may be accomplished by a molded metal or rubber arch support, or by a snug plaster of paris boot. This should be done, but the results are by no means certain. As a last resort, operative excision of the chronically inflamed tendon sheath offers the most certain promise of success.

RUPTURE OF PERONEAL RETINACULUM

The peroneal grooves on the posterior aspect of the lateral malleolus are sometimes quite shallow. Sudden extension of the foot may displace

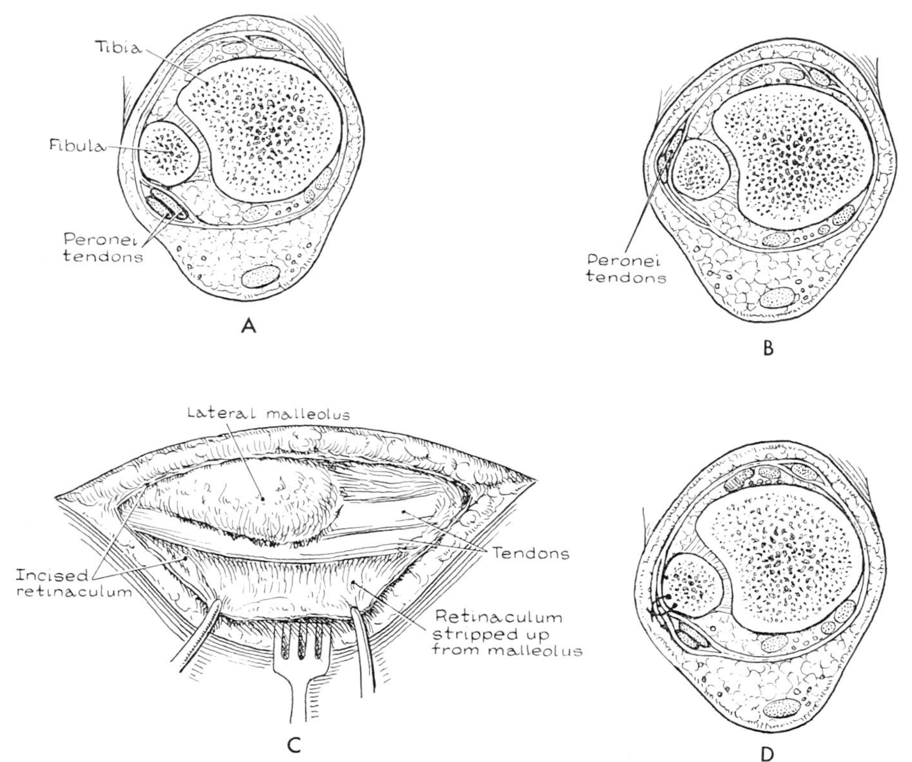

Figure 11–6. Rupture of the peroneal retinaculum and repair.
A. Normal cross section just above the ankle joint.
B. Retinaculum ruptured and peronei tendons displaced forward.
C. Operative exposure and replacement of peronei tendons in their grooves.
D. Retinaculum repaired, tendons in place. In addition to repair of the retinaculum, it is sometimes necessary to deepen the peroneal grooves in the fibula.

the peroneal tendons forward, rupturing the fibrous retinaculum which restrains them in their respective grooves (Fig. 11–6, *A*, *B*). The tendons slip forward over the lateral malleolus on dorsiflexion and eversion of the foot, and return to normal position as the foot is plantar flexed or inverted. These phenomena are visible and palpable.

Treatment

Following the initial episode, the foot should be immobilized in a plaster of paris walking-boot for six to eight weeks. The prospects for adequate fibrous healing are good. Chronic recurrent subluxation of the peroneal tendons from their fibular grooves becomes irreversibly established very rapidly, if immobilization is not provided within a short time after the first injury. Operative reconstruction of the injured retinaculum (Fig. 11–6, *C*, *D*) may then be necessary for relief of the intermittent symptoms of "buckling" of the ankle, which occur with each subluxation.

SPRAIN OF THE FOOT

Sprain of the foot most commonly consists of an injury to the ligaments supporting the intertarsal or tarsometatarsal joints. Avulsion of small chips of bone by the overstretched ligaments is common, and the condition should not be considered or treated as a fracture. Any displacement of one tarsal bone on another represents a complete ligament tear and an incomplete dislocation, and should not be considered or treated as a simple sprain.

A true sprain results from a wrenching or twisting injury, often a misstep, and is manifested by early and extensive swelling and ecchymosis, principally on the dorsal surface of the foot, and wincing tenderness on pressure and pain on motion, centered at the location of the injured ligaments. The roentgenogram reveals nothing, except for the common presence of a small separated chip of bone from some articular edge in the neighborhood of the center of trouble noted clinically.

Treatment

The early treatment of a sprained foot should consist of rest and protection of the injured ligaments, according to the dictates of pain and swelling. In short, treatment is predicated upon symptoms. Resumption of motion and weight bearing should be allowed when and as tolerated. Persistent pain on walking, after subsidence of the acute injury, is an indication for the use of a rigid arch until the repair of injured mid-foot ligaments has matured sufficiently for the longitudinal arch to be supported without pain.

INJURIES OF THE TALUS (ASTRAGALUS)

A major portion of the talus, like the scaphoid of the wrist, is intra-articular and surfaced by articular cartilage. Most of the vascular supply enters the distal segment, so that fractures through this bone carry a risk of avascular necrosis of the proximal fracture fragment similar to that encountered with fractures in the neck of the femur and in the carpal scaphoid. Most of the nutrient vessels enter the talus at the location of ligament attachments and, in the assessment of an injury, damage to these ligaments must be considered to be synonymous with damage to their associated nutrient vessels.

In order of importance the vascular nourishment of the talus is as follows:

1. From the posterior tibial artery, a branch behind the medial malleolus enters the talus close to the tibiotalar portion of the deltoid ligament and just below the cartilaginous facet, which articulates with the medial malleolus.

2. A branch of the dorsal artery of the foot enters a nutrient foramen on the superior surface of the neck of the talus.

3. Vessels enter the inferior surface of the talus from the sinus tarsi in company with the interosseous ligaments connecting the calcaneus and the talus.

4. Small nutrient vessels gain access to the talus with the posterior and lateral talocalcaneal ligaments.

DISLOCATION OF THE TALUS

Complete dislocation of the talus without fracture, which may be marked by talar displacement in relation to the tibia, calcaneus, or

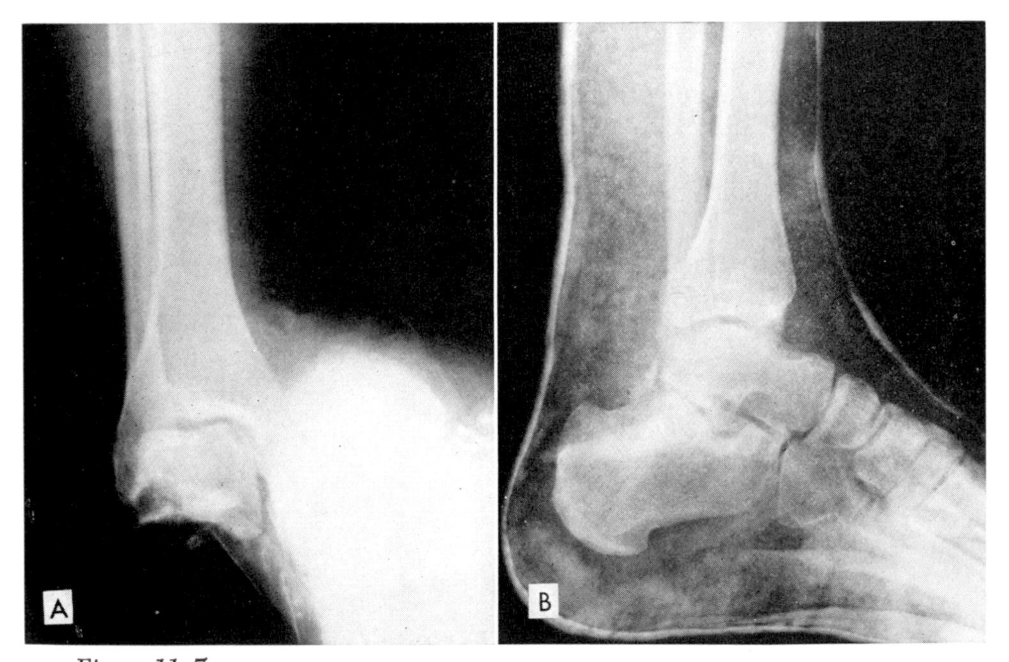

Figure 11–7.

A. Open dislocation of the foot at the talonavicular and talocalcaneal joints, foot medialward, complete.

B. Position after debridement and open reduction.

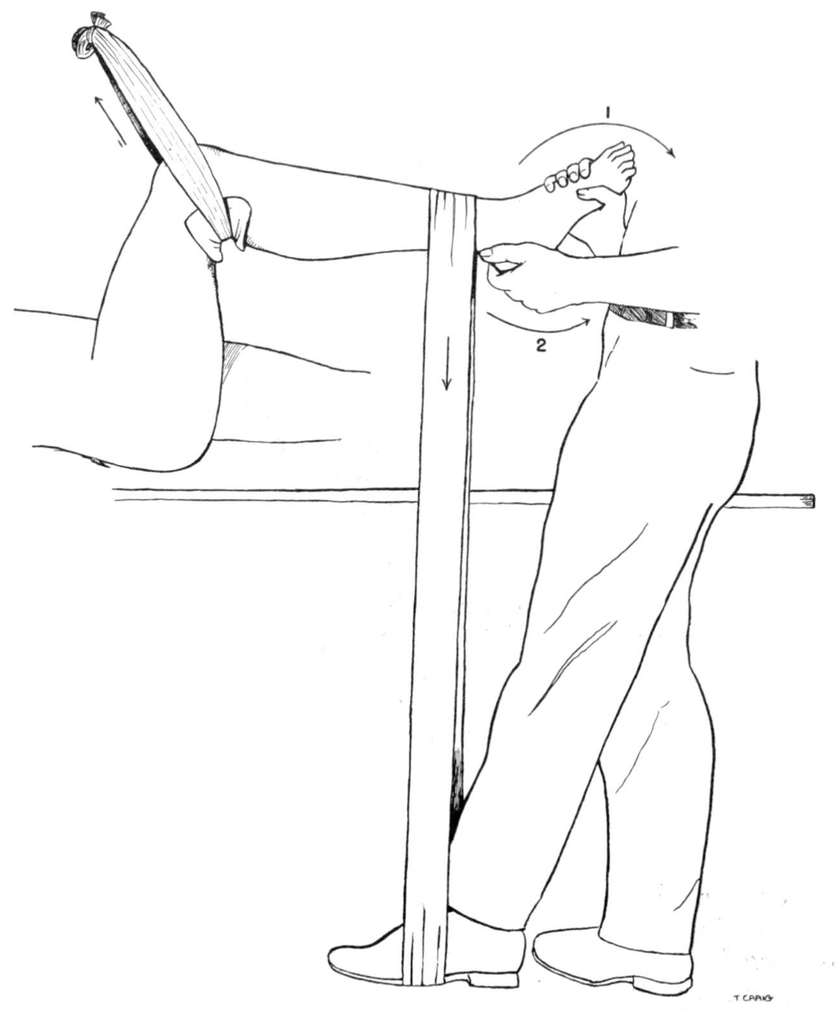

Figure 11–8. A useful method for reduction of many injuries about the ankle joint, including a posterior dislocation of the talus. The gastrocnemius is relaxed by flexing the knee to 90 degrees and plantar flexing the foot (1). The tibia is held by the loop around its lower third, while the foot is lifted upward (2) and maintained by dorsiflexion of 90 degrees. To prevent recurrence of the posterior dislocation by gastrocnemius spasm, the knee must be immobilized in flexion.

navicular, is exceedingly uncommon. At the ankle the talus may dislocate in any direction from the malleolar mortise. The calcaneus may be displaced in any direction from its normal relationship to the talus, as may also the navicular (Fig. 11–7).

Posterior Dislocation of the Talus

Posterior dislocation of the talus from the ankle mortise is the displacement most commonly encountered. A force which drives the plantar-flexed foot backward may produce this displacement with relative ease, since in plantar flexion the narrowest portion of the talar tenon (see Fig. 12–2, page 334) is engaged in the malleolar mortise. Rupture of the deltoid ligament occurs, and destruction of the posterior malleolar nutrient artery to the talus must be presumed. Relatively little damage may be done to the remaining sources of talar nourishment, however, and, if the dislocation is reduced quickly, avascular necrosis of the talus is unlikely.

Diagnosis. The foot is displaced backward on the leg, as viewed from the side. The heel is lengthened and unduly prominent. The heel cord is curved, with the convexity forward. The malleoli can be felt to be intact and in normal position. The foot is fixed in plantar flexion. The unduly prominent anterior edge of the lower end of the tibia can be seen and palpated.

Treatment. Flexion of the knee to a right angle in order to relax the calf muscles and increased flexion of the foot are prerequisites to reduction (Fig. 11–8). Traction is applied to the foot with countertraction at the knee. A forward lift of the foot, coincident with a backward thrust against the anterior surface of the lower tibia, replaces the talus under the tibia.

Fixation requires the knee to be immobilized in flexion in order to maintain calf muscle relaxation, and the foot should be dorsiflexed so that the wide anterior portion of the talar wedge is engaged between the malleoli. Splints should extend from toes to upper thigh but, after about four weeks, may be reduced to the level of the tibial tubercle. After six to eight weeks the splints may be removed and unsupported motion permitted.

Anterior Dislocation of the Talus

The dorsiflexed foot is driven forward from the tibia, and the displacing talus usually fractures the anterior lip of the tibia. Both collateral ligaments are damaged, but the talonavicular and talocalcaneal ligaments remain intact. Avascular necrosis of the talus is an uncommon sequel to this injury.

Diagnosis. The heel is shortened and the heel cord appears flattened. The body of the talus can be palpated as it projects forward under the anterior lip of the tibia. Otherwise, little in the way of obvious deformity is present, and the diagnosis must be confirmed by roentgenogram.

Treatment. When a single fragment has been fractured from the anterior lip of the tibia to allow forward subluxation of the talus, open reduction with internal fixation of the fracture is the most certain method for maintaining reduction of the dislocation.

When the tibial lip is comminuted, reduction of the dislocation is easily accomplished merely by pushing the foot backward until the talus once again becomes seated in the mortise. Under these conditions, however, maintenance of reduction may be very difficult. The talus tends to slip forward into a subluxed position with great ease, and the penalty of any talar displacement is eventual painful arthritis. Immobilization should be applied with the foot and knee in moderate flexion, and maintained for four to eight weeks, depending upon the stability of the talotibial relationship.

Lateral Dislocation of the Talus

This injury is uncommon. The medial collateral and both anterior and posterior capsular ligaments of the ankle are disrupted widely, and the talus swings out of the malleolar mortise on the hinge of the intact lateral collateral ligaments. Similar injuries with medial dislocation (see Fig. 12–*11*, page 345) are even more uncommon. It is obvious in such injuries that all nutrient vessels to the talus, except those entering its plantar surface and possibly an intact dorsalis pedis branch, are completely disrupted. Nevertheless, in the few cases that have been encountered, in which reduction was performed at once, avascular necrosis has not supervened. Immediate reduction is mandatory, not only for preservation of

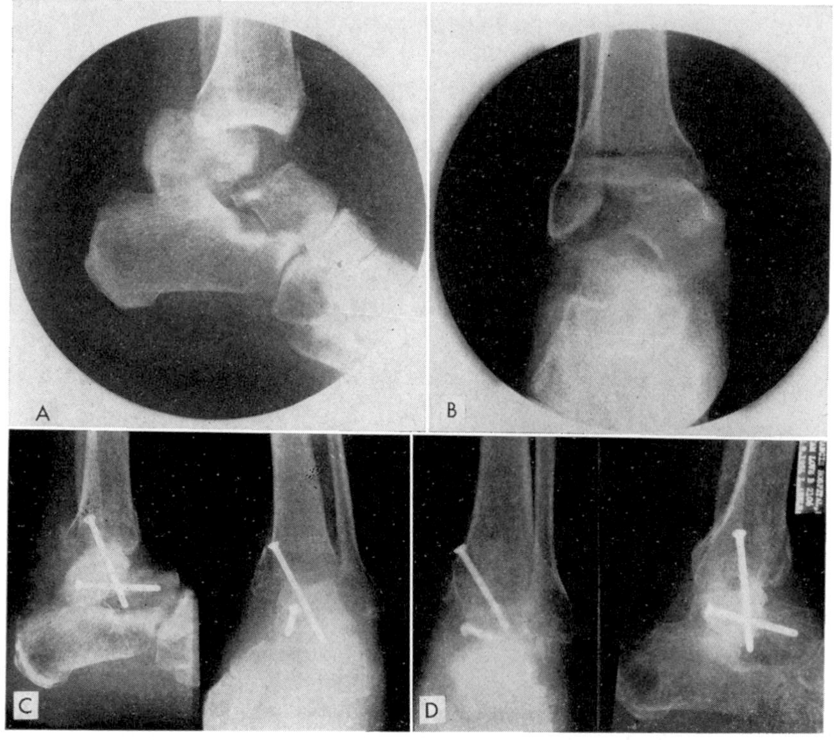

Figure 11–9.

A, B. Extrusion of the body of the talus from the ankle joint. Edema, hemorrhage, and pressure caused rapid destruction of the overlying skin. Any attempt at closed reduction should be done in the operating room, with preparation for open reduction. In this case three attempts at closed reduction had been made, following which open reduction was delayed for weeks because of infected blebs.

C. Open reduction with screw fixation. Since the violence of the injury had destroyed all circulation to the body of the talus, channels for revascularization were opened by removing the cartilage barrier from the inferior surface of the tibia and the superior surface of the talus, and from the apposed surfaces of talus and calcaneus. The increased density shows aseptic necrosis of the body of the talus six months later.

D. Two years later, showing a successful pan-talar arthrodesis with the foot in good position, and the body of the talus becoming revascularized.

nutrient vessels to the talus but, more important, for preservation of the blood supply to the foot.

Total Dislocation (Extrusion) of the Talus

All, or a major portion, of the talus may be separated from its soft-part connections to the tibia, calcaneus, and navicular. As a rule, a fragment of the head of the talus remains attached to the navicular. The remainder of the talus is extruded from the ankle joint and comes to rest in a subcutaneous position. An open wound commonly accompanies such a violent injury. Under any circumstances, rapid deterioration of the tense skin over the extruded talus is to be expected.

Treatment. Unless the extruded talus is replaced in the ankle at once, great swelling of all the tissues and bleb formation on the skin surface is likely to prevent active treatment for a considerable period, during which the viability of the entire foot remains jeopardized (Fig. 11–9, *A*, *B*). The extruded bone is avascular, and replacement into the ankle by manipulation merely removes the danger of vascular privation of the foot and allows a little extra time in which to prepare for definitive treatment. Operative repair should be done as soon as possible. The loose talus should not be discarded. Its cartilage should be removed, and a pan-talar arthrodesis carried out in all cases in which the loose bone is devoid of soft-part attachments (Fig. 11–9, *C*, *D*).

DISLOCATION ON THE TALUS (SUBTALAR DISLOCATION)

The remaining tarsals may be dislocated from the talus by an injury combining great force with severe torsion of the foot. The talus remains in the ankle mortise, and the dislocation occurs at the talonavicular or talocalcaneal joint, or at both. An adequate blood supply to the talus is preserved, but may remain seriously compromised until the dislocation has been reduced.

The foot is obviously deformed, swollen, tender, painful, and relatively immobile. The details of the damage cannot be educed accurately by clinical examination, but must be documented by roentgenogram. The calcaneus alone may be dislocated from the talus and the cuboid bones (Fig. 11–*10*), or the calcaneus and the navicular may dislocate from the talus (Fig. 11–*11*).

Treatment. Manipulative reduction under adequate anesthesia should be carried out. These grossly displaced lesions are notorious for the frequency with which reduction may be easily accomplished. Almost before the manipulator knows it, the objective of his manipulations has been achieved. When this does not happen, strong traction on the foot with countertraction against the flexed knee should be employed and maintained while the heel is pushed and molded into normal position. As a rule, when complete reduction cannot be accomplished easily by manipulation, soft tissue structures are interposed between the displaced bones and must be extricated by operation before complete reduction can be accomplished.

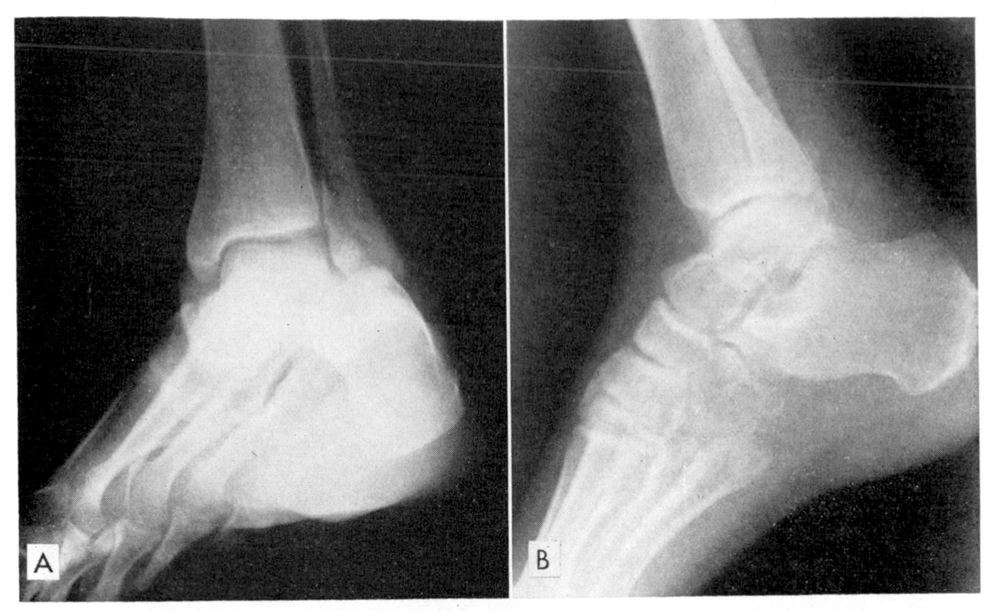

Figure 11–10.

A. Dislocation at talocalcaneal and calcaneocuboid joints, calcaneus lateralward. Open reduction was required.

B. Roentgenogram three months later does not show aseptic necrosis or disuse atrophy. The patient admitted returning to active duty truck driving four weeks after injury, having removed his plaster without authorization.

Following reduction the foot and lower leg should be immobilized in a plaster of paris boot or molded splints for at least six weeks. Ambulation in a weight-bearing walking-boot, or the removal of splints for warm soaks and gradual resumption of motion, is then permissible and safe. A stiff foot with mild symptoms must be expected. Significant pain in the arch of the foot may be reduced by the use of a molded rigid arch support.

Dislocation at the Talonavicular Joint

This rather uncommon injury results from violent torsion of the forefoot while the hindfoot (and the talus) is fixed. Most often the displacing force moves the foot lateralward on the talus. The talar head ruptures through the talonavicular joint capsule which, on occasion, may become interposed between the dislocated bone to prevent reduction by manipulation. The anterior tibial tendon displaces with the forefoot, and may slip under the neck of the talus while the foot is displaced, to prevent reduction (Fig. 11–*11*).

The diagnosis is not obscure since the deformity is obvious and the unduly prominent head of the talus is easily palpated. Roentgenograms should be studied for additional injuries, since gross displacement between talus and navicular occurs only in event of subluxation and often marginal fractures at either the talocalcaneal or calcaneocuboid joints (Fig. 11–*11*).

Treatment. Realignment of the forefoot coincident with pressure against the talar head effects reduction with reasonable ease, unless the

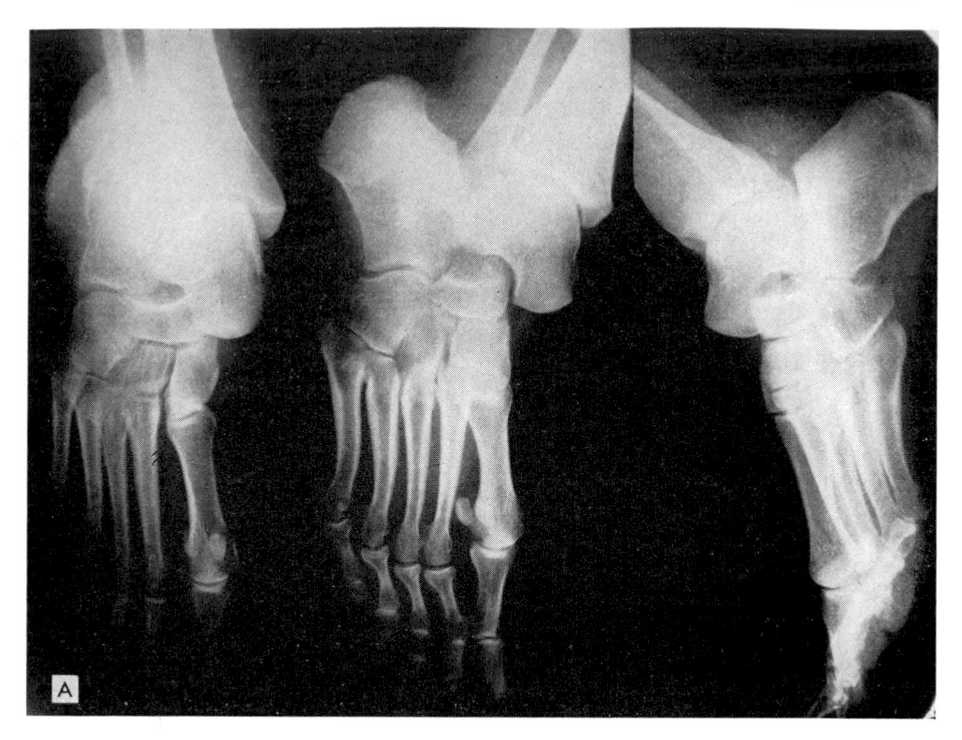

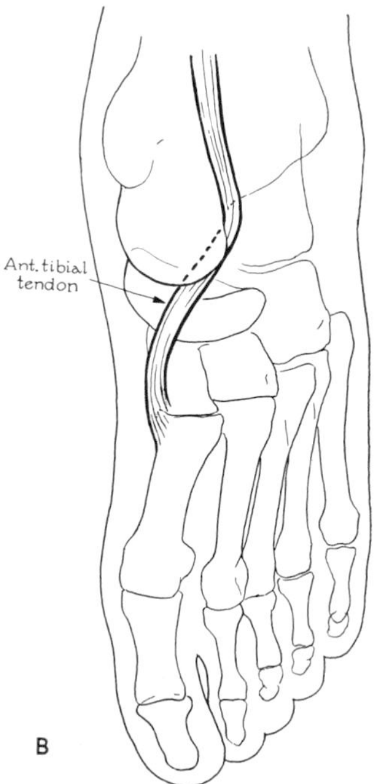

Figure 11–11.

A. Roentgenograms showing dislocation of the calcaneus at the talocalcaneal joint, calcaneus backward and outward.

B. The tendon of the tibialis anticus muscle displaces outward with the dislocated forefoot, and may slip under the neck of the talus and prevent reduction by manipulation.

Displaced fractures usually require open reduction, but manipulative reduction is sometimes possible, and a trial manipulation prior to operation is justified. The more posterior the fracture line, the greater is the danger of avascular necrosis of the posterior fragment. Accurate reduction and secure fixation is necessary if this fragment is to survive. Weight bearing should be deferred until union is complete and the bone density of the jeopardized fragment approaches that of the adjacent bones. Evidence of progressing avascular necrosis warrants consideration of tibiotalar arthrodesis, because, once avascular necrosis becomes established, it is probable that arthrodesis will be required sooner or later.

Fracture of Posterior Tubercle of Talus

The posterior tubercle of the talus commonly presents as an ununited center of ossification which simulates a fracture in the roentgenogram. Occasionally a true fracture of this process is produced by a sudden flexion injury. The injury is followed immediately by pain and a mild swelling behind the ankle, and deep tenderness on pressure under each side of the Achilles tendon. Since the talar tubercle is in close proximity to the flexor hallucis longus tendon, pain in this area is usually produced by motion of the great toe.

Pain is the only significant penalty of an injury to the posterior talar tubercle, and is almost always relieved by a short period of rest and immobility of the foot.

OSTEOCHONDRITIS DISSECANS OF TALUS

Separation and sequestration of a small segment of subchondral bone along with its covering of articular cartilage is not uncommon and usually affects the central portion of the dorsomedial or dorsolateral edge of the body of the talus (Fig. 11–*16*). The sequestered fragment may heal to the donor cavity by a creeping replacement type of repair (Fig. 11–*17*), or may remain avascular and become completely separated from the talus.

Diagnosis

The patient complains of a painful ankle. Detailed interrogation often educes a history of transient sudden painful episodes suggestive of "buckling" of the ankle. There may be a mild limp. Motion is normal or only slightly restricted, but motion to the maximum limits produces poorly localized pain, usually at the inner side of the ankle. When the foot is plantar flexed the inner or outer edge of the talus is tender. Swelling is minimal. The final diagnosis must depend upon the roentgenographic findings.

Treatment

If the diagnosis is made and the foot immobilized and protected from weight bearing prior to the development of sclerosis, healing may occur

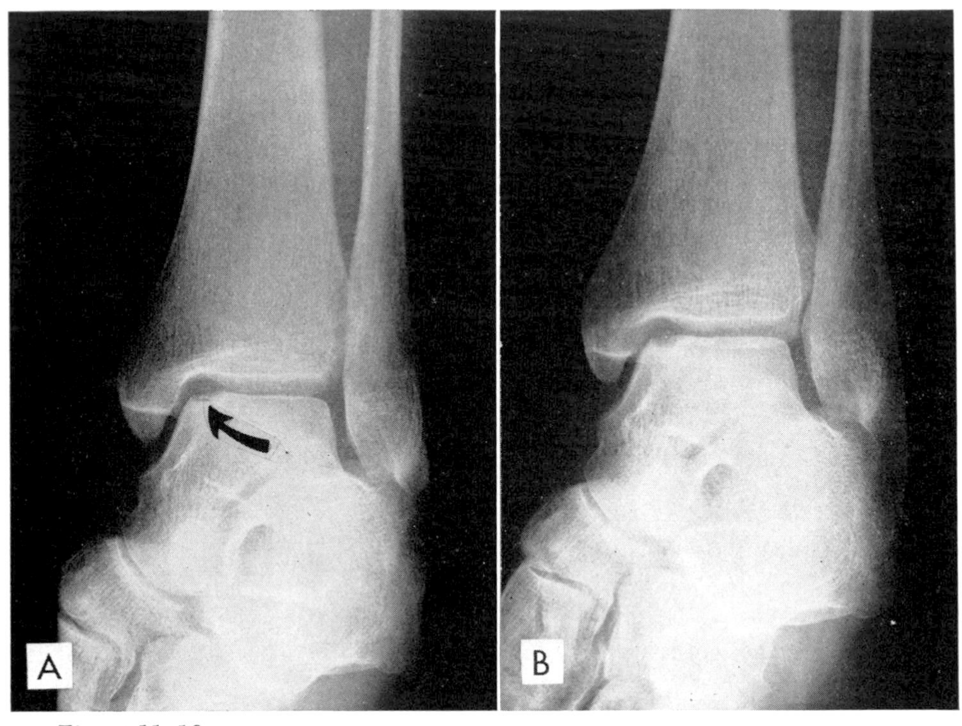

Figure 11–16.
A. Osteochondritis dissecans. Note the small separated bone fragment (arrow).
B. The sequestrated small fragment has been excised.

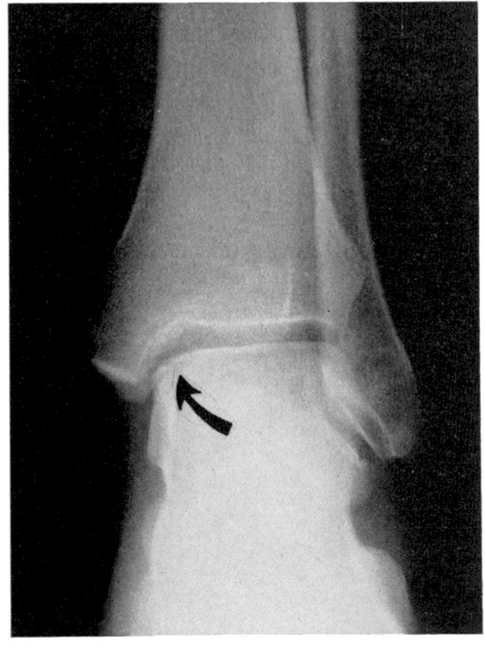

Figure 11–17. Osteochondritis dissecans of the talus (arrow), partially healed two months after injury. Eventual sound healing occurred under observation.

spontaneously. However, the symptoms which bring the patient to the surgeon are usually reflections of separation and sequestration. The separated fragment should be removed, and the donor cavity saucerized. A short period of immobilization should follow the operation. The results are very satisfactory.

FRACTURES OF THE CALCANEUS

The common cause of a calcaneus fracture is a fall from a height, with the patient landing on his feet. The height does not have to be great, and a fracture may result from merely jumping from a chair to the floor. Similarly, a sudden blow against the plantar surface of the heel compresses and may fracture the calcaneus (Fig. 11–*18*, *A*). The location and character of the fracture will depend upon the force of the injury, the exact point of impact, and the position of the foot. Under any circumstances, pain in the heel following a fall in which the patient landed on his feet is highly suggestive of a fractured calcaneus.

It must be remembered, moreover, that landing on the feet is invariably accompanied by an instinctive flexion of the spine, and as invariably some of the impact is transmitted through the skeleton to the spine. In almost 30 per cent of patients in whom fracture of the calcaneus occurs a compression fracture of a vertebra in the lumbodorsal region is simultaneously produced. The heel fracture is visible, spectacular, and exceedingly painful. Frequently the attention both of the patient and of the surgeon is so attracted to this obvious injury that the spine fracture

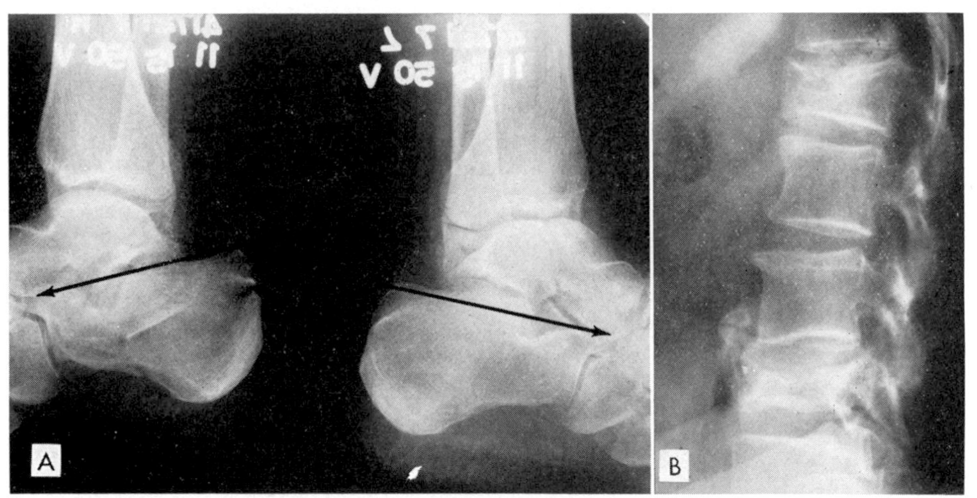

Figure 11–18. Typical injuries resulting from a fall, landing on the feet.

A. A comminuted fracture of the right calcaneus, and a fracture through the body of the left talus.

Note that the subtalar joint is well above a straight line between the anterior and posterosuperior tips of the uninjured left calcaneus, but level with, and largely below, a similar line on the other side.

B. Concomitant compression fracture of the first lumbar vertebra, which is a frequent occurrence, and a long-standing antecedent lesion of the fourth lumbar vertebra.

is missed. Lateral films of the lumbar spine should be made in every patient who has a fractured heel (Fig. 11–*18*, *B*).

Nothing more than localized pain and tenderness with mild to moderate swelling may mark the minor fracture of the calcaneus which does not involve the body of the bone. Motion may remain relatively unimpaired, and without adequate roentgenograms the injury may easily pass for a sprain. When the body of the bone is fractured the diagnosis is obvious. The heel is thickened, the posterior malleolar sulci are flattened, and the entire hindfoot is swollen, tender, and exquisitely painful. Adequate roentgenograms are necessary to localization and detailed assessment of the bone damage.

Interpretation of the roentgenogram is not always easy. Fracture of the calcaneus is reflected in a crushing and compression of cancellous bone. Often clear-cut fracture lines are absent, and the diagnosis must be predicated upon alterations in the outline of the bone. These alterations are characteristic and consistent, vary only in degree, and may be recognized and estimated in two ways.

1. A straight line from the superior extremity of the tubercle to the superior tip of the anterior end of a normal calcaneus is, for the most part, inferior to the subtalar joint; in fractures through the body of the calcaneus the subtalar joint is at or below this line (Fig. 11–*18*, *A*).

2. The angle between the axes of the tuberosity and body of the calcaneus, known as the *tuber-joint angle*, is normally about 40 degrees (Fig. 11–*19*, *A*); reduction or reversal of this angle, as measured on the

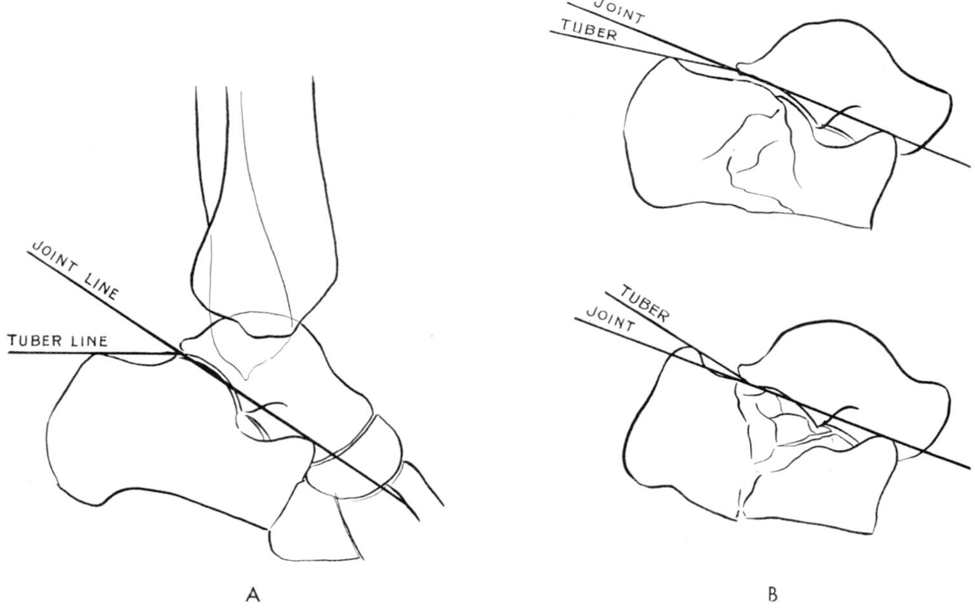

Figure 11–19.

A. The axis of the calcaneal tuberosity (tuber line) and that of the calcaneal body (joint line) form the tuber-joint angle. *This is usually about 40 degrees.*

B. Vertical compression of the calcaneus and upward displacement of the tuberosity is measured by the amount of reduction or reversal of the tuber-joint angle.

roentgenogram, reflects the amount of proximal displacement of the tuberosity resulting from vertical compression fractures (Fig. 11–*19*, *B*).

CLASSIFICATION OF FRACTURES OF CALCANEUS

The clinical significance and therapeutic difficulties to be expected of a broken heel depend upon the location of the injury and the presence or absence of involvement of the subtalar joint. Watson-Jones has proposed a simple and logical classification of these fractures.

FRACTURES OF CALCANEUS NOT INVOLVING SUBTALAR JOINT

Vertical Fracture of Calcaneal Tuberosity

The medial aspect of the heel is struck a glancing blow from below while the foot is in a valgus position. The medial prominence of the calcaneal tuberosity is sheared from the bone, but is rarely displaced (Fig. 11–*20*, *A*). Immobilization in a plaster walking-boot until the fracture unites is usually followed by an excellent result. Union in

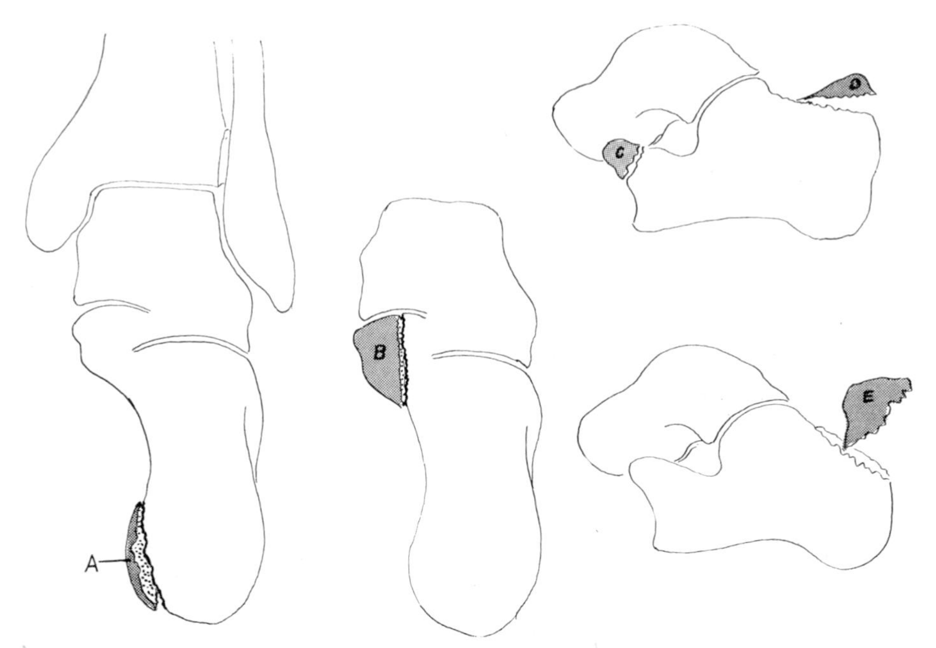

Figure 11–20. Fractures of the calcaneus not involving the subtalar joint.

A. Vertical tuberosity fracture—rarely displaced; usually heals well, but may produce painful pressure areas on weight-bearing surface of heel.

B. Fracture of sustentaculum tali—rarely displaced; usually heals rapidly and well.

C. Fracture of anterior tip of calcaneus—a concomitant of a midtarsal sprain; should be treated according to the symptoms it may produce.

D. Horizontal tuberosity fracture—tilted only, and above the insertion of the tendo achillis; not to be confused with the fracture shown in E.

E. Large horizontal tuberosity fracture with rotation or retraction in addition to tilting, may represent tendo achillis avulsion, and warrants operative repair.

malposition may produce painful pressure points, necessitating shoe corrections for relief of pain.

Horizontal (Beak) Fracture of Calcaneal Tuberosity

A triangular segment of the tuberosity is fractured and displaced upward by a shearing blow. When the fragment is merely tilted upward (Fig. 11–*20, D*) the insertion of the tendo achillis is not involved in the injury, and if the foot is put in plantar flexion the fragment may be pushed back into place. When the fragment is rotated as well as tilted (Fig. 11–*20, E*), or retracted upward, the injury should be considered a partial or complete avulsion of the tendo achillis, and operative repair should be done.

Fracture of Sustentaculum Tali

This uncommon fracture usually occurs as a result of downward impact of the talus against the calcaneal sustentaculum process, but may be produced by a glancing blow against the inner side of the foot. The fracture line is vertical (Fig. 11–*20, B*), and the fragment, held up by the sling of the long flexor tendons of the toes, is rarely displaced. Immobilization in a walking-boot for about six weeks is followed by union of the fracture and a good clinical result.

Fracture of Anterior Superior Tip of Calcaneus

This injury is not uncommon and is a concomitant of a midtarsal sprain resulting from a violent twisting injury. Rapid subsidence of symptoms and sound union of the small triangular fracture fragment (Fig. 11–*20, C*) is the rule.

FRACTURE OF CALCANEUS INVOLVING SUBTALAR JOINT

Almost all fractures of the body of the calcaneus involve the subtalar joint either directly or indirectly. Attempts have been made to catalogue these fractures, and to postulate both treatment and prognosis upon the absence or the presence and degree of joint involvement. This is an undependable classification in that the roentgenogram is a poor measure of subtalar joint involvement, and derangement of this joint is only one of the five or six conditions productive of pain and disability following calcaneus fracture.

PATHOLOGY OF COMPRESSION FRACTURE OF CALCANEUS

Vertical compression produces consistent fracture and deformity patterns in the calcaneus which vary only in degree. The tuberosity is driven upward; the middle articular facet, which articulates with the talus, is driven toward the plantar surface. The main fracture line traverses the body of the bone obliquely from the medial plantar region to the lateral and superior aspect of the bone, as viewed from behind (Fig. 11–*21*, *B*). As a rule, the fracture enters the subtalar joint, but sometimes appears to emerge just lateral to the joint. It is this roentgen illusion which may stimulate a false hope that the subtalar joint has not been injured. Two main fracture fragments are thus produced; a small superior medial fragment including the sustentaculum tali, and the mesial portion of the subtalar joint, and a large lateral plantar fragment containing the tuberosity and the lateral aspect of the subtalar joint. The latter fragment almost invariably assumes a varus position (Fig. 11–*21*, *B*).

Continuation of the impacting force subsequent to the production of this fracture drives the tuberosity fragment further upward, while the talus is driven downward, like a wedge, into the central portion of the bone. The articular facet for the talus is impacted into the substance of the calcaneus, which shatters into many fragments, and the normally concave plantar surface flattens in profile, or the curve is reversed

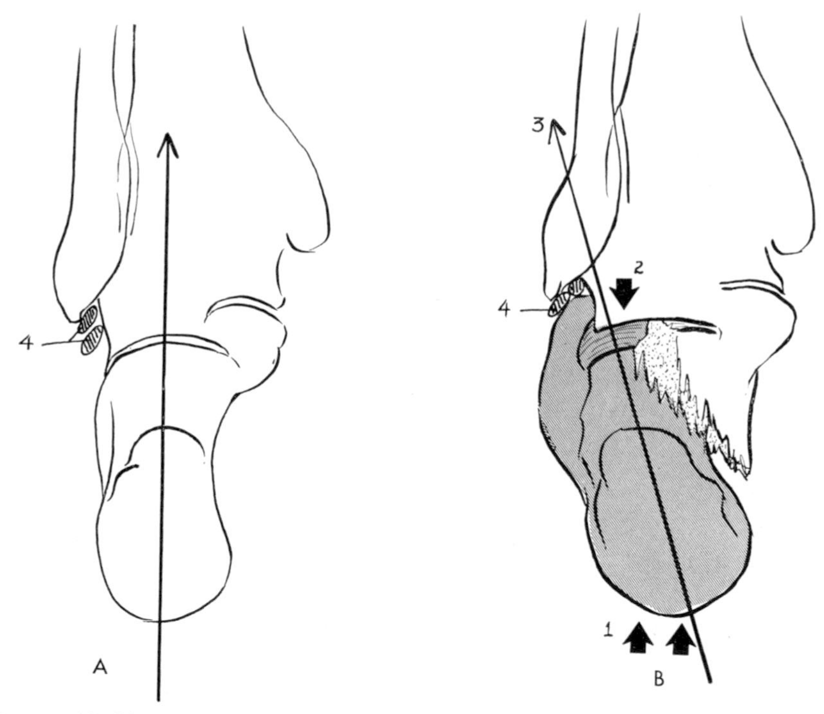

Figure 11–21.

A. When the foot and ankle bones are viewed from behind the calcaneus should appear neither varus nor valgus. The peroneal tendon–tendon sheath mechanism (4) is not crowded.

B. Fracture of the calcaneus. Vertical compression between 1 and 2 produces an oblique fracture beginning on the plantar medial surface and extending upward and laterally to enter (or at least involve) the subtalar joint. Continued force compresses the talar facet into the midportion of the calcaneus at 2. The tuberosity fragment usually assumes a varus deformity (3). The superolateral aspect of the calcaneus is driven upward and laterally to encroach upon the lateral malleolus and the peroneal tendons at 4.

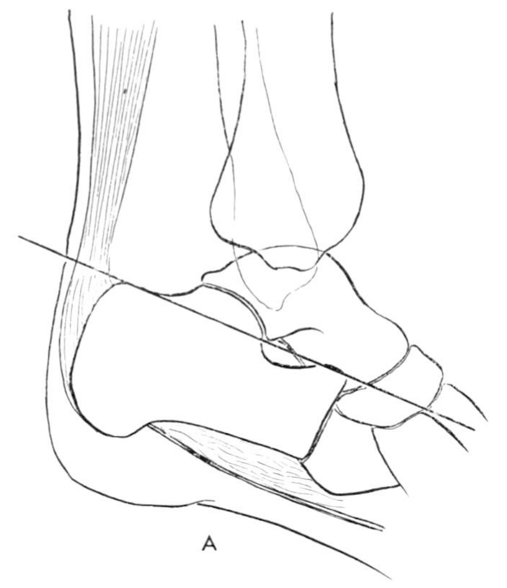

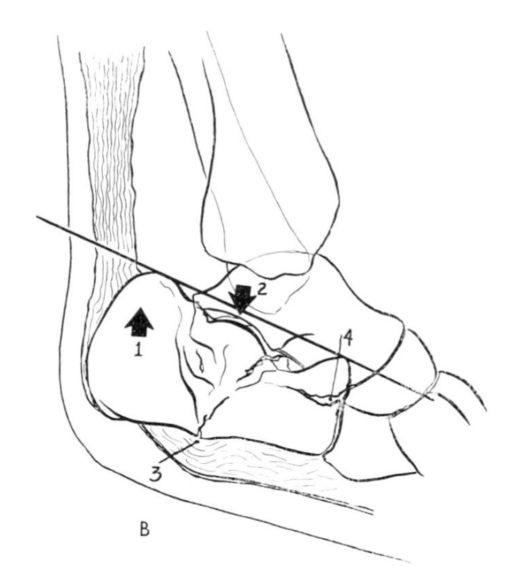

Figure 11–22.

A. The normal calcaneus viewed from the side is such that a straight edge between its anterior and posterosuperior extremities is well below the subtalar joint.

B. Vertical compression fracture of the calcaneus drives the tuberosity upward (1) to produce relative lengthening of the tendo achillis, the middle articular facet downward (2) into the body of the bone, which shatters to produce a reduction or reversal of the normal plantar curve (3). Extension of the fracture into the calcaneocuboid joint (4) deranges this structure. The subtalar joint is below the line drawn from the tuberosity to the anterior tip of the calcaneus.

(Fig. 11–22). Frequently the main fracture line extends to the anterior extremity of the calcaneus to involve the calcaneocuboid joint.

The preceding rather consistent pattern of pathology should be considered in the light of its potentials for the production of a painful and disabled foot. Injury to, followed by arthritis of, the subtalar joint, although probably the most common cause of pain, is but one of the causes for an unsatisfactory result.

CAUSES OF LATE PAIN AND DISABILITY AFTER COMPRESSION FRACTURE OF CALCANEUS

Lengthening of Tendo Achillis

Malunion with upward displacement of the tuberosity is synonymous with lengthening of the tendo achillis. Calf muscle power is correspondingly reduced. The patient walks with a flat-footed gait, and is unable to take off from or stand on his toes. Eventual compensatory shortening of the calf muscles usually results in a final gait that is reasonably satisfactory.

Spastic Flat Foot

Crowding of the peroneal mechanism under the lateral malleolus (Fig. 11–*21*, *B*) often is productive of chronic peroneal spasm. Despite the consistent varus deformity of the calcaneal tuberosity, such spasm produces a valgus deformity of the forefoot, and a painful spastic flat foot. When pain and tenderness under the lateral malleolus are centered at and coincide with motion and tension of the peroneal tendons, the essential offending lesion may consist of a chronic stenosing tenosynovitis of these tendons. The simple procedure of incision of the constricted tendon sheaths may result in relief of pain, and should be considered seriously before other more major procedures are attempted.

Impingement of Thickened Calcaneus upon Lateral Malleolus

With or without coincident peroneal tendon–tendon sheath derangement the displaced lateral surface of the calcaneus (Fig. 11–*21*, *B*) or an exuberant outgrowth of reparative callus or scar in this area may impinge upon the lateral malleolus and produce pain on motion, which is easily mistaken for subtalar joint pain.

This pain occurs mainly on flexion and extension; subtalar joint pain occurs with inversion and eversion. The lateral mass of displaced bone or reparative tissues is palpable and tender, and is the center of pain on motion. When no other source of pain can be recognized, removal of excess bone sufficient to allow clearance by the lateral malleolus warrants consideration. Incision of the peroneal tendon sheaths should be carried out simultaneously.

Plantar Fasciitis

Malunion with reversal of the plantar curve of the calcaneus, as viewed from the side (Fig. 11–22), often produces a painful spot on the weight-bearing surface of the heel. Weight should be diverted from the painful area by an excavation in the shoe and the use of soft rubber soles. When this does not produce relief, incisional release of the plantar fascia from its calcaneal attachment may be done, but is followed by somewhat uncertain results.

Derangement of Calcaneocuboid Joint

The calcaneocuboid joint involved by a fracture of the calcaneus may, in itself, be a significant source of pain. Talocalcaneal arthrodesis should be reserved for those fractures which do not involve the calcaneocuboid joint; otherwise arthrodesis of the talonavicular and calcaneocuboid joints should be done as well.

Derangement of Subtalar Joint

The subtalar joint and/or its supporting ligaments are involved in every compression fracture of the calcaneus. Even when the fracture does not enter the subtalar joint cavity the ligaments are damaged, become host to hemorrhage and chronic edema, and eventually are implicated by fibrosis, which inevitably produces a marked defect in subtalar joint motion. When the fracture enters the joint, as is usually the case, ligament damage is augmented by joint surface derangement and the formation of intra-articular adhesions. The potential of joint surface damage for the production of pain is not directly proportional to the severity of the damage. On the contrary, the more damaged the joint, the more likely it is that it will eventuate with a painless spontaneous fibrous ankylosis. However, the consummation of a spontaneous ankylosis may not be complete for a year or more. In the presence of a grossly disrupted joint, which appears predestined to such an end, the surgeon may well consider the propriety of surgical arthrodesis as a time-saving procedure attended by more certain results than could be expected of the natural processes of repair. Early arthrodesis, by election, should be delayed for two or three weeks after the injury.

TREATMENT OF COMPRESSION FRACTURE OF CALCANEUS

The management of a compression fracture of the calcaneus must be tempered by recognition of the following: Immobilization is not necessary to bony union; the fracture will heal with or without treatment; immobilization is invariably productive of a stiff foot; a stiff foot is frequently a painful foot.

Reduction and Immobilization

Immobilization, in the absence of a perfect reduction, is simply the surgical preservation of deformity, without which motion might mold the shattered joint surfaces into an improved congruity. A perfect reduction rarely, if ever, can be obtained by any means. Treatment by fixed skeletal pin traction serves only to bring the tuberosity back down to its proper level, and does little to improve the position of the damaged subtalar joint surfaces (Fig. 11–23, *A*). Operative reduction can accomplish little, except for an improvement of the joint surface by elevation and support of the depressed facet. Combined open reduction maintained by fixed skeletal traction has produced excellent roentgen films (Fig. 11–23, *A*), but the clinical results are as uncertain as with other methods of attempted reduction and fixation, most of which have been discarded. It is impossible to foretell with certainty which fracture of the calcaneus will require eventual arthrodesis of the subtalar joint. These facts leave the surgeon in a quandary, from which his only escape is the knowledge that, when he is not certain that one of these treatment methods should be used, he should not use it.

There are but three clear-cut indications for the reduction of a compression fracture. The tuberosity which is displaced upward an excessive amount should be transfixed with a pin and pulled down to its normal level. The lower tibia is transfixed with a second pin. Both pins are incorporated into a circular plaster dressing, or some mechanical device such as the apparatus devised by Stader, and this fixation is maintained until healing occurs.

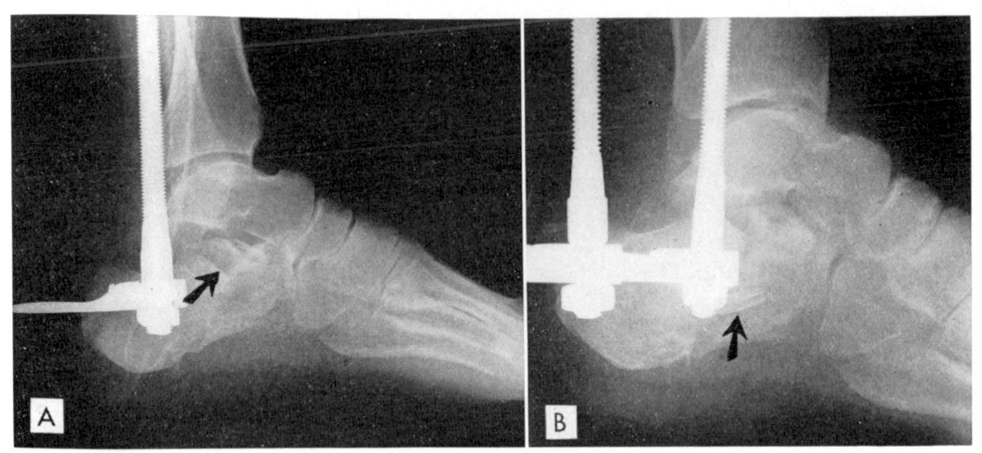

Figure 11–23.

A. Fixed skeletal traction, by some mechanical device (here a Stader apparatus) or by incorporation of traction pins in a plaster boot, succeeds in returning the displaced tuberosity to its proper level, but does not often effect replacement of the depressed lateral portion of the subtalar joint (arrow).

B. Fixed skeletal traction maintains the tuberosity in place. The depressed subtalar joint surface has been elevated into position, and the resulting gap in the crushed underlying bone is filled with bone grafts (arrow).

A grossly widened calcaneus, or one in which the lateral fragment is jammed up under and against the lateral malleolus, should be compressed manually, or with a clamp such as that devised by Böhler, until the width of the bone approximates that on the normal side. Immobilization with fixed skeletal traction is almost always mandatory to secure fixation.

Operative elevation of a depressed articular facet, which has been driven into the body of the bone, without significant comminution, is justified. Bone grafts should be inserted under the elevated facet and the reduction supported by fixed skeletal traction (Fig. 11–23, *B*) until the fracture heals.

Mobilization without Reduction

The modern trend is to reduce and immobilize fewer and fewer calcaneus fractures. This has evolved naturally from the high incidence of unsatisfactory results from this method of treatment. Instead, a pressure dressing is applied to the injured foot and the patient is put to bed for a few days until the acute tissue reaction subsides. The deformity is ignored. Motion is encouraged from the start, and weight bearing with crutches is permitted as soon as it is tolerated. Recovery occurs more rapidly than and is as good as that achieved by any method of reduction and immobilization. When treated by immobilization few patients return to full work short of a year after injury; when mobilized from the start, most patients can return to gainful occupation within a few months.

Primary Subtalar Arthrodesis

Spontaneous fibrous ankylosis of the subtalar joint following fracture often is not consummated for a year or more. The foot is then fairly comfortable and useful. Much time could be saved by early elective surgical arthrodesis of the joint. In other cases fibrous ankylosis may not occur spontaneously. The foot remains painful. Surgical arthrodesis is required eventually. Unfortunately, there are no reliable criteria by which the surgeon may anticipate these eventualities, and the indications for or against early elective arthrodesis must be predicated upon his experience and judgment.

FRACTURES OF THE NAVICULAR, CUBOID, AND CUNEIFORM BONES

Fracture of Navicular Bone

The navicular is virtually enveloped in strong ligaments and, except when fracture accompanies a talonavicular dislocation, displacement of fragments of this bone is rarely more than minimal. Most navicular fractures are the result of a crushing injury, and the body of the bone is compressed in an anteroposterior plane, and comminuted. The joint surfaces are almost always implicated, and late traumatic arthritis is almost certain. However, the tolerance of the talonavicular joint to arthritis without serious symptoms is great.

Treatment. When the fracture fragments are displaced the shape of the bone should be restored as well as possible by manual molding. After reduction adequate splints should be used until swelling subsides, after which ambulation may be allowed in a snug plaster walking-boot for six to eight weeks. Residual midfoot pain with unsupported weight bearing is greatly reduced by the use of a molded rigid arch.

Fractures of Cuboid and Cuneiform Bones

Fracture of these smaller tarsal bones does not often occur as an isolated injury, but is almost always a concomitant of a dislocation or a severe crushing injury. The amount of motion at their associated joints is small, hence the penalty of joint incongruity or late arthritis is relatively unimportant. Reduction is difficult, and at times impossible, except by operation, when significant displacement is present. As a rule, treatment of the associated injuries provides ample fixation and time for consolidation of fractures of these bones.

DISLOCATION OF TARSOMETATARSAL JOINTS

These injuries are commonly the result of a wheel passing over the forefoot. The first metatarsal is dislocated much less frequently than the other four, possibly due to its greater size. Any combination of the other metatarsals may be displaced in any except a medial direction. They should be replaced by manipulation, and immobilized for three or four weeks. When manipulative reduction fails, an interposed fragment of bone or tongue of joint capsule is the usual offending lesion, and such an obstruction should be removed surgically.

Unstable reductions often cannot be maintained securely by plaster immobilization alone. Transfixion of the replaced bones by removable small pins supplemented by plaster dressings is the simplest and most certain method for preventing loss of position until healing occurs. The pins may be left projecting from the skin for easy removal, or may be cut off just below the skin surface.

FRACTURES OF METATARSALS AND PHALANGES

Fracture of Base of Fifth Metatarsal

This is the most common metatarsal fracture. The base of the tuberosity is avulsed by the peroneus brevis, coincident with a sudden inversion strain. Displacement is uncommon. The relatively undisplaced fracture has an appearance similar to the normal epiphysis of the immature fifth metatarsal, and the two should not be confused. The only treatment required is control of the painful symptoms until healing occurs. In some instances this requires the use of a plaster walking-boot for several weeks. Complete recovery is the rule.

Fracture of Metatarsal Neck

Metatarsal neck fractures usually are multiple and are characterized by a consistent deformity. The metatarsal heads are depressed toward the plantar surface of the foot. Malunion in this position may create an extremely painful spot on the weight-bearing surface of the sole of the foot. The depressed metatarsal head must then be removed. This should not be done through a plantar incision, but can be accomplished with ease through the dorsal surface. Prevention of malunion is difficult. Open reduction and transfixion of the displaced head fragment by longitudinal medullary pins, or the use of traction through the toes by an outrigger attached to a well-fitted plaster boot, may be required for preservation of a satisfactory alignment of the small and relatively uncontrollable head fragment.

"March" Fracture of Metatarsal Shaft

No history of injury is educed. The patient complains of pain and tenderness in the region of the second, third, or fourth metatarsal, and a lump may be present at the tender area. Roentgenograms show a fusiform mass of new bone formation surrounding the shaft or neck of the bone. A clear fracture line is not often visible. The lesion may be mistaken for a sarcoma. Treatment by a snug plaster walking-boot is followed by firm union of the fracture, and complete subsidence of pain.

Fractures of Phalanges of Toes

Anatomically, the displacing forces acting upon fractures of the phalanges of the toes are identical to those described in the section on finger fractures. Theoretically the mechanics of treatment should be similar to those which obtain in fractures of the fingers. Practically, this is difficult, and it is usually impossible of accomplishment. The average broken toe may be treated for its symptoms, stabilized by binding it to an adjacent toe, if necessary, and a satisfactory result can be expected. Late complications are uncommon, and their successful management is much simpler and more certain than would be any formal method of treatment for the original fracture.

Fracture of Sesamoid Bones

An incorrect diagnosis of sesamoid fracture is frequently made. A fragmented appearance of the sesamoids in the roentgenogram is common, but fracture is rare.

Diagnosis. After any injury to the plantar surface of the first metatarsal head there may be exquisite tenderness, marked swelling, and complete inability to bear weight on this area. In order to differentiate between a fracture of the sesamoid and a simple contusion there should be visible in the roentgenogram a fine fracture line, not present in comparable films of the other foot, increasing in width after one or two weeks, and not having rounded corners.

Treatment. The only treatment possible is palliation of the painful symptoms and interdiction of weight bearing until all pain subsides. A metatarsal bar for diversion of weight from the metatarsal head area should be used when walking is permitted. Persistent pain may necessitate subsequent excision of the injured sesamoid.

CHAPTER 12

INJURIES OF THE ANKLE

By HARRISON L. McLAUGHLIN, M.D.

THE ANKLE consists of the lower leg, which sits atop the foot like a man on horseback. Its seat in the saddle of the talus is stabilized by the malleoli, each of which is connected to the foot by ligaments which act like stirrups (Fig. 12–*1*). Good horsemanship requires the rider to remain in the saddle, and no less important to good ankle function is maintenance of correct relationship between tibia and talus. This was emphasized as long ago as the 1st Century A.D. by A. Cornelius Celsus. A torn collateral ligament is a serious injury, reducing ankle stability to the same precarious state as that of a man with a broken stirrup, astride a galloping horse. This was recognized and emphasized by Jean Louis Petit in 1723. Today

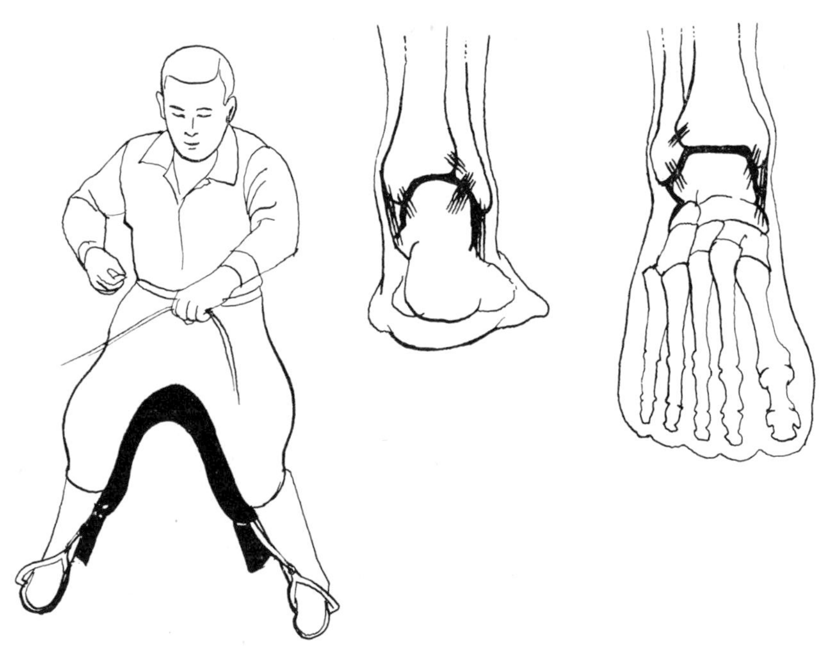

Figure 12–1. The ankle mechanism is comparable to a man on horseback—the malleoli grasp the talar saddle like the legs of a horseman, and each is connected to the foot by collateral ligaments, which function like stirrups.

failure to recognize and treat ligament injuries, or failure to restore and maintain a normal relationship between tibia and talus, probably accounts for the majority of the poor results following ankle injuries.

ANATOMY

The talar saddle is broader anteriorly than posteriorly, and the bone articulates within a mortise formed by the malleoli (Fig. 12–2). This wedge-shaped tenon and mortise prevents posterior displacement, and limits dorsal flexion of the talus. Short, strong interosseous ligaments bind the fibula firmly to the tibia and provide a slight resilience to the mortise. These ligaments allow a little upward excursion of the fibula to augment this resilience, and provide for a slight increase in the transverse capacity of the mortise when the talar wedge is forced between the malleoli by dorsal flexion of the foot.

The medial ligament is large and strong (Fig. 12–3), investing the medial malleolus on three sides as it blends with tibial periosteum. Distal to the malleolus it spreads fan-like to insert diffusely into the talus, navicular, and calcaneus. The lateral ligament is weaker and more subject to injury. It is comprised of three main fasciculi, originating jointly at the lateral malleolus, and inserting separately into the talus and calcaneus. The middle (calcaneal) fasciculus is intimately associated with the peroneal tendons, their sheath, and the retinaculum distal to the tip of the malleolus.

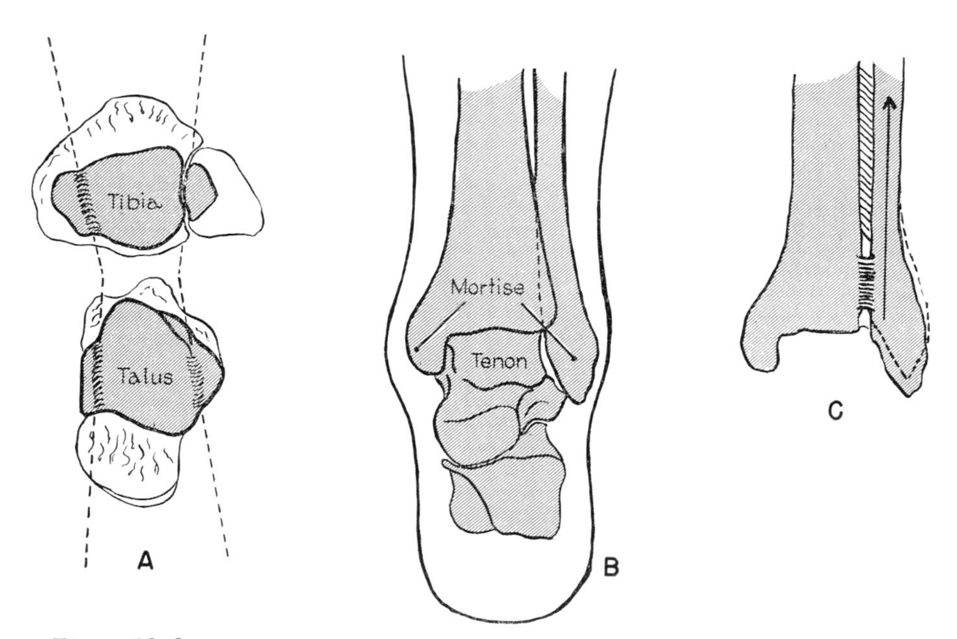

Figure 12–2.

A. The articular surface of the talus is broader in front than it is behind.

B. The talus fits between the malleoli as a tenon in a mortise.

C. When dorsal flexion of the foot forces the wider anterior portion of the talus between the malleoli, the interosseous ligament permits slight upward movement of the fibula to increase the transverse capacity of the malleolar mortise.

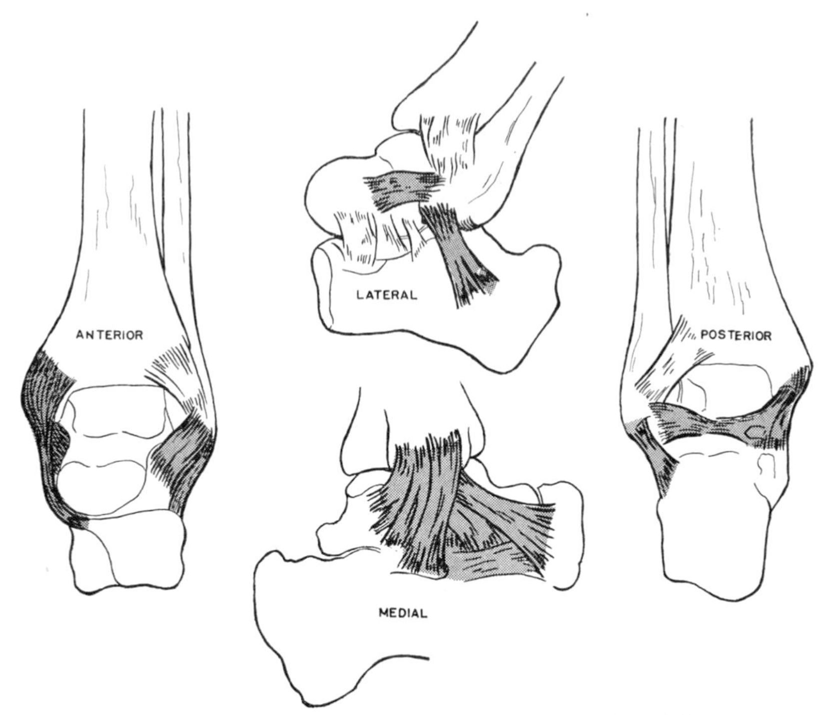

Figure 12–3. The collateral ligaments of the ankle.

Roentgen Implications of Ankle Anatomy

The ankle ligaments do not stretch. Therefore, every displacement of the talus away from an intact malleolus represents some ligament damage, and gross displacement is pathognomonic of ligament disruption (see Fig. 12–*16*). By the same token, tilting of the talus within the malleolar mortise indicates rupture of a collateral ligament (see Fig. 12–*9*). Widening of the malleolar mortise without fracture signifies a rupture of the interosseous ligaments, and a fracture of the fibular shaft above the ankle, except when caused by direct violence or accompanied by a fracture of the tibial shaft, should be considered to represent interosseous ligament rupture (see Fig. 12–*13*), until it is proven otherwise. Fracture of one or of both malleoli, or interosseous ligament disruption, is implicit in posterior displacement of the talus. In routine anteroposterior roentgenograms the malleoli of a normal ankle embrace the talus snugly enough so that at least one malleolus appears to overlap the talus. The exceptions to this may occur in full plantar flexion, which places the narrowest portion of the talar wedge in the mortise so that no overlap is seen, and in full dorsal flexion, when both malleoli may overlap the talus.

A transverse malleolar fracture occurs at or below the level of the ankle and is an avulsion injury with special implications. An oblique or spiral lesion occurs at or above the level of the ankle and is a shearing fracture caused by impact of the talus (see Fig. 12–*14*). Inability to achieve perfect reduction of an avulsed malleolus usually signifies interposition of soft tissues between the fragment and bone and foreshadows delayed or fibrous union (see Fig. 12–*14*). Inability to reposition the talus exactly against an intact malleolus should excite suspicion that the collateral ligament has been avulsed and become interposed between these two bones (see Fig. 12–*18*).

LIGAMENT INJURIES

SPRAIN OF ANKLE LIGAMENTS

Inversion Sprain of Lateral Collateral Ligament

A sprained ankle results from a stumble or fall which throws the body weight on the inverted foot, and the brunt of the force on the anterior and middle bands of the external ligament. A true sprain leaves the continuity of the ligament intact, merely rupturing some of its fibers. The stability of the talus is not jeopardized, and the extent of ligament damage can be estimated only by the degree of early ecchymosis and swelling (not to be confused with later edema resulting from spasm and continued dependency of the foot).

Diagnosis. The differential diagnosis requires exclusion of lesions commonly simulating or accompanying a simple sprain. These include

(1) a complete rupture of the external ligament;
(2) a rupture of the interosseous ligaments without fracture;
(3) an injury to the anterior inferior tibiofibular ligament;
(4) a fracture at the base of the fifth metatarsal;
(5) an undisplaced fracture of the lateral malleolus;
(6) a fracture of the medial malleolus.

The positive findings include pain, swelling and tenderness localized (early) and centered (late) just below and in front of the lateral malleolus, increased pain in this area when the foot is inverted but not when it is gently abducted or externally rotated, a stable talus, and absence of roentgenographic findings. If pain and spasm preclude clinical demonstration of talar stability, fluoroscopic examination and inversion stress roentgenograms, facilitated when necessary by anesthesia, should be made in all equivocal cases.

Treatment. TREATMENT BY LOCAL ANESTHESIA AND CONTINUED FUNCTION should be reserved for mild sprains. The manual application of some counterirritant is a universal home remedy and it is well known, especially in athletic circles, that the benefit of such measures is only temporary unless the function of the injured part is maintained. The injection of 5 to 15 ml. of procaine hydrochloride through a surgically cleansed skin surface into the center of the swollen and painful area has attained some measure of popularity. The resultant obliteration of pain and spasm allows the patient to resume ambulation, and he is encouraged to continue normal activities. Recurrence of pain often requires repetition of the injection, but in properly selected mild sprains a rapid subsidence of symptoms and disability may be expected within a few days to a week. Surface anesthesia by ethyl chloride may be employed to accomplish the same end. A preliminary coating of some greasy substance should be applied to prevent burning of the skin. The area of the subjective center of pain is then sprayed up to, but not beyond, the point of skin blanching. Coincident gentle massage soon relieves the pain at this spot. Progressive motion, weight bearing, and finally ambulation is carried out, each successive pain center being sprayed as it is localized by the patient. In mild sprains the results are similar to those obtained with procaine hydrochloride. None of these anesthetic, analgesic, or counterirritant drugs is apt to be of much help in severe sprains.

Some of the basic physiological effects of trauma suggest a rationale for expecting rapid cure of a mild sprain if it can be made possible for the patient to continue normal function of the injured part, and also for expecting a therapeutic failure if these measures are employed in more severe injuries. Regardless of the drug employed, the denominators common to success are relief of pain and continuance of function. Relief of pain interrupts the cycle of afferent-efferent nerve impulses (Fig. 12–4) and,

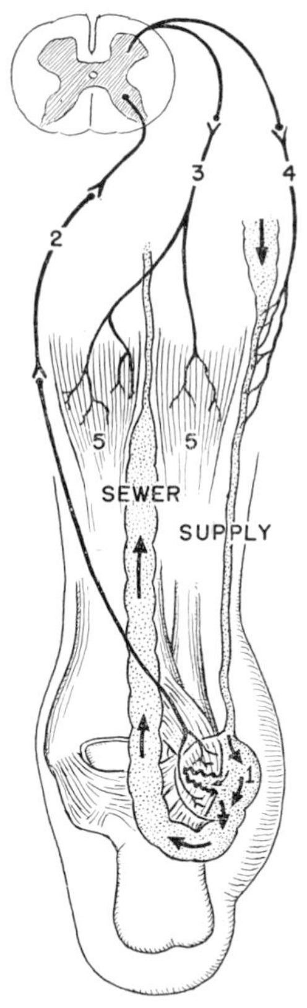

Figure 12–4. One result of injury is stagnation at the site of local tissue damage. From the region of injury (1) afferent pain stimuli (2) are carried to the spinal cord. Efferent stimuli (3) return to cause spasm in the muscles of the extremity (5), and thereby reduce to a minimum their pumping action upon the venous and lymphatic return flow. Sympathetic stimuli (4) produce arterial spasm in the extremity to reduce the blood supply to the injured part. Any measure which interrupts this vicious cycle of afferent-efferent impulses tends to re-establish the efficiency both of the arterial supply and of the venous and lymphatic sewer.

ipso facto, relieves muscular and vascular spasm throughout the involved extremity. A blood supply adequate to ensure an efficient flushing effect through the region of previous local stasis at the site of the tissue damage is restored. Continuance of function re-establishes the pumping effect of the musculature upon the veins and lymphatics, which are the sewers draining the affected area. In short, any interruption of the vicious cycle of afferent-efferent nerve impulses restores an efficient vascular pump and drainage system for the orderly elimination of the waste products of protein catabolism. In direct response to this, local inflammation subsides and local osmotic balance is rapidly re-established. Acceleration of healing and disappearance of edema are but two of the objective manifestations of this phenomenon. However, in more severe injuries, the primary offending factor (tissue damage) is a powerful enough stimulus so that the cycle cannot be broken for more than a short time by any local agent.

TREATMENT BY EXTERNAL SUPPORT AND CONTINUED FUNCTION is appropriate for the ankle sprain without marked swelling, that is, for mild or moderately severe lesions, before edema occurs or after it has been eliminated. The objectives of treatment include protection against re-injury, relief of pain, prevention of edema, and restoration of function.

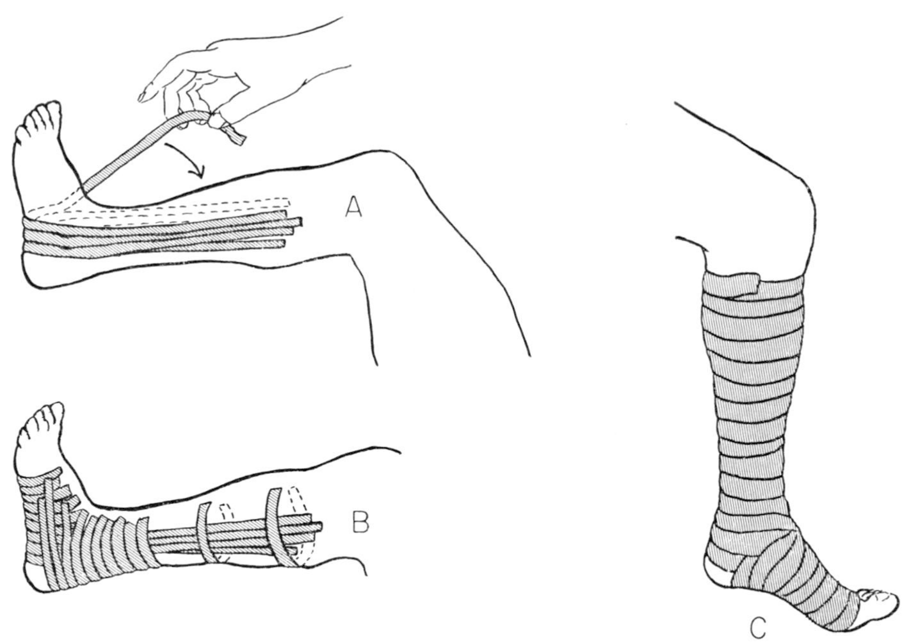

Figure 12–5. Ankle sprain without marked swelling.

A. Narrow (1-inch) strips of adhesive are applied parallel to the course of the collateral ligaments from the level of the tibial tubercle, around the foot, and up to the same level on the other side of the leg. The foot must be maintained in the weight-bearing position.

B. The main adhesive straps are held in position by semicircular strips, none of which completely encircles the extremity.

C. An elastic bandage is applied over the adhesive support from the base of the toes to just below the knee.

These can be provided for by an adequate adhesive support to the ankle and the temporary use of a cane or crutches. An inadequate adhesive dressing usually does more harm than good. The adhesive support must be applied so that upon it will fall the functional demands of motion and weight bearing normally accepted by the injured ligament (Fig. 12–5). The skin is shaved and painted with tincture of benzoin. The adhesive is applied in overlapping narrow (1-inch) strips, since smooth conformity to the contour of the limb is much more difficult to achieve with wider strips. Each strip should start and end at the level of the tibial tubercle. None of the shorter stabilizing strips should completely encircle the extremity, lest a partial tourniquet be formed. During the entire time such a support is applied, the foot should remain at right angles to the leg, and be neither inverted nor everted. An elastic compression bandage is applied over the adhesive, extending from the base of the toes to just below the knee. Properly applied, such a support should allow the patient to get both foot and dressing into his own shoe, and to ambulate with safety and reasonable comfort while his injured ligaments are healing.

TREATMENT OF SEVERE SPRAIN. The markedly swollen and painful sprain will not respond satisfactorily to treatment by local anesthesia, or to support and continued function. The aim of primary treatment should be to reduce pain and swelling by some combination of rest, elevation, and gentle heat, and an efficient compression dressing. When complete rest and elevation cannot be carried out, a compression dressing and crutches without weight bearing should be insisted upon, and the foot should be elevated at every opportunity. When pain and swelling have subsided to a point compatible with application of an adhesive dressing, weight bearing may be resumed and crutches gradually discarded. Occasionally ambulation is mandatory under conditions precluding the use of crutches. A plaster walking-boot, carefully applied over an elastic compression bandage, may then be used, but the vascular status of the toes must be checked frequently if the walking-boot is applied in the early stages after injury. The patient should elevate the foot as much as possible lest increased swelling under the plaster embarrass the circulation of the foot. Prolonged (six to eight weeks) immobilization of this type is good treatment for any sprain serious enough to cast suspicion upon the stability of the talus, but under ordinary circumstances the boot should not be applied until swelling has been controlled.

Complications. PERONEAL TENOSYNOVITIS FOLLOWING SPRAIN OF LATERAL COLLATERAL LIGAMENT. A painful derangement of the peroneal tendons occasionally results from cicatrization following an injury to the calcaneal fasciculus of the external ligament. Two forms of this condition are encountered, a diffuse stenosing tenovaginitis and a localized constriction of the tendon sheath (Fig. 12–6). Both produce symptoms simulating recurrent subluxation of the talus, but without talar instability. Prolonged restriction of motion due to peroneal spasm may produce a stiff foot. Localized constriction of the sheath eventually may result in a bulbous enlargement of one or both tendons just distal to the constricted area and

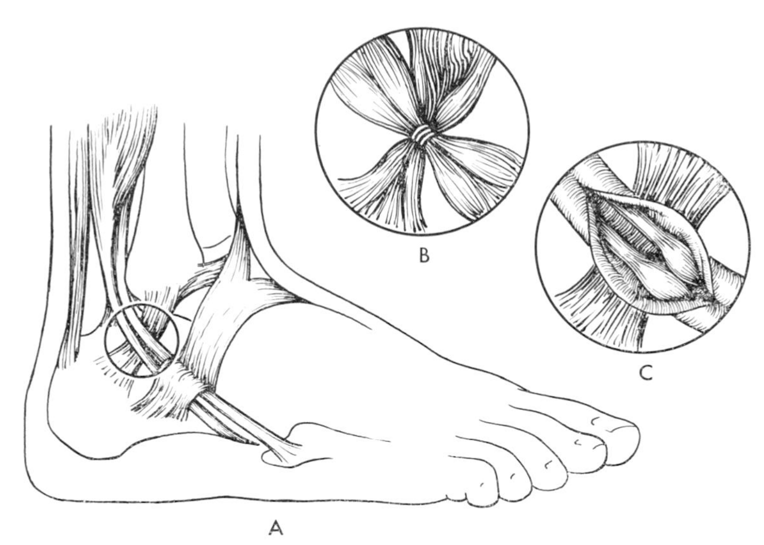

Figure 12–6. Peroneal synovitis following sprain of lateral collateral ligament.

A. The peroneal tendons, tendon sheath, and retinaculum are intimately associated with the calcaneal fasciculus (middle band) of the external collateral ligament.

B. Fibrous tissue healing and cicatricial contracture following an injury to the middle band of the external ligament may secondarily involve the peroneal mechanism.

C. Longitudinal incision of the peroneal tendon sheath and retinaculum may be required to relieve the symptoms of stenosing tenosynovitis or "trigger" tendon.

the production of a "trigger" phenomenon with motion. Mild, but fairly constant, peroneal spasm is almost always present. Pain, tenderness, and, occasionally, a little edema are present just distal to the tip of the lateral malleolus. This lesion may produce significant chronic symptoms and disability, but when necessary these can be relieved rapidly and completely by incision of the peroneal tendon sheath and retinaculum throughout the stenotic area.

External Rotation (Skier's) Sprain of Anterior Tibiofibular Ligament

Skiing enthusiasts, especially those less adept at the sport, are peculiarly susceptible to violent external rotation injuries of the ankle. The brunt of this force falls first upon the anterior inferior tibiofibular ligament and, after this structure gives way, upon the interosseous ligament or the lateral malleolus (Fig. 12–7). The clinical picture of an external rotation sprain is grossly similar to that of a simple inversion sprain. However, the center of pain and swelling is in front of and just above, rather than below, the tip of the lateral malleolus, and external rotation or eversion of the foot accentuates the pain, whereas inversion may be painless. The treatment is the same as that described for inversion sprain.

Complications. HERNIATION OF ANKLE CAPSULE FOLLOWING SPRAIN OF ANTERIOR INFERIOR TIBIOFIBULAR LIGAMENT. The injured anterior tibiofibular ligament may heal imperfectly, leaving a defect in the arcuate veil of

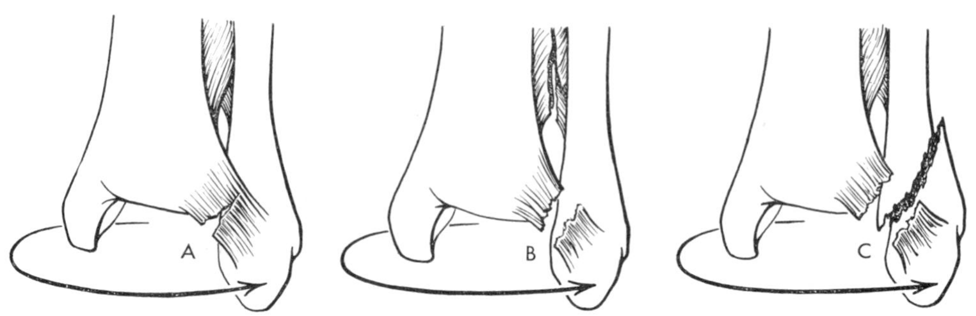

Figure 12–7. Forcible external rotation of the foot (skier's injury) first ruptures the anterior inferior tibiofibular ligament (A), and next disrupts either the interosseous ligament (B) or the lateral malleolus (C).

ligaments supporting the anterior ankle joint capsule. Occasionally the synovial membrane may herniate into the resulting hiatus to become pinched on dorsal flexion of the foot. The diagnosis depends upon the history of an external rotation sprain, tenderness, and at times a palpable ganglion-like prominence on the anterolateral surface of the ankle, and pain localized to the same area on dorsal flexion of the foot. The treatment is herniorrhaphy (Fig. 12–8).

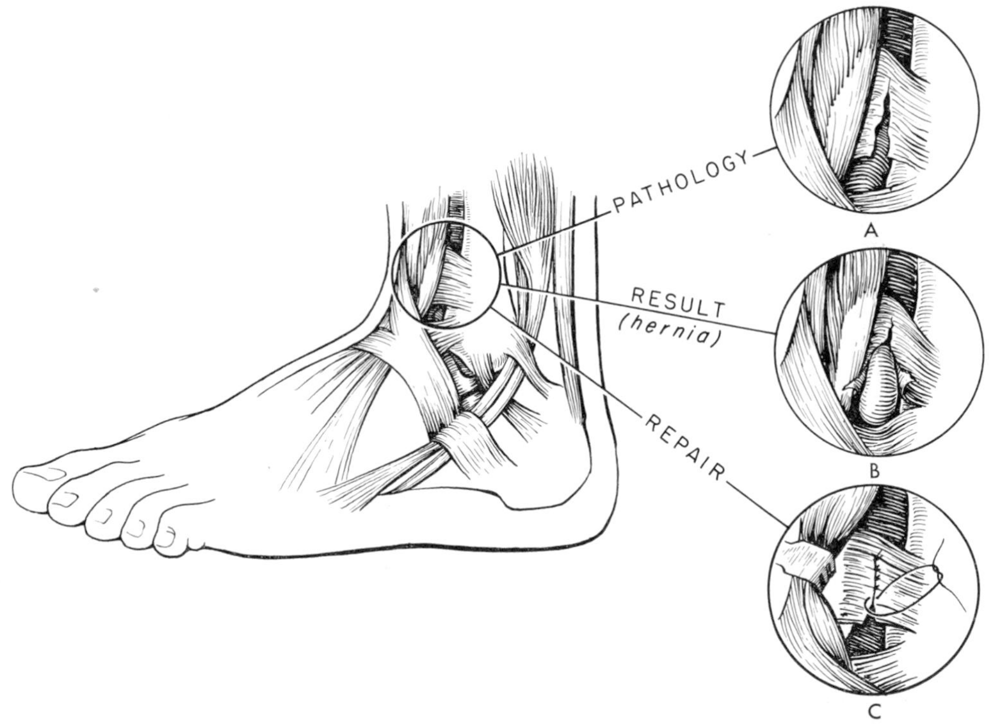

Figure 12–8. Rupture of the anterior inferior tibiofibular ligament (A) may heal imperfectly, leaving a weak spot through which the joint capsule herniates (B) on dorsiflexion of the foot to produce symptoms of pain and tenderness, and necessitating herniorrhaphy (C).

RUPTURE OF ANKLE LIGAMENTS

Rupture of the interosseous, internal, or external ligament of the ankle is not uncommon. Coincident rupture of the internal and interosseous ligaments is fairly common. Rupture of the external ligament usually, and of the internal ligament rarely, occurs as a solitary lesion. Ligament ruptures escape recognition more often than any other form of ankle injury. When they are unaccompanied by fracture of the ankle bones the common mistake is to consider and treat the injury as a sprain. At other times attention is apt to be centered on coincident obvious fractures to the exclusion of the more subtle ligament tear. The penalties of these common mistakes are serious. A painful ankle, due to talar instability, is inevitable, and in neglected cases the advent of arthritis eventually precludes all therapy except arthrodesis. It is a simple matter of great importance to test the integrity of these ligaments in every ankle injury, even when nothing more serious than a simple sprain seems to be present.

Rupture of Lateral Ligament

The function of the lateral ligament is to hold the talus against the lateral malleolus and prevent it from inverting within the mortise. In a simple sprain, which leaves the continuity of the ligament intact, talar stability is not jeopardized. When the anterior band is ruptured some excess mobility of the talus accompanies inversion of the foot, the talus subluxes (inverts) slightly on the tibia, and the patient may complain of repeated sprains or "locking" episodes. The usual history is that of an original inversion injury, treated as a simple sprain, but followed by repeated similar episodes throughout the ensuing months. The patient will explain that ever since the original injury the ankle has "turned" easily. When both anterior and middle bands of the ligaments are ruptured, the talus is almost devoid of lateral stabilizers and tends to tilt out of the malleolar mortise on inversion of the foot. The usual history is of a severe sprain which never fully recovered, leaving the patient with an ankle prone to buckle under him with little or no provocation, especially when walking on rough ground.

Diagnosis. The articular edge of the talus is palpable just in front of the lateral malleolus. Normally, when the ankle is stabilized with the examiner's hand in such a way that the thumb palpates both this talar edge and the malleolus, and the foot is inverted, it will be found that the talus does not move. All the inversion occurs in the subtalar joints. However, if the ligament is torn, it will be obvious that the talus participates in the inversion in direct proportion to the extent of the tear. If only the anterior band is torn, excess talar mobility will be slight, but if the middle band is also disrupted the talus can invert enough to create a palpable and sometimes visible sulcus between its lateral border and the fibula. This test is a dependable criterion of ligament damage if the lesion is chronic and without undue pain or peroneal spasm. In a recent injury, pain and swelling militate against dependable clinical estimation of the extent of the tear.

ROENTGEN DIAGNOSIS. The functional status of the external ligament

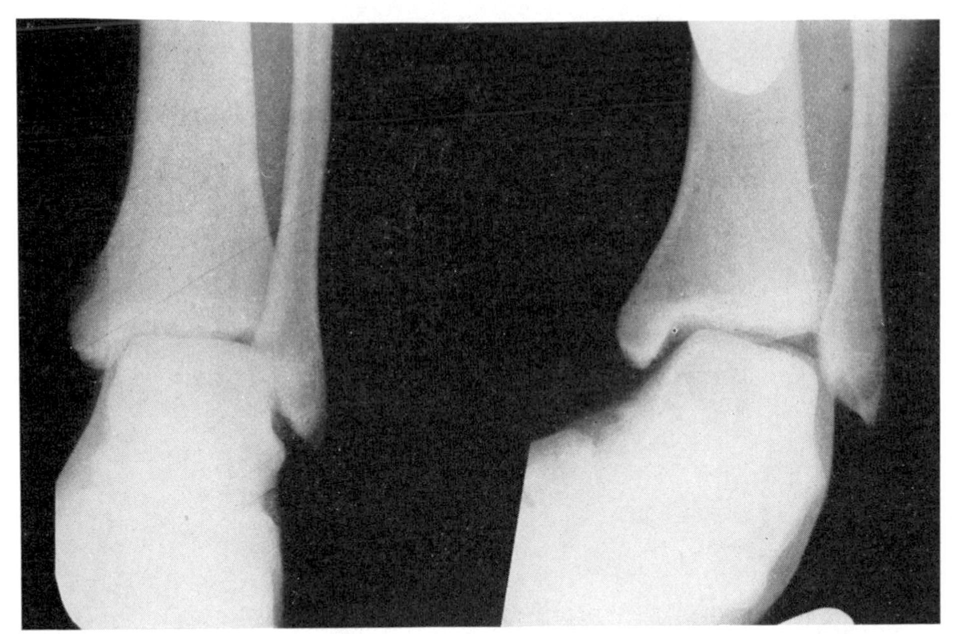

Figure 12–9. The clinical evidence indicated a severely sprained ankle. An ordinary anteroposterior roentgenogram (left) is negative. Inversion stress roentgenogram (right) discloses a complete rupture of the external ligament, without which no such tilting of the talus could be produced by inverting the foot.

can be determined accurately by fluoroscopic or roentgenographic examination, carried out with the foot strongly inverted. Anesthesia sufficient to relieve pain or peroneal spasm may be required, and will prove well worth while since small excesses of talar mobility, although difficult to recognize by clinical examination, are quite apparent roentgenographically if pain and spasm are overcome (Fig. 12–9). Little tilting of the talus occurs in a normal ankle. When the findings seem equivocal they should always be compared with those in the uninjured ankle.

Treatment. A small amount of excessive talar mobility can be compensated for by the peroneal muscles. Conservative treatment is indicated after a recent injury in which the ligament damage permits less than 15 degrees tilt of the talus. A non-padded plaster walking-boot, replaced at intervals appropriate to ensure a continued snug fit as swelling recedes, is worn for at least eight weeks. The prognosis should be guarded, since the damaged ends of the ligament may heal imperfectly or not at all, regardless of the duration of immobilization. Elevation of 3/16 of an inch on the lateral edge of the heel may reduce, but will not abolish, the symptoms of residual talar instability. Continuance of significant symptoms and disability after a period of conservative treatment justifies operative replacement of the damaged ligament.

Operative treatment requires specialized surgical ability and facilities. The entire length of the peroneal tendons and the lateral aspect of the ankle joint are exposed. Repair or re-attachment of the broken ligaments by suture is usually impractical, and a substitute ligament must be

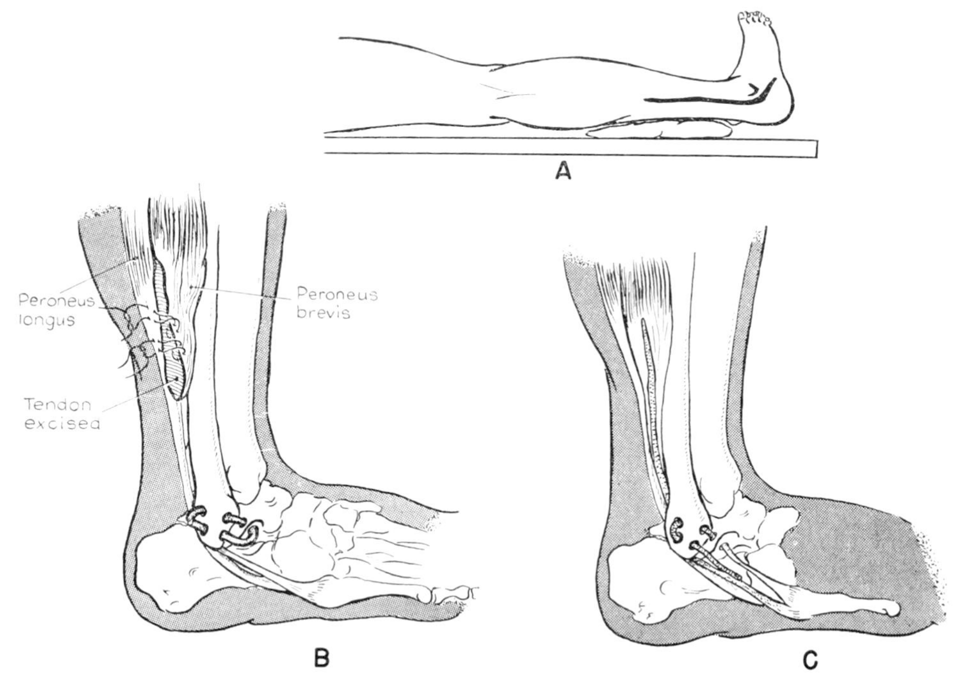

Figure 12–10. Operative replacement of ruptured external ligament.

A. Incision

B. Operative technique (Watson-Jones), utilizing the entire peroneus brevis tendon, and suturing the muscle belly to the peroneus longus.

C. One half of the peroneus brevis tendon is used to replace the torn ligament, leaving the other half to carry on its normal function.

provided. All or part of the peroneus brevis tendon is used for this purpose. Whenever possible, and especially in young patients and athletes, it is advisable to use only a part of the tendon (Fig. 12–*10*), leaving the remainder to carry on the normal function of the muscle. After healing of the incision, a plaster walking-boot is worn for six to eight weeks, following which normal ambulation is gradually resumed. Maximum rehabilitation occurs within three or four months, and the results are good, provided operation is done before arthritis becomes established in the ankle. This procedure consistently has restored talar stability sufficient to allow a return to heavy labor; one patient resumed a career as a professional hockey player.

Extensive Rupture of Anteroposterior and Lateral Ligaments

Occasionally violent inversion combined with internal rotation and a forward thrust of the foot on the leg will wrench the talus from the mortise solely at the expense of the soft parts. Ordinarily the internal ligament remains intact in continuity and, although it may be partially peeled from the tibia, acts as the hinge upon which the foot swings off the leg. The extent of the soft part damage in such a lesion (Fig. 12–*11*) is obvious. Usually the skin splits over the lateral surface of the ankle before complete

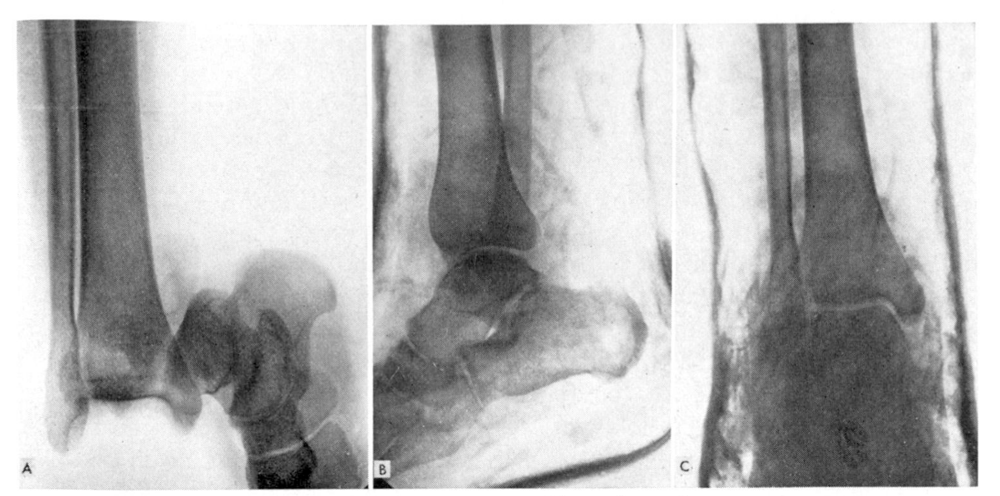

Figure 12–11. Complete dislocation of ankle without fracture.

A. The talus has rotated out of the mortise on the hinge of the partially intact medial collateral ligament. All other ankle joint ligaments are completely ruptured.

B, C. X-ray films following manipulative reduction. Immobilization was continued for three weeks. The talus remained viable.

Examination fifteen years later disclosed an excellent result.

(Roentgenograms courtesy of Dr. George Curry.)

dislocation can occur, and the lower ends of the leg bones become grossly contaminated as they are driven into the ground. If, perchance, the skin remains intact, a manipulative reduction followed by immobilization in a plaster dressing should be carried out. The circulatory status of the foot must be constantly supervised until its integrity becomes certain. Any associated wound should be excised and cleansed. The talus is then replaced in the malleolar mortise, and the soft part damage repaired or not, according to the dictates of the local pathology. Skin coverage must be obtained whenever possible by tension-free primary suture, or by a free split-thickness skin graft, since all such structures as periosteum, tendons, or ligaments will undergo rapid surface necrosis if they are left exposed. The ankle should be immobilized for at least eight weeks by a circular plaster dressing applied to the level of the tibial tubercle.

Rupture of Interosseous Ligaments

External rotation injuries, which disrupt the interosseous ligaments without fracture (see Fig. 12–*13*), undoubtedly occur much more often than is generally appreciated. The clinical picture simulates that of a severe sprain. However, careful examination demonstrates the center of pain, tenderness, and swelling to be over the anterior rather than the lateral surface of the ankle, and, whenever symptoms permit manipulation of the foot, excess lateral mobility of the talus can be demonstrated by pushing the foot from side to side with the leg held immobile.

Diagnosis. Roentgen examination often is the only certain diagnostic procedure. Excess lateral mobility of the talus that is equivocal on clinical examination becomes obvious on adequate roentgen examination. Under the fluoroscope the talus can be seen to shift lateralward, and the fibula to spring apart from the tibia as the foot is pushed outward. Both the talar shift and the diastasis can be well portrayed in the roentgenogram (Fig. 12–*12*). However, both fluoroscopic examination and roentgenography are apt to be unrevealing so long as the ankle is at rest, and should always be performed with the leg stabilized and lateral stress applied to the foot (Fig. 12–*13*). Both should also be carried out with the leg in about 20 degrees internal rotation, rather than in the true anteroposterior projection, as this projection will bring the fibula out from behind the tibia and demonstrate both the talar shift and the diastasis to best advantage.

Treatment. Early reduction of the diastasis is essential. Otherwise, organizing blood clot quickly fills the space between the bones to make manipulative compression of the widened mortise difficult or impossible. Following reduction, constant firm compression of the malleoli must be maintained until the ligaments heal, or the certain recurrence of slight diastasis will result in eventual talar instability. Closure of the diastasis is accomplished by manual compression of the malleoli under general anesthesia. The foot must be at right angles as this is carried out, for dorsiflexion prevents complete closure of the mortise. A snug, well-molded but unpadded plaster boot is applied in such a way that the compression is maintained, and this must be replaced at appropriate intervals to ensure

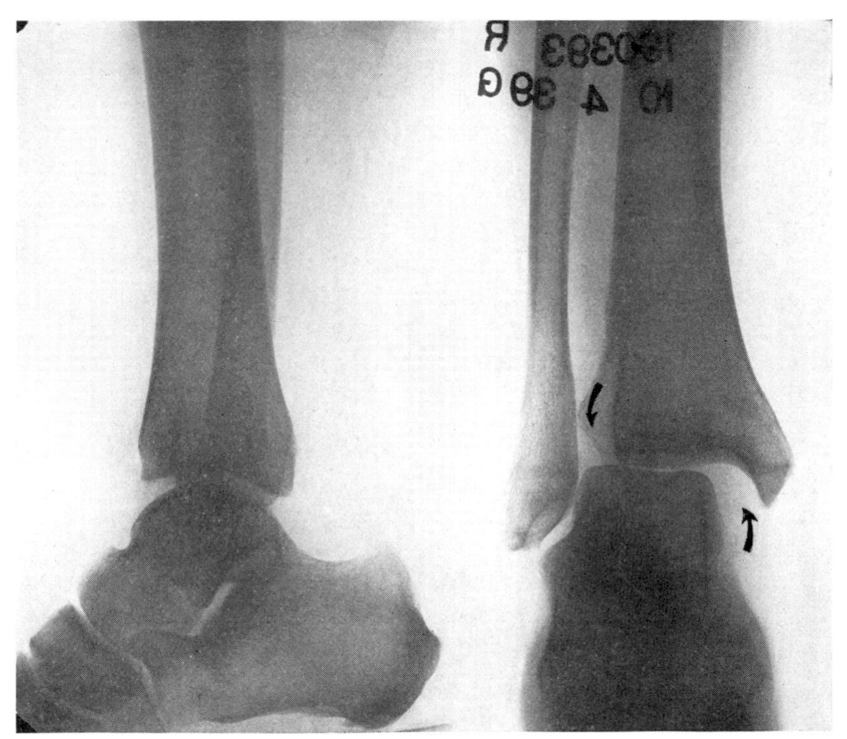

Figure 12–12. Ordinary roentgenograms, portraying complete rupture of interosseous and internal ligaments. More often than not ordinary roentgenograms fail to disclose such an injury (see Figure 12–13, A).

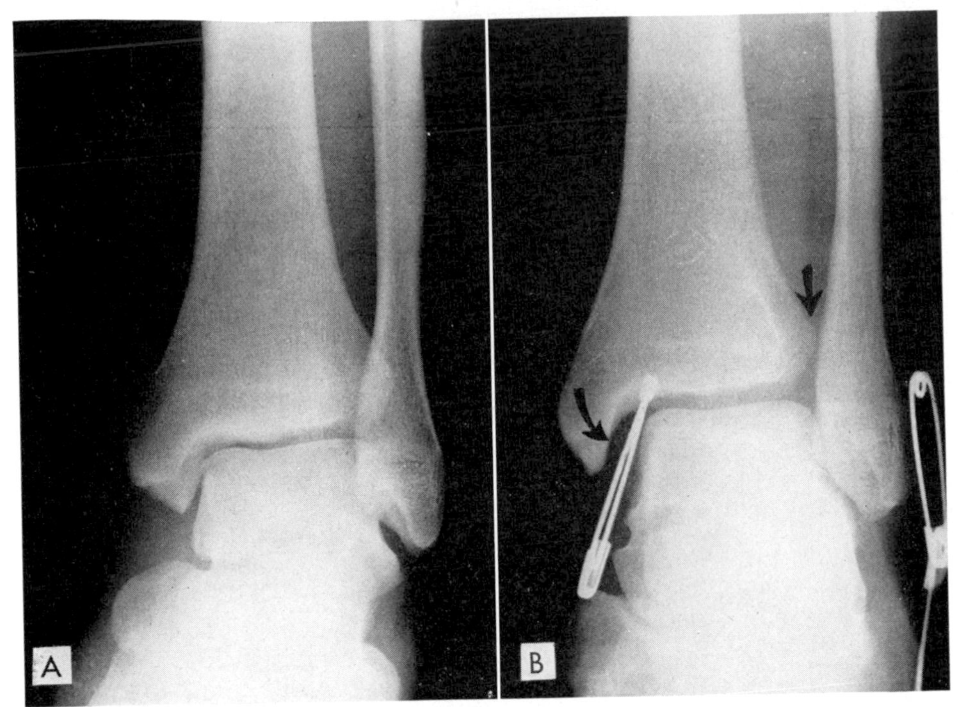

Figure 12–13. Interosseous ligament rupture without fracture.
The clinical examination indicated a severely sprained ankle.
A. Ordinary anteroposterior roentgenogram is negative.
B. Stress roentgenogram (foot thrust lateralward) discloses rupture of the interosseous ligament and damage to the internal ligament, allowing both talus and fibula to shift lateralward on the tibia.

a continued snug fit. Immobilization without weight bearing is continued for two months, at which time the ligaments are healed by fibrous union. Because such fibrous healing is apt to stretch under strain, full weight bearing should not be permitted until a minimum of four months after the injury. Provided the diastasis is adequately reduced and the reduction maintained, this program produces excellent results. The disability period is prolonged and full recovery seldom occurs within six months from the time of injury. Open reduction and internal fixation of a recent diastasis reduces the period of disability, but does not produce better final results. Diastasis of more than a few days' duration becomes noncompressible, and all such lesions of more than a week's duration deserve operative treatment.

FRACTURES OF THE MALLEOLI

Time-honored classifications of malleolar fractures based upon etiology lend little to comprehension of the intrinsic structural damage or to the management of these lesions. It is more useful to remember that every fractured malleolus is pushed by the talus, or pulled, by means of the collateral ligaments, from its parent bone (Fig. 12–*14*). When the malleolus is avulsed the fracture is transverse and situated at or below the level of

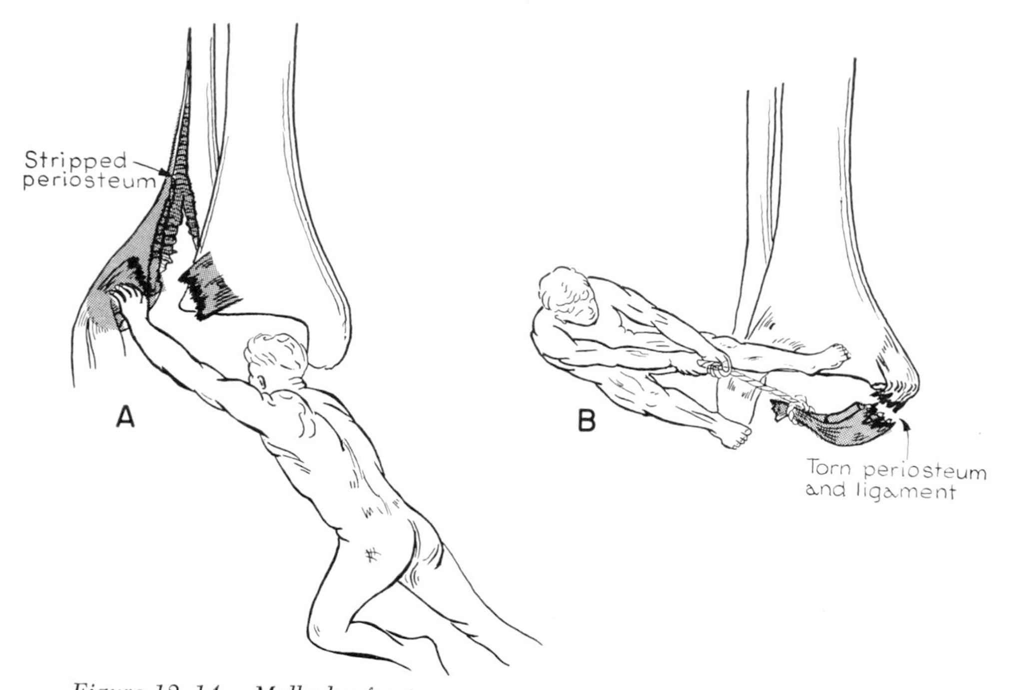

Figure 12–14. Malleolus fractures.

Every fractured malleolus is either pushed (A) or pulled, by means of the collateral ligaments (B), from the parent bone by the talus.

the ankle joint, but when injury is caused by direct talar impact the fracture is oblique and at or above the ankle joint level. As mentioned previously, a violent external rotatory twist of the foot may also fracture a malleolus, and when torsion is added to direct talar impact the resulting fracture is spiral as well as oblique. In any event, the primary offending force in every malleolar fracture is some abnormal motion of the talus. Talar mobility sufficient to produce gross displacement of a malleolar fracture prerequires that either the contralateral malleolus or collateral ligament gives way. It follows, therefore, that in every instance of an unstable fracture of one malleolus, the contralateral ligaments should be considered ruptured until it is proved otherwise (see Fig. 12–*17*).

Pathology

In a spiral or oblique fracture, the periosteal sleeve, although peeled from the proximal fragment (Fig. 12–*14*), rarely becomes interposed between the fragments. Usually these extra-osseous soft parts are more of a help than a hindrance to reduction and fixation of the fracture. Transverse fractures are a different matter. The periosteal and ligamentous investment of the avulsed malleolus is stretched, shredded, and torn transversely in a ragged manner (Fig. 12–*14*). The lacerated soft parts curl inward as they are pulled across the fracture surfaces and usually become interposed between the fragments. This makes accurate reduction difficult, and delayed or fibrous union is common.

Fibrous Union of Medial Malleolus

The implications of fibrous union pertain commonly to the medial and, rarely, to the lateral malleolus. Failure of a medial malleolar fracture to unite by bone often is indicted unjustly as a cause of ankle pain. The true significance of such a lesion comes into proper focus when the basic function of the malleolus (stabilization of the talus) is considered. When the level of the fibrous union is sufficiently distal to the ankle that an intact shoulder of malleolar base remains to prevent medial shift of the talus, little or no functional defect occurs (Fig. 12–15, *A*). When, however, it is at or proximal to the ankle joint level, the elasticity of the fibrous union potentially allows some medial shift of the talus, ankle instability, chronic symptoms, and eventually painful arthritis (Fig. 12–15, *B*). Occasionally elongation of the malleolus allows subtalar instability (Fig. 12–15, *D*). The roentgenogram indicates whether or not a fibrous union is at a level potentially apt to cause trouble. Clinical evidence of talar or subtalar

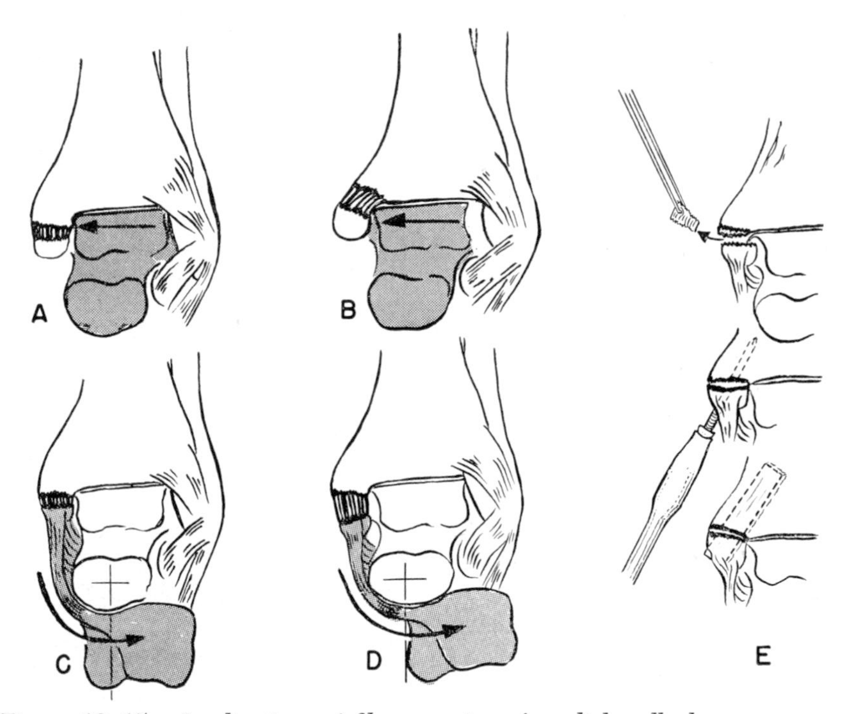

Figure 12–15. Implications of fibrous union of medial malleolus.

A. When the pseudoarthrosis is distal to the ankle level, an intact shoulder of malleolus remains to prevent the talus from slipping medialward; the ankle is stable.

B. When the lesion is at or proximal to the level of the ankle joint, the talus may shift medialward; the ankle is unstable.

C. When the medial malleolus is not elongated, the function of the internal ligament is normal.

D. When the pseudoarthrosis elongates the malleolus, undue eversion of the heel may produce symptoms; the subtalar joint is unstable.

E. Treatment is by excision of the pseudoarthrosis, and fixation of the fragments by screw, nail, or bone peg.

instability indicates that the lesion is causing trouble. The degree of symptoms and disability determines the necessity for treatment, which should consist of operative removal of the fibrous union, re-approximation of the fragments, and fixation by a screw or bone graft until bony union is obtained (Fig. 12–*15*, *E*). In neglected lesions of this type the advent of arthritis may necessitate arthrodesis for relief of pain. Fibrous union often must be prevented by operation, or accepted as inevitable at the time of reduction. The factors influencing such a decision are discussed on page 355.

Stable Fracture of One Malleolus

This is a minor injury. Absence of displacement and stability of the talus certify that both the contralateral ligaments and the soft tissues adjacent to the fracture are intact. This makes immobilization relatively unnecessary to maintenance of position of the fragment. Comfort, protection against re-injury, and maintenance of function are required, and, although these sometimes can be provided adequately by an adhesive dressing which prevents abduction and adduction of the foot (see Fig. 12–5), the use of a walking-boot for two to four weeks is simpler and safer. Immobilization, by a molded splint, and elevation may be required until subsidence of swelling makes the application of supportive dressings appropriate. Continued ambulation is desirable, but may require the aid of a cane or crutches during the first week or two. Rapid union is the rule. An undisplaced fibular malleolus heals strongly in about two weeks, and the medial malleolus within three or four weeks. The results are uniformly excellent, except when complicated by overtreatment. Immobilization or abolition of function until roentgen evidence of bony union has been obtained incurs a penalty of atrophy, atony, stiffness, and pain much more serious than would ordinarily follow complete neglect of a single undisplaced malleolar fracture.

Unstable Fracture of One Malleolus

Such a lesion, which may or may not be displaced in the original roentgenogram, has potentially serious implications. Gross instability or displacement of a sheared-off malleolus signifies rupture of the opposite collateral ligament (Fig. 12–*16*). Any instability of the fragment requires exclusion of contralateral ligament rupture from the diagnosis (Fig. 12–*17*). Contralateral ligament rupture rarely, if ever, accompanies an avulsion fracture, but a displaced avulsion fracture of the medial malleolus often is accompanied by a rupture of the interosseous ligament (Fig. 12–*16*, *E*) and requires treatment for diastasis.

Treatment. In the absence of contralateral ligament rupture the instability of a single malleolar fracture is small in amount. Nevertheless, accurate reduction is important, since even a slight residual displacement of the talus is a disabling condition. An anesthetic which allows digital manipulation of the fragment and certification of talar stability is advis-

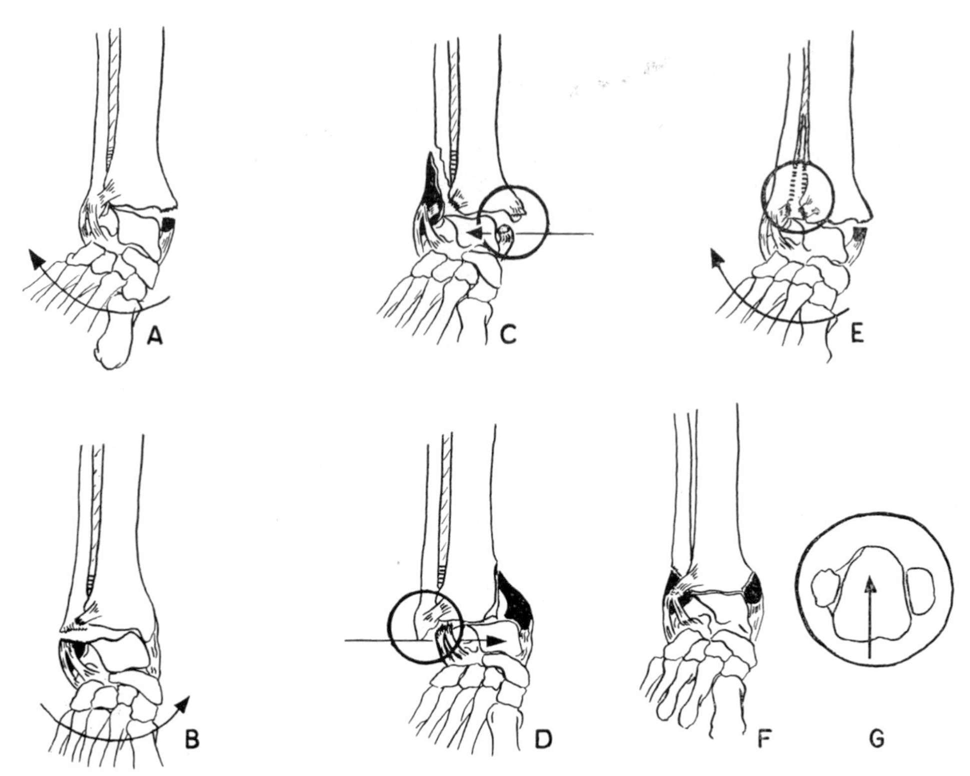

Figure 12–16. Fracture of one malleolus.

Commonly missed soft part lesions (circled) which accompany single malleolar fractures.

A, B. It is theoretically possible, but extremely rare, to encounter displacement of an avulsed malleolar fragment unaccompanied by contralateral malleolar fracture or interosseous ligament tear.

C. A displaced shearing fracture of the lateral malleolus is usually accompanied by disruption of the internal ligament.

D. A displaced shearing fracture of the medial malleolus is often accompanied by disruption of the external ligament.

E. Displacement of an avulsed fragment of the medial malleolus is often accompanied by disruption of the interosseous ligament.

F. A fracture of either or both malleoli, unaccompanied by ligament damage, may result from a force which jams the talar wedge backward between the limbs of the malleolar mortise (G).

able. Molded splints to the level of the tibial tubercle provide adequate fixation. The healing time is longer than with similar but undisplaced lesions, since the surrounding soft tissues are damaged. Splints may safely be replaced by a plaster walking-boot within two to four weeks after injury, but unprotected ambulation should not be allowed for six weeks. Healing may be rapid with bony union, or delayed with fibrous union, depending not only on the type of fracture and its displacement but also on the accuracy of reduction and efficiency of immobilization. Barring interposition of soft tissues and poor therapeutic technique, the results are uniformly good and late arthritic changes rare.

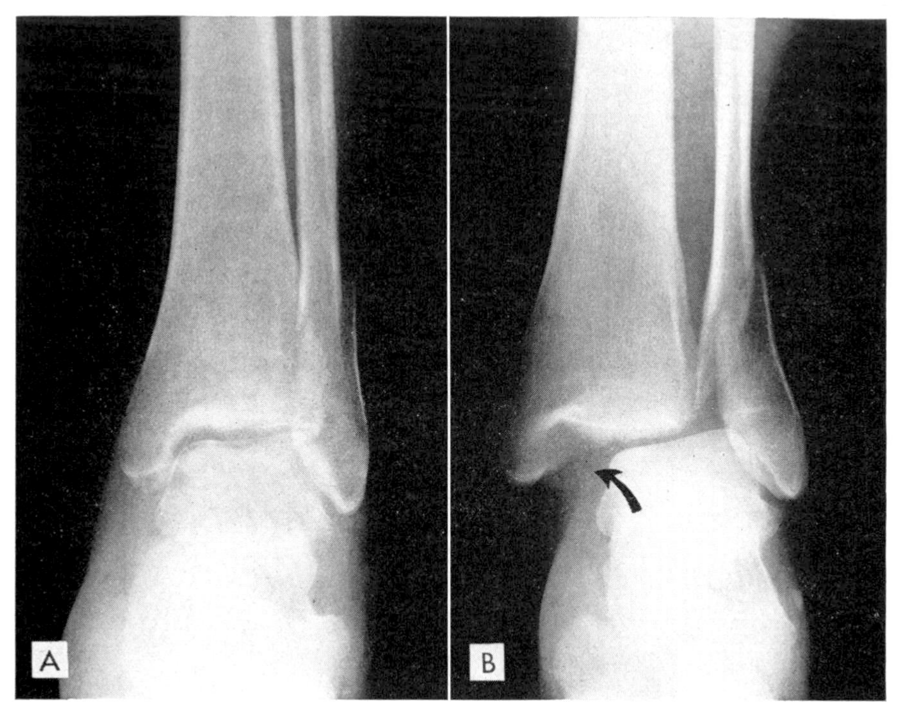

Figure 12–17. Unstable fracture of one malleolus.

A. Roentgenogram without stress shows nothing but a fracture of the lateral malleolus with slight displacement.

B. Stress roentgenogram reveals, in addition, a complete rupture of the medial collateral ligament (arrow).

In the presence of gross displacement and, ipso facto, contralateral ligament rupture, primary operative treatment gives the most certain results and deserves serious consideration. However, this does not imply that conservative treatment should be abandoned, for if manipulative reduction is exact and the ensuing immobilization efficient and prolonged (at least eight weeks), a good result may be expected. The uncertainty of conservative treatment stems from ignorance of whether the disrupted ligament is avulsed from the malleolus or shredded and torn through its own substance, whether repositioning of the talus re-approximates the ends of these torn tissues, or whether the ligament is curled up into a position making healing impossible. In any event, the relatively avascular ligament ends are subjected to a continual bath of joint fluid, which deters healing and justifies a guarded prognosis.

The indications for operative treatment include a failure to obtain or maintain anatomical reduction. The position of the talus is all important. Unless it can be restored and held exactly in normal relationship to the intact malleolus, the torn ligament has little or no chance to heal adequately, and operative repair should be carried out as early as possible. Delayed operation is always difficult because of progressive softening and friability of the torn ligament, and of swelling and inelasticity of all the surrounding soft tissues. The medial ligament should be repaired by suture or, if it is avulsed, by re-attachment to the malleolus. The external ligament rarely can be repaired in this manner and usually requires replacement (Fig. 12–*10*). Coincident open reduction, extirpation of interposed soft tissues when necessary, and internal fixation of the fractured malleolus should also be done. Precise reduction of this fracture enhances the prospects for a perfect result, and its fixation by screws or nails acts as protec-

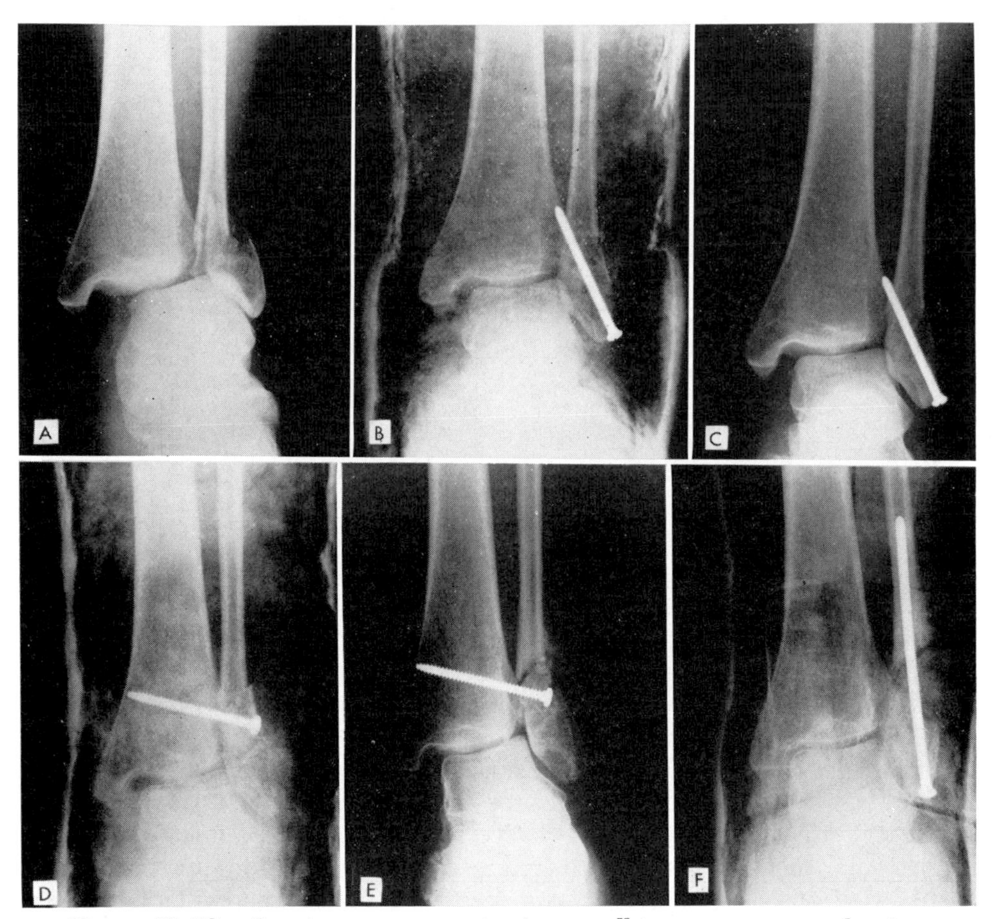

Figure 12–18. Roentgenograms portraying an all-too-common tragedy of errors.

A. Original diagnosis was a fracture of the lateral malleolus; it is obvious that the internal ligament is also ruptured.

B. The decision to operate followed multiple failures at attempted closed reduction. Note the incomplete reposition of the talus shown in this postoperative film.

C. Two weeks after operation, the deformity recurred in plaster.

D. Three months after injury, the fibula was osteotomized, and an unsuccessful attempt was made to manipulate the foot into normal position.

E. One month after osteotomy, the deformity remains.

F. Eight months after injury, the nature of the injury was recognized, the ruptured internal ligament was removed from between the talus and the medial malleolus, and sutured to the tibia. The fibula was osteotomized and fixed.

The final result was good.

tion for the repaired or replaced contralateral ligament. Ambulation in a walking-boot is then permissible and safe shortly after the operative incisions are healed. The boot is discarded after eight weeks and progressive resumption of unprotected function is allowed. The results will be uniformly good, provided treatment has been early and adequate; late and inadequate treatment invites disaster.

A typical and all-too-common tragedy of errors and temporization is illustrated by the roentgenograms (Fig. 12–*18*) of a young woman patient who was diagnosed as having fracture of the lateral malleolus. Several manipulative reductions were attempted, none of which quite satisfied her surgeon. Several weeks later he did an open reduction of the malleolus and fixed it with a single screw. Two weeks later the original deformity had recurred, despite plaster immobilization. Various wedgings and changes of plaster failed to correct this displacement. Three months after her injury her continuing problem was blamed on malunion of the fibula, and this bone was accordingly osteotomized and screwed to the tibia. One month later the original deformity was again present. Eight months, many manipulations, two operations, and several surgeons later, the rupture of the internal ligament finally was recognized. She was again operated on, and the avulsed ligament extricated from between the talus and the medial malleolus, where it had remained from the start to defy all attempts to replace the talus in normal position. The ligament was sutured to the malleolus, the fibula was straightened and fixed by a screw, and the patient finally regained a useful extremity.

Bimalleolar Fractures

Bimalleolar injuries consist of a shearing and an avulsion fracture (Fig. 12–*19*). Because both arms of the malleolar mortise are broken, gross displacement is often present, and, more often than not, the avulsion lesion is complicated by interposition of soft tissues between the fragments. Conservative management is made difficult by the characteristic instability of the ankle as a whole, and success or failure depends upon small details of therapeutic technique. Manipulative reduction may be a simple matter, but manual maintenance of the reduced position during the application and setting of plaster splints is a task for the most expert member of the operating team.

Reduction. Adequate anesthesia is essential. The knee should be flexed to a right angle to eliminate the pull of the calf muscles. The first step consists of replacing the foot in normal relationship to the leg, where it must be held firmly while each malleolar fragment is manipulated into place. At this point the avulsed malleolus should be tested for the presence or absence of bony crepitus. Absence of crepitus signifies the interposition of soft tissues, which at times may be worked out of the fracture site by to-and-fro manipulation of the malleolar fragment. When this cannot be done, an immediate decision between acceptance of a potential fibrous union and open reduction, preceded by operative removal of the interposed soft tissues, must be made.

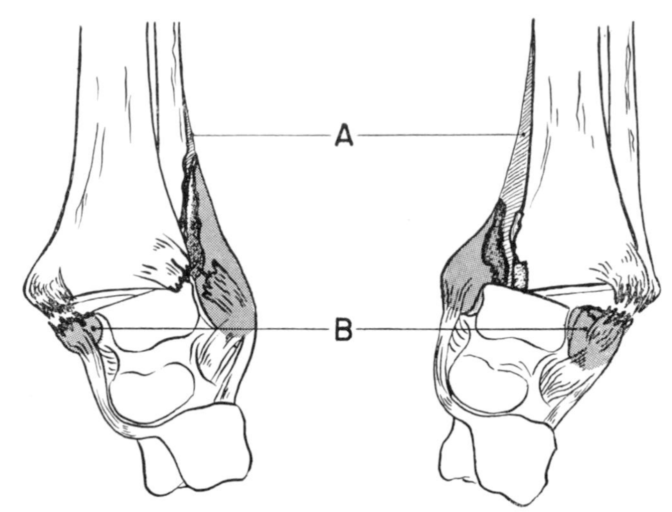

Figure 12–19. Bimalleolar fractures.

One fracture is an avulsion lesion, the other is caused by talar impact.

A. The shearing (direct impact) fracture tends to peel the periosteal sleeve from the parent bone. Interposition of tissue is rare.

B. The avulsion fracture lacerates the ligamentous and periosteal investment of the malleolus in a ragged manner. Interposition of these tissues between the fragments is common.

Indications for and against Open Reduction. The decision between operative and closed treatment for an avulsed malleolus, complicated by interposition of soft tissues, calls for mature surgical judgment and an assessment of the following points:

1. Fibrous union is often unassociated with symptoms and disability (see page 349).
2. Closed reduction and immobilization require a minimum of facilities.
3. Safe and successful operative treatment requires not only a specialized technical ability of the surgeon but also a surgical environment of maximum efficiency.
4. The penalties of inadequate operative technique or postoperative infection are much more severe than those of fibrous union.
5. Examination of avulsed fractures often reveals multiple loose particles of bone and cartilage in the ankle joint. This debris is not visible in roentgenograms, and unquestionably contributes to or may be the most important cause of unexpected and otherwise unexplainable arthritic sequelae in certain cases. Operation permits removal of all such debris.
6. Operative treatment, in addition to eliminating certain complications and predisposing to others, allows perfect reduction, and internal fixation minimizes the extent and duration of external immobilization required.
7. If the avulsed malleolus is explored, the other malleolar fracture also should be treated by open reduction and internal fixation. Otherwise, all the risks of operation are accepted without avoidance of the disadvantages of prolonged external fixation.

Aftercare. When a conservative régime is elected, the reduced fracture is immobilized with the foot in a position of maximum function, neither inverted nor everted, and neither plantar flexed nor dorsiflexed. The plaster dressing must be molded around the replaced malleoli with care and should extend from toes to upper thigh, holding the knee sufficiently flexed (Fig. 12–20) to prevent rotational displacement at the ankle. Within a month sufficient healing is present to permit reduction of the extent of the dressing to the level of the tibial tubercle so that knee motion may be resumed. Within another two weeks ambulation in a plaster walking-boot is permissible and safe. All immobilization may be discarded within eight weeks of reduction, and progressive weight bearing commenced. After removal of the plaster dressings considerable edema and stiffness are usually present. This is most marked in the foot. A program of soaks, exercises, and elevation almost always must be followed during this stage of rehabilitation. Some permanent defect in motion of the small joints of the foot, especially the subtalar mechanism, is common, and the patient should be warned to expect some evening edema for a year or more.

THE EXTENT OF IMMOBILIZATION. This must be dictated by the indi-

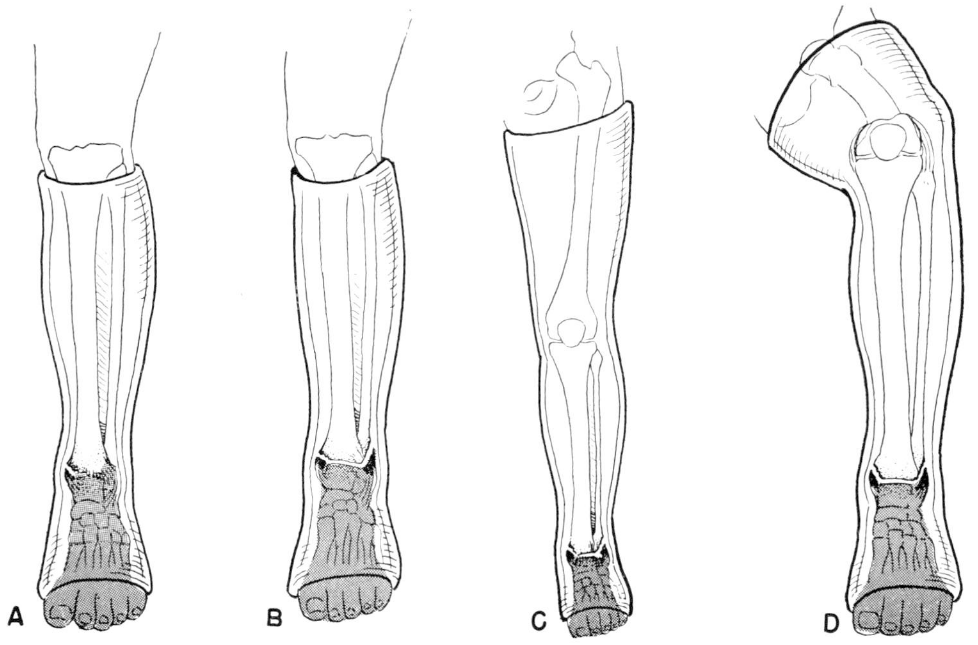

Figure 12–20. The extent of immobilization for ankle fractures.

The immobilizing dressing should extend from the toes to the level of the tibial tubercle, or to the groin.

A. When a single malleolus is fractured, and the other malleolus with its ligament is intact, there is little danger of rotatory displacement of the foot on the leg. A short plaster is adequate.

B, C. When both limbs of the ankle mortise or one malleolus and the contralateral ligament are broken, the foot can rotate on the leg in a short plaster, and even in a high plaster, if the knee is straight.

D. Control of rotatory displacement requires a high plaster with the knee flexed.

vidual characteristics of the lesion. Every plaster dressing should extend either to the level of the tibial tubercle, or to the upper third of the thigh. In deciding which to use, the injured ankle in question should be considered as a break in the continuity of the extremity as a whole, with the foot and malleolar fragments as the distal entity and the remainder of the extremity as the proximal entity (Fig. 12–*20*). When only one malleolus is fractured, the other, along with its soft-part attachments to the foot, acts as an efficient bulwark against a rotational displacement of these two entities. In such instances plaster fixation to the level of the tibial tubercle, which prevents shift or tilt of the foot on the leg, is adequate. When both malleoli are fractured, rotation is not controlled by a tubercle-high dressing; neither, for that matter, is it controlled by a groin-high plaster, if the knee is straight (Fig. 12–*20*). Bimalleolar fractures, therefore, must be immobilized by a dressing extending to the upper thigh and holding the knee sufficiently flexed (about 135 degrees) so that the extremity cannot rotate within the plaster.

Operative treatment should replace accurately and fix firmly each malleolus. It is then possible (when the weight-bearing elements of the joint are intact) for the patient to commence protected ambulation when the operative wounds heal and the local reaction subsides. This protection should be a plaster walking-boot or a low-leg brace, which is worn until the fractures are healed, a matter usually of four to six weeks. An alternative program is the use of crutches, without weight bearing, and local protection by splints which are removed frequently for exercises, soaks, and other measures designed to maintain function pending union of the fractured fragments.

FRACTURES OF WEIGHT-BEARING SURFACE OF TIBIA

The lesions considered up to this point have involved not the weight-bearing elements of the ankle but only the structures serving to maintain a correct relationship between the foot and the leg. A fracture of the weight-bearing surface of the tibia, resulting from direct impact by the talus, is a common complication of any injury which disrupts the mortise sufficiently to allow displacement of the talus. The character and location of such a complicating lesion and the displacement involved depend not upon the presence of specific malleolar or ligamentous injuries, but only upon the force and direction of displacement of the talus.

Fracture of Posterior Lip of Tibia

This fracture is by far the most common injury to the weight-bearing mechanism, since in most ankle injuries a forward momentum of the body tends to drive the tibia forward on the foot (and so on the talus), which is fixed to the ground at the moment of injury. The wedge-shaped talus cannot move backward through an intact mortise, except when the foot is in extreme plantar flexion. Consequently these fractures are almost synonymous with some disruption of the mortise from diastasis or malleolar injury. In the absence of any malleolar fracture the presence of a diastasis must be assumed until it is disproved. The posterior lip fragment is pushed into its displaced position by the talus and, therefore, its displacement is synonymous with actual or potential posterior subluxation of the talus. Above all else the goal of treatment for every ankle injury is to ensure a stable talus (which requires an intact mortise), and a normal relationship between the tibia and talus (which is incompatible with any talar subluxation). As set forth in the following paragraphs the prerequisites for simultaneous correction of displacement of the posterior lip and disruption of the mortise often prove paradoxical.

Paradoxical requirements for correction of talar subluxation and mortise disruption. The calf muscles maintain the talus and posterior lip fragment in a displaced position, and this force must be neutralized. It can be reduced by flexion of the knee, but plantar flexion at the ankle may be required for its neutralization. On the other hand, both the talus and the posterior lip fragment are inaccessible and can be manipulated only through their soft tissue attachments to the remainder of the foot. It is frequently necessary to dorsiflex the foot in order to pull the lip fragment down to a level where the tibial articular surface is restored to a continuous curve. Under these circumstances maintenance of reduction may require continuous fixation in dorsiflexion. This tightens the calf muscles and may cause talar subluxation and redisplacement of the lip fragment, either at the time of reduction or later, within plaster dressings.

Dorsiflexion maneuvers necessary for reduction of the posterior lip fragment may also derange the mortise. Anatomical restoration of a disrupted mortise requires that fractured malleoli be replaced or a diastasis compressed with the foot in a normal weight-bearing position, neither plantar flexed nor dorsiflexed. If these maneuvers are carried out with the foot in plantar flexion (for complete relaxation of the calf), it is possible for the mortise to heal in a state that is too narrow for proper acceptance of the talar tenon; if they are carried out with the foot in dorsiflexion (for complete reduction of the posterior lip fragment), the mortise may heal in a widened state and allow eventual talar instability. In short, the surgeon may find himself unable to effect by manipulation, and maintain by external immobilization, a simultaneous reduction of the talar subluxation and restoration of an intact mortise. Both are essential, but an accurate replacement of the posterior lip fragment is not always necessary. Analysis of the end-results in a large series of cases, treated over a 20-year period, disclosed data of some value in determining the clinical and therapeutic significance of posterior lip fractures, regardless of the lesions which accompanied them (Fig. 12–*21*).

Some of these data are as follows:

1. Two out of every three patients in whom a residual posterior subluxation of the talus was found complained of a painful ankle. Only one of every five patients whose talus was in normal position in the lateral roentgenogram complained of pain. The earliest and most severe arthritic changes consistently developed in ankles with talar subluxation, regardless of its degree. No common denominator could be educed to correlate

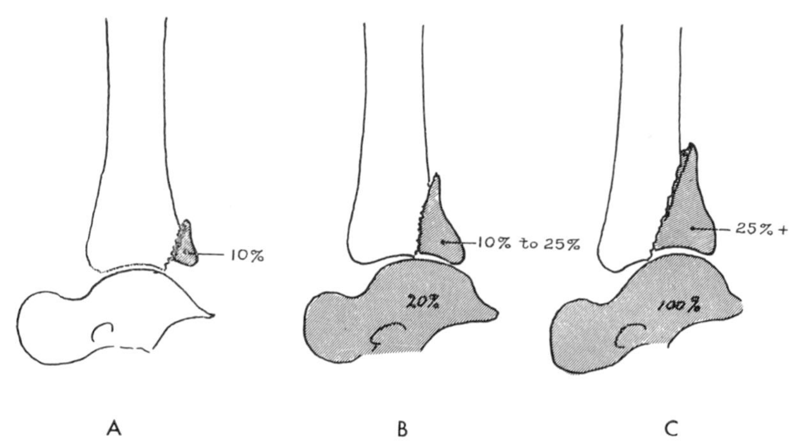

Figure 12–21. Subluxation of the talus.

A. When the posterior lip fracture represents 10 per cent of the total articulating surface of the tibia, subluxation of the talus does not occur, and it is immaterial whether or not the fragment is reduced.

B. When the fragment represents 10 to 25 per cent of the tibial surface, the talus subluxates slightly in about 20 per cent of cases, despite exact reposition of the fragment and all attempts to maintain this position by external immobilizing devices. A slight talar subluxation is as certain a harbinger of eventual painful arthritis as is gross displacement.

C. When the fragment constitutes 25 per cent or more of the tibial articular surface, it is virtually impossible to maintain a perfect reduction, except by internal fixation. Without this, secondary displacement of both fracture fragment and talus is to be expected. The inevitable result is a painful arthritis.

painful end-results and other pathologic or therapeutic factors, such as the number and type of coincident lesions or the quality of their care. As Celsus pointed out in the 1st Century A.D., accurate replacement and maintenance of the talus in its normal position remains the most important single prerequisite to a happy result.

2. Residual displacement of the posterior tibial lip was found to produce no harmful effects, except when it permitted posterior subluxation of the talus. Subluxation was not present in any case in which the posterior lip fragment involved less than 10 per cent of the tibial articular surface, regardless of the residual position of the lip fragment. Eventual subluxation was present in 20 per cent of all cases with a lip fragment involving between 10 and 25 per cent of the tibial surface, regardless of the perfection of the original reduction or the trouble taken to maintain it by external immobilizing dressings. When the posterior lip involved one fourth or more of the tibial surface some posterior subluxation eventuated in every case treated by manipulative reduction and external immobilization.

The prerequisites to a happy result in these more complicated injuries, therefore, include the coincident restoration and maintenance of both an intact mortise and an absolutely normal relationship between the tibia and the talus. When both of these objectives cannot be accomplished and maintained simultaneously, open reduction and internal fixation should be done. Operative fixation has proved to be the only method consistently productive of a stable painless ankle in the injuries with posterior lip fractures which involved 25 per cent or more of the tibial articular surface. This statement may be received with skepticism in some quarters, but will be supported by surgeons who have kept in touch with their patients for more than two years. Minor displacements, subluxations, and instability of the talus have notorious sequelae; the ankle may remain in excellent condition for the first year or two after injury, only to disintegrate and become host to a crippling disability several years later.

Fracture of Both Malleoli and Posterior Lip of Tibia

It has been pointed out that fractures of one or both malleoli, without damage to the weight-bearing surface of the tibia, require treatment designed to ensure an adequate mortise and a stable talus. A large proportion of malleolar fractures are accompanied by a fracture of the posterior weight-bearing surface of the tibia. Treatment for these common injuries, which have become widely known as "trimalleolar" fractures, must provide and maintain, in addition to a restored mortise and a stable talus, an exact replacement of the talus under the articulating surface of the tibia. The difficulties and sometimes paradoxical requisites involved in the simultaneous accomplishment of all these objectives have been discussed. Manipulative reduction and adequate fixation by external immobilizing devices are extremely difficult and often impossible, yet anything short of perfection augurs for a poor result. When a perfect reduction can be maintained, immobilization should be continued until the weight-bearing posterior lip fragment has healed completely. When a perfect reduction cannot be produced by manipulation or maintained by plaster dressings, open reduction and internal fixation must be done

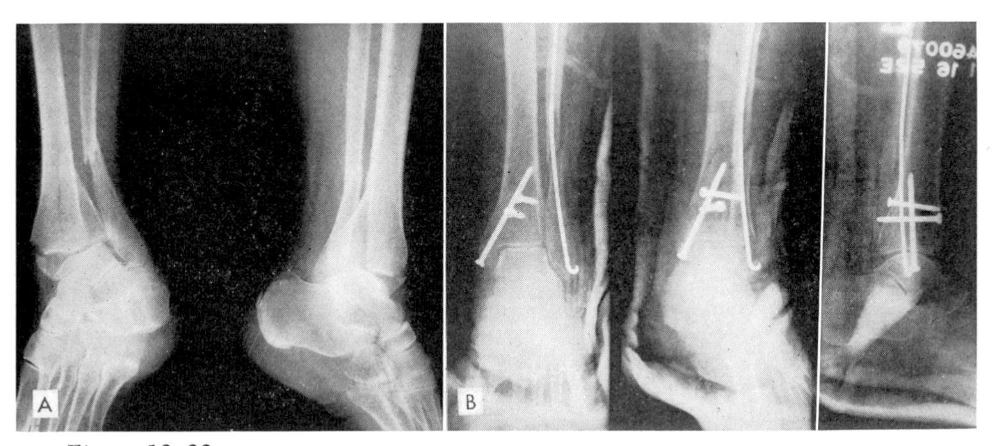

Figure 12–22.

A. The talus, posterior tibial lip, and lower fragment of the fibula have displaced from the leg, accompanied by the avulsed medial malleolus. The posterior lip involves almost 50 per cent of the weight-bearing surface of the tibia in the lateral view. A perfect reduction could be obtained by manipulation, but could not be maintained by plaster.

B. Open reduction and internal fixation obtains and maintains a perfect reduction. A good result is certain.

if a satisfactory result is to be obtained (Fig. 12–22). The decision brooks no delay. If an injured ankle requires operation it must be done quickly, before tissue tension and hypoxia so deplete the resistance of all the tissues to infection that it becomes unsafe to subject them to any operative insult until one or two weeks later, after the acute local reaction has subsided.

Fracture of Anterior Lip of Tibia

This injury is not common. It is caused by talar impact, usually consequent to a fall from a height, landing on the dorsiflexed foot. Comminution of the tibia is much more common than in fractures of the posterior tibial lip, and the talus is usually displaced forward from its normal seat in the malleolar mortise. Reduction by manipulation is difficult and, even when effected, can be maintained only by immobilization with the foot in a position of extreme plantar flexion. This presents a paradox, the reverse of that encountered with posterior lip fractures, for, although the plantar-flexed position helps to maintain the tibial fragment in a reduced position by traction through the anterior joint capsule and ligaments, this position also delivers the narrow posterior segment of the talus into the ankle mortise and predisposes to easy anterior talar subluxation. Open reduction with internal fixation of the tibial fragment is usually the treatment of choice.

Fracture of Lateral Lip of Tibia

An isolated fracture of the anterolateral lip of the tibia results from a fall on the dorsiflexed and everted foot. It is quite uncommon and, because the fracture fragment is small, is displaced only a slight amount, and is almost always impacted into the parent tibia, this lesion frequently is not recognized. More often than not failure to recognize or treat such an injury is followed by serious disability of indefinite duration, because, although the fracture fragment is small and not grossly displaced, it is, nevertheless, situated in a position to derange all three elements of the ankle mechanism, namely, the tibiofibular syndesmosis, and the tibiotalar and fibulotalar articulations. All such fractures with appreciable displacement of the small impacted tibial fragment should be explored and the fragment either replaced in normal position or removed.

Shattered Fractures of Lower Tibia Involving Ankle Joint

The lower end of the tibia may be shattered into many small fragments with a virtual disappearance of any remaining clean-cut articular surface in the roentgenogram. These are problems more of salvage than of reduction and immobilization of the fracture. Normal length and alignment of the limb must be maintained. Fixed skeletal traction (see Fig. 13–*10*, page 376) is required to prevent collapse and shortening of the shattered segment of tibia. This is incorporated into circular plaster dressings, which maintain the alignment of foot and leg. Prolonged immobilization is mandatory. Little residual ankle motion should be expected. Persistent ankle pain may require subsequent arthrodesis and, indeed, there are occasionally some valid indications for primary ankle arthrodesis in these severe injuries.

CHAPTER 13

INJURIES OF THE LEG

By HARRISON L. McLAUGHLIN, M.D.

THE SOFT PARTS

THE MUSCLES OF THE LEG are housed within three fascial chambers, two of which also contain the nerves and vessels serving the foot (Fig. 13–*1*). The anterior tibial artery enters the anterior fascial compartment through an aperture in the upper end of the interosseous membrane, at which point it is relatively immobile and easily damaged by injuries to adjacent bone (see Fig. 13–*5*). The fascial compartments have a fixed capacity and the main blood vessels, as the most compressible of their contents, are the first structures to suffer from the effects of increased subfascial tension. Muscles arise from only the proximal half of the tibia. The remainder of this bone is surrounded by relatively avascular connective tissue structures separated by loose areolar tissues, which produce an environment poorly suited to the elaboration of extra-osseous callus for fracture healing. When a modern motor vehicle strikes a pedestrian the leg is almost always a primary point of impact. The subcutaneous location of the tibia predisposes to an open wound, complicating all fractures

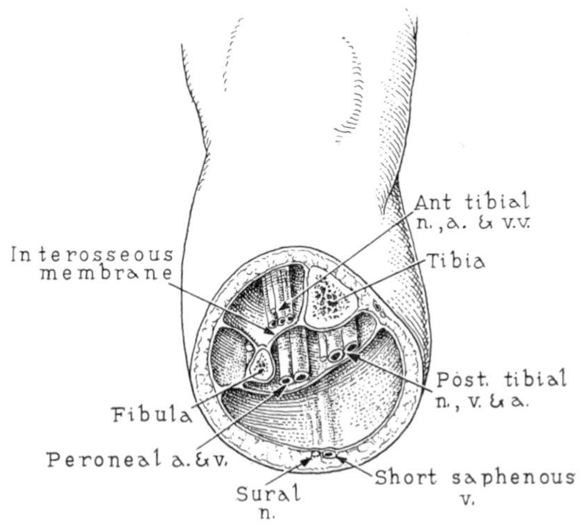

Figure 13–1. The fascial compartments of the leg and their neurovascular contents.

caused by direct violence. Consequently injuries to the leg are common, usually serious, and often difficult treatment problems.

Anterior Compartment of the Leg

The motors for dorsiflexion of the foot and toes (tibialis anterior, extensor hallucis longus, and extensor digitorum longus) are compressed into the anterior interosseous space by a strong expanse of deep fascia (Fig. 13–*1*). The small and inconstant peroneus tertius, which may be considered a distal segment of the extensor digitorum longus, contributes to dorsiflexion and eversion of the foot. All four muscles are supplied by the anterior tibial (deep peroneal) nerve, which enters the anterior compartment after winding around the outer surface of the neck of the fibula. The anterior tibial artery travels the length of the anterior compartment deep to the tibialis anterior muscle, and becomes the dorsalis pedis artery of the foot.

Lateral Compartment of the Leg

The lateral compartment, having only one rigid wall and containing no large vessels (Fig. 13–*1*), is relatively immune to the penalties of subfascial tension. It houses the peroneus longus and brevis muscles, both of which are supplied by the superficial branch of the peroneal nerve. These are the muscles of foot eversion.

Peroneal nerve. The common peroneal nerve emerges from behind the protective cushion of the biceps femoris and divides into superficial and deep branches which wind around the outer surface of the upper fibula, covered by little except skin and subcutaneous tissues (Fig. 13–2). At this level one or both branches may be stretched by a varus strain of

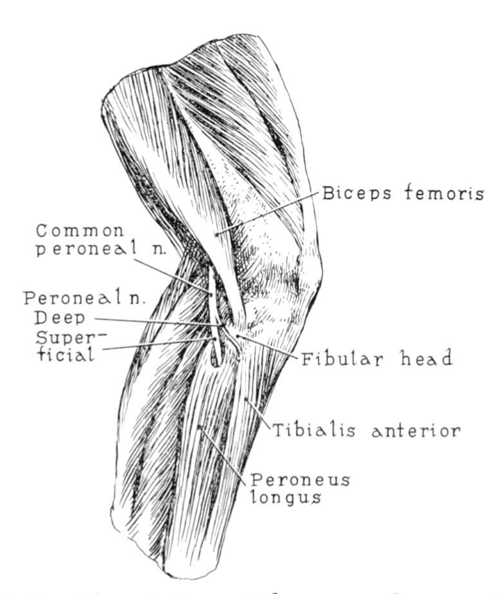

Figure 13–2. The relations of the peroneal nerve at the knee.

the knee, contused or lacerated by a contiguous fracture, or compressed secondarily to trauma by fibrous tissue or callus.

INJURY OF THE PERONEAL NERVE. Delayed peroneal nerve palsy, characterized by progressive weakness of the muscles of dorsiflexion and eversion of the foot, following an injury at or about the neck of the fibula, deserves exploration and neurolysis. Peroneal nerve palsy commencing immediately after injury usually recovers spontaneously, except when due to stretch. Nerve injury by stretch rarely, if ever, benefits from an operation. Consequently, early peroneal palsy warrants temporization. The foot is supported by a light spring brace, and the patient is warned that spontaneous recovery, while probable, may not be complete for many months.

Treatment is the most common cause of peroneal palsy. Every surgeon has confirmed the vulnerability of his own peroneal nerve by crossing his knees in a fashion which produced numbness in the peroneal sensory distribution. He should, therefore, be aware that the upper edge of a plaster of paris dressing, the constriction of a circular bandage, the misplaced pressure of a suspension apparatus, a misused tourniquet, the sandbag or rolled sheet under the knee of an anesthetized patient, and even the chronic extended leg posture of a bedfast patient, all constitute every-day causes for compression of the peroneal nerve, against which he must remain constantly on guard.

Posterior Compartment of the Leg

The posterior fascial compartment of the calf, containing the muscles of plantar flexion and inversion, as well as the peroneal and posterior tibial vessels and the posterior tibial nerve, is subdivided by a continuation of the posterior intermuscular septum (Fig. 13–*1*). The superficial chamber contains the plantaris, soleus, and gastrocnemius muscles, which converge distally to form the tendo achillis. The other calf muscles and the major nerves and vessels are compressed into the deep interosseous space by the posterior intermuscular septum.

Rupture of the tendo achillis. A healthy heel cord may be cut, but does not rupture. Severance by accidental incision warrants immediate suture. The tendon ends are healthy, secure repair can be accomplished by mattress type sutures, and a normal result may be anticipated, provided disruption of the suture line is prevented by immobilization in a position of knee flexion and plantar flexion of the foot for a period of four to six weeks.

Rupture of the tendo achillis takes place through a diseased or degenerated segment of tendon, and is the result of some sudden contraction of the calf muscles against resistance. Frequently clinical examination will suggest that the rupture is incomplete because some power of plantar flexion is preserved. Usually this is a false hope. The tear almost always is complete, and the persisting plantar flexion power results from calf muscle pull on an intact fragment of tendon sheath, or from the action of the smaller posterior compartment muscles. The patient walks flatfooted and cannot stand on his toes. A palpable sulcus traverses the tendon in the early stages after rupture, and later this may be camouflaged by a palpable tumor, which is the swollen end of the retracted proximal fragment.

Only two alternatives are available: the patient must learn to live with his flatfooted gait and a complete inability to stand on his toes, or submit to operative repair of the rupture. Attritional degeneration of the tendon is the usual lesion predisposing to spontaneous rupture and, consequently, most patients who sustain this injury are past middle age. Some of them are content to put up with the resulting disability of gait.

OPERATIVE REPAIR is made difficult by the poor quality of the tissues through which the rupture occurred. The ends of the tendon fragments are fragile and fibrillated. To attempt a direct suture of these tendon

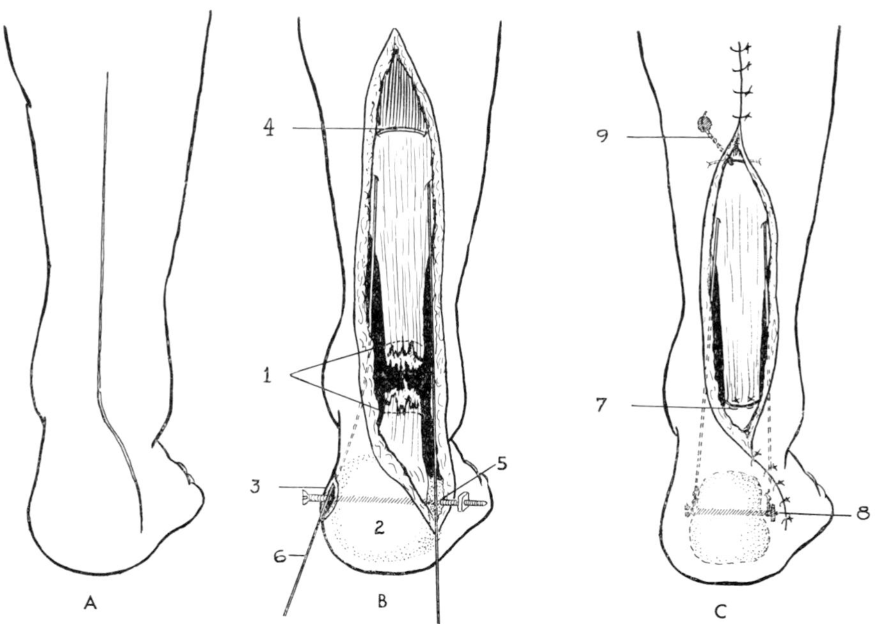

Figure 13–3. Repair of ruptured tendo achillis by removable suture.

A. A midline incision is made which curves laterally in its distal portion to avoid shoe pressure upon the scar.

B. The tendon ends are not only separated, but frayed and fragile. Each must be trimmed back to reasonably healthy tissue (1). A drill hole is made through the calcaneus (2), and a stab wound made at its point of emergence (3). A long heavy wire mattress suture is placed at the musculotendinous junction (4). A long screw is passed through the drill hole in the os calcis (5) and the proximal tendon fragment is pulled down into position by the two ends of the wire suture (6), which are then fastened to the projecting ends of the screw.

C. With retraction thus counteracted, the trimmed tendon ends may then be sutured (7). The superfluous portion of the screw is cut free and removed (8). A twisted wire (9) with a split lead shot (for palpable localization of the mattress suture at the time of removal) is attached to the proximal portion of the wire suture. (From McLaughlin, H. L., in Cole's Operative Technic in General Surgery, 2nd ed., 1955. Courtesy of Appleton-Century-Crofts, Inc.)

ends is like attempting to sew the ends of two paint brushes together, and is about as effective. The diseased or degenerated tissue at the rupture site must be removed (Fig. 13–3, *B*). A hiatus, usually measuring 5 to 10 cm. in length, is thereby produced between the trimmed tendon fragments. This can be eliminated by flexion at the ankle and knee, but special measures are necessary to neutralize the pull of the calf muscles after repair has been effected. A removable wire suture, which maintains a fixed distance between the muscle bellies and the calcaneus (Fig. 13–3, *C*) serves this purpose efficiently. This is removed after eight weeks, in which time the tendon is healed sufficiently to permit unprotected ambulation.

Rupture of the plantaris tendon. The plantaris muscle is functionally insignificant. Spontaneous rupture of its long, thin, string-like tendon, which stretches the entire length of the calf, may occur suddenly from the exertion of any strenuous activity. The clinical picture is constant. The patient whirls around to see who hit him in the calf with a stone or other missile. The entire calf becomes painful, tender, swollen, and, within several days, ecchymotic. Function of the calf muscle is impeded by pain, and the lesion may be misinterpreted as a ruptured gastrocnemius muscle or a rupture of the tendo achillis. Complete recovery occurs within several weeks. The only treatment required is relief of pain. Use of a ½-inch heel raise and a cane, with support of the calf by an elastic bandage, will make continued ambulation less uncomfortable during the early painful period which follows this insignificant injury.

"Tight calf" due to penetrating wounds. Subfascial tension in the calf demanding urgent measures in its own right does not often complicate fractures of the leg bones. As a rule, excessive tension in the posterior compartment then is decompressed spontaneously through the injured bones and interosseous membrane. However, small penetrating wounds of the calf which implicate the peroneal or posterior tibial arteries may produce an alarming syndrome characterized by an intensely swollen, board-like calf, which is exquisitely tender and painful, and a cold, white, immobile foot with some vascular insufficiency. Arterial spasm may progress retrograde and implicate the anterior tibial artery. A lumbar sympathetic block should be done, but more often than not will prove ineffectual. Elevation, in the face of vascular insufficiency, may do more harm than good. The posterior compartment should be decompressed by incision of its fascial walls within a few hours, if the foot remains devoid of any signs of returning circulation.

Volkmann's ischemic paralysis in the leg. This dread complication is not limited to injuries of the elbow, but occurs in the leg much more frequently than is generally appreciated. It has been the writer's distressing experience to sit helplessly by and observe the development of ischemic paralysis in the fractured leg of a boy afflicted with hemophilia, because the risks of fasciotomy were considered insurmountable. An unrelieved "tight calf" may produce irreversible muscle damage by anoxia within a few hours. A similar, but circumscribed, ischemic catastrophe occasionally follows prolonged subfascial tension localized to the anterior compartment of the leg. The risks of decompression by fasciotomy, even in experienced hands, may be accepted gratefully as an alternative to such an irreversible and crippling lesion.

VOLKMANN'S ISCHEMIA CAUSED BY TREATMENT. The majority of ischemic complications in the leg are caused by treatment. There is little excuse for this deplorable fact, because ischemic paralysis is invariably heralded by a period of intense unremitting muscle pain, accompanied by obvious signs of vascular depletion in the foot. These warning signs demand that a circular plaster dressing be split at once and, unless improvement follows rapidly, removed completely. Any suspension apparatus capable of constricting or pressing upon the calf or popliteal area must be examined and adjusted regularly and frequently. Bryant's traction (p. 415) is a cause of ischemic paralysis, more often than not affecting the uninjured leg. The injured leg is slightly shortened at the fracture, all muscles remain in some steady spasm, and the vascular tree is not stretched by the traction. Not only is the uninjured leg stretched to full length but, in the infant ordinarily treated by this method, the knee is also hyperextended. Constant stretch of the popliteal vessels by this combination of traction and hyperextension, often accentuated by too-tight bandages holding the traction strips to the skin, are the factors potentially capable of producing ischemia of the leg in every case. The uninjured leg should be protected from this danger by the application of a plaster splint which maintains the knee in slight flexion, before traction is commenced.

The application of a traction device to a lower extremity, injured or uninjured, should be accompanied by orders to assess the color, temperature, mobility, and vascular state of the toes at regular and frequent intervals. *Ischemic paralysis of the leg is heralded by warning signs, usually results from negligence, and can be prevented by diligence.*

Decompression of subfascial tension by incision. The anterior and lateral compartments of the leg are subcutaneous and may be decompressed at any point through a longitudinal incision in skin and fascia. The posterior compartment is deep in the calf, and both subdivisions must be opened to ensure adequate release of subfascial tension. The skin is incised along the proximal two-thirds of the palpable posteromedial edge of the tibia. The deep fascia is incised to open the space between the soleus and gastrocnemius muscles. The medial (tibial) origin of the soleus muscle is then divided sufficiently to open the sub-soleus space, which contains the large vessels and nerves. Control of the posterior tibial artery at this proximal point is a useful preliminary to localization and management of an injury to this artery at some more distal point in the calf.

THE FIBULA

This long thin bone bears no weight. Both ends are bound securely by ligaments, and the shaft by an interosseous membrane, to the adjacent tibia. The proximal end, by virtue of continuity with the external collateral ligament, is essential to stability of the knee joint (Fig. 14–*1*). The distal malleolus is essential to stability of the ankle (Fig. 12–3). The intervening shaft is almost completely surrounded by vascular muscle tissues. Fractures usually unite rapidly and well, with or without treatment. The shaft of the fibula is expendable, and large segments can be removed for use as a bone graft, or in the ablation of infection or neoplasm, without fear of any significant functional defect.

Use of Fibula as Bone Graft

The shaft of the fibula is well adapted to serve as a strong cortical bone graft. Full-thickness segments make eminently satisfactory bone pegs for use as medullary grafts in the treatment of ununited fractures of the femoral neck. Half-thickness segments are admirably suited for use as cortical onlay grafts in the treatment of nonunion of the smaller bones. Partial or complete removal of a segment of the shaft incurs no significant penalty, and, since the fibula bears no weight, ambulation may be resumed quickly and without the potential risk of fracture through the donor site that may follow removal of a graft from the shaft of the tibia. Fibular grafts should be removed from the middle third of the bone. If a graft is taken from the proximal third, the peroneal nerve may be damaged; if one is taken from the lower third, the lateral malleolus may tilt and the ankle become unstable. The distal stump of fibular shaft remaining after removal of a full-thickness graft should extend at least 4 inches proximal to the level of the ankle joint in order to ensure a stable malleolus.

The fibular shaft is exposed through a lateral incision of the skin and fascia over the peroneal muscles, which are then retracted forward from

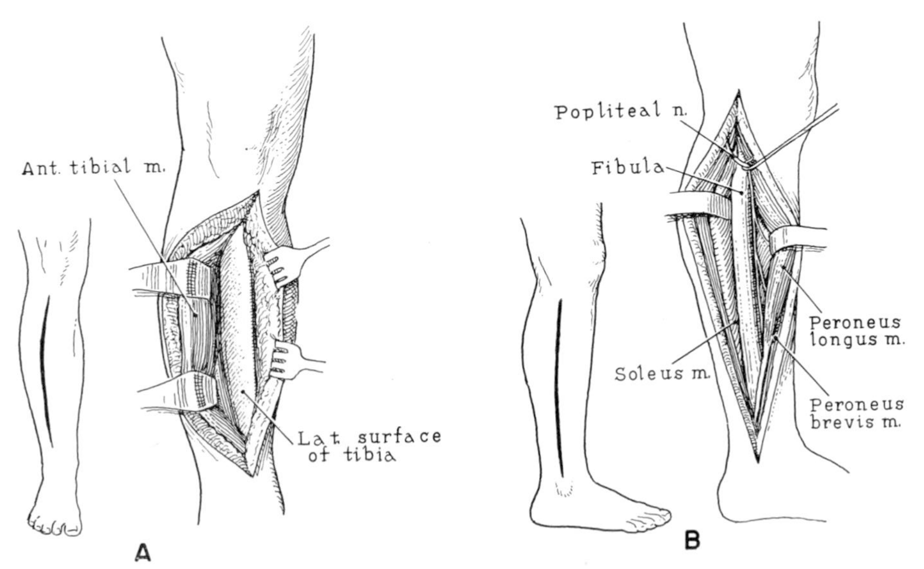

Figure 13–4. Exposure of the shafts of the tibia (A) and the fibula (B).

the posterior intermuscular septum (Fig. 13–4). When a graft composed of only half of the circumference of the bone is to be removed, the bone should first be cut longitudinally, for the length of graft desired, with a motor saw. When the half-thickness graft is removed, the continuity of the fibula then remains intact. Ambulation with the leg dressed in an elastic bandage may be permitted as soon as the incision heals.

Solitary Fracture of Shaft of Fibula

The roentgenogram which reveals only a fracture of the shaft of the fibula often is a diagnostic trap. An isolated fracture of the fibula above the level of the ankle joint can be caused only by a direct blow against the outer side of the leg. Some evidence of the direct injury should be visible, and the fracture should be transverse, sometimes shattered, and almost always without gross displacement. These injuries are neither common nor serious. Temporary assistance in walking by cane or crutches, with the painful leg supported by an elastic bandage, is followed by complete recovery within a short period.

Oblique or spiral fractures are caused by some combination of leverage and rotation. Above the level of the ankle the fibula is immune to both forces so long as the tibia and the interosseous connections remain intact. It follows that a spiral fracture of the fibular shaft, in the absence of a fracture of the tibial shaft, must be considered to be accompanied by a disruption of the inferior tibiofibular syndesmosis until proved otherwise. Fractures at the head of the fibula are usually caused by a direct blow against the outer side of the knee. The valgus strain consequent to such an injury may simultaneously rupture the internal collateral ligament of the knee. This potentially serious soft part injury should be excluded from the diagnosis in all fractures of the head of the fibula.

THE TIBIA

Each end of the large, strong, weight-bearing tibia is composed of richly vascularized cancellous bone within a thin cortical shell, which is perforated by many small nutrient vessels. The intervening shaft has a small vascular medullary canal surrounded by a thick and virtually avascular cortex (Fig. 13–5), which is perforated by a single nutrient artery. Soft tissues provide a vascular extra-osseous environment propitious to the growth of callus only in apposition to the proximal portions of the posterior and lateral tibial surfaces. The remainder of the tibia is apposed to a loose areolar stroma and to avascular connective tissue structures. Adult periosteum plays little or no part in bone repair. Consequently, it is logical that fractures of the distal tibia should heal more slowly and imperfectly than similar injuries to other bones and fractures of other parts of the tibia, since in this region all the fundamental physiological and anatomical requisites to bone repair are at a minimum.

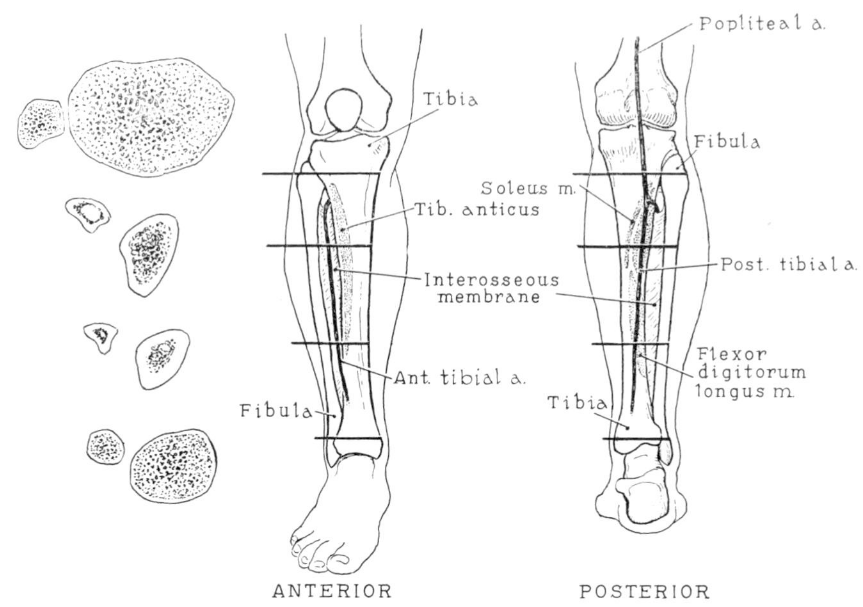

Figure 13–5. The tibia and its main muscle attachments.

Each end of the tibia is composed of cancellous bone which heals rapidly and well. The distal shaft of tibia is composed of thick avascular cortex with a small medullary vascular space, and this segment of the bone is almost devoid of circulation-bearing muscle attachments. Healing is slow and poor at best.

Significance of Nutrient Artery in Fracture Repair

The notoriously slow or imperfect union common to fractures in the distal shaft of the tibia is commonly, and erroneously, attributed to interruption of the nutrient (medullary) blood supply by the fracture, and vascular privation of the proximal end of the distal bone fragment. This theory is supported neither by operative findings nor by the vascular dynamics of the tibia, nor by what is known about the processes of bone repair. Avascular necrosis is rare. Interruption of the nutrient artery to the shaft has little effect upon interosseous hemostatic pressure, since both fragments retain an ample medullary circulation by virtue of the many nutrient vessels entering the cancellous bone at each end (Fig. 13–6, *B*). Furthermore, these fractures unite primarily by extra-osseous callus, the elaboration of which is essentially independent of medullary circulation. Probably only completely separated, loose and segmented fragments of bone are significantly affected by separation from the medullary circulation (Fig. 13–6, *C*). Even under these circumstances avascular necrosis is uncommon and union often proceeds uneventfully.

Solitary Fracture of Shaft of Tibia

An isolated tibial shaft fracture is not uncommon in young children in whom the fibula is quite resilient. Shortening is prevented by the intact fibula. Displacement is prevented by interosseous connections. The

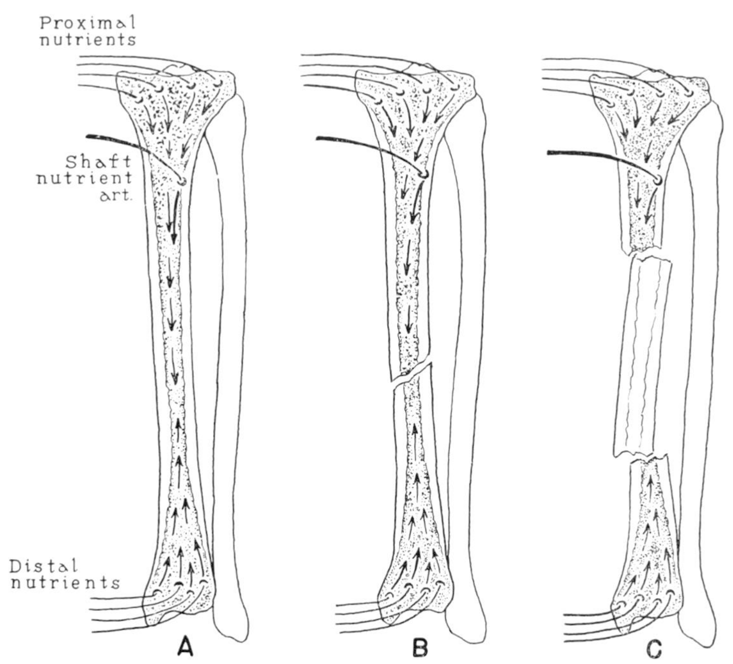

Figure 13–6. Medullary circulation of the tibia.

A. The nutrient artery to the shaft of the tibia is not the sole source of medullary circulation, but is augmented by many smaller vessels entering each cancellous end of the bone.

B. Fracture of the shaft of the tibia separates the distal fragment only from the blood supply donated by the nutrient artery to the shaft; the distal fragment remains viable.

C. Segmental fractures deprive the intermediate fragment of all medullary sources of circulation.

extremity should be immobilized in a circular plaster dressing which extends from toes to groin. The knee should be flexed sufficiently so that the toes swing clear of the ground when walking with crutches. Immobilization should be continued until sound union is present. The results are uniformly excellent.

An isolated fracture of an adult tibia is not common, for the force required to break such a large bone is usually sufficient to fracture the fibula as well. Displacement of the fragments is slight and follows a consistent pattern of angulation toward the intact fibula. Especially in transverse or short spiral fractures this mild deformity may have serious implications (Fig. 13–7). Recurrence of the deformity, despite the best of plaster dressings, is frequent. Persisting angulation precludes good approximation of the fragments, except at their medial edges; the lateral edges, due to maintenance of length by the intact fibula, remain distracted. Slow union and a mild varus deformity are common.

Treatment. Treatment should be influenced by the absence, or by the presence and degree of persisting angular deformity. A fracture with less than 15 degrees of angular deformity and adequate approximation

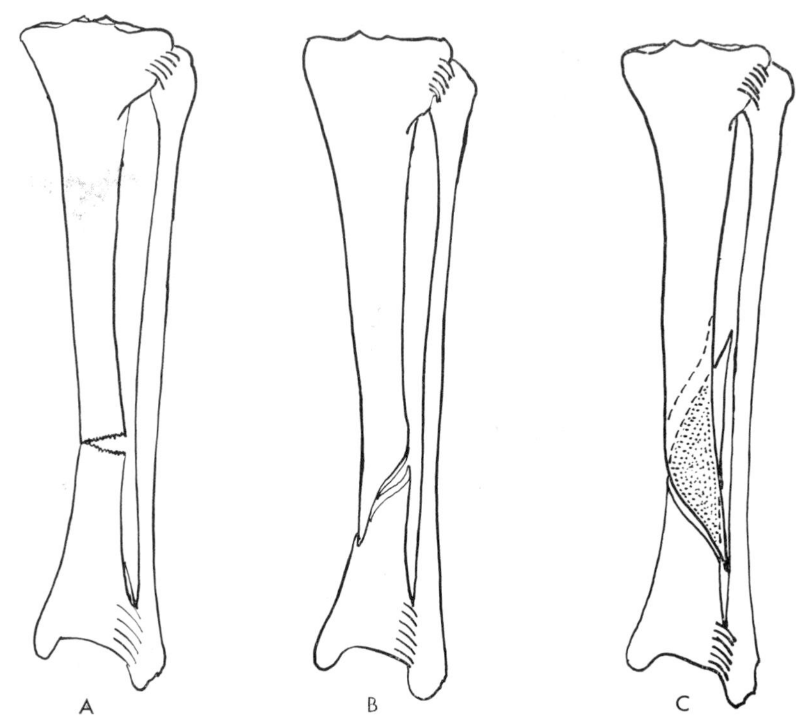

Figure 13–7. *Isolated fracture of the adult tibia.*

All isolated tibial shaft fractures tend to angulate toward the intact fibula.

A. When the fracture is transverse, distraction obtains between a large area of the broken bone surfaces. Healing is slow and uncertain.

B, C. The more oblique the fracture line, the larger is the area of apposed raw surfaces, and the better are the prospects for uneventful repair of the fracture.

of the fracture surfaces may be treated in a snug circular plaster dressing which includes the thigh, until the bone is united. A recurring or persisting angulation in excess of 15 degrees, or one which prevents good approximation of fracture surfaces, is an indication for open reduction and internal fixation. Continuance of external immobilization in the face of gross angulation is poor treatment. Complete consolidation of the fracture under such circumstances may be delayed for a year or more.

FRACTURES OF THE TIBIA AND FIBULA

Stable Fractures of Tibia and Fibula

The stability of fractures of tibia and fibula can be established in no other way than by trial and error. Following reduction of a fracture of both bones of the leg, if length and alignment of the limb and adequate apposition of the bone ends can be maintained securely by a plaster dressing (Fig. 13–8), the fractures are stable. Uneventful union and a happy result can be expected, if the fractured bones are securely immobilized until healing occurs.

As a rule, little in the way of manipulative reduction is required, since

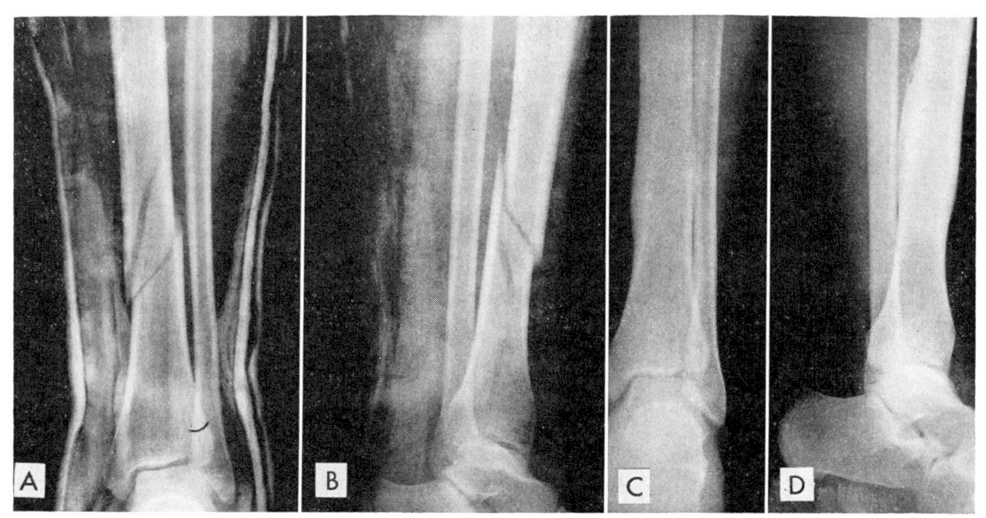

Figure 13–8. Stable fractures of tibia and fibula.

A, B. When normal length and axis and good apposition of the broken fragments can be maintained by plaster dressings the fractures are stable. (The fracture in the proximal portion of the fibular shaft is not shown in these roentgenograms.)

C, D. Secure immobilization until union occurs leads to a good result.

the inherent stability of such a fracture prevents more than a small amount of displacement. If the injured leg is allowed to hang from a bent knee over the edge of a table, gravity provides normal length and alignment of the broken bones. All that is required, in addition, is manual correction of existing displacement of the tibial fragments. The fibular fracture should be ignored. Plaster dressings should be applied to the level of the tibial tubercle while the leg hangs free. This portion of the immobilization should not be performed with the leg held in a horizontal position. If it is, some sag of the fracture into recurvatum is almost certain. After this plaster dressing has been well molded to the contour of the leg and the plaster has set, the dressing should be extended to include the upper thigh, the knee being held in moderate flexion in order to preclude the rotatory displacement of the fracture fragments that might occur in a plaster boot alone.

Role of compression by weight bearing in tibial shaft fractures. It is well documented that distraction of fracture fragments is detrimental to bone repair, and that a certain amount of compression of the fragments may enhance the speed and quality of union of cancellous and membranous bone fractures. There is no evidence that compression has any beneficial effect upon the healing of cortical bone fractures, except by providing a more secure apposition of the bone ends, and undue compression ends in bone necrosis. Nevertheless, the use of a walking-boot for the treatment of fractures of both bones of the leg has gained a measure of popularity. This is based upon a postulate that the repeated impacts of weight bearing "stimulate" bone union. Objective examination of this theory cannot reconcile repeated minute traumas to any healing

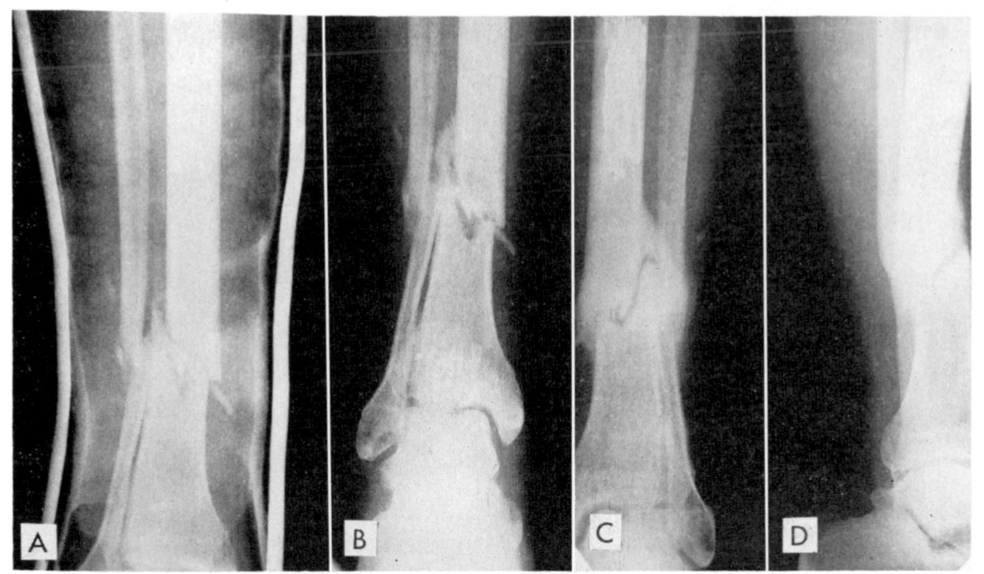

Figure 13–9. Stable fractures of tibia and fibula.

A. At time of treatment, in a plaster walking boot.

B. Five months after injury–some callus, but little or no evidence of union of the fracture.

C, D. Eight months after injury–excessive callus, but the fracture line is still visible and the fracture clinically ununited. Eventual clinical union without roentgen evidence of complete consolidation of the fracture finally occurred many months later.

area with an acceleration of repair, but only with an increased area of tissue damage in which eventual repair must take place, and, ipso facto, a larger mass of reparative tissues, including both fibrous tissue and new bone formation. This is confirmed consistently by clinical experience. Intermittent compression of a tibial fracture by weight bearing in a walking-boot, even as the false motion of a similar fracture permitted by inadequate fixation of any type, is usually productive of excessive extra-osseous callus formation, but not always of union of the fracture (Fig. 13–9, *C*). It is probable that the most logical function of a plaster walking-boot in the treatment of fractures of the lower leg is as an instrument which permits safe ambulation, after the fractures have healed soundly enough to withstand the repeated traumas of protected weight bearing, and until union is strong enough to allow weight to be borne without support.

Unstable Fractures of Tibia and Fibula

A fracture of the tibia is unstable when adequate reduction, alignment, and length of the bone cannot be secured and maintained by manipulative reduction and external immobilization. But the criterion of adequacy is not perfection. Frequently it is necessary or advisable to create some shortening of the tibia in order to ensure good apposition of the bone ends. Malunion with tibial angulation, not in excess of 15 degrees, and in all except varus deformities, is functionally insignificant. Complete apposition of the fragments is desirable, but is not necessary to union. Clinically significant instability and its influence upon treatment, therefore, must remain a relative matter to be estimated according to the individual characteristics and requirements of each case. Regardless of the degree of instability, however, the tibial fracture which cannot be treated satisfactorily by reduction and external immobilization must then be treated by some form of continuous traction or by internal fixation.

Treatment of shattered fractures by fixed skeletal traction. A shattered fracture of the tibia containing many small bone fragments cannot be stabilized adequately by internal fixation. Alignment can be maintained by plaster splints alone, but length cannot. Some form of traction must be used. Incorporation of transfixion pins into a well-fitted plaster dressing (Fig. 13–*10*) answers both requirements and permits ambulation on crutches throughout convalescence.

This method of treatment has been decried as one which causes a delay in union of the fracture by distraction of the bone ends. Distraction, of course, must be scrupulously avoided; instead, the fracture should be

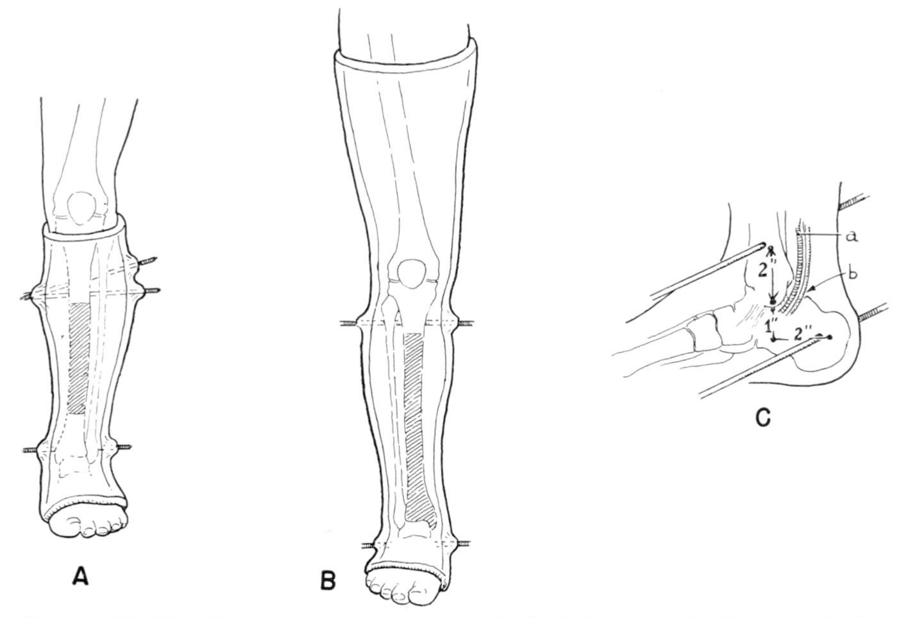

Figure 13–10. Treatment of comminuted tibial fractures by "pins and plaster."

A. Fixation of shattered fracture (shaded segment) of tibia by transfixion pins and plaster boot. Two proximal pins are required, otherwise the proximal fragment would pivot upon a single pin. The two proximal pins should not be parallel. Knee motion can be maintained while the fracture heals.

B. If only a single proximal pin is used, the plaster dressing should be extended to the upper thigh.

C. The distal pin may be inserted through the distal tibial fragment or the calcaneus. The relation of the pin sites to the tip of the medial malleolus should be such that the pins will not endanger the neurovascular structures (a), or the tendons (b), passing behind and under the medial malleolus.

permitted to collapse a small amount in length prior to incorporation of the pins in the plaster dressing. Delayed union in tibial fractures treated by properly applied continuous traction is a statistical figment which ignores the fundamental fact that fractures which are sufficiently shattered to require treatment by traction are likely to suffer from delayed union under any circumstances.

Screw fixation supplemented by plaster immobilization. Fixation of uncomminuted spiral or oblique tibial fractures by one or two screws, followed by the use of external immobilization, is common practice, but rarely an operation of necessity. Many fractures so treated are inherently stable and would unite, a little more slowly perhaps, if treated by manipulative reduction and plaster immobilization alone. This is "internal suture" by election, and accepts all the risks of operation without escaping the penalties of prolonged immobilization. Nevertheless, there is no doubt that, in fractures in which mature surgical judgment and experience dictate a guarded prognosis for an uneventful spontaneous recovery, this procedure enhances the prospects for accelerated and certain bony union.

Fixation by some such "internal suture" may be a matter of necessity. Certain comminuted fractures are so unstable that reduction cannot be maintained by plaster alone or by traction, and require some supplemental internal fixation (Fig. 13–*11*). The least amount of foreign material necessary to ensure position and apposition of the bone ends should be used. The reduction is merely steadied by the internal fixation sufficiently so that it can then be maintained adequately by external immobilizing dressings. Use of more than the amount of foreign material necessary to

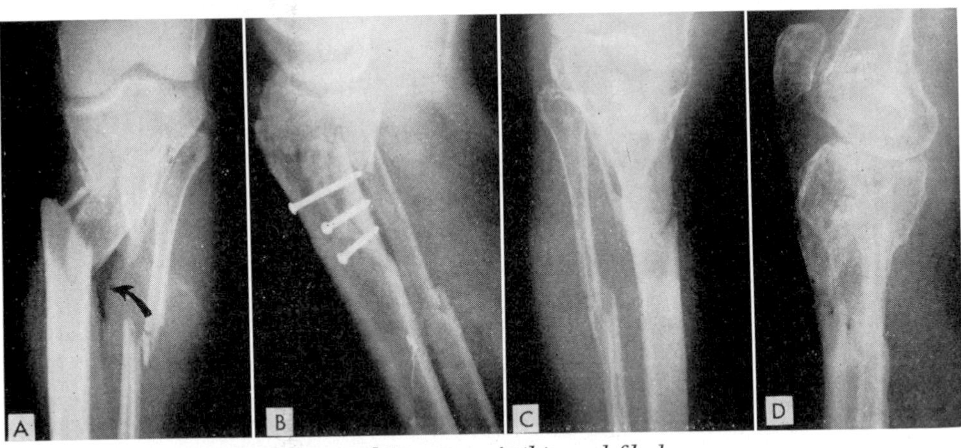

Figure 13–11. Comminuted fracture of tibia and fibula.

A. The distal fragment of the tibia protruded through a large wound in the calf. Note the air in the tissues (arrow). Reduction was quite unstable, even with a combination of plaster splints and traction.

B. "Internal suture" by necessity. The large anterior fragment of the tibia which was persistently displaced by the quadriceps pull was fastened to the large loose posterior fragment by the proximal screw, and the posterior fragment in turn was fastened to the shaft by the other screws. Reasonably normal gross alignment and position could then be preserved by plaster splints.

C, D. The result, a comfortable, useful leg with a mild varus deformity at the knee.

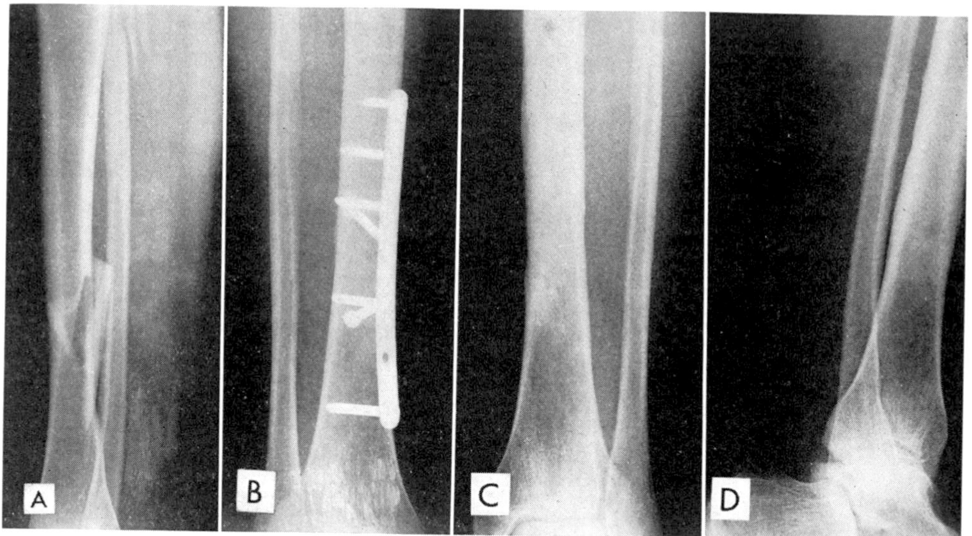

Figure 13–12. Fixation by plate and screws.

A. An unstable fracture of tibia and fibula. There is a longitudinal split in the loose intermediate fragment of tibia

B. The intermediate fragment was fixed to the main tibial fragments by two screws, but the reduction remained potentially unstable. The plate was added. The missing screw had penetrated the longitudinal fissure in the loose fragment and was removed. Aftercare was by removable splints and maintenance of gentle function

C, D. The result following removal of the plate which, by the nature of the fracture, was necessarily applied to the subcutaneous surface of the bone. By choice, plate fixation should be applied to the lateral surface of the tibia.

serve this purpose does not appreciably increase the security of the total fixation provided.

Fixation of fractures with intermediate fragment by plate and screws. A large number of tibial fractures are characterized by a triangular intermediate fragment. The fibula is almost always fractured at its neck, and the tibial fracture is inevitably quite unstable. Often the loose fragment can be used as a bone plate, fastened to each of the main fragments by one or two screws, and the reduction maintained by plaster splints. Equally often this amount of internal fixation proves to be inadequate. A plate should then be added, the more securely to maintain a fixed relationship between the two main fragments (Fig. 13–*12*). Secure fixation of this type reduces the amount and duration of supplemental external immobilization required to maintain reduction. Protected motion and use of the soft tissues can be commenced while the fracture is uniting, to the end that, when the bone has healed, the limb is prepared to resume its normal function, and a post-healing period of rehabilitation designed to overcome the penalties of prolonged immobilization is avoided.

Fixation by an intramedullary device. Medullary fixation of tibial shaft fractures has gained a measure of popularity. Unlike the other long bones, through which a straight medullary fixation instrument can be passed with ease, the tibia requires a curved fixation device which must always be inserted with skillful precision, a maneuver which is sometimes attended with considerable difficulty, and is never without risk of serious complications consequent to some defect in technique. Once the device is inserted, medullary fixation preserves tibial length and alignment very satisfactorily, but shortening may occur if the fracture is comminuted, and rotational displacement is not often prevented adequately. Supplemental plaster immobilization until the fracture unites is always required. That a high plaster walking-boot may be utilized within several weeks after the operation is a precarious excuse for subjecting any patient to all the risks of an operation which may be attended by particularly serious complications, without avoiding the penalties of plaster immobilization, when there is available any less dangerous method of adequate treatment. Medullary fixation is justified for segmental fractures, which heal poorly with other methods of treatment (Fig. 13–*13*, *A*). Except in the hands of a surgeon expert in its use, it cannot often be justified for a fractured tibia amenable to treatment by simpler and safer methods (Fig. 13–*13*, *B*).

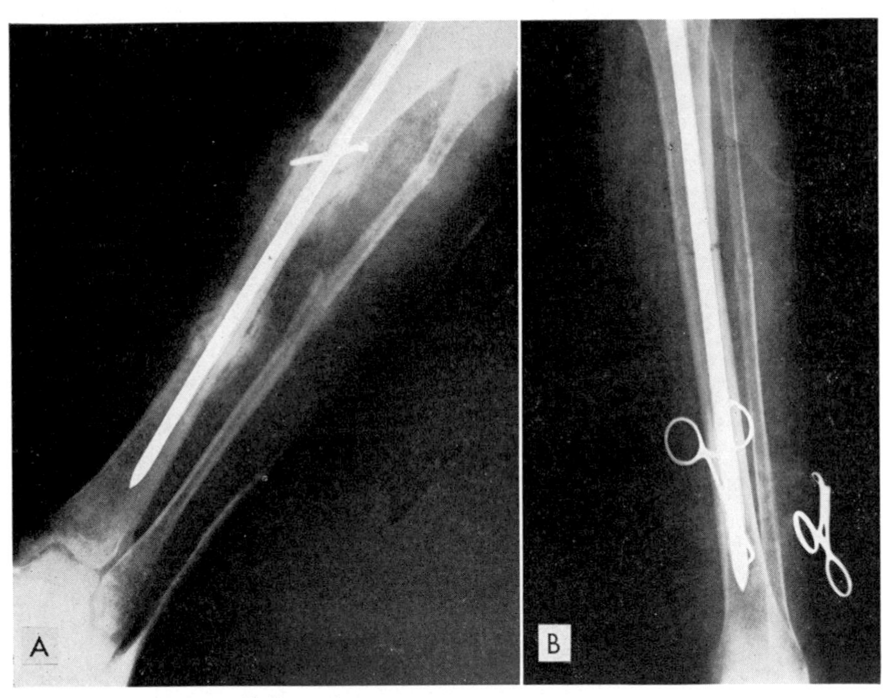

Figure 13–13. Medullary fixation.

A. Medullary fixation by necessity. A severe segmented fracture for which there is presently no consistently good method of fixation, except by an intramedullary device. Films three months after primary bone grafts to each fracture and fixation by the instrument devised by Lottes.

B. Is this medullary fixation necessary? An open but stable fracture amenable to treatment by manipulative reduction and plaster immobilization, screw fixation and supplemental plaster dressings, or plate and screw fixation followed by a minimum amount of external immobilization. The medullary device failed to control rotation, plaster immobilization was required, and the contaminated area was extended for the entire length of the medullary canal. That the result was good does not vitiate the preceding facts.

BONE GRAFT IN TREATMENT OF TIBIAL SHAFT FRACTURES

As a Primary Procedure

Delayed union and nonunion are the most common complications attending a fracture of the shaft of the tibia. Undue delay or established failure of union usually necessitates a late bone grafting operation, followed by an additional prolonged program of immobilization and disability. The risk of these complications is greatest in those fractures requiring primary open reduction and internal fixation. It is only logical, therefore, that faulty spontaneous union should be anticipated at the time of the first operation. Bone from a bone bank or autogenous bone from the ilium or the adjacent tibia itself may be removed and packed around the reduced and fixed fracture. The quantity of bone used in this manner must not be sufficient to interfere with wound closure. This is a good procedure which can do no harm and may prove of inestimable assistance to the local processes of bone repair. It is recommended for a closed tibial shaft fracture which is to be treated by operation. However, bone grafts should not be added to similar fractures which are associated with open wounds, except at the dictates of mature surgical judgment based on a large experience in the management of accidental injuries.

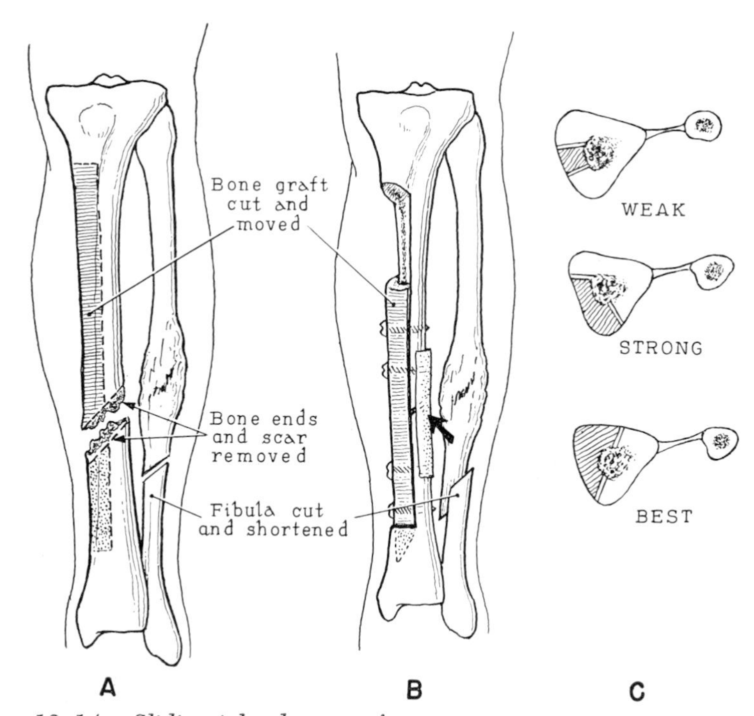

Figure 13–14. Sliding inlay bone graft.

A. The graft (shaded) is cut. The pseudoarthrosis is excised. The fibula is cut.

B. The fracture is reduced. The long graft is moved to bridge the fracture and secured by screws. The short graft may be used as an "onlay" (arrow).

C. Sliding inlay grafts must also provide fixation. They should be large and strong and include one angle of the tibia.

For Delayed Union or Nonunion

Undue delay in healing or established failure of union necessitates operative treatment designed to re-establish the local circumstances of a new fracture under conditions of reduction and fixation suitable for union, or to provide assistance to the repair processes by the use of bone grafts, or both. The technique for implementation of these objectives must be adapted to the characteristics of the fracture. Success or failure will depend not so much upon what type of bone grafting operation is done, but upon how well it is done. Under any circumstances, rehabilitation of the soft tissues surrounding the fracture is an essential feature of the operative procedure. Implanting a bone graft in a fibrotic avascular environment, in a leg that has been reduced to skin, bones, and scar by prolonged immobilization, and expecting union to occur, is comparable to planting grain in dry and barren soil and expecting to reap a crop. Prior to every bone graft operation the regional soft tissues must be reconditioned until they constitute as fertile an environment as possible for reparative tissue growth. Toward this end it is often necessary to excise avascular scars and resurface the operative area with healthy skin prior to doing a bone graft operation on the subcutaneous tibia.

There is no single best type of bone graft for any fracture. Frequently, a mere excision of the pseudoarthrosis and freshening, re-apposition, and secure fixation of the bone ends is sufficient to promote union. There are, however, common characteristics inherent to the ununited tibia which

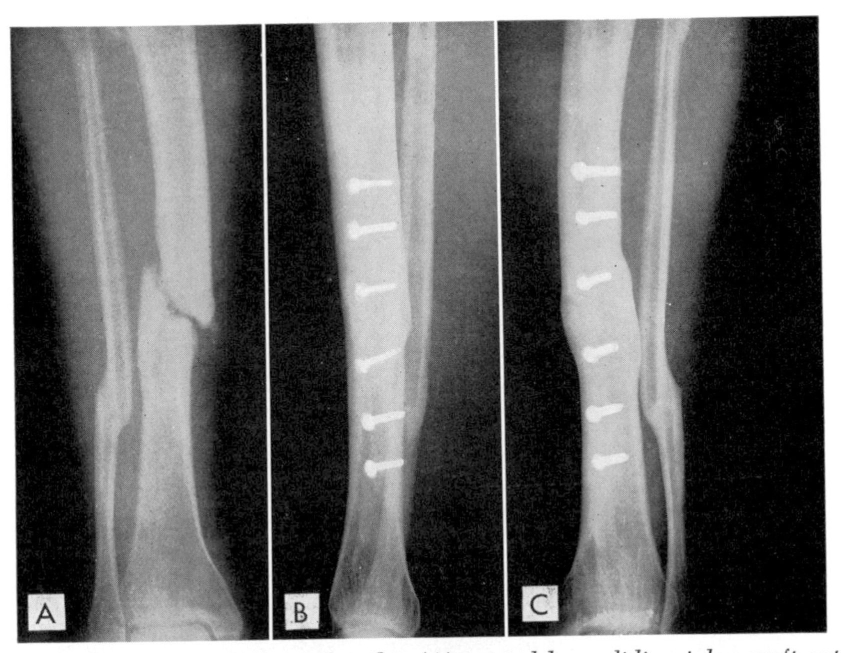

Figure 13–15. Nonunion of the tibia (A) treated by a sliding inlay graft cut from the anteromedial tibial surface and fixed in place by six screws (B, C). The pseudoarthrosis was firm and allowed only a small amount of motion. Therefore, it was not removed, except at the graft site, but utilized as additional fixation. Except when the pseudoarthrosis is removed completely, it is not necessary to cut the fibula.

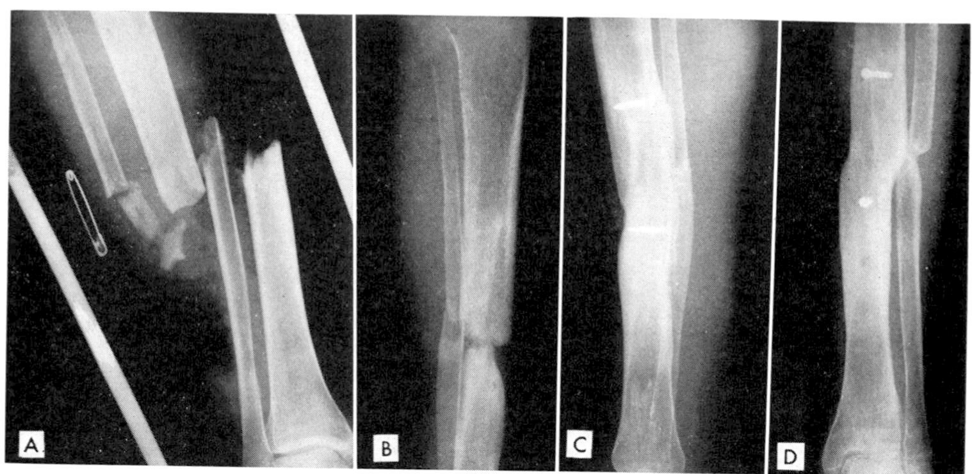

Figure 13–16. *A severe open fracture (A) which went on to nonunion of both tibia and fibula (B). Devitalized scar covered the anterior surface of the pseudoarthrosis. Treated by posterior sliding inlay graft (C, D), using a posterior incision through healthy soft tissues.*

warrant the use of "sliding inlay graft" (Fig. 13–*14*) in preference to some type of "onlay graft." Adequate onlay grafts may so increase the circumference of the tibia that wound closure becomes difficult or impossible. An onlay graft which permits tension-free wound closure is perforce so small that it cannot be utilized as an instrument for fixation. Appropriate inlay grafts do not jeopardize wound closure, and they provide adequate internal fixation of the fracture. Depending on the condition of the skin and the optimum site for an operative incision, an inlay graft may be cut from the posteromedial angle, or from the anteromedial or anterolateral surface of the tibia with equal prospects of success (Figs. 13–*15*, 13–*16*). The graft should include one angle of the tibia for added strength, and its cut edges should be accurately fitted and firmly fixed to the cut edges of both fragments (Fig. 13–*14*, *C*).

CHAPTER 14

INJURIES OF THE KNEE AND THIGH

By HARRISON L. McLAUGHLIN, M.D.

Injuries of the Knee

THE FEMUR AND THE TIBIA form an imperfect and unstable bony hinge, articulating only at two inconstant points, where the rounded femoral condyles bear against the flat and horizontal table of the tibia. Motion and weight subject this incongruous hinge to the leverage exerted by the two longest and strongest bones in the body. The functional stability of the knee is almost entirely dependent upon its muscular and ligamentous supports.

THE LIGAMENT SUPPORTS OF THE KNEE

THE MEDIAL (TIBIAL) COLLATERAL LIGAMENT

Arising from the adductor tubercle at about the pivot point of knee motion, and passing down and forward as a broad straplike thickening in the joint capsule, the medial collateral ligament is so firmly attached to the rim of the medial meniscus that an injury to one of these structures usually is accompanied by damage to the other. After spanning the joint interval, the ligament finally inserts into the anterior and medial surface of the upper tibia in concert with the tendons of the semimembranosus, semitendinosus, and gracilis muscles (Fig. 14–*1*).

The medial collateral ligament defends against abduction of the tibia from the femur. However, this defense is absolute only when the knee is in full extension; in other positions some laxity (in direct proportion to the amount of flexion) is permitted. It has been postulated that certain segments of the medial ligament are tight in all positions. To be sure, certain segments are tighter than others, according to position, but the ligament as a unit is functionally tight only in full extension. This is of some significance in assessment of the integrity of the ligament after injury. The ligament may be considered to be intact if no "give" into abduction of the fully extended tibia from the femur can be educed. Complete extension of a recently injured knee is rarely possible. Some

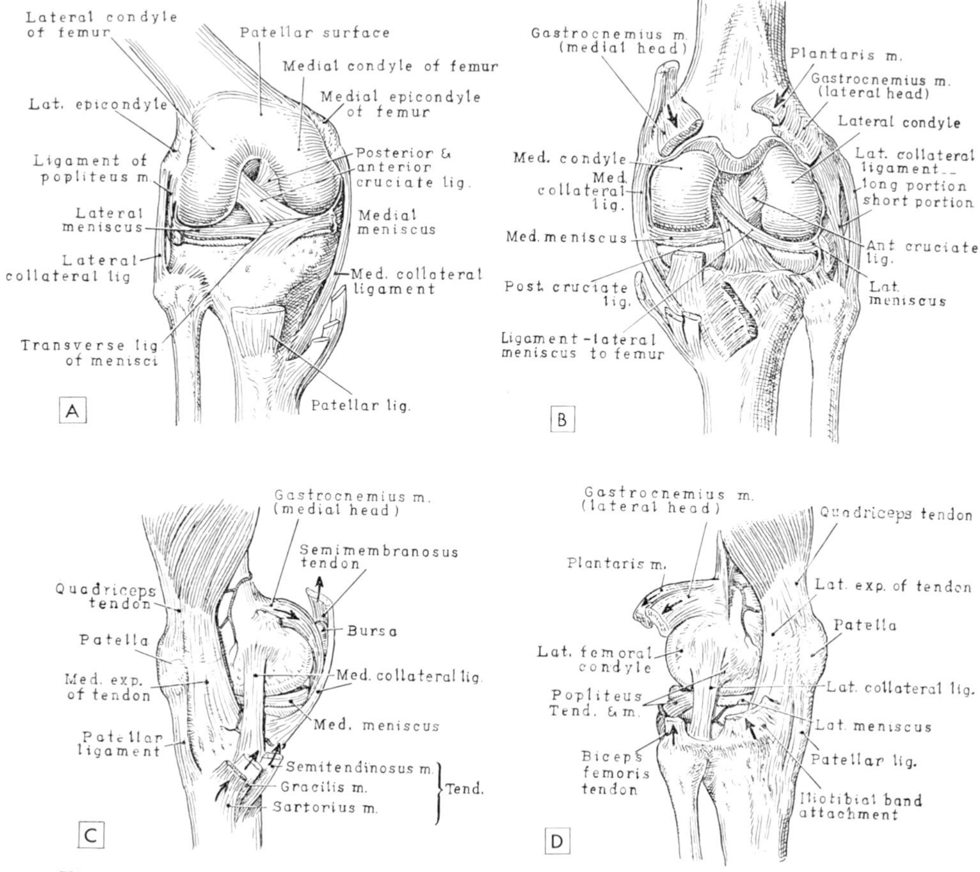

Figure 14–1. The ligaments and muscle attachments at the knee.
A. Anterior view.
B. Posterior view.
C. Medial view.
D. Lateral view.

abduction of the tibia can be produced in a normal knee if it is slightly flexed. Both knees must be tested for stability in exactly the same position before any comparison is valid.

Sprain of the Medial Collateral Ligament

Rupture of some of the fibers of the medial collateral ligament by an abduction force is the most common injury of the knee. This is the "sprained knee," which recovers without subsequent symptoms of joint derangement.

Early clinical picture. Because of the frequent coincidence of damage to both the medial ligament and the medial meniscus, early anatomical diagnosis is usually difficult or impossible. Such injury is attended by a tense hemarthrosis, which may require aspiration before adequate examination is even possible. Ecchymosis at the inner side of the knee justifies a presumption of ligament damage, but does not exclude a meniscus tear. Increased pain at the inner side of the knee when the tibia is abducted is indicative of ligament injury. An absence of this response, or an increase of pain when the tibia is adducted, is more suggestive of meniscus injury. The tenderness of a sprained medial ligament extends in a vertical line from the adductor tubercle to a point well below the medial joint line; that produced by a damaged meniscus extends in a horizontal line which is limited to the joint interval. Both injuries produce a small painful defect in extension. In the early stages after an abduction injury the entire inner side of the knee is diffusely swollen, painful, and tender. A firm diagnosis should be deferred until the period of acute pain has passed.

Treatment of medial collateral ligament sprain. A tense hemarthrosis should be aspirated in order to relieve pain and facilitate examination. The knee should be rested in a plaster splint, and a gentle compression dressing may be applied. Non–weight-bearing quadriceps drill should be practiced from the start. Weight bearing should be delayed until it can be done without more than mild discomfort. Recovery within four to eight weeks, depending on the extent of ligament damage, may be expected. The prognosis should be guarded, for a concomitant meniscus tear may not produce symptoms of internal derangement until after function has been regained.

Complications of medial collateral ligament sprain. OSSIFICATION ADJACENT TO ADDUCTOR TUBERCLE (PELLEGRINI-STIEDA). The ligament may be incompletely avulsed from its site of insertion on the femur, in which event repair not infrequently is characterized by the formation of an ossified plaque adjacent to the adductor tubercle. The tubercle may look and feel enlarged, and remain tender to palpation and painful when the ligament is stretched. Recovery is delayed, but the symptoms subside gradually and eventually disappear. Operative removal of the bone plaque is rarely, if ever, necessary.

LAX MEDIAL COLLATERAL LIGAMENT. When the amount of ligament damage has been underestimated and the knee inadequately protected against the strain of weight bearing, or when weight bearing has been permitted before the quadriceps muscle has been reconditioned, the ligament may become stretched and slightly elongated. The knee is unstable. The medial meniscus and the articular surfaces of the joint are subjected to repeated minor mechanical insults. Medial joint line pain and tenderness persist, and eventually buckling episodes may supervene. The medial meniscus usually must be removed, abraded areas of articular cartilage excised, and the lax medial ligament shortened or supported before comfortable and efficient knee joint function can be restored.

Rupture of Medial Collateral Ligament

The medial collateral ligament may be disrupted in continuity by a violent abduction injury. The ligament may be avulsed from the femur or tibia, or ruptured through its substance at any point. A concomitant rupture of the anterior cruciate ligament is the rule, and more often than not

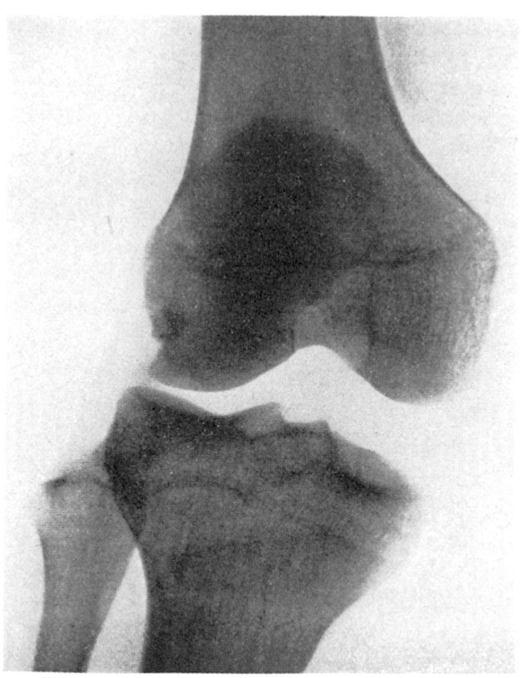

Figure 14–2. Complete rupture of the medial collateral ligament. There is no roentgenological evidence of injury unless the film is taken with the knee joint in abduction. (From Smillie, I. S.: Injuries of the Knee Joint, E. & S. Livingstone, Ltd., 1946.)

the medial meniscus is lacerated or pulled loose from its coronary ligament attachments. Not uncommonly an avulsed tongue of ligament is drawn into the medial joint space to become interposed between the femur and tibia.

Clinical picture. There is a rent in the medial joint capsule through which intra-articular bleeding is decompressed spontaneously. A tense hemarthrosis is, therefore, uncommon, but, by the same token, early and extensive periarticular swelling and ecchymosis are the rule. Gentle manipulation reveals that the extended tibia can be abducted from the femur with ease, but pain and spasm may camouflage this finding. Ordinary roentgenograms appear normal and produce false negative evidence. Films taken with abduction stress applied to the knee reveal the medial side of the joint to be abnormally open (Fig. 14–2) and confirm the diagnosis. Anesthesia should be used to facilitate the taking of such stress films in all equivocal cases. When the extended tibia can be abducted from the femur more than 15 degrees, the ligament rupture may be considered complete and suitable for operative repair; abduction of less than this amount is indicative of ligament damage that will probably recover satisfactorily with immobilization.

Treatment. NONOPERATIVE TREATMENT OF MEDIAL COLLATERAL LIGAMENT TEAR. The extended extremity should be dressed in a well-fitted circular plaster encasement extending from groin to ankle. Immobilization without weight bearing should be continued for at least two months.

Quadriceps drill should be done from the start. Weight bearing should be interdicted until the quadriceps is in good condition, for without the protection of strong muscles the healed ligament will surely stretch under the load of body weight. Maximal recovery often does not occur for six or more months after the injury.

OPERATIVE REPAIR OF RUPTURED MEDIAL COLLATERAL LIGAMENT. The best time for operative repair is in the first few hours after injury. A short delay is permissible when there is massive established swelling, but the lacerated ligament fibers become soft and friable, and are difficult to identify and suture with great rapidity. End-to-end suture or reattachment to bone usually is a simple matter, owing to the bulk and strength of the ligament. Repair of the concomitant anterior cruciate rupture is not necessary, but may be done when the circumstances are favorable; otherwise, this ligament may be excised. The medial meniscus is usually damaged or loose and should be removed. The postoperative program is similar to that outlined for the nonoperative management of less extensive ligament injuries.

THE LATERAL (FIBULAR) COLLATERAL LIGAMENT

Unlike its broad, strong intracapsular medial counterpart, the lateral collateral ligament is an extracapsular ligamentous rope which extends from a ridge on the lateral femoral condyle to the head of the fibula (see Fig. 14–*1*). Its course is paralleled, and its function as a defense against adduction of the extended tibia from the femur is supported, by the tendon of the biceps muscle and the iliotibial band. It is relaxed and relatively immune to adduction injuries, except in extension, when it is protected by the other leg.

Rupture of Lateral Collateral Ligament

Rupture occurs only as a result of great violence, and usually is reflected in avulsion of a fragment of the fibular head by the ligament and the biceps tendon. The iliotibial band and the lateral knee joint capsule may also be torn. Neglected ruptures often do not incur a serious penalty in terms of knee joint instability or dysfunction, but the peroneal nerve is almost always ruptured or damaged by overstretch, and the peroneal and anterior tibial muscle groups are paralyzed. The prognosis for recovery of muscle function in the face of such an injury is poor. Arthrodesis of the ankle and subtalar joints is often necessary for management of the drop-foot deformity. The ruptured ligament and nerve should be sutured early whenever possible, but the results of nerve repair are uncertain. When operative repair is not done, the knee should be immobilized in extension until the ruptured tissues have healed and the quadriceps muscle is reconditioned.

THE ANTERIOR CRUCIATE LIGAMENT

The ligament extends from the posterior and lateral surface of the intercondylar notch to the anterior portion of the medial tibial condyle (see Fig. 14–*1*). It is tight only in full extension, and relaxes progressively as the knee is flexed. In full extension it prevents, and in other positions it limits, forward displacement of the tibia from the femur. The importance of this function is commonly overemphasized. This ligament is the least important of the multiple defenses against forward displacement of the tibia from the femur. Complete absence of the anterior cruciate ligament produces no demonstrable adverse effect upon the stability of the knee, if the collateral ligaments and the quadriceps muscle are intact.

Fallacy of Anterior Cruciate "Drawer Test"

This test for anterior cruciate ligament function, as commonly carried out and interpreted, is fallacious. It consists of estimating, in comparison with the uninjured knee, the amount which the flexed tibia can be moved forward from the femur. Excessive anterior mobility, which has been accepted as and taught to be an indication of defective function of the anterior cruciate ligament, is, in fact, a reflection of weakness of the total muscular and ligamentous support of the knee. Operative findings consistently confirm that a complete rupture of the anterior cruciate ligament produces no such instability when the quadriceps muscle and the medial collateral ligament are intact. This is of some significance in evaluating the propriety of the many operations which have been devised for repair or replacement of the anterior cruciate ligament. So long as the medial collateral ligament is intact, rehabilitation of the quadriceps will almost always make such an operation unnecessary.

Avulsion of Tibial Spine by Anterior Cruciate Ligament

It has become widely accepted that avulsion of the tibial attachment of the anterior cruciate ligament is an injury generally restricted to children and adolescents. This is not true in the writer's experience, in forty-two such injuries seen, twenty-one patients being less, and twenty-one patients more, than 17 years of age. The clinical picture was characterized by a history of injury which, in the majority of cases, was a direct blow to the front of the femur, with a rapid and tense hemarthrosis which, when aspirated, was often noted to contain fat droplets, and roentgen confirmation of an elevated fragment of bone from the intercondylar surface of the tibia. Tenderness and pain at the medial collateral ligament were present in about half these cases. The predominant disabling finding in neglected cases was not excessive anterior mobility of the tibia from the femur, but a mechanical block to complete knee joint extension.

Treatment. In a dependable and cooperative patient nondisplaced lesions may be treated by aspiration of the hemarthrosis and maintenance of motion, but the strain of weight bearing should be abolished by the use of crutches for about six weeks. Otherwise, the extended knee must be immobilized for a similar period. Displaced fractures must be reduced. In early cases this usually can be accomplished under adequate anesthesia by hyperextending the knee and pushing the tibia backward under the femur. When complete extension can be obtained by this maneuver, reduction is adequate whether or not it appears to be complete in the roentgenogram. The knee is then immobilized in complete extension for eight weeks. When complete extension cannot be obtained, and in neglected cases where replacement of the avulsed bone fragment is prevented by scar tissue, operative replacement and suture, or removal, of the bone fragment must be done.

POSTERIOR CRUCIATE LIGAMENT

The posterior cruciate ligament extends from the medial surface of the femoral notch to the posterior aspect of the tibia (see Fig. 14–*1*). It is tight and defends against posterior displacement of the tibia when the knee is fully flexed; in other positions it prevents undue posterior motion of the tibia from the femur. Its position is such that it also becomes tight in full extension of the knee. Isolated injuries to this ligament occur, but are quite uncommon. Complete rupture is rare, except as a concomitant of dislocation of the knee joint.

COMBINED FUNCTION OF CRUCIATE LIGAMENTS

The tibia glides upon the femur, forward in extension and backward in flexion. The synchronized contributions of the cruciate ligaments in limiting excessive forward and backward motion of the tibia have been discussed. The tibia also rotates upon the femur, internally in flexion and externally in extension. In flexion, when the collateral ligaments are relatively lax, the cruciate ligaments twist around each other to produce some increased stability in the center of the joint, and to limit excessive internal rotation of the tibia from the femur.

RUPTURE OF COLLATERAL AND CRUCIATE LIGAMENTS (DISLOCATION OF KNEE)

Dislocation of the knee is rare and results only from gross violence sufficient to disrupt both collateral and cruciate ligaments. Usually some of the muscles spanning the joint are also lacerated, and the great vessels and nerves of the popliteal space are damaged or in great jeopardy. Immediate replacement of the tibia under the femur is imperative. This requires adequate anesthesia, and should be preceded by strong but steady traction. Inability to replace the tibia should arouse a suspicion that the medial hamstring tendons have slipped into the open joint and become caught in the femoral notch. A ruptured popliteal artery seldom can be sutured successfully, but may be amenable to bridging with some form of vessel graft. The results of early or late nerve repair are uncertain. Amputation is indicated only when it is impossible to maintain adequate circulation to the lower leg but, once this catastrophe becomes clearly established, should be done without delay. Otherwise, the limb should be securely immobilized with the knee at 180 degrees extension for a period of three months. The results are surprisingly good.

THE MUSCLES SUPPORTING THE KNEE JOINT

The ligaments of a joint protect it only against abnormal motions. In all phases of normal knee joint motion stability is primarily and mainly dependent upon muscle support. This is provided by the gastrocnemius, the hamstring, and the quadriceps muscles (Fig. 14–3).

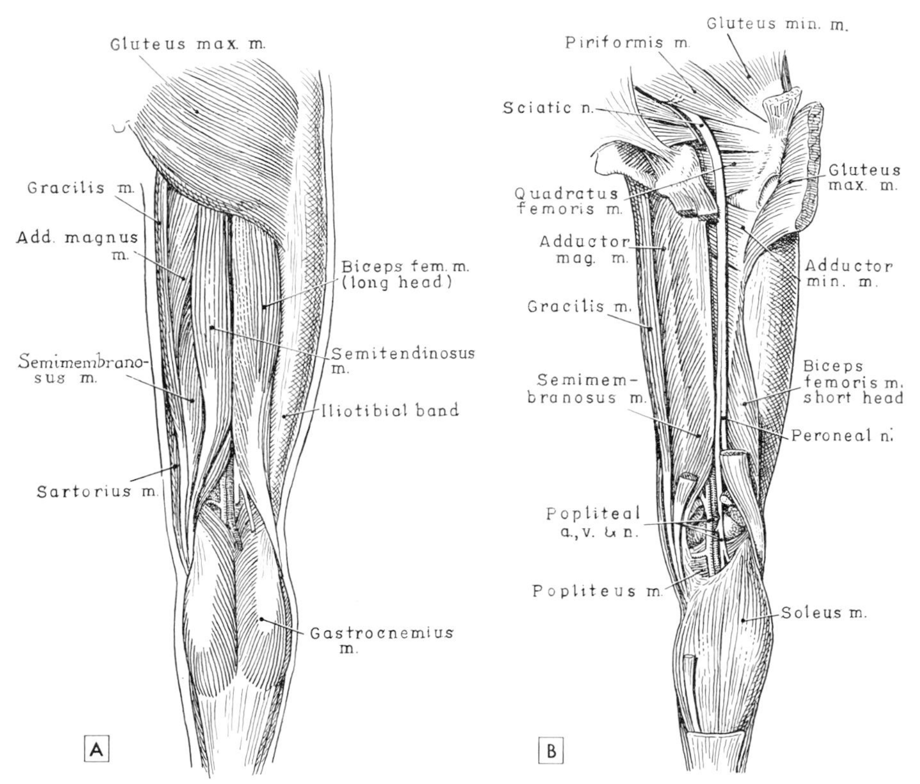

Figure 14–3. The hamstring and calf muscles.
A. Superficial muscles.
B. Deep muscles.

THE GASTROCNEMIUS

This large muscle, which arises from dual origins at the posterior and superior aspect of each femoral condyle (see Fig. 14–*1*), proceeds downward and, in concert with the soleus muscle, forms the calf of the leg, and motivates the tendo achillis. Plantar flexion of the foot, however, is not its sole function. It is also a motor which participates in flexion, and is a strong defense against hyperextension of the knee. The small associated plantaris muscle is functionally insignificant.

THE POPLITEUS MUSCLE

This muscle arises from the side of the lateral femoral condyle, just in front of the fibular collateral ligament, and passes downward and medially between this ligament and the knee joint capsule (see Fig. 14–*1*) and across the back of the knee to insert into the posterior and medial surface of the tibia. It acts as a small transverse motor which internally rotates the tibia from the femur as the knee flexes, and guards against excessive external rotation of the tibia in extension of the knee.

THE HAMSTRING MUSCLES

This large powerful muscle group, including the biceps femoris, semimembranosus, and semitendinosus muscles (Fig. 14–*3*), spans the posterior knee joint space, constitutes the main instrument for knee joint flexion, and, along with the gastrocnemius, is a strong defense against hyperextension.

THE QUADRICEPS EXTENSOR MECHANISM

The secret of good knee joint function, despite unstable and incongruous articulating surfaces, is in the quadriceps extensor mechanism (Fig. 14–*4*). Functional integrity of this musculotendinous unit is the sine qua non of knee joint stability. The aponeurotic inserting tendon cuff embraces the front and both sides of the knee joint (see Fig. 14–*1*), encloses the patella as a sesamoid bone, and extends from a broad tibial attachment to a level several inches proximal to the knee joint, where it becomes continuous with its massive muscle motors, the rectus femoris, and the vastus intermedius, lateralis, and medialis. Each of these muscles enjoys

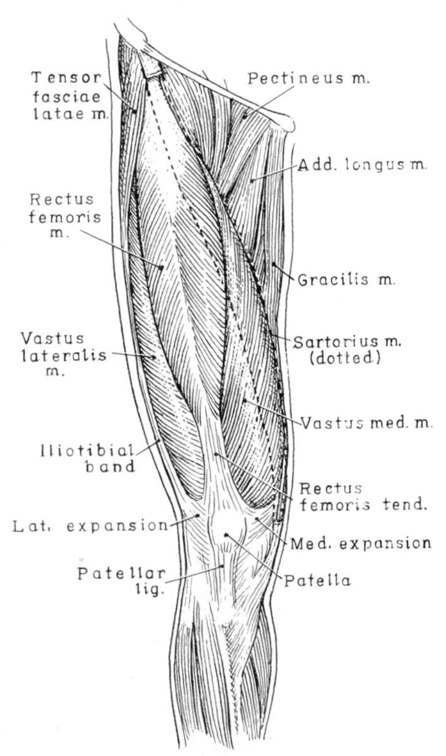

Figure 14–4. The quadriceps extensor mechanism.

individual functions; together they act as a synchronized unit to produce extension and stability of the knee.

The vastus medialis was the last segment of the quadriceps to evolve in man, and is an important factor in his unique ability to attain and maintain complete knee joint extension. In conditions of injury or disease man first loses those functions which were last evolved. This is of some clinical significance. Following an injury to the knee, atrophy and dysfunction (reflected by inability to lock the knee securely in complete extension) invariably appear first in the vastus medialis muscle. This association between vastus medialis dysfunction and incomplete extension is consistent enough to suggest that this muscle is of paramount importance in locking the joint into its only stable position, that of complete extension.

Quadriceps Atrophy and Rehabilitation

Selective atrophy and atony, sometimes amounting to a total reflex inhibition of muscle contractions and limited to the quadriceps, are common to all injuries and operations at the knee. Although muscle wasting occurs first as a recognizable entity in the vastus medialis, it soon involves the entire quadriceps mechanism. Associated disuse may secondarily produce atrophy of the remaining muscles, but the predominant evidences and penalties of muscle wasting remain centered in the quadriceps. Defective quadriceps function is synonymous with an unstable knee, which in turn is productive of additional symptoms in its own right. Recovery cannot occur until the quadriceps has been reconditioned. Pain-producing conditions amounting to a continuing inhibition of quadriceps function often must be eradicated by operation before this can be accomplished. Under any circumstances, the quality of the result will depend upon the degree to which quadriceps function can be restored by a program of non–weight-bearing exercises. These should include quadriceps clenching and maintenance of the contraction for a few seconds without knee motion, straight leg raising against gravity, and active extension of the knee against the resistance of progressively increasing weights tied to the ankle. The surgeon should provide detailed instructions in the proper technique for these exercises, which should remain within the limits of pain and fatigue, and be practiced for a few minutes at a time, *every hour, on the hour, all day long.* Progressive weight bearing and resumption of normal use should be graduated according to the recovery of muscle function.

Of all injuries, arthrotomy of the knee is prone to produce rapid and spectacular quadriceps wasting. This should be anticipated by the institution of intensive quadriceps drill preparatory to operation whenever possible, and by a resumption of exercises immediately after operation. The degree and intractability of postoperative quadriceps dysfunction are generally proportionate to the surgical insult imposed upon the tissues, and to the duration of abolition of physiological function following operation. The surgeon whose technique is precise and gentle, and whose patients suffer minimal postoperative pain and enjoy an early return of function, will invariably produce the most rapid and best results in all types of knee surgery.

Injuries to the Quadriceps Extensor Mechanism

The quadriceps extensor mechanism extends from the pelvis to the tibia and may be injured at various levels. In addition to intrinsic atrophy and dysfunction caused by a knee joint injury, and fixation of the vastus intermedius to the femur following a fracture, such injuries include the following:

(1) avulsion of the rectus femoris from or with the antero-inferior spine of the ilium, which is considered in Chapter 16, Injuries of the Pelvis;

(2) rupture (usually incomplete) through the quadriceps muscle bellies;

(3) rupture through or avulsion of the quadriceps tendon from the upper pole of the patella;

(4) rupture through or avulsion of the patellar tendon from the lower pole of the patella;

(5) rupture through the patella;

(6) avulsion of the tibial tubercle.

Incomplete Rupture (Hematoma) of Quadriceps Muscle

A heavy blow to the front of the thigh while the quadriceps is tense often produces rupture of many muscle fibers over a poorly circumscribed area. Usually a large hematoma occurs. The anterior thigh is greatly swollen, exquisitely tender, and devoid of adequate quadriceps function. Large and well-localized hematomas should be aspirated if seen within thirty-six hours after injury; after this time the hematoma will be clotted sufficiently to prevent aspiration of more than a small amount of fluid. A compression dressing, rest, and relative immobility of the limb should be used until the hematoma becomes organized and replaced by scar. Gentle heat may be applied for palliative purposes, but massage and exercises should be interdicted in all but minor injuries.

A gross injury of this type may produce a massive muscle belly rupture. Operative repair is unwarranted and adequate accomplishment is usually impossible, except when the disruption has occurred at the musculotendinous junction of the quadriceps mechanism. Treatment should be similar to that outlined for less severe injuries. Spontaneous repair is characterized by a palpable defect in the quadriceps mass, but there is reasonably good recovery of quadriceps function.

Complications of quadriceps hematoma. When the quadriceps muscle fibers adjacent to the femur are ruptured the consequent hematoma is prone to ossify. Whether this is called **ossifying hematoma** or **myositis ossificans** is academic. Usually the extra-osseous new bone mass eventually becomes confluent with the femur. What is important for the surgeon to appreciate is that the mass of new bone is surrounded by unossified fibrous tissue which extends in all directions, often for a considerable distance. The quadriceps mechanism is stuck securely to the femur and serves as a checkrein to prevent knee joint flexion. It is during the early stages of this progressive condition that great harm can accrue from therapy designed to combat the steadily increasing defect in knee flexion. There is a great temptation to passively stretch the knee, or to institute a program of forceful active flexion exercises. All such treatments serve but to accelerate the formation of new bone and accentuate the penalties of quadriceps fixation. *Passive stretching is to be condemned.* Active function should remain within the limits of pain, and within the motion range easily available. Time and abstinence from active treatment will, in the long run, produce the best result. Unless it is chronically irritated by treatment or overuse, the heterotopic bone mass will eventually reduce in size and may disappear, but some defect in flexion usually remains.

Rupture or Avulsion of Quadriceps Tendon

A rupture through the quadriceps tendon or an avulsion of the tendon from the patella may be considered together. As is the case in all spontaneous ruptures of the extensor mechanism, the cause is a violent contraction, against body weight, while the knee is flexed, of the muscles constituting the quadriceps mechanism. However, a normal quadriceps or patellar tendon does not rupture; instead, the patella fractures. Almost all tendon ruptures occur in patients over 45. In the writer's experience, tissues taken from the ruptured areas consistently have revealed antecedent weakening of the tendon by neoplasm or attritional degeneration.

Diagnosis. The diagnosis is often missed because only the quadriceps tendon is ruptured, and the adjacent vastus tendons provide surprisingly full but weakened extension power of the knee. A hiatus is always palpable just above the patella. Proximal to the hiatus the curled and retracted proximal tendon fragment feels like a small tumor. In more extensive ruptures involving the vastus tendons, extension of the knee against gravity is weak and incomplete, or absent. Lateral roentgenograms usually reveal the patella to be at a lower level than normal. When the quadriceps ruptures at the level of the patellar tendon, lateral films will reveal the patella to be retracted to a level higher than normal.

Treatment. Since the tendon rupture usually occurs through diseased or degenerated fibers, and since retraction is the rule, spontaneous repair rarely, if ever, occurs. Immobilization is neither necessary nor useful, except when the rupture is so small that full extension of the knee is maintained. The tear should be repaired when extension is defective. The torn tendon fibers are tattered and frayed out into strings, and one is often completely frustrated in attempts to suture them together or to the patella. The fibrillated fibers should be excised back to tendon of sufficient toughness to hold a suture. At times a considerable gap is produced by excision of these useless tissues. Special techniques for closing the gap and overcoming the retraction of the muscle bellies are advisable (Fig. 14–5). Following repair the limb is protected by a circular plaster dressing for

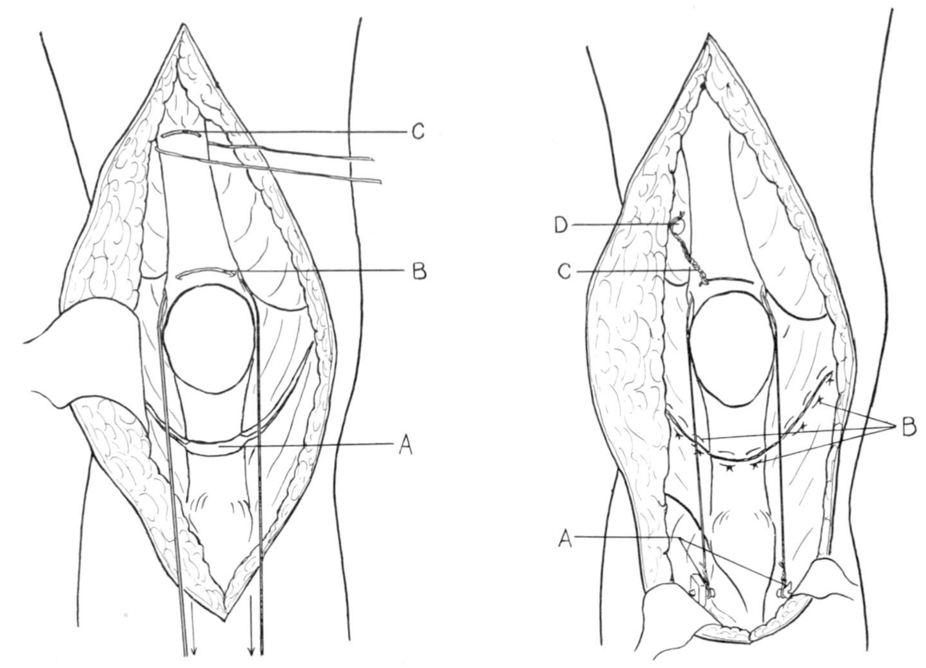

Figure 14–5. Repair of ruptured infrapatellar tendon by removable suture.

Left. Exposure by a median parapatellar incision. A, rupture through infrapatellar tendon. The devitalized edges of the tear have been excised and the fragments are held in apposition by traction on B, the main traction suture. C, placement of main suture in ruptures through the quadriceps tendon, for neutralizing muscle pull following surgical removal of the patella.

Right. A bolt (A) is passed through the tibial crest at the level of the tubercle. An ordinary bone screw, cut off lateral to the nut at the desired length, may be used. The ends of the main suture are wound around either end of the bolt. B, exact apposition of the tendon ends is ensured by use of a few fine silk sutures. C, a removing wire is attached to the main suture. D, a split lead shot is clamped to the end of the removing wire. This remains palpable through the skin after wound closure. (From McLaughlin, H. L., in Cole's Operative Technic in General Surgery, 2nd ed., 1955. Courtesy of Appleton-Century-Crofts, Inc.)

about eight weeks. The knee does not stiffen if the patient walks during this period.

Rupture or Avulsion of Patellar Tendon

The problems of diagnosis and treatment for patellar tendon injuries are similar to those for injury of the quadriceps tendon. This injury is uncommon. Extension of the knee against gravity is absent, but quadriceps contractions can be felt to tug on the patella. The rupture is reflected in a palpable tendon defect just below the patella, and the lateral roentgenogram reveals the patella to be riding higher than normal. The principles of operative repair (Fig. 14–5) are similar to those for repair of a ruptured quadriceps or other tendon (see also Fig. 13–3).

Rupture through the Patella

A transverse or avulsion fracture of the patella is a rupture of the quadriceps extensor mechanism. The bone breaks because it is weaker than the quadriceps and patellar tendons. The vastus tendons may escape injury, or may be ruptured by horizontal extensions of the patellar tear.

Avulsion fracture of patella without retraction. Only the sesamoid patella is broken. The quadriceps tendon cuff remains intact in continuity. Extension is painful and weak, but preserved. The tendon cuff investments of the cracked patella serve as precise and secure instruments for internal fixation of the bone fragments, so that, barring a re-injury which ruptures the vastus tendons, displacement cannot occur. Optimal treatment must provide relief from pain, protection against re-injury (which can occur only by sudden flexion of the knee), and maintenance of function.

A tense hemarthrosis should be aspirated. Quadriceps drill should be commenced as soon as tolerated. Both protection and maintenance of function are provided by a circular plaster dressing from ankle to upper thigh for four to six weeks. The patient is enjoined to carry on his normal activities as much as possible during this period. Complete recovery may be expected.

Comminuted fracture of patella without retraction. A direct blow may shatter the patella into many fragments but, unless the adjacent vastus tendons are torn across by coincident quadriceps contraction, little or no displacement can occur. Healing will occur as in an unretracted avulsion fracture, but with roughening of the articular surface at each point where one of the many fracture lines involved the deep surface of the bone. Subsequent arthritis at the patellar-femoral articulation is almost certain.

TREATMENT. The patella may be excised (*total patellectomy*) without undue sacrifice of normal function, provided the resulting hiatus between the quadriceps and patellar tendons is repaired securely. This is the operation of choice for patellar-femoral arthritis, for pain consequent to malunion of a patellar fracture, and when a smooth patellar articulating surface cannot be obtained or maintained following a recent fracture.

Partial patellectomy is sometimes indicated when a small fragment of the upper or lower pole of the bone has been avulsed. The small bone fragment represents only a small part of a rupture of the quadriceps tendon cuff. It may be comminuted, or difficult to replace accurately and hold securely in place. Probably most uncomminuted fragments representing more than 30 per cent of the total bone should be securely sutured to the other fragment. Whether or not smaller fragments should be excised and the tendon end sutured to the remaining fragment has been the subject of some argument. The practical surgeon who finds that utilization of such a fragment facilitates his repair of the quadriceps rupture will leave it in place; otherwise he will excise it.

Avulsion fracture of patella with retraction. Not only the patella, but also the vastus tendons are torn, and the proximal fragments of bone and tendons are retracted. The amount of retraction is proportionate to the extent of the tear. The knee cannot be extended actively. Immobilization is fruitless, and operative repair is necessary. The lacerated vastus tendons must be sutured securely. Reduction and suture of the bone fragments should also be done in order to re-establish and preserve a smooth patellar articulating surface. An ideal repair not only maintains a precise reduction of the fracture fragments but also re-establishes continuity of the quadriceps mechanism as a whole. Aftercare then requires nothing more than the provision of comfort, protection against disruption of the repair, and maintenance of function until healing occurs.

Dislocation of the patella. The quadriceps tendon, containing the patella, rides in the anterior intercondylar furrow of the femur just as a rope, containing a bearing, rides in a pulley. A sudden valgus strain sufficient to tear the medial capsule or collateral ligament, or a direct blow against the inner side of the patella when the knee is slightly flexed, may displace the tendon rope over the lateral edge of the femoral pulley. The deformity is obvious. There is a large bony lump at the outer side of the knee, which is the displaced patella. Active motion is impossible until the knee is extended passively, at which time the patella snaps back into place spontaneously.

Traumatic dislocation of the patella in an adult almost always is accompanied by a significant rupture of the vastus medialis tendon and the medial joint capsule, and usually is complicated by an injury to the articular cartilage of the patella, the lateral femoral condyle, or both. Not infrequently the edge of the lateral femoral condyle is fractured by the displaced patella. Such an injury to the outer edge of the femoral pulley, or relaxation of the medial capsular structures, may predispose to recurrent patellar dislocations or subluxations.

TREATMENT. Spontaneous reduction of the displaced patella, sometimes aided by a gentle push, occurs as soon as the leg is fully extended. Rapid and marked swelling may require aspiration. The extended limb should be protected by a walking plaster encasement from ankle to upper thigh for about six weeks. The prognosis should be guarded, since recurrent episodes or derangement of the patellar-femoral articulation may subsequently necessitate surgical treatment.

Subluxation of the patella. This condition may be accentuated, but is not caused, by trauma. It is usually encountered in female adolescents, but occurs in males and in adult life with sufficient frequency to create a diagnostic trap for the unwary surgeon. The subluxing episodes, which occur as an abnormally small or high patella slips toward a lateral femoral condyle having an edge lower than average, may be described by the patient in such a way that differentiation from the locking episodes produced by a medial meniscus tear is impossible.

THE APPREHENSION TEST is a useful method for indicting a loose patella as the cause of locking episodes. With the knee fully extended, the patella is displaced outward as far as it will go. While the patella is held in lateral displacement, the knee is flexed slightly so that the patella is forced to snap back into the intercondylar groove. This maneuver reproduces the pathological mechanism of a patellar subluxation. If the symptoms are in fact the product of recurrent subluxations, there will be great apprehension of an impending painful episode as the knee is flexed, and a minor reproduction of the offending symptom as the patella snaps back into place.

The usual recurrent subluxation of the patella occurs in a chubby adolescent girl with some knock-knee deformity. The patella is more mobile than normal, and often can be displaced manually to the very edge of the lateral femoral condyle. The apprehension test is positive. When the history describes, on the lateral side of the knee, a "bump" which the patient has learned to push back into place after each episode, the diagnosis is confirmed beyond doubt. The roentgenogram may reveal a patella that is smaller and higher than usual, and a relatively flattened lateral femoral condylar rim, but these findings are by no means constant.

TREATMENT should be predicated upon the frequency of the subluxations and the amount of symptoms and disability they produce. Not infrequently these symptoms cease spontaneously when the adolescent reaches maturity. Significant or persistent symptoms warrant operative stabilization of the patella.

Avulsion of the Tibial Tubercle

Avulsion of the tibial tubercle rarely, if ever, occurs as an isolated lesion in an adult, but it is a not infrequent concomitant of a comminuted fracture of the upper tibia. A separate bone fragment containing the tibial tubercle is tilted forward and upward by quadriceps pull on the patellar ligament. Flexion of the knee increases this angular displacement, and the limb must either be immobilized in extension or the loose fragment secured in position by some form of internal fixation (see Fig. 13–*11, B*).

Avulsion of the apophysis of the tibial tubercle may occur as an isolated injury. Usually gross retraction is prevented by intact attachment of the vastus tendon to the tibia, and uneventful healing may be expected if the limb is immobilized in extension for about eight weeks. Grossly retracted fragments of apophyseal bone and cartilage should be sutured back in place.

Epiphysitis of Tibial Tubercle (Osgood-Schlatter Disease)

This condition is not a disease, but merely the accumulated penalties of continuously repeated mechanical insults to the apophyseal cartilage of the tibial tubercle by quadriceps action. For this reason it is almost always encountered in an active adolescent boy, and only rarely in a girl. Roentgen evidence of irregularity or fragmentation of the tibial tubercle ossification centers is commonly bilateral, commonly seen in asymptomatic knees, and of questionable significance. The tibial tubercle is enlarged, tender to palpation, and painful with stretch or contraction of the quadriceps. Pain and tenderness consistently are accentuated by activity and somewhat reduced with rest. The problem is to keep an adolescent boy from playing games and using his legs strenuously. If this can be done, the symptoms will subside; if not, they will surely persist and become more severe. Enforced inactivity by immobilization of the limb in a plaster dressing is sometimes necessary. The duration of inactivity or immobilization must be governed by the behavior of the symptoms. Operative procedures are almost never necessary. This is a temporary and self-limited condition of adolescence. Complete recovery eventually occurs spontaneously, regardless of the absence, or presence and type, of treatment.

THE GLIDING MECHANISMS OF THE KNEE

At first glance the rather simple hingelike structure of the knee would seem to require little in the way of a synovial gliding mechanism, but,

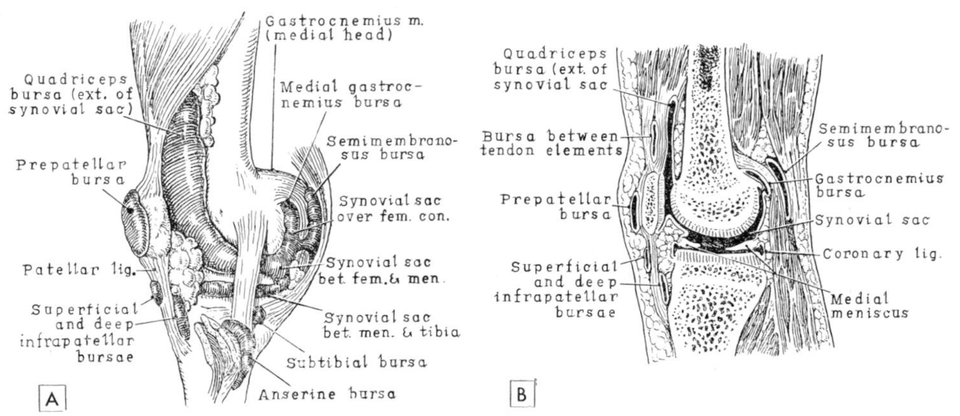

Figure 14–6. The synovial gliding mechanisms of the knee.
A. Distended.
B. In section.

when the multiplicity of extra-articular moving structures is considered, it is clear that many points of friction require lubrication. Gliding synovial structures are to be found at each friction point (Fig. 14–6). Each constitutes a potential source of pain and disability.

THE SYNOVIAL CAVITY OF THE KNEE JOINT

The synovial cavity of the knee is the largest of any joint, and contains the articulating surfaces of the femur, tibia, and patella. A large pocket of this synovial sac extends upward to separate the quadriceps tendon from the femur. Effusion into the knee distends this pouch (Fig. 14–6, *A*), and floats the patella from its normal seat on the anterior surface of the femur. Pressure upon such a floating patella educes a characteristic "patellar click" against the femur, which is a dependable sign of excessive fluid in the knee joint.

Aspiration of the Knee Joint

Aspiration of fluid from the knee is best done through the quadriceps pouch or bursa. If the patella is considered as the face of a clock, a needle can be inserted into the quadriceps pouch at any point above 9 and 3 o'clock. Below these two points the needle may be inserted into the infrapatellar fat pad, or a loose fold of synovial membrane may be sucked across the needle end and prevent withdrawal of fluid. Ideally, the needle should be inserted at 10 or 2 o'clock in relation to the circle of the patella, and passed into the interval between the femur and the floating patella.

EXTRA-ARTICULAR SYNOVIAL CAVITIES

Many synovial bursae are interposed between the moving structures about the knee (Fig. 14–6). All are apposed to friction points in the tendons which span the joint. Any of these tendons may become host to an inflamed deposit of amorphous calcific material (Fig. 14–7). The life cycle and management of painful calcium deposits about the knee are similar to those described for identical lesions which occur so much more frequently in the shoulder tendons (see Chapter 10, page 281). Any of the extra-articular synovial bursae about the knee may become inflamed, secondarily as a result of proximity to deposit which excites irritation, or primarily as a result of injury or disease.

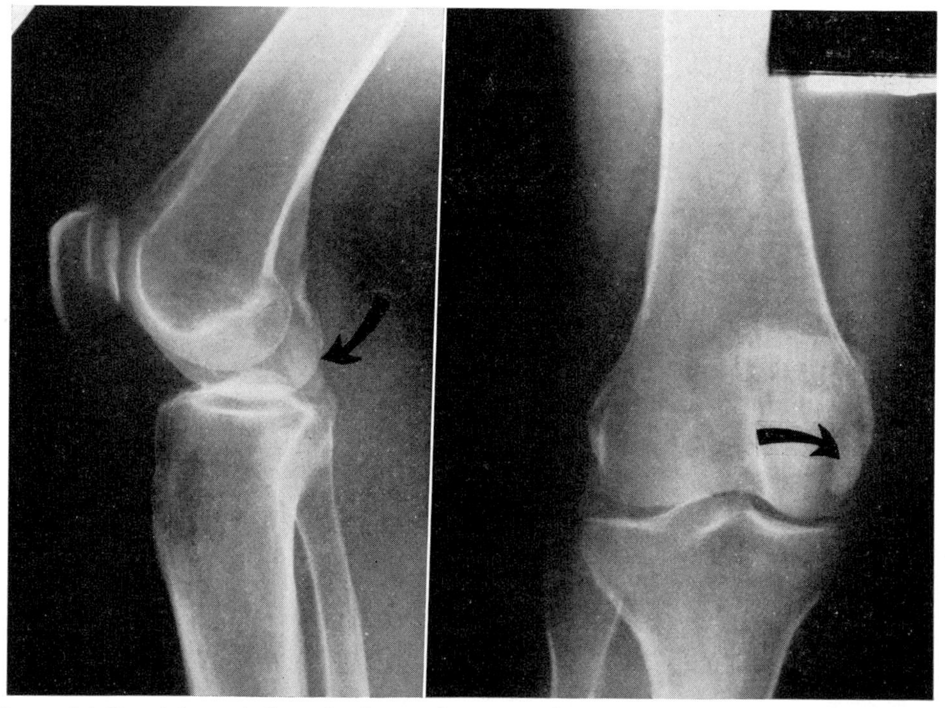

Figure 14–7. A large inflamed calcium deposit in the semimembranosus tendon (arrow). The anserine bursa was secondarily involved by the inflammatory process.

Prepatellar Bursitis (Housemaid's Knee)

The subcutaneous prepatellar bursa (Fig. 14–6) is vulnerable to direct trauma and to chronic mechanical irritation consequent to a person's working on hands and knees. Immediate swelling over the patella after a direct blow signifies distention of this bursa by blood, but fracture of the underlying patella should always be excluded by adequate roentgenograms. Aspiration should be done, followed by a compression dressing and rest of the limb. Chronic mechanical irritation initiates and perpetuates a serous bursal effusion, and promotes fibrosis of the walls of the bursa. Under such circumstances repeated aspiration or incisional drainage is to be condemned as a precursor of infection. The cause should be identified and removed, after which excision of the bursa may be required if spontaneous recovery does not ensue.

Suppurative prepatellar bursitis not infrequently follows an infected abrasion on the front of the knee. The infected bursa should be incised, left open, and allowed to heal by secondary intent, appropriate antibiotic

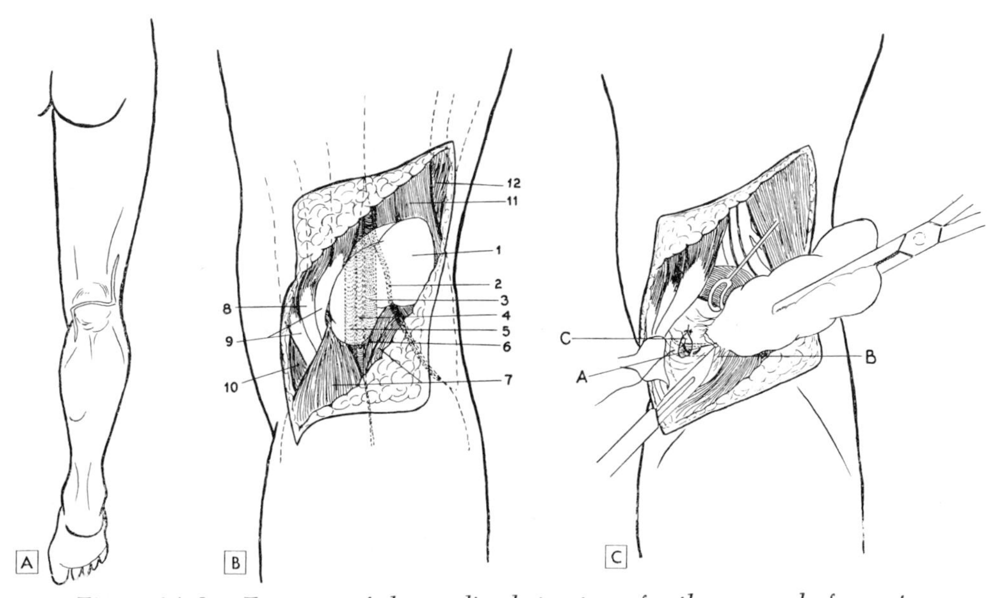

Figure 14–8. Exposure of the popliteal structures for the removal of a cyst.

A. A step-cut incision gives an excellent exposure and avoids the risk of contractures common to vertical incisions across the flexion crease.

B. The skin flaps are reflected at the level of the fascia and the popliteal structures exposed: 1, *the cyst;* 2, *common peroneal nerve;* 3, *tibial nerve;* 4, *popliteal vein;* 5, *popliteal artery;* 6, *plantaris muscle;* 7, *gastrocnemius;* 8, *semitendinosus;* 9, *semimembranosus;* 10, *gracilis;* 11, *biceps, long head;* 12, *biceps, short head.*

C. Removal of a popliteal cyst. The tumor is dissected free from its surrounding structures by sharp dissection. A, *its point of origin is identified and divided, flush with the connective tissue from which it arose.* B, *all connections with the point of origin should be divided and a portion of the connective tissue surrounding the base of the tumor should be removed.* C, *any communication with the knee joint cavity should be obliterated by suture. (From McLaughlin, H. L., in Cole's Operative Technic in General Surgery, 2nd ed., 1955. Courtesy of Appleton-Century-Crofts, Inc.)*

drugs administered, and the limb maintained at rest until the infection has been overcome. An effusion into the knee joint is a frequent concomitant of suppurative prepatellar bursitis and constitutes a pitfall for the unwary surgeon. Diagnostic aspiration of the joint through cellulitic superficial tissues should not be done lest a sterile knee joint (as is usually present) become infected. By the same token such a sympathetic joint effusion must be watched with great care, and decompressed immediately if firm evidences of suppurative arthritis supervene.

Semimembranosus Bursitis (Baker's or Popliteal Cyst)

Effusion into the semimembranosus bursa (Fig. 14–6) results in a popliteal tumor, which at times may be difficult to differentiate from a solid neoplasm or an aneurysm. The history usually provides no information of diagnostic value. If the enlarged bursal sac becomes sufficiently distended, mechanical interference with the adjacent popliteal structures is to be expected, but, even before this occurs, the slowly growing and relatively asymptomatic popliteal mass demands histological identification. The distended bursa should be removed and any communication with the knee joint cavity closed securely (Fig. 14–8).

THE MENISCI

Two semicircular menisci are situated at the periphery of the knee joint and somewhat improve the poor fit of the rounded femoral condyles against the flat upper surface of the tibia (Fig. 14–9; see also Fig. 14–*10*, *A*). Their anterior and posterior extremities are firmly attached to the tibia, and the middle segment of the medial meniscus is firmly attached to the medial collateral ligament. They function as mobile washers which

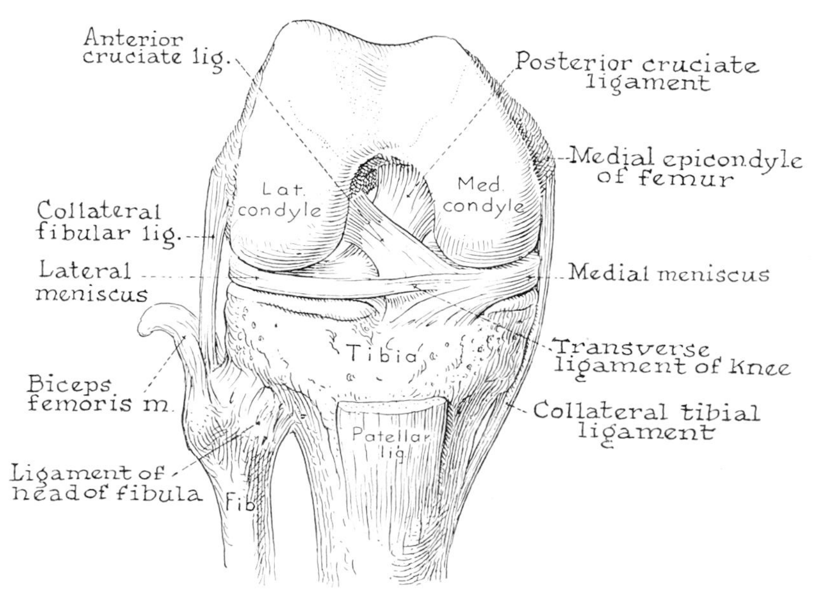

Figure 14–9. Cruciate ligaments and semilunar cartilages. (Modified from Anson.)

glide freely with the tibia against the femur. Except at their fixed attachments, there is also some mobility of each meniscus in relation to the tibia.

Each meniscus moves with the tibia in relation to the femur, forward and into external rotation with extension of the knee, and backward and into internal rotation with flexion. Except at their fixed attachments, each is mobile enough to enter the joint and become pinched between the femur and tibia.

Meniscus Tear

Mechanism of meniscus tear. At the limits of flexion, extension, and rotation the mobile menisci normally are squeezed toward the periphery of the joint between the femur and tibia, in much the same manner as a moist watermelon seed is squeezed out from between two fingers. Excessive peripheral displacement is checked by the coronary ligaments connecting the rim of each meniscus to the underlying tibia. Laceration of a meniscus occurs when, instead of being extruded to the periphery of the joint, it becomes trapped between the weight-bearing surfaces of the bones. A meniscus cannot be torn by a direct blow against the knee; such injury results only if the patient twists the knee or falls as a result of the blow. While the usual cause of a meniscus tear is a twisting

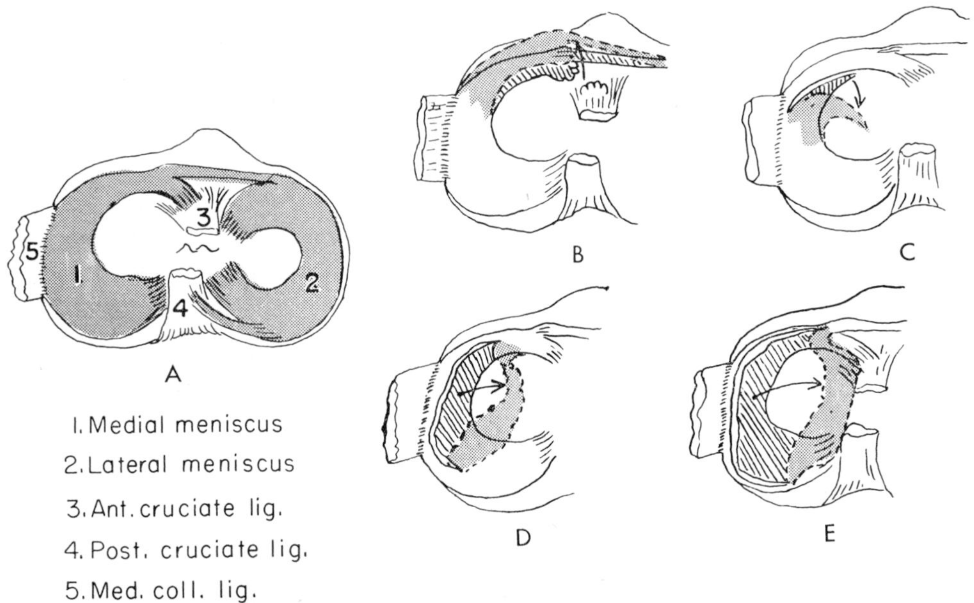

Figure 14–10. Types of meniscus tear.

A. Normal structure.

B. Avulsion of anterior tibial attachment of the medial meniscus–the loose anterior horn (stippled) swings in and out of the joint interval.

C. Single pedicle tear–the hypermobile fragment swings in and out of the joint.

D. A splitting tear–the torn fragment swings in and out of the joint on a double pedicle.

E. A locked bucket handle tear–a major portion of the meniscus becomes trapped in the femoral notch.

injury to a flexed knee which is bearing weight, laceration of the posterior horn of either meniscus may be produced merely by arising awkwardly from a squatting position. Most knee joint injuries are associated with a valgus strain, which tends to suck the medial meniscus into the opened medial joint space. For this reason, and due to its greater mobility, the medial meniscus is injured much more frequently than is the lateral.

Pathology of meniscus tear. The injury may be limited to an avulsion of the anterior tibial attachment (Fig. 14–*10, B*). The hypermobile anterior horn of the meniscus enters the joint more than normally when the knee flexes, and is thereby vulnerable to pinching as the knee-joint hinge closes in extension. Many tears commence as a longitudinal split. The torn fragment may swing in and out of the joint space on a double pedicle, or break free at one end and displace around the pivot of a single pedicle (Fig. 14–*10, C*). Long, double-pedicle ("bucket handle") tears (Fig. 14–*10, D*) may be characterized by displacement of the torn fragment into the femoral notch (Fig. 14–*10, E*), where it remains as a continuing obstacle to complete extension. In any event, the chronic symptoms and disability produced by a torn cartilage are essentially the result of persistent or intermittent interposition of the hypermobile torn fragment between the femur and the tibia.

Diagnosis of medial meniscus tear. *The history* of a torn medial meniscus reveals an adequate twisting injury, followed by pain and tenderness over the inner side of the knee, abolition of full extension due to pain and, within a few hours, a tense swelling of the entire joint. This history, however, is common to most knee joint injuries. The most frequent knee injury is a sprain of the medial collateral ligament (see page 384), which is firmly connected to the medial meniscus at the joint line. Either structure, or both of them, may be damaged by identical injuries, and early clinical differentiation between a sprained medial ligament and a torn medial meniscus is always difficult, never dependable, and often impossible.

Hemarthrosis is evidence of nothing more than damage to and hemorrhage from some structure in the knee joint capsule or cavity. A tense or painful effusion, which prevents motion, should be aspirated. The ensuing relief of pain often permits a detailed assessment of the injury. Whether or not a firm diagnosis can be made, the limb should then be rested until the acute reaction from the injury has subsided.

All such injuries at first appear to be serious. Many will recover spontaneously within a short time. In the absence of a definite diagnosis, treatment should be governed by the symptoms and their rate or failure of subsidence. An elastic compression dressing should be used until the hemarthrosis is no longer present. Non–weight-bearing quadriceps drill should be commenced as soon as pain permits, and continued until recovery occurs. Crutches should be used until gradually increasing weight can be borne without pain. Within a short period recovery will occur, or signs and symptoms diagnostic of the offending lesion will become clear.

"Locking" episodes usually occur. These are the symptoms which occur when the hypermobile torn fragment becomes pinched between the femur and the tibia. Interrogation must not, however, be limited to the use of

this medical colloquialism. The patient should be asked if the leg buckles, catches, caves in, lets him down, slips, gives way, or collapses. Depending upon his subjective interpretation of the symptoms, he will rise to the bait for one of these expressions. He should then be asked to describe exactly what occurs. Intermittent and sudden but usually transient painful episodes, with or without actual collapse or a sense of impending collapse of the knee, will be described. Immediate or rapid relief of the pain upon removal of weight from the limb, and tentative motion or manipulation of the knee, strengthens the presumption that some hypermobile body is catching between the bones. Temporary mild swelling following each episode makes this presumption fairly certain. When the roentgenogram fails to reveal a loose body in the knee, and subluxation of the patella can be ruled out, the most probable offending agent is a torn medial meniscus.

Absence of a locking history is not uncommon, and should not be accepted as evidence against a medial meniscus tear. Tears of the posterior horn of the medial meniscus do not often produce true locking episodes, but are more likely to be reflected in painful twinges which occur when weight is borne on the flexed knee, and only sometimes in a sense of impending collapse. An absence of locking may weaken, but should not exclude, the diagnosis of medial meniscus tear.

Physical findings of meniscus tear. There are visible atrophy and palpable hypotonicity of the quadriceps most marked in the vastus medialis muscle. There is tenderness, limited to the medial joint interval. Medial joint line discomfort is sharply accentuated by forcible external rotation of the flexed tibia on the femur, but not by abduction of the extended tibia. Medial joint line pain and tenderness usually are accentuated by forced extension of the knee. The collateral ligaments are functionally intact. The patella is not hypermobile and shows no tendency to subluxation. There is no roentgen evidence of a loose body in the joint.

Posterior horn tears of the medial meniscus often are attended by a nondescript history, devoid of true buckling episodes, and containing little of diagnostic significance. It is when the history is vague that it is most important to verify the integrity of all other components of the knee joint mechanism, and then to concentrate the examination on the posterior segment of the medial meniscus. The posterior half of the medial joint line can be palpated adequately only when the knee is flexed in excess of 90 degrees. Palpation reveals tenderness at most posterior horn tears. The "click" described by McMurray, which occurs as a hypermobile posterior torn fragment locks and unlocks from between the condylar surfaces as the fully flexed tibia is rotated on the femur, is not always present, and requires some skill and experience on the part of the examiner for its production.

Locked bucket handle tear of the medial meniscus is characterized by displacement of all, or a major part, of the meniscus into the femoral notch. The early history is characteristic of a meniscus tear, but the subsequent clinical picture is attended by a persistent painful elastic block to the last 10 or 15 degrees of extension. When extension is forced passively and then released suddenly there is a slight "rebound spring" into flexion. Because the meniscus is trapped in the femoral notch the history is usually free from intermittent buckling episodes.

Tear of the lateral meniscus is much less frequent than injury to the medial meniscus. The pathology of the tear and the resultant clinical picture are similar to those attending a medial meniscus tear, are not confused by concomitant collateral ligament damage, and are centered in the lateral joint interval.

Cyst of the lateral meniscus is frequently encountered, as a result of mucoid degeneration of the substance of the lateral meniscus adjacent to a small injury. The soft degenerated tissues are extruded from between the bones toward the periphery, to produce a cystlike protrusion from the joint interval, which is tense and prominent in extension, but which disappears with flexion of the knee. This characteristic appearance or disappearance of the cystic tumor according to posture is a useful test by which a cyst of the lateral meniscus can be dependably differentiated from a ganglion or a solid tumor, neither of which is affected by posture.

Indications for treatment. The menisci enjoy a significant blood supply only at their peripheral attachments. Only when a tear is peripheral can union occur, and then only if the torn surfaces are precisely apposed and remain apposed for four to six weeks.

Apposition of the torn surfaces can be promoted only by complete extension of the knee, and never is certain. Prolonged immobilization is essential to maintenance of apposition, which is never certain or secure. Prolonged immobilization produces not only a stiff knee, but marked quadriceps atrophy, despite the best of quadriceps drill. In short, this "conservative" treatment for a torn meniscus is, in its own right, productive of serious and prolonged disability, and offers no assurance that it will not later be necessary to remove the damaged meniscus. When the diagnosis is beyond doubt, continuing symptoms and disability warrant operative removal of the meniscus. This is particularly true in the presence of locking episodes. Each such episode is synonymous with a bruise and an abrasion of the articular cartilage adjacent to the tear. The inevitable result of these continued mechanical insults is a painful arthritis.

Expectant treatment and maintenance of quadriceps tone should be continued until the diagnosis is certain, or maximal spontaneous recovery has taken place. Then, even in the absence of a clear diagnosis, if neoplasm, infection, and metabolic causes can be excluded, and if continuing mechanical signs and symptoms warrant treatment, exploratory arthrotomy of the knee should be done and the offending meniscus excised.

Removal of torn meniscus. A tourniquet may be used, but is not necessary. A transverse curved incision paralleling the rim of the medial femoral condyle permits access to both the anterior and posterior joint cavities, and is much less likely to sever branches of the infrapatellar division of the internal saphenous nerve than is any type of vertical incision. The capsule is incised in the line of its fibers from the mid-point of the patella to the tibia. The front half of the medial meniscus is then visible, and the infrapatellar fat pad, the anterior cruciate ligament, and the articular surfaces of femur and patella may be inspected. The medial meniscus should be excised, even if no tear can be seen. As often as not the tear will be found in the invisible posterior horn. The meniscus is severed from its coronary attachments by sharp dissection. The entire meniscus must be removed. This can rarely be done with certainty, precision, and adequate hemostasis through a single anterior opening in the capsule. A second incision of the capsule behind the medial collateral ligament makes it possible to remove the posterior meniscus segment completely and under direct vision.

Aftercare. The quality of the result following removal of a meniscus and the speed with which it is attained do not depend on the use of splints, pressure dressings, early or delayed motion, or lumbar sympathetic blocks during the postoperative period. They depend, rather, upon precise dissection, gentle handling of all tissues, and complete hemostasis at the operation. Given these requisites, quadriceps contractions will be regained rapidly, effusions requiring aspiration will be uncommon, and the great majority of patients will walk comfortably with crutches within 48 hours after operation, discard their crutches after another 48 hours, and walk out of the hospital in good condition within 10 days. Quadriceps drill should be continued, and strenuous activities deferred until the quadriceps muscle has been reconditioned.

TIBIAL CONDYLES

Fractures of Tibial Condyles

Body weight driven through the femur coincident with a forceful valgus strain is transmitted to the tibia through the lateral femoral condyle. In young persons with resilient bones, fracture is uncommon, and the result is usually a rupture of the medial collateral ligament; however, in persons past middle age, having more brittle bones, the lateral tibial condyle may be crushed by femoral impact. Almost all such fractures are accompanied by some damage to the medial collateral ligament, but complete rupture is uncommon. Nevertheless, regardless of the absence, presence, or amount of ligament damage, compression of a tibial condyle is productive of a "wobbly" knee in its own right, and this hypermobility of abduction is highly suggestive to the casual observer of medial ligament rupture. It is the equivalent of a lax ligament, and must be compensated by the quadriceps. The muscles of a person past middle age can be reconditioned only with difficulty and by prolonged perseverance in quadriceps drill. Once rehabilitated, the quadriceps compensates for residual valgus deformity and moderate medial ligament laxity with surprising efficiency.

Fractures of the lateral tibial condyle are of two main types: clean-cut fractures involving the entire condyle and without comminution or gross derangement of the weight-bearing surface, and comminuted fractures in which the crushed central portion of the condyle is driven down into the substance of the tibia and a relatively intact peripheral shell of bone is pushed outward by the femur. Similar injuries to the medial tibial condyle rarely occur as isolated lesions and, since they are produced by body weight without a valgus strain, are almost always accompanied by compression of the lateral tibial condyle.

Uncomminuted fracture of lateral tibial condyle. The entire condyle is depressed and impacted into the soft bone of the upper tibia (Fig. 14–*11, A*). The articular cartilage is essentially intact. The net effect is the production of a valgus deformity. The medial ligament may be stretched, but remains intact in continuity. A tense hemarthrosis is present. A valgus deformity of 15 degrees or less needs no reduction. Greater deformities should be corrected by manipulation. Adequate anesthesia is essential. The knee should be forced into complete extension, and, while it is in this position, the depressed condyle disimpacted by strong adduction of the tibia, and the horizontal plane of the tibial articular surface restored. Immobilization must preserve both complete extension and tibial adduction, if reduction is to be maintained, and must continue for a minimum of three months. Quadriceps drill must be practiced from the start, and weight bearing delayed until complete healing has occurred.

Not infrequently the depressed tibial condyle is so firmly impacted into the upper tibia that adduction of the lower leg fails to loosen the condylar fragment. Bone clamps and crushing implements designed to disimpact the fragment forcibly, as a rule, serve but to comminute the bone

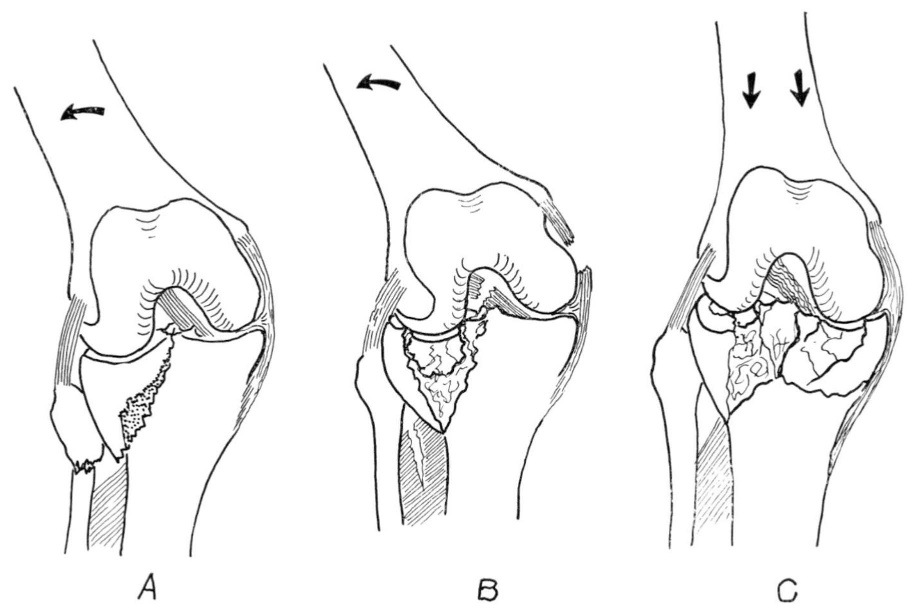

Figure 14–11. Fractures of tibial condyles.

A. Depressed fracture of lateral tibial condyle without comminution. The articular cartilage remains intact.

B. Comminuted fracture of lateral tibial condyle. The articular cartilage is fragmented. The central portion of the tibial plateau is depressed more than the peripheral shell. Some combination of cruciate and collateral ligament damage is usual.

C. Depressed fractures of both tibial condyles are comminuted but, as a rule, devoid of gross displacement.

and make matters worse. Inability to disimpact and elevate the condylar fragment by manipulation is an indication for operative reduction of the fracture, followed by internal fixation of the fragment in normal position.

The resultant valgus deformity produced by many of these fractures is less than 15 degrees and requires no reduction. If immobilized immediately, the knee becomes extremely, and sometimes intractably, stiff. The hemarthrosis should be aspirated. The knee then may be supported in a balanced suspension device, and gentle gravity-free motion encouraged until the acute reaction subsides and a moderate range of flexion and extension is regained (usually within a period of 7 to 14 days). The limb then may be immobilized for the necessary three months at a greatly reduced price in terms of stiffness.

Occasionally, mildly depressed and firmly impacted fractures of this type may, in an intelligent and cooperative patient, be treated without immobilization. Use of crutches, abstinence from weight bearing, and quadriceps drill must be continued until the fracture has consolidated.

Comminuted fracture of lateral tibial condyle. The lateral tibial condyle is not only depressed but is also shattered into many fragments (Fig. 14–*11, B*). Usually the central portion of the weight-bearing surface has been driven down into the tibia much more than the peripheral shell of the condyle. The articular surface is irregular, and much of the articular cartilage is destroyed by the injury. The lateral meniscus is damaged, and any combination of collateral and cruciate ligament ruptures may occur. Manipulative reduction is not often possible, since the depressed central fragments serve as a wedge to prevent replacement of the split-off peripheral shell. Occasionally, when the rim of the broken condyle is tilted grossly outward, this central wedge must be elevated from below before any semblance of a horizontal joint line can be restored. From the roentgenogram, the knee seems ruined beyond repair, but restoration of a reasonably level, if irregular, joint line, prolonged immobilization, and faithful reconditioning of the quadriceps will usually produce an astonishingly comfortable and useful knee.

Fracture of both tibial condyles. These relatively uncommon injuries are produced by femoral impact without coincident valgus strain. Almost always both tibial condyles are fractured, but the force of femoral impact is diffusely distributed, and gross depression of the fracture fragments is uncommon (Fig. 14–*11, C*). In the absence of comminution, the tibial condylar fragments tend to split apart and often justify operative reduction and fixation by a transverse bolt. When the upper tibia is comminuted, significant displacement is uncommon, and prolonged immobilization is the treatment of choice.

Injuries of the Femur

STIFF KNEE FOLLOWING FRACTURE OF FEMUR

The inevitable penalty of a fractured adult femur is stiffness of the knee. This is not difficult to understand when one considers the structures involved by fibrous adhesions to form an inelastic checkrein between the femur and the patella (Fig. 14–*12*). Even a fractured hip, which involves neither the quadriceps muscle nor pouch directly, but merely by immobility, when treated by traction is consistently complicated by a stiff knee. All treatments for fractures of the adult femur, therefore, should be planned so as to preserve as much knee joint mobility as is possible and safe throughout the healing period. Neither this therapeutic requisite nor the danger of a stiff knee obtains for fractures of the femur in children.

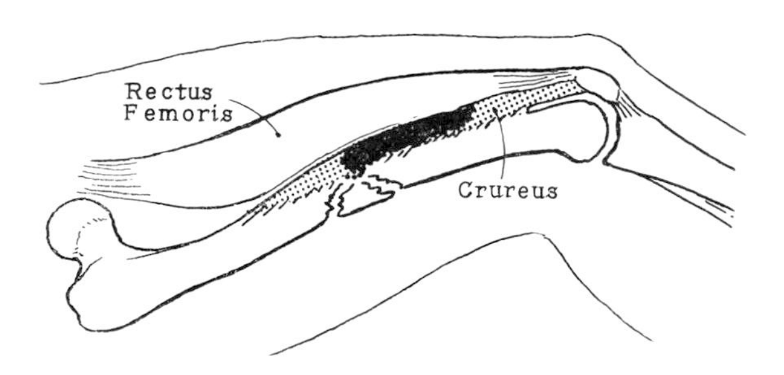

A. CRUREUS M. FIXATION

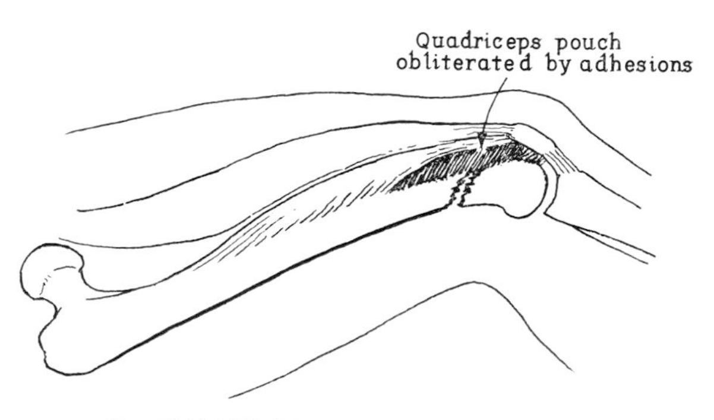

B. FIXATION OF PATELLA

Figure 14-12. Fractures of femur.

A. Hemorrhage, edema, and laceration of the components of the quadriceps muscle which surround the fractured femoral shaft eventuate in fibrosis. The resulting inelastic checkreins from femur to patella effectively prevent motion of the knee.

B. In fractures of the lower femur treated by immobilization or traction, the patella becomes fixed to the femur by the adhesions which abolish the quadriceps pouch. An immobile patella is synonymous with a stiff knee.

SUPRACONDYLAR FRACTURE OF FEMUR

A purely supracondylar fracture of the adult femur is uncommon, for the force required to break the massive lower end of this bone is so great that the condyles also are apt to be shattered or split apart. When such a fracture does occur, it is transverse and the deformity is constant. The gastrocnemius flexes the distal fragment on the tibia, for, except for the popliteus, this is its sole attached muscle motor (Fig. 14–*13*). The sharp

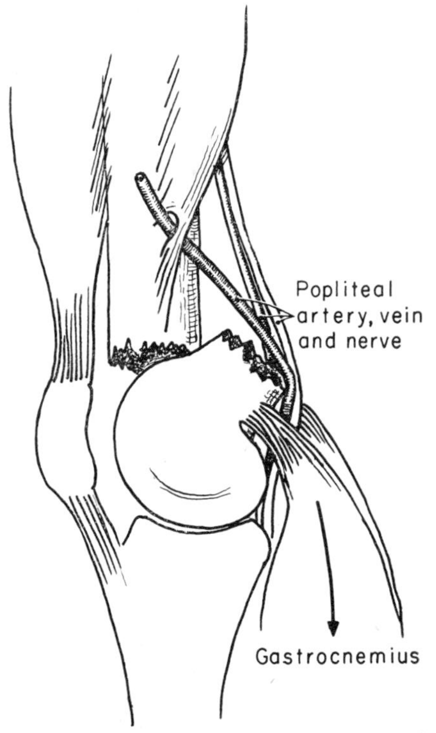

Figure 14–13. The short distal fragment of a supracondylar fracture is flexed by the gastrocnemius and, unless this muscle force is neutralized by knee flexion, the popliteal structures may be injured.

broken end of the fragment is then directed backward to place the great popliteal vessels in dire jeopardy. The danger of damage to the popliteal structures is increased by traction to the extended limb, and by pressure against the popliteal region.

Treatment

Immobilization by plaster may suffice when the displacement is minimal and easily corrected by manipulation, and when the reduction is stable. A good reduction is necessary. Malunion with a small valgus deformity may be compensated for by a good quadriceps muscle, but a corresponding varus deformity produces a real disability. Malunion in recurvatum, which is the penalty of immobilization without sufficient knee joint flexion, is the forerunner of a painful, unstable knee. The surgeon must make certain that the reduction is marked by normal alignment in both planes, and that the immobilizing dressing is snug and secure, and applied with the knee joint flexed at least 25 degrees. The immobilization should be maintained until firm union occurs, usually a matter of eight weeks or longer. The quadriceps bursa becomes obliterated by adhesions, efficiently fixing the patella to the fracture area. Following union the knee is very stiff, and many weeks of intensive stretching exercises are required before motion is regained.

Treatment by traction may be necessitated by comminution of the fracture which precludes the use of plaster or internal fixation. Flexion of the knee is as essential to this form of treatment as to external immobilization. Russell traction, which exerts pressure against the popliteal area, should not be used. The limb may be placed in balanced suspension in a Thomas splint and a Pearson low-leg attachment. The knee must be flexed enough to neutralize the displacing effect of the gastrocnemius. The amount of flexion required for this purpose can be determined only by trial and error, and roentgen examinations. A pin is passed through the upper end of the flexed tibia, and an appropriate amount of traction applied in the longitudinal axis of the femur.

Open reduction with internal fixation is an exacting and major procedure calling for the utmost in surgical skill and facilities, but when done wisely and well it promises the most rapid, economical, and best results. Two fixation devices are in common use. The reduced fracture may be stabilized by a pair of resilient medullary pins, such as those devised by Rush, which are inserted from within the knee joint through

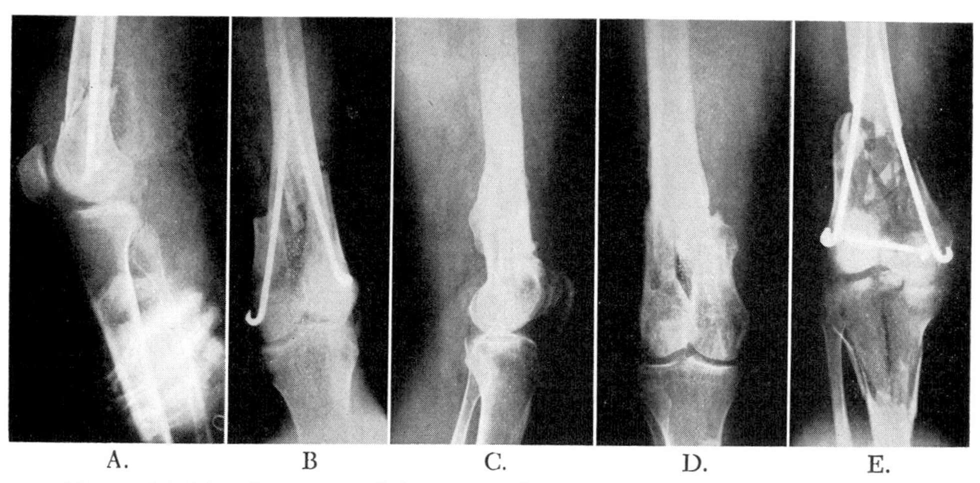

A. B C. D. E.

Figure 14–14. Comminuted fracture of both femoral condyles.

A, B. Views following fixation by Rush pins. It will be noted in the anteroposterior projection that if the pins had been placed more nearly parallel to the cortices of the condylar fragments (as in E), the existing separation of these fragments would have been reduced. This simple technical point often is overlooked, as in this case.

C, D. The end result, a comfortable and mobile knee.

E. Fixation by Rush pins and a bolt facilitated treatment of the associated fracture of the tibia.

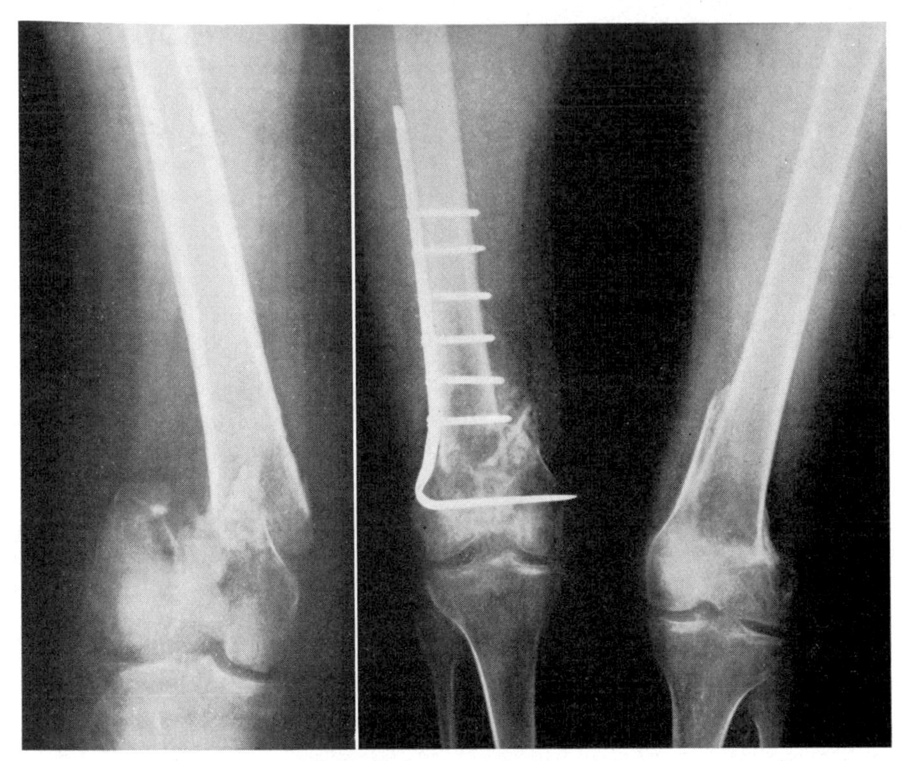

Figure 14–15. Supracondylar fracture of femur.

Left. A comminuted supracondylar fracture which was too unstable to be managed by external immobilization or traction.

Right. Fixation by a blade plate, following which treatment in balanced suspension with continued gentle knee motion was employed. A similar, but stable, injury in the other leg was treated by traction in balanced suspension.

the distal fragment and well up into the medullary canal of the femur (Fig. 14–*14*); or the blade plate devised by Moore and Blount for fixation of hip fractures may be molded to the contour of the lower femur, the blade driven horizontally through the condylar fragment, and the plate screwed to the femoral shaft (Fig. 14–*15*). With either device a period of several weeks with the limb in balanced suspension is required after the operation. Depending upon the security of fixation obtained, some knee motion usually may be maintained throughout this period, and the patient may leave hospital on crutches in four to six weeks. Weight bearing should not be allowed until the fracture has healed firmly. The results are excellent, and, when the required surgical skill and facilities are available, open reduction with internal fixation is the treatment of choice for displaced supracondylar fractures of the femur in adults.

FRACTURES OF THE FEMORAL CONDYLES

Fracture of a Single Condyle

A violent valgus or varus strain of the knee may fracture a femoral condyle instead of the apposed tibial plateau. This is an uncommon injury.

The cracked-off condylar fragment is often undisplaced and is seldom displaced more than a small amount. Its soft tissue attachments remain essentially intact, so that the broken fragment is usually quite stable. After a short period of immobilization, progressive knee motion may be commenced, but weight bearing should be delayed until the fracture unites. When the condylar fragment is grossly displaced the surrounding soft tissues are disrupted; the fracture is no longer stable and should be reduced accurately and fixed in place with screws.

Fractures of Both Condyles (T or Y Fractures)

This is the most common fracture of the lower end of the adult femur. An associated wound often is present. The femoral condyles are split apart and comminuted by the shaft fragment, and the knee mechanism is grossly disorganized. The comminuted fracture is almost always so unstable (Fig. 14–*14*) that treatment by external immobilization is of no avail. Skeletal traction, followed by compression of the spread condyles, occasionally succeeds in maintaining satisfactory alignment until healing occurs. Often the two condyles must be bolted together before any semblance of stability is obtained. Frequently the bolt may be passed through the distal screw hole in a plate, which is then molded and screwed to the femoral shaft so that the entire fracture is fixed with sufficient stability to permit some knee motion in balanced suspension at an early date. At other times, gross alignment may be maintained by some form of medullary fixation (Fig. 14–*14*).

INJURIES OF LOWER FEMORAL EPIPHYSIS

Violent hyperextension injuries may displace the lower femoral epiphysis forward from the metaphysis. As in supracondylar fractures, the epiphyseal fragment is flexed on the tibia by the gastrocnemius, but, unlike supracondylar fractures, it is the posterior projection of the femoral shaft that protrudes into the popliteal area and presses upon the vessels to the foot and leg. Fortunately, the sheared-off surfaces are broad and smooth, and fit perfectly. Reduction is easily secured by strong and steady traction, followed by backward pressure against the displaced fragment. Flexion of the knee, by creating tension upon the intact anterior soft parts, then holds the reduction securely. The knee may safely be flexed to an angle of 90 degrees, provided the circulation of the foot is watched carefully, but *flexion must not be employed until after the fragments have been replaced;* otherwise the popliteal vessels may be pinched and occluded. The optimal amount of flexion to be employed may be stated as the least amount that will maintain the reduction without embarrassing the circulation to the foot and leg.

Violent varus or valgus forces may also displace the lower femoral epiphysis. These lesions are much less stable than those produced by hyperextension. The displaced epiphysis almost always is accompanied by a triangular fragment of the metaphysis, and some disturbance of growth resulting in a varus or valgus deformity is fairly common. Growth between the triangular fragment and the displaced epiphysis proceeds normally, and any retardation of growth at the sheared-off portion of the epiphyseal plate results in some knock-knee or bowleg. Nevertheless, a satisfactory reduction can almost always be effected by manipulation. When this is not the case, or when the reduction cannot be maintained by plaster, skeletal traction through the upper end of the tibia may be necessary.

Regardless of the cause or character of the injury, the reduced epiphysis should be immobilized in a circular plaster dressing whenever possible. Immobilization with the knee flexed an appropriate amount should be maintained for eight weeks. Especially when the epiphysis has been displaced in a medial or lateral direction and is accompanied by a metaphyseal fragment, parents of the patient should be warned of the possibility of growth disturbance. This complication is rarely of clinical significance in adolescents, but premature closure of all or part of the injured epiphysis in a small child is a catastrophe.

FRACTURES OF SHAFT OF FEMUR

Fractures of Shaft of Femur in Children

Birth fractures of the femoral shaft are not uncommon. Reduction is not required. Union occurs with great rapidity. Even gross malunion and shortening are corrected by growth within one or two years. The broken thigh may be flexed against and bound to the abdomen or stabilized by a simple board splint, or the two legs may merely be bound together for two or three weeks. The prognosis is consistently excellent.

Childhood fractures of the femoral shaft are common. The majority occur in children between two and six years of age. These fractures consistently are followed by a temporary stimulation of growth in the injured bone. The overgrowth averages 1 to 4 cm., occasionally reaches 6 cm., and appears directly proportional to the total amount of original tissue damage. Fractures which heal with normal bone length are subsequently attended by some overgrowth, and a permanent discrepancy in the length of the lower limbs; those which heal with slight overriding of the fragments are more likely to eventuate with normal length. Therefore, although normal alignment is desirable, the surgeon should not attempt to regain full length of the broken bone. The realigned limb should be immobilized in a plaster spica for about six weeks, after which union by exuberant callus is almost always present. All but rotational deformities will be obliterated by subsequent growth.

Bryant's skin traction is in common use for the treatment of femoral shaft fractures in small children. It should not be used for any child who weighs more than 50 pounds. Both legs are hung by adhesive skin traction from an overhead frame, so that the buttocks are just lifted from the mattress. The vascular status of both limbs, but especially of the uninjured extremity, must be determined frequently and carefully, for there is a constant risk of Volkmann's ischemic paralysis of the lower legs. The pathomechanics of this catastrophic complication are discussed on page 367. The greatest danger is to the uninjured limb, in which hyperextension of the knee should be prevented by application of a molded plaster splint before traction is instituted.

The dangers inherent in Bryant's traction are such that it should not be used by the novice, or by anyone without a compelling reason. It is a useful device when an actual or questionable visceral injury necessitates frequent examination of the abdomen at the same time the fractured femur is being treated, but for the average fracture of the femoral shaft in a young child, in which normal length of the bone is neither necessary nor desirable, the indications for traction in any form are open to question.

Fractures of Shaft of Femur in Adults

Fractures of the adolescent or adult femoral shaft usually are bridged by a soft extra-osseous callus in three to four months, but are not consolidated completely until some time between six and twelve months after injury. This means that few patients can afford to be treated by traction, or by any other method which requires hospitalization throughout the healing period.

The problem is not one of obtaining union of the fracture, for the femur and its surrounding tissues are richly endowed with vessels, and union almost always occurs except when the processes of repair are overwhelmed by tissue destruction, infection, or some other adverse factor

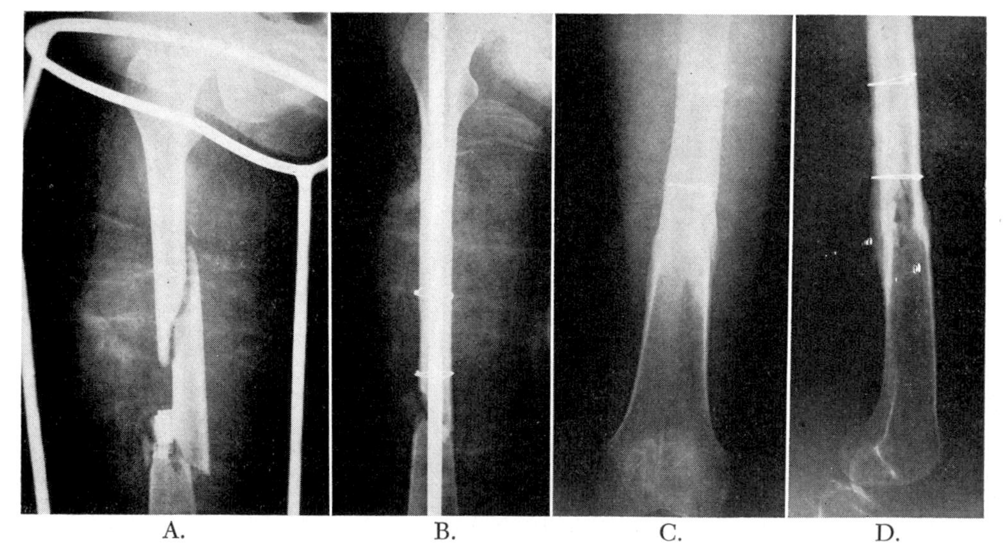

A. B. C. D.

Figure 14–16. Segmental fracture of femur.

A, B. Views of a shattered segmental fracture before and after fixation with a medullary device. The intermediate bone segment was found to be split longitudinally; hence the supplemental support of two circular wires.

C, D. The result following bony union and removal of the medullary fixation device.

such as distraction of the bone fragments. However, the strong muscle forces influencing the fracture must be neutralized continuously for the prolonged period required for complete union. The powerful abductor muscles constantly exert an abduction force on the proximal fragment, and the adductor muscles an adduction force on the distal fragment. As a result, a gross angular deformity, apex outward, occurs within the best of plaster dressings. This may be prevented by traction, but will inevitably occur at a late date if the traction is removed before union is complete; and, more often than not, angulation will occur with breakage or disruption of plate fixation in fractures of the middle third of the femur. All fractures in this segment of the femur should be reduced by open surgery and fixed by a strong medullary device whenever possible (Fig. 14–*16*). This is the only way, except by a prolonged and prohibitively expensive hospitalization program, that the adverse muscle forces can consistently be neutralized until the fracture heals completely.

Plate and screw fixation of femoral shaft fractures has been largely superseded by use of intramedullary fixation devices, except in specific circumstances. One of these may obtain in fractures through the lower third of an adolescent femur in which the grasp of a medullary fixation device is reduced by the presence of an open lower femoral epiphysis, and is insecure owing to a progressive increase in the capacity of the medullary canal. If plate fixation is elected, the plate should be at least six times as long as the diameter of the bone, the screws should engage

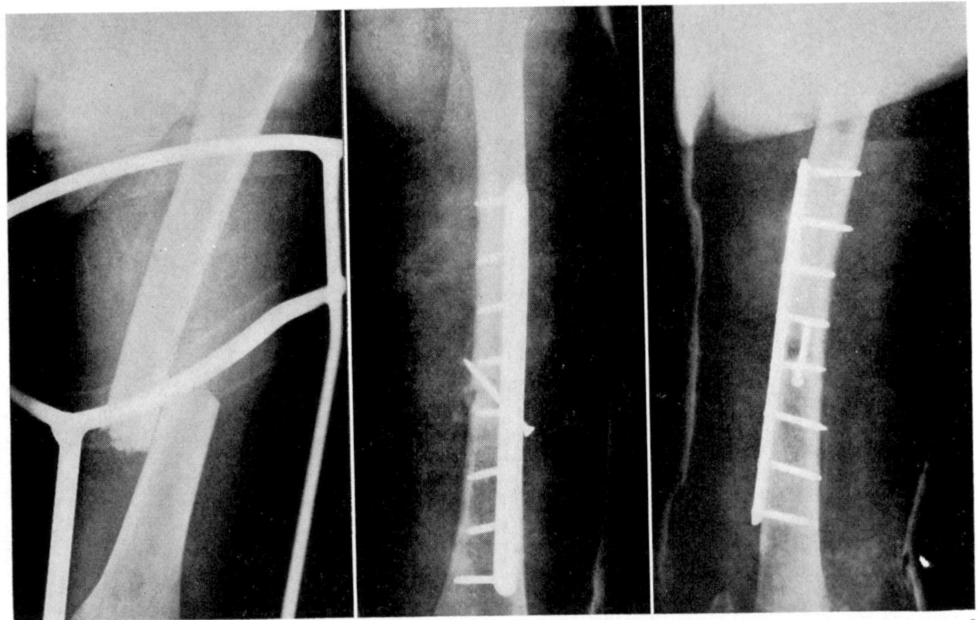

Figure 14–17. Films before and after fixation of an open fracture in the lower third of an adolescent femur. The plate is at least six times longer than the diameter of the bone, and screws engage both cortices, a transfixion screw provides a defense against torque forces, and this internal fixation is supported by a plaster dressing.

both cortices, and an additional screw or screws should be inserted in such a way that two-plane fixation is provided (Fig. 14–*17*). It is probable that, even when applied with technical perfection, plate and screw fixation should be supported by supplemental plaster immobilization until the fractured femur unites.

CHAPTER 15

INJURIES OF THE HIP

By CHARLES S. NEER, II, M.D.

THE HIP JOINT is the keystone to ambulation. It is subjected to trauma throughout life. Fortunately it is an extremely powerful structure and is capable of withstanding severe mechanical stress. Nevertheless, the upper femur is susceptible to injury at two stages of life. First, from infancy until closure of the epiphysis, the ossification center for the head of the femur constitutes a weak point. Secondly, in the declining years following middle life, the bone undergoes the changes of senility and is easily fractured. Most traumatic disruptions, therefore, occur at the two extremes of life. In the middle years the bone is generally more powerful than the ligaments, and during this period fractures are uncommon, but the joint is occasionally dislocated. Three groups of injuries should, therefore, be considered:

(1) epiphyseal separations;
(2) fractures of the upper femur;
(3) dislocations.

EPIPHYSEAL SEPARATIONS

SURGICAL ANATOMY AND PHYSIOLOGY

The secondary ossification center for the *head of the femur* appears within the first six months of extrauterine life, and shortly thereafter is subjected to the strain of ambulation. It obtains most of its blood supply from branches of the medial circumflex femoral and gluteal arteries reflected under the posterior capsule of the neck of the femur in the retinaculum of Weitbrecht. The intramedullary and ligamentum teres arteries are less important sources of nutrition in the young. During childhood these vessels supplying blood to the capital epiphysis may be damaged, producing avascular necrosis and resulting in collapse and flattening of the femoral head (coxa plana, Legg-Calvé-Perthes disease). After the tenth year of life the cartilage between the head and the neck begins to take up more calcium in preparation for ossification and closure. During these years, between the ages of 10 and 14, the epiphyseal line is brittle and easily fractured (slipping of the upper femoral epiphysis).

Although the epiphysis of the head of the femur is the major site of injuries in childhood, avulsion of one of the *traction epiphyses*, present in adolescence, occasionally occurs; for example, avulsion of the ischial tuberosity by the hamstrings, or of the anterior inferior spine by the rectus femoris (Chap. 16, pp. 478, 479). The lesser trochanter is occasionally avulsed by the iliopsoas, or the greater trochanter by the abductor muscles.

COXA PLANA

Coxa plana is a flattening of the head of the femur due to compromised supply of blood to the ossification center. It occurs in children between the ages of 4 and 10 years, and predominantly in boys. It was described independently by Legg of Boston, Calvé in France, and Perthes in Germany. Any pathological condition which interferes with the blood supply during childhood, such as osteomyelitis, Gaucher's disease, and neoplasms, may result in coxa plana. The immediate etiological factor involved in coxa is trauma.

Pathology

The ossified portion of the developing femoral head depends upon its blood supply for nutrition. The overlying cartilage is nourished by the synovial fluid. When the blood supply is reduced sufficiently, necrosis of the bony center occurs (the stage of fragmentation—see Fig. 15–*1*, *B*). During this stage the overlying articular cartilage is not affected, but remains healthy until the supporting bone collapses. Weight-bearing stress may crumble the necrotic bone, resulting in distortion of the overlying cartilage. If the articular surface becomes flattened and irregular, it will wear unevenly, and degenerative changes are accelerated. Then follow the changes of hypertrophic osteoarthritis, consisting of fibrillation and pitting of the articular surface, synovitis and thickening of the capsule, and marginal exostosis formation and lipping. In this instance advanced degenerative changes are often present in early adult life. On the other hand, if the articular surface retains its normal shape throughout the period of avascular change and until the dead bone has been completely replaced with living bone by Axhausen's "creeping substitution," which occurs concomitantly with the phase of fragmentation as well as during the stage of repair, one might expect to find a normal joint which would stand up under strain. Unfortunately, the process of replacement of necrotic bone with living bone requires many months. Avoidance of weight-bearing stress through this period of revascularization and repair forms the basis for the present concept of therapy.

Diagnosis

Good therapeutic results depend upon early diagnosis, before collapse of the head and distortion of the articular cartilage occur. There is usually no clear history of trauma. The most common complaint is the presence

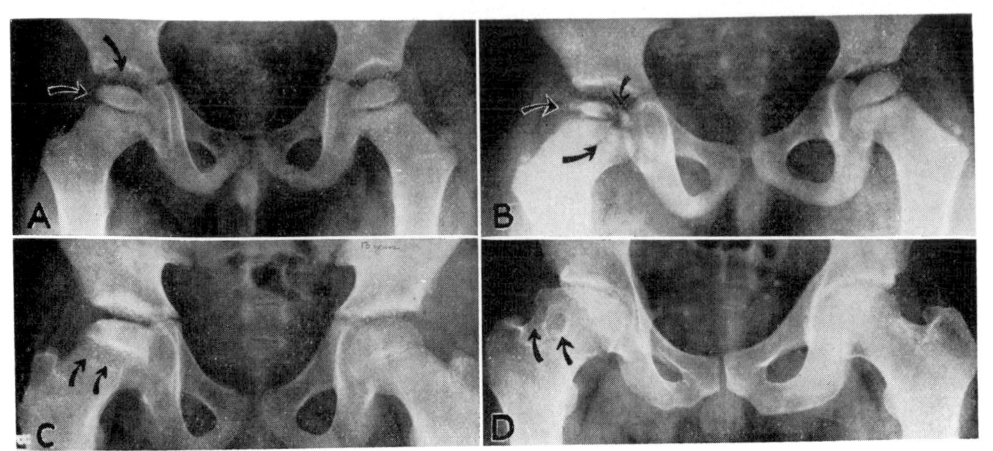

Figure 15–1. Roentgenographic changes in coxa plana.

A. At 4½ years of age, within three months of injury and onset of limp. Note widening of right joint space and slight flattening of femoral head (arrow).

B. At 5 years of age–fragmentation of head with widening and cystification (arrow) in the epiphyseal zone.

C. At 13 years of age–revascularization of the head.

D. At 32 years of age–residual stage. The distortion of the femoral head and incongruity of hip joint might have been averted by early recognition and treatment.

of a limp noted by the parents. The child may have pain, and, if so, it is often referred to the knee region. In the early stages physical examination will reveal muscle spasm which limits movement of the hip, particularly internal rotation, hyperextension, and abduction. Atrophy of the muscles is usually present. In the later stages, if deformity of the head and contracture occur, there may be a fixed adduction and flexion deformity. The roentgen findings (Fig. 15–*1*) are quite characteristic in the later stages, when fragmentation and flattening of the dense epiphysis, broadening of the neck, and widening of the joint space make the diagnosis apparent. The earlier roentgenographic signs are more important, however, and consist of areas of resorption at the femoral neck adjacent to the epiphyseal plate, slight thinning or flattening of the ossification center, and, perhaps, beginning fragmentation. The laboratory is helpful in the differential diagnosis. The blood count, sedimentation rate, and Mantoux test all are within normal limits.

Differential diagnosis. Since coxa plana is a manifestation of avascularity, an underlying cause for the loss of blood supply must be considered. A focus of *osteomyelitis* in the neck of the femur, an infarct due to *sickle cell anemia,* and replacement of the femoral neck by *Gaucher cells* or *neoplasm* are some of the possibilities. Early *tuberculosis* of the hip joint must be excluded. The elevation of the sedimentation rate, the positive Mantoux test and narrowing of the joint space roentgenographically (space is wider in coxa plana) are invaluable aids. *Rheumatic fever* and *rheumatoid arthritis* generally involve multiple joints and produce a different laboratory picture. Certain *normal variants* occurring in ossification may resemble early coxa plana roentgenographically, and in these questionable cases the treatment should be the same as for coxa plana until the cause is established.

Treatment

The primary aim is to remove the strain of weight bearing. If pain and muscle spasm are severe, the child should be placed upon a régime of bed rest and skin traction to the limb until the acute symptoms disappear (usually within two weeks). Weight bearing should be avoided throughout the stage of repair, and this can generally be accomplished efficiently by the use of a sling (Fig. 15–2) and crutch walking. It should

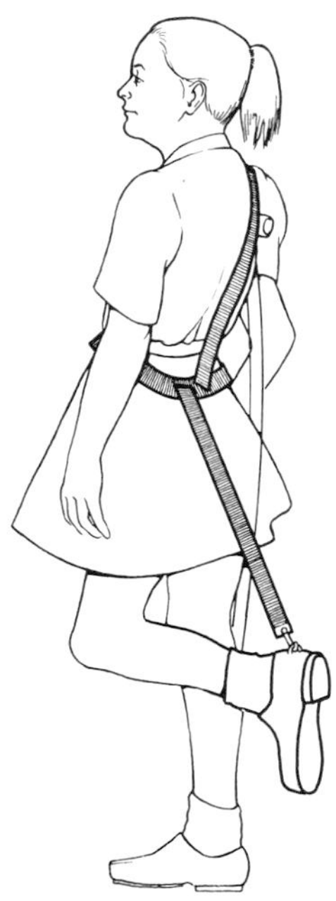

Figure 15–2. Sling used in treatment of unilateral coxa plana. (Left crutch not shown.)

be remembered that occasionally both hips become involved in coxa plana, and the "good hip" should be evaluated repeatedly throughout the crutch-walking period. Contractures can be avoided by hyperextension exercises. Twelve to 24 months or more may be required before roentgenograms reveal the end stage of repair. The vulnerable femoral head should be spared the stress of weight bearing throughout this period. Attempts at speeding revascularization by drilling the epiphyseal zone have not improved the results and may do more harm than good. The use of plaster immobilization generally has been abandoned. Rigid immobilization of this sort over a period of months produces bone atrophy and may affect the eventual development of the extremity. The walking caliper splint is in use in many clinics; however, this does not remove strain from the femoral head as effectively as the sling and crutch method.

In old cases, with secondary osteoarthritic changes associated with pain, the choice lies between arthroplasty and arthrodesis.

SLIPPING OF THE UPPER FEMORAL EPIPHYSIS

Displacement of the capital femoral epiphysis may follow severe trauma as a so-called "acute slip," but more commonly is of gradual onset occurring over a period of months from chronic stress. It is seen between the ages of 10 and 16 years, more commonly in boys. These youngsters are either of the obese "Fröhlich type," or of the rapidly growing, tall, "bean-pole" variety. The high incidence of slipping in the obese group is probably the result of load and mechanical strain rather than of an inherent "endocrine effect." The tall, lanky child has just finished a spurt of growth, and the epiphyseal plate is becoming more calcified in preparation for closure. In this instance the brittle, hypercalcified zone of cartilage, such as is normally present immediately before the blood vessels invade the plate for final ossification and closure, may fracture. There may be a complete fracture or a gradual disintegration following repeated minute fractures. Theories involving low-grade infection and hypofunction of the pituitary are less logical and lack substantiation.

Pathology

The "acute slip." Complete and sudden disruption through the hypercalcified cartilage results in the same sort of displacement as is seen in other fractures of the neck of the femur. Pain produces spasm in the muscles which cross the joint. The long muscles pull the shaft upward so that the head appears to be displaced into a varus position in relation to the neck. The external rotators of the hip joint are more numerous and powerful than are the internal rotators. The shaft is externally rotated, causing the head to lie posterior to the neck. The head appears to have been displaced downward and posteriorly. The blood supply to the head may be destroyed, except for the ligamentum teres vessel. The important vessels within the retinaculum of Weitbrecht may be severed. Avascular necrosis of the capital ossification center, with subsequent collapse and distortion of the articular cartilage, occurred in five of nine cases (55 per cent) of acute disruption encountered by the writer.

The "gradual slip." Gradual epiphyseolysis begins with fragmentation at the hypercalcified zone of the epiphyseal plate, producing what is widely termed a "pre-slipped" stage. These minute fractures are accompanied by the normal hyperemic response to injury. This hyperemia accounts for the decalcification of adjacent bone and the irregular widening of the epiphyseal line seen roentgenographically at this stage. Subsequent muscular pull and weight-bearing stress may cause the head gradually to migrate. As the head slowly moves downward and backward two processes are occurring simultaneously: additional minute fractures at the epiphyseal plate, and repair. Granulation tissue, fibrosis, cartilage, osteoid, and new bone form locally in natural physiological repair. These tissues accumulate along the anterior and inferior portion of the neck, causing it to become widened. Since the head is migrating posteriorly and inferiorly, the new bone causes the neck to appear bowed and twisted. Microscopic sections through the region of slipping show every stage of fracture repair, i.e., hemorrhage, small fragments of necrotic bone, granulation tissue, fibrosis, cartilage, new bone, and maturing bone. Small areas of fresh fracture are mixed with the various stages of repair. The vascular retinaculum becomes shortened as the head moves backward, and is then particularly susceptible to injury if the head is forcibly replaced.

Diagnosis

Patients with an acute slip usually present a history of trauma. The symptoms of a gradual slip are insidious, and commence with fatigue, limp, and pain. Pain usually is referred to the knee region, and may be lacking at the hip. This may focus attention upon the knee and often leads to a mistaken diagnosis. Physical examination consistently reveals a limitation of internal rotation. It is often difficult to distinguish restriction of movement based upon muscle spasm from that produced by bony deformity. If the femoral head has migrated any appreciable distance, some shortening of the extremity will be present and the limb will rotate externally and tend to abduct when flexed. Acute displacements are more painful and produce the signs of a fracture of the neck of the femur. The roentgenographic findings (Fig. 15–3) vary between four major patterns: pre-slip, acute-slip, gradual slip, and residual. The important characteristic of the pre-slip stage is the irregular widening of the epiphyseal line. In acute displacements there is a displaced fracture through the epiphyseal line, and no evidence of new bone formation or repair. Gradual epiphyseolysis demands study of both hips in the anteroposterior and lateral planes. If the displacement is slight, one sees widening of the epiphyseal line, minimal tilting of the femoral head, and a trace of thickening of the neck. If marked displacement has occurred, torsion and widening of the neck, formation of a beak of bone at the inferior aspect of the neck adjacent to the epiphyseal plate, end-to-side position of the head, and avascular changes may be observed. Late cases may show residual deformity of the neck, malposition and avascular necrosis

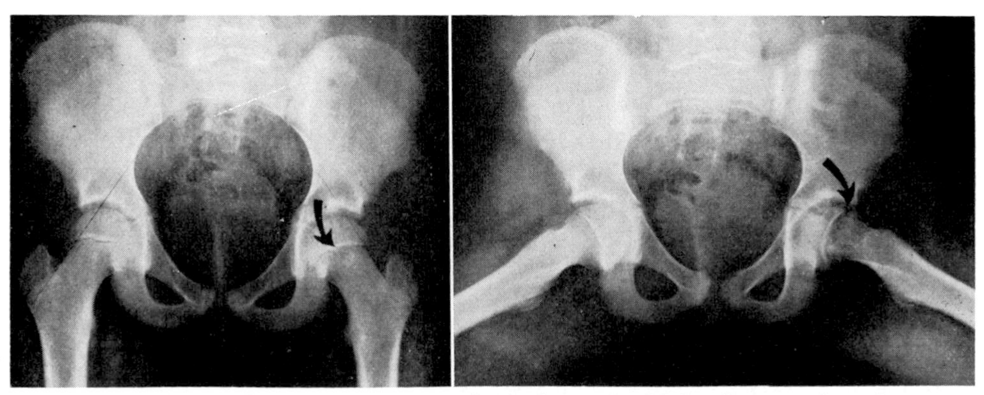

Figure 15–3. Slipped upper femoral epiphysis should be diagnosed at this stage, when migration is minimal. Note widening of the epiphyseal zone (arrow) and, in the lateral view, slight posterior displacement of the head (arrow).

of the head, and secondary osteoarthritis. Laboratory studies are not helpful. The incidence of bilateral involvement is about 25 per cent.

Differential diagnosis. Any complaint of pain in the hip or knee in an adolescent should suggest the diagnosis of slipped upper femoral epiphysis. Roentgenographic examination of both hips in the anteroposterior and lateral views is indicated. The roentgen picture is diagnostic. Old residual deformities may be confused with other conditions producing coxa vara in childhood. The early pre-slipping stage can be confused with early tuberculosis or osteomyelitis, and examination should include determination of blood count and sedimentation rate, and Mantoux test, to exclude these possibilities.

Treatment

The treatment of an acute slip follows general fracture principles with special emphasis upon the threatened loss of blood supply to the proximal fragment. The injured extremity should immediately be immobilized in a Thomas splint for transportation to relieve pain and to minimize damage to the soft part attachments of the femoral head. The reduction should be as atraumatic as possible. Closed manipulative reduction may succeed, and many surgeons favor this method and use it in conjunction with blind nailing. The writer prefers open reduction, believing it to be more accurate, sure, and gentle. Forceful repeated manipulations may sever any remaining nourishing attachments, and should be avoided. Reduction is followed by internal fixation. Plaster immobilization generally has been discarded, because it is a less certain means of controlling reduction, roentgen appraisal is made difficult, and prolonged immobilization may affect the development of the limb. The patient is taught crutch walking, and weight bearing is forbidden until the epiphysis has closed. If avascular necrosis supervenes, it is advisable to extend the non–weight-bearing period until the necrotic bone has been revascularized, or until it is certain that revascularization will not occur. The articular cartilage is nourished by synovial fluid, and will remain healthy unless it is distorted by collapse of underlying bone. Unfortunately, 18 to 24 months may be required before revascularization by "creeping substitution" has been complete. The treatment of acute displacement differs in no way from that of a fracture of the neck of the femur in an adult; however, the patient's youth makes it doubly important to leave no stone unturned which might further the chances of obtaining a durable hip.

The results of treatment in patients with gradual slipping are much better when therapy is instituted before marked displacement of the head has occurred. When displacement of the head is less than 1 cm., it is better to accept the existing deformity than to attempt to replace the femoral head in normal position. At this stage, the objective is to obtain bony union between the head and the neck, and to prevent further slipping until this has occurred. Weight-bearing stress should be removed immediately, and the patient admitted to a hospital. One cannot depend upon crutch walking alone to stop the progression of slipping. The head

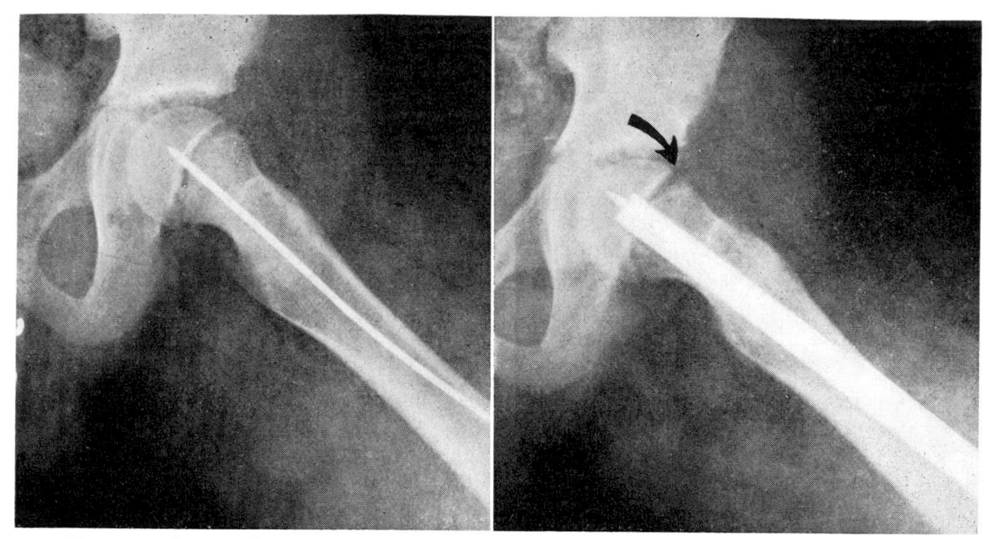

Figure 15–4. Slipped femoral epiphysis with minimal displacement.
Left. Error of failing to adequately transfix the head prior to nail insertion.
Right. Note displacement of the head produced by impact of the nail (arrow).

should be securely fixed to the neck with a tri-flanged Smith-Petersen nail. Some surgeons prefer the multiple pins of Moore, because they believe this method inflicts less trauma on the femoral head. However, displacement of the head by the impact of the Smith-Petersen nail (Fig. 15–*4*) can be prevented by transfixing the neck, head, and acetabulum with a stiff guide wire before inserting the nail. Internal fixation prevents further displacement and maintains alignment until the epiphysis is closed. Howorth advocates the insertion of multiple iliac bone pegs across the epiphyseal plate to accelerate closure. If secure internal fixation is obtained, the patient may be ambulated on crutches within a few days after operation, provided the condition of the opposite hip permits. Bone pegs alone do not supply secure fixation, and when this method is used an eight-week postoperative bed stay is necessary before crutch walking is instituted. In either instance, weight bearing is not allowed until the epiphyseal line has closed. Treatment of the slipping of mild degree makes possible a simpler operative procedure with an excellent prognosis. Avascular necrosis is uncommon, provided the position of the head is not disturbed at the time of operation.

When the displacement has progressed beyond 1 cm. the problem becomes more difficult. Displacement is a precursor of traumatic arthritis. Gross malposition of the head necessitates correction of alignment, which is accompanied by further damage to the blood supply of the head, and avascular necrosis frequently compromises the result. The vessels along the postero-inferior aspect of the neck remain as the major source of nutrition to the head, and these shorten as the neck shifts forward and upward. They are disrupted by forceful manipulation or improper surgery. New bone formation has increased the length of the neck. Carefully performed wedge resections through the callus (Fig. 15–5, *A*) may be

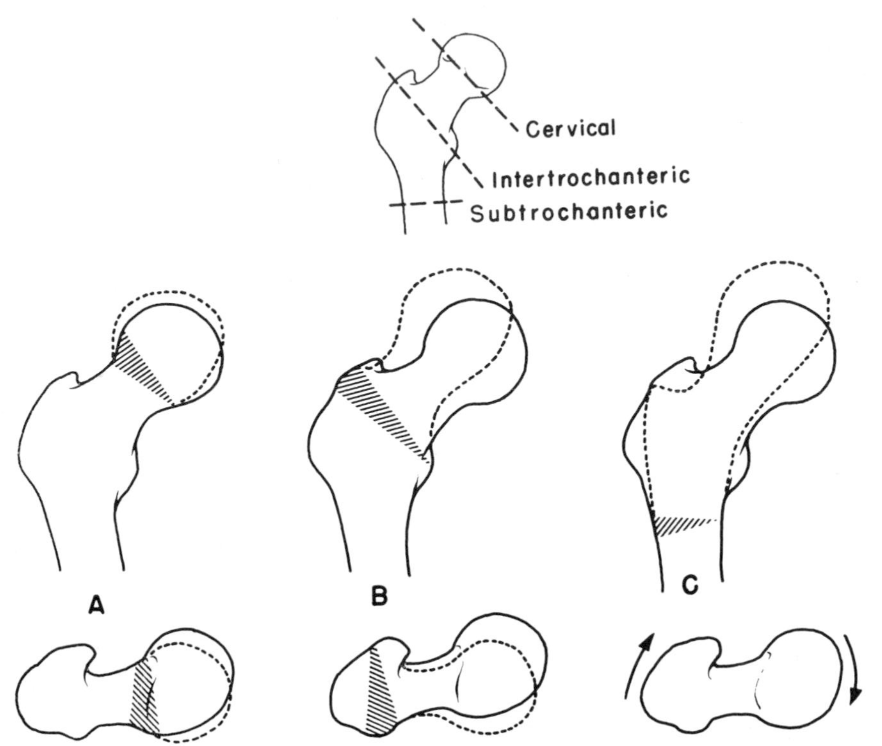

Figure 15–5. Osteotomies used for correction of slipped capital femoral epiphysis with significant displacement.
A. Cervical.
B. Base of neck.
C. Subtrochanteric.

successful, if the neck is shortened sufficiently to permit repositioning of the head without exertion of tension on the posterior vascular retinaculum. An osteotomy through the base of the neck (Fig. 15–5, *B*) has been favored by some, because there is less risk of injuring Weitbrecht's retinaculum. Subtrochanteric osteotomy (Fig. 15–5, *C*) has been used to correct internal rotation and adduction; however, although this method preserves the nutrition of the head, it has the disadvantage of rendering complete correction difficult. Each of these types of osteotomy is followed by internal fixation to maintain alignment. The Smith-Petersen nail alone is adequate for the cervical wedge resection (Fig. 15–6), but in the two other types of osteotomy attachment of the nail to the femoral shaft is required. These procedures demand gentleness, skill, anatomical knowledge, and attention to detail. They can be classed with the most difficult operations of skeletal surgery. Improperly executed osteotomy, forceful manipulation, and misdirected fixation invite failure and permanent disability. The major early complication is avascular necrosis of the head, and under ideal circumstances this still occurs in about 30 per cent of these patients. Even if the nutrition proves adequate, arthritis may develop later because of incongruity. Since osteotomy with internal fixation is a relatively new procedure

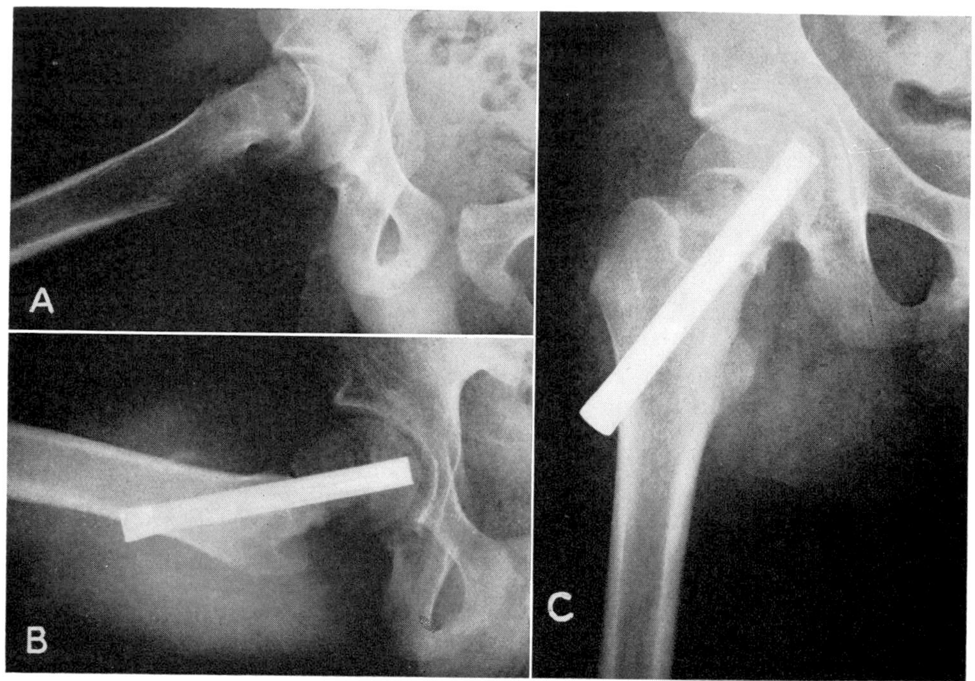

Figure 15–6. Correction of epiphyseal displacement by osteotomy through the base of the **neck.**

A. Preoperative view showing 55 degrees retroversion.

B, C. Anteroposterior and lateral views showing correction. The ten-year result is excellent.

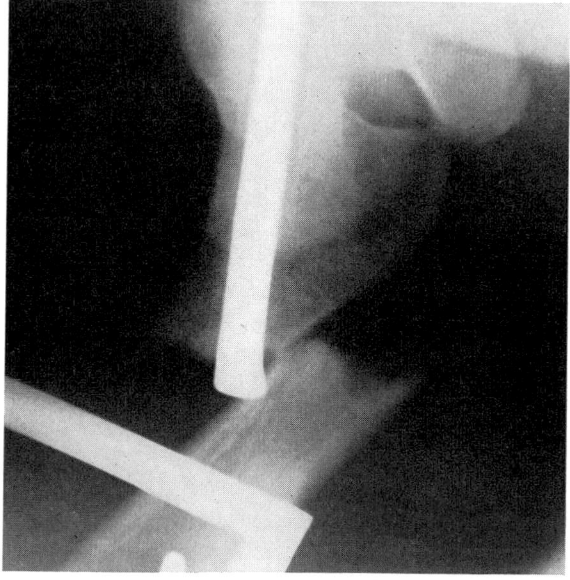

Figure 15–7. This fracture occurred at the base of the nail three years after successful treatment of a slipped epiphysis. The metal is rigid, compared with the bone, and should be removed following epiphyseal closure.

and was not performed until about 18 years ago, much more time will be required for the full evaluation of the results of its different variations and modifications. In any case, the nail should be removed after the epiphysis has closed (Fig. 15–7).

When the displacement has existed for more than two years, and narrowing of the joint or other evidences of arthritic change have appeared, treatment must consist of an arthroplasty or arthrodesis at such time as symptoms demand. In this event, no attempt at realignment of the head is indicated. A recent operation, consisting of simple removal of the bony prominence from the anterior aspect of the neck, is of interest but has not been fully evaluated.

AVULSION OF EPIPHYSES AT THE HIP

Avulsion of the Greater Trochanter

Most fractures of the greater trochanter are produced by direct violence. Occasionally detachment and retraction are produced by the gluteus medius and gluteus minimus. This ossification center appears earlier than do the other traction epiphyses, being present at four years of age. It remains open until age 17. Surgical repair or plaster immobilization is rarely, if ever, indicated. Crutch-walking ambulation and progressive function have consistently produced excellent results with a minimal disability period.

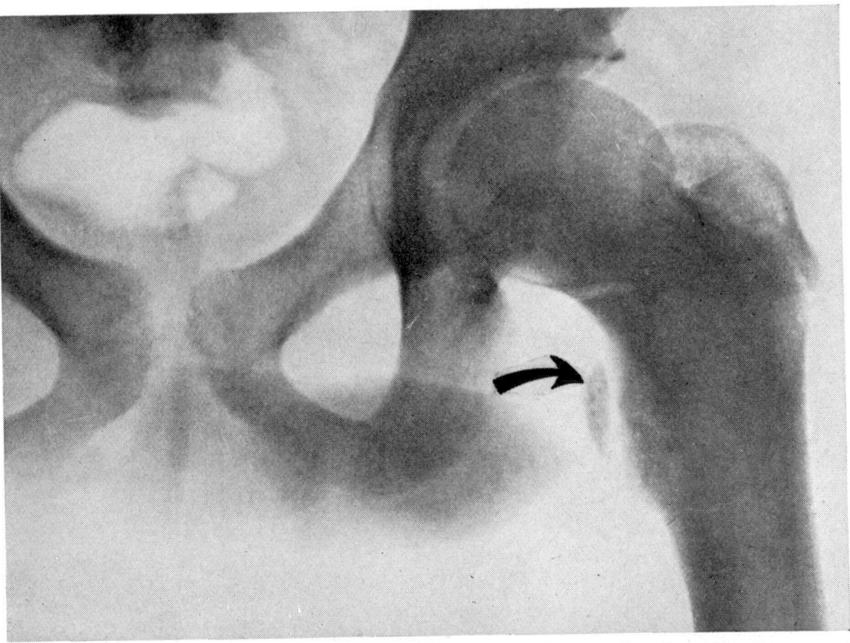

Figure 15–8. Avulsion of epiphysis of lesser trochanter by iliopsoas (arrow). These injuries are usually seen in boys of about 15 years of age, just prior to closure of the epiphysis.

Avulsion of the Lesser Trochanter

This epiphysis is sometimes avulsed by the iliopsoas muscle (Fig. 15–8). Since the attachment of the iliopsoas tendon includes a portion of the femur distal to the epiphysis, the displacement is usually limited, and surgical replacement is unnecessary. Crutch walking may be desirable for the first two weeks, at which time symptoms usually have subsided sufficiently for the resumption of normal ambulation.

FRACTURES OF THE HIP

A sprained hip in an individual past middle life must be considered to be a fracture until it is proved otherwise. Fractures of the neck and trochanteric portion of the femur are seen with equal frequency. They form the most common and important group of hip problems. They usually occur in elderly persons, in whom bone changes of the declining years are present.

GENERAL CONSIDERATIONS

Classification

It is necessary to differentiate hip fractures into several categories in order to understand individual problems. It is essential to apply a simple

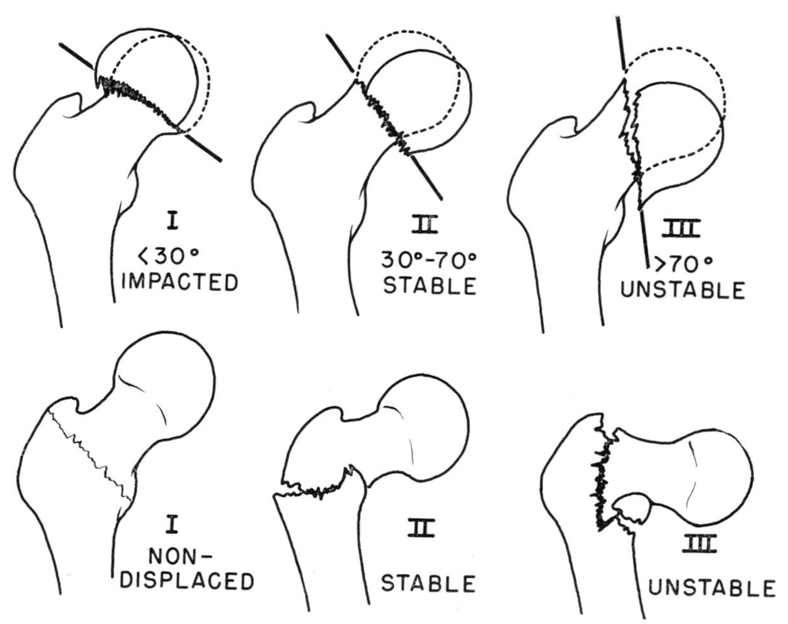

Figure 15–9. Classification of hip fractures.

Upper. Intracapsular group: type I, "impacted valgus" (10 per cent); type II, "transcervical" (25 per cent); type III, "vertical subcapital" (18 per cent). (Degrees indicate angle of incidence of fracture line.)

Lower. Intertrochanteric group: type I, "nondisplaced" (15 per cent); type II, "stable" (6 per cent); type III, "comminuted" (29 per cent).

TABLE 15–1. INCIDENCE OF RESULTS IN INTRACAPSULAR AND EXTRACAPSULAR FRACTURES

	Intracapsular	*Extracapsular*
Avascular necrosis	40%	Nil
Nonunion	20%	Nil
Mortality	4%	20%

working classification to a discussion of diagnosis, treatment, and prognosis. The diagrams (Fig. 15–9) schematically illustrate the salient roentgen criteria and the incidence of these important groups. In general, it may be stated that intracapsular fractures produce less morbidity and mortality than do extracapsular lesions. The former are splinted by the capsule. On the other hand, nonunion and avascular necrosis of the femoral head frequently complicate certain intracapsular fractures, but rarely are seen in the extracapsular group (Table 15–*1*).

There are three main types of intracapsular fractures (Fig. 15–9). Pauwels emphasized the importance of these categories in so far as the prognosis for union was concerned. It is, of course, apparent that these considerations have direct bearing upon diagnostic criteria and the rationale of treatment, as well as the eventual prognosis.

Extracapsular fractures include those involving the base of the neck (within ligamentous attachments), and intertrochanteric and subtrochanteric lesions. Although these fractures cause little concern with regard to avascular necrosis and nonunion, the displaced fractures of this group produce severe systemic effects and high mortality. In addition, in the unstable comminuted type there is an overwhelming tendency toward varus rotation, resulting in significant shortening of the extremity. Displaced intertrochanteric fractures are serious injuries, and should not be confused with the simpler nondisplaced fractures. The differences depend on the extent of the soft part trauma and bony comminution.

Blood Supply of the Femoral Head

The articular cartilage is nourished by synovial fluid, and is not dependent upon a blood supply. The underlying bone cannot survive critical vascular privation. Extensive division of nourishing vessels is followed by death of bone. If the necrotic bone is subjected to weight-bearing stress it will collapse, and then the overlying articular surface becomes deformed. Traumatic arthritis results from this incongruity of weight-bearing surfaces.

Why is avascular necrosis a common sequela of type II and type III intracapsular fractures when it rarely follows type I lesions? Do extracapsular fractures ever cause avascular necrosis of the femoral head? A knowledge of the blood supply to the upper femur is essential. There are three main sources: (1) intramedullary arteries coming through the neck of the femur, which for the most part do not cross the point where the epiphyseal plate had previously been situated and are, perhaps, the least

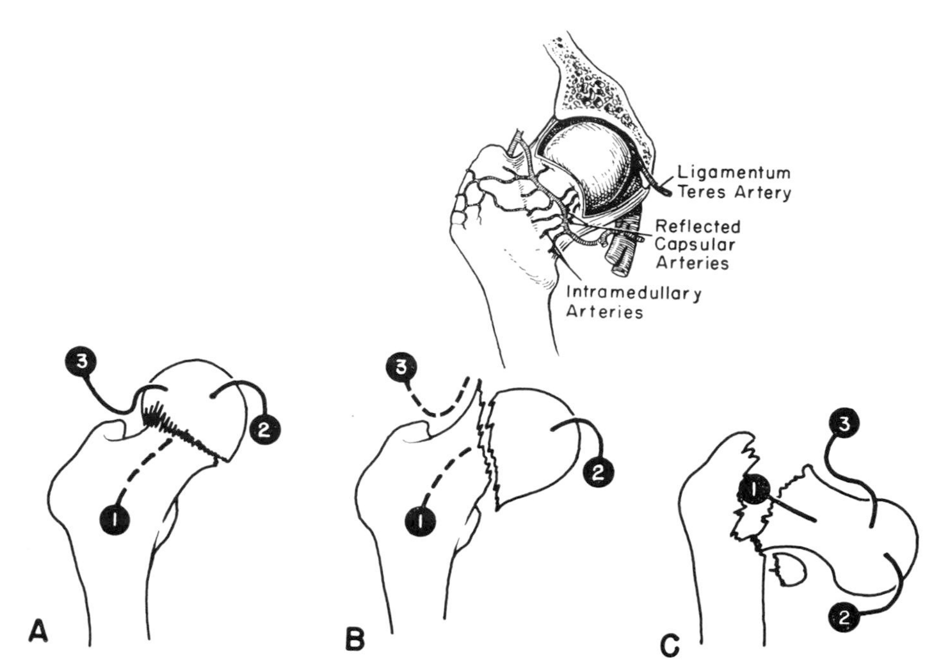

Figure 15–10. Blood supply to the head of the femur: (1) intramedullary arteries, (2) ligamentum teres artery, (3) reflected capsular arteries.

A. Avascular necrosis of the femoral head is an infrequent complication of an impacted lesion of the femoral neck.

B. It frequently occurs after a displaced intracapsular fracture.

C. Avascular necrosis is never seen after a trochanteric fracture.

important; (2) the ligamentum teres artery, which is derived from the obturator artery or medial circumflex femoral vessel, or both, and is of variable importance; and (3) capsular vessels, which are branches of the gluteal and medial circumflex femoral arteries and are especially prominent along the posterior aspect of the head and neck, forming the major source of blood supply. Avascular necrosis does not follow extracapsular fractures (Fig. 15–*10*), and it does not often complicate impacted valgus (type I) lesions, because in this situation the important vessels coming through the reflected capsule remain intact. Half of the type II and type III intracapsular fractures produce enough vascular damage to cause definite roentgen evidence of avascular necrosis.

Sherman and Phemister have emphasized that replacement of necrotic areas of bone by Axhausen's "creeping substitution" requires many months and continues after bony union of the fracture. Throughout this period the articular cartilage remains healthy, provided the shape of the head is not distorted by weight bearing. Histological facts indicate that, even though avascular necrosis has occurred, traumatic arthritis might be avoided if weight bearing could be eliminated until complete replacement of bone has occurred. Unfortunately, it is usually impossible to effect a prolonged non–weight-bearing régime in this age group.

Shearing Force

Thrust is transmitted from the shaft of the femur to the acetabulum via the angulated neck. This change in direction of mechanical force places leverage upon the neck and trochanteric regions. Muscle spasm following fracture continues to exert force upon the lever. This leverage accounts for the instability of vertical fractures of the neck, and the varus rotation common to comminuted intertrochanteric lesions. Impacted valgus fractures are horizontal, and an impacting pressure results, promoting prompt union. The intracapsular type III fracture often tends to slip after reduction because the head lacks purchase on the neck. In this event the head fragment must be well balanced on the neck before internal fixation is carried out, or subsequent motion at the fracture may occur in spite of the nail. This motion results in resorption of the neck, and nonunion. Seventy-five per cent of the nonunions in 500 hip fractures studied occurred in type III intracapsular lesions.

Extracapsular fractures pass through a vascular part of the femur and union is not a problem. However, before union occurs, shearing occurs, shearing leverage collapses comminuted fragments and often produces disabling amounts of shortening. Nondisplaced and stable intertrochanteric fractures do not tend to shorten.

Treatment of Aged Patients with Hip Fractures

The systemic effect of the injury is related to the extent of soft-part damage and bony comminution, for example, extracapsular fractures generally produce greater morbidity than do intracapsular lesions. Another factor is pain. Nearly all hip fractures produce pain. Pain, in its own right, has decidedly undesirable effects upon elderly patients. It prevents rest and leads to fatigue. It produces a disinclination on the part of the subject to take nourishment, and dehydration may result. Pain immobilizes the patient as a whole, and thus predisposes to thrombophlebitis, cystitis, decubitus ulcer, and pneumonia. Shock is unusual without concomitant injury. However, when definitive treatment is delayed, elderly people with hip fractures rapidly deteriorate into a state of exhaustion and dehydration. It is clear that the best way to reverse this process is to abolish pain by internal fixation of the fracture at the earliest possible time.

When should the operation be performed? Generally, these subjects are at their physiological normal when injured. From then on adverse changes occur. With few exceptions, these patients are in optimal condition to withstand surgery at the instant they fall. As each hour passes, the risk increases. There are only four specific situations in which delay is justified.

1. Diabetic acidosis should be rectified.
2. Cardiac failure and arrhythmias merit full digitalization.
3. Acute myocardial infarction or fresh cerebral hemorrhage demands evaluation.
4. The fracture has been neglected for over 24 hours, and dehydration

and exhaustion give evidence that the advantages of immediate operation have been lost.

Unless one of these specific contraindications is present, reduction and internal fixation should be performed without delay. There is no place for "prophylactic" digitalization. There is no "fluid balance problem" unless the operation has been unduly delayed. There is no need for prolonged medical study. Adequate appraisal should be accomplished within a few hours after the patient's arrival in the hospital. The majority of patients with hip fracture should be operated on within a few hours after admission; in only 20 per cent should surgery be delayed for one day or longer. If one of the four causes for delay is present, the internist should work with the surgeon in aggressive preparation of the patient. The fracture should be treated concomitantly with the medical problem so far as is possible.

Should the patient remain at absolute bed rest for several days after the operation? With specific exceptions it is neither wise nor kind to permit this indulgence to comfort. The patient should be urged to get into a wheelchair within 24 hours after surgery. It is often necessary to assist these activities during the first few days. However, the patient must participate, and is not lifted bodily into a chair like a knight in armor. Repeated and detailed instructions in how to get out of bed are followed by insistence that the individual perform these movements with minimal assistance (Fig. 15–*11*). This spartan program is designed to maintain total physiology and muscle tone. It has been a constant observation that prolonged inactivity so weakens the musculature of old people that few become safe crutch walkers. There are, of course, special problems, such as cardiac disease, uncontrolled diabetes, and recent cerebral accident,

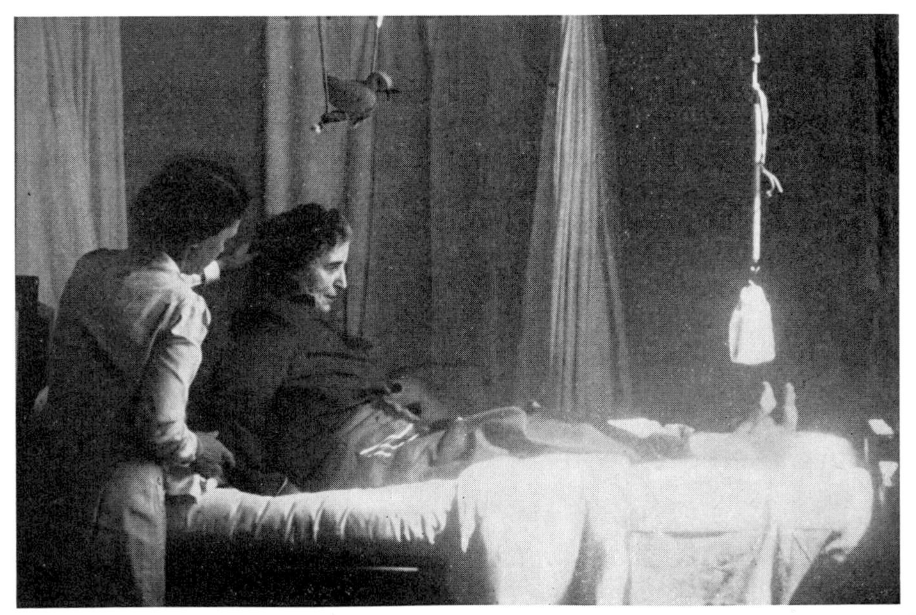

Figure 15–11. Detailed instruction is essential to mobilization of the patient. This patient is pushing herself to the sitting position with her arms, not being lifted like a knight in armor!

which may interdict this program. However, these are relatively uncommon. Ambulation in a walker and on crutches is encouraged as rapidly as it can safely be done.

When should weight bearing be allowed? Sherman and Phemister have emphasized the need for delaying weight bearing when impaired blood supply has rendered the femoral head unsound. Collapse of the head may occur, which otherwise might have been prevented had time been permitted for replacement of necrotic bone. The implementation of this principle is not a simple matter when dealing with aged subjects. Furthermore, the decision as to when union has occurred is often difficult. Roentgenograms and clinical appraisal give no unfailing answer to these questions, and many elderly persons will bear weight when so inclined, regardless of warnings to the contrary.

Does replacement prosthesis have a place in the treatment of fresh fractures? These procedures are considered in detail subsequently in this chapter (p. 453). The immediate insertion of a metal replacement for intracapsular fractures in aged and inactive patients may be indicated. This eliminates the long period necessary for healing, and is useful in situations where life expectancy is not great, or where the patient's ability to ambulate is limited by other causes, such as paralysis, Parkinsonism, or blindness. In general, the use of such appliances as initial treatment is unjustified in younger patients because many years must pass before the late results of these operations will be known. At the present time, primary replacement arthroplasty should be a salvage procedure designed to meet the patient's requirements, and not to treat the fracture.

INTRACAPSULAR FRACTURES OF NECK OF FEMUR

Mechanism of Injury

Most femoral neck fractures (type II and type III) are caused by indirect violence, such as a twisting force, or a misstep on a stairway or uneven ground. Shearing force exerts sufficient leverage so that trivial injury may disrupt senile bone (Fig. 15–*12*). On rare occasions these fractures occur in young adults, but only if the force is severe. Indirect violence displaces the femoral neck upward, producing a varus deformity. The pain of the fracture causes muscles crossing the joint to go into spasm, and the more powerful external rotators pull the shaft into external rotation. Type I lesions (20 per cent of the intracapsular group) are produced by a direct blow on the greater trochanter. The neck is impacted into the head, rolling the proximal fragment into valgus (Figs. 15–*12*, 15–*13*). There is little displacement.

Diagnosis

Every individual in middle life or over who complains of pain in the hip, thigh, or knee following an injury, however trivial the injury might be, should be considered to have a fractured hip until it is proved otherwise by roentgenogram. The fact that the patient is able to walk after the

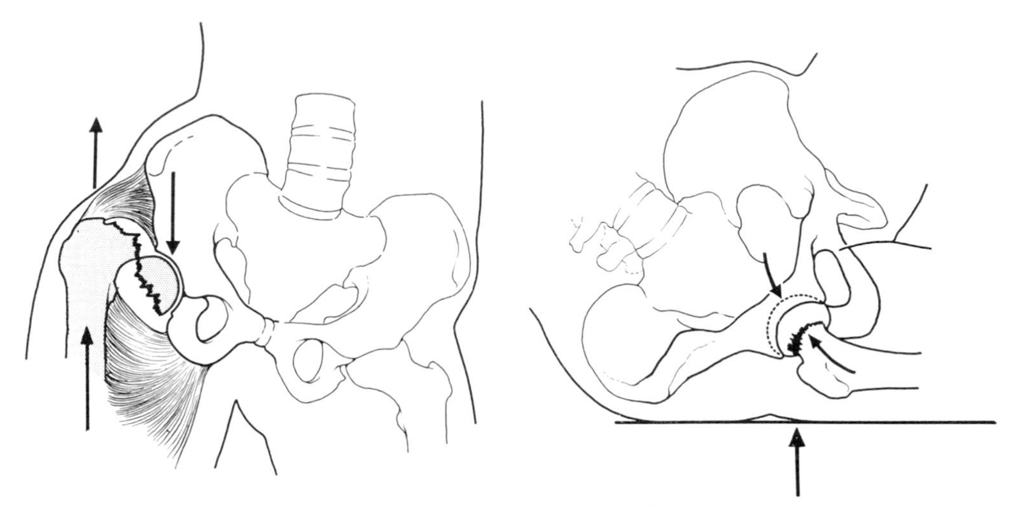

Figure 15–12. Mechanism of injury in femoral neck fractures.
Left. Indirect shearing force producing varus displacement of the head.
Right. Direct blow on the trochanter with resultant valgus impaction.

accident does not rule out a broken hip. Patients with type I (impacted valgus) lesions may walk into the examining room and present no physical signs other than slight muscle spasm. Displaced fractures (type II and type III) are relatively easily diagnosed. External rotation of the extremity, shortening, compared with the opposite side, when measured from the anterosuperior iliac spine to the medial malleolus, tenderness directly over the hip joint, and indirect tenderness on attempted motions of the hip or tapping of the heel are constant findings. Two other signs of little more than academic interest are narrowing of the base of Bryant's triangle, and the presence of the greater trochanter above Nélaton's line. *Nélaton's line* extends from the anterosuperior iliac spine to the ischial tuberosity. Normally the tip of the greater trochanter is on this line, but with displacement of the neck the trochanter comes to lie above it. *Bryant's triangle* is formed by dropping a line from the anterosuperior iliac spine perpendicular to the table with the patient supine, and a second line from the anterosuperior spine through the tip of the greater trochanter with the table as the base. If the trochanter is displaced proximally, the base of this triangle is narrowed in comparison with the normal side.

Accurate diagnosis is dependent upon adequate anteroposterior and lateral roentgenographic studies. These should be obtained *without delay.*

Treatment

Treatment of type I (impacted valgus). The fracture is stable and in ideal position (Fig. 15–*13*). No reduction is necessary. Obviously, any strenuous manipulation would only serve to injure blood supply, and to disrupt impaction, and for these reasons is distinctly undesirable. The aim is to maintain the existing position of the fragments throughout the healing period. If the diagnosis is missed, or if inadequate protection is given

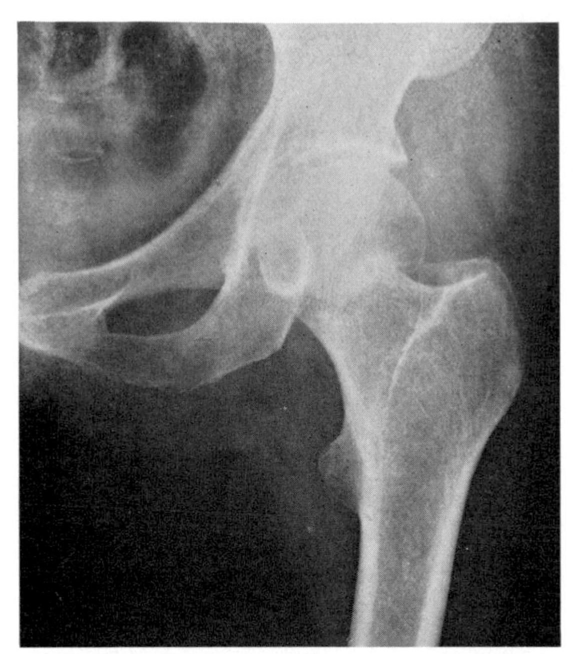

Figure 15–13. Roentgenogram of type I femoral neck fracture. Note the valgus displacement of the head and impaction of the upper corner of the femoral neck fragment into the head fragment.

during convalescence, the fracture may become unimpacted and displaced. Protection and support must be provided until union occurs. This may be accomplished by bed rest with traction or balanced suspension. After eight weeks the patient is taught crutch walking and non–weight-bearing ambulation is begun. Weight bearing is allowed about four months after injury. Satisfactory results are usually obtained with this method. However, when one considers the effect of prolonged immobilization upon the geriatric patient from the systemic, social, and economic views it becomes apparent that a better way to accomplish the objective in view is by internal fixation (without altering the position of the fragments), early crutch ambulation, and maintenance of normal physiology.

TECHNIQUE OF "BLIND" NAILING. A 9-cm. incision is made over the lateral aspect of the greater trochanter from its tip downward. This is deepened through tensor fascia femoris tendon and vastus lateralis muscle to bone. The ridge of origin of vastus lateralis at the lateral aspect of the trochanter is found. The nail will be inserted 3 cm. below this point (Fig. 15–*14*). A three-flange cut is made in the lateral femoral cortex with a drill and small osteotome. This step makes it possible to feel the guide wire in cancellous bone for accurate insertion, and later reduces the risk of the nail catching and carrying the wire with it. If the limb is rotated inward 20 degrees, the femoral neck is horizontal. The largest Kirschner wire that can be passed through the cannula of a Smith-Petersen nail is selected. The wire is *pushed* by sense of touch into the neck of the femur to the greatest distance possible at an angle of 45 degrees from the femoral

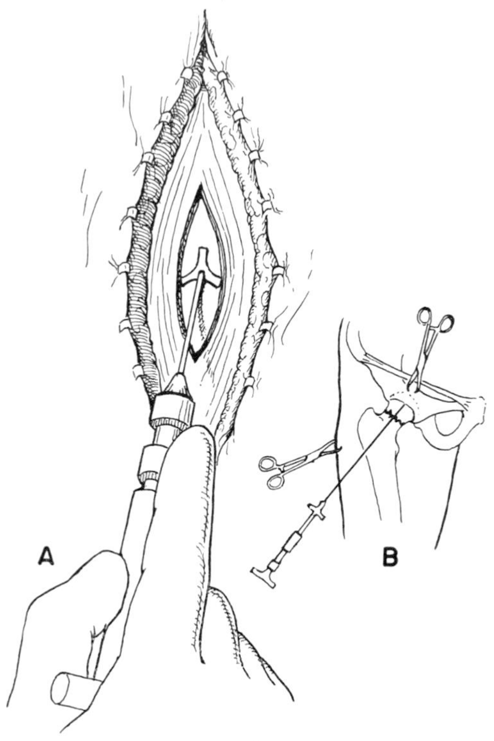

Figure 15–14. Technique of blind nailing.

A. Tri-flange opening in cortex made 3 cm. below trochanteric ridge facilitates free palpation of the interior of the neck with the guide wire.

B. Guide wire inserted at a 45 degree angle with the shaft, with towel clamp 1 inch below center of Poupart's ligament, is a guide. Femur is internally rotated 15 degrees and wire held parallel to the floor for proper anteroposterior alignment.

shaft. Often the sides of the neck of the femur can be palpated with the point of the wire from within for determination of direction. The wire is then drilled through the fracture lines, through the head of the femur, and into the acetabulum. Resistance is encountered at each of these three levels. The stiff wire transfixes the head to the neck and acetabulum so that the fracture will remain impacted when the nail strikes the head (Fig. 15–*15*). Prior to insertion of the nail roentgenograms are taken in two planes to check the position of the guide wire. If the first wire does not pass through the center of the head, a second wire is inserted at a corrected angle to the first. The length of nail is determined by measuring the amount of guide wire outside of the bone in comparison with a wire of identical length. The amount within the bone is thus known, and the roentgenogram taken for checking the position of the wire can be used to indicate proper nail length. The nail is passed over the wire and pushed through the cortical opening. It is then driven home with sharp, firm blows. If the nail is passed through the outer cortex by hand, there is little danger of the wire becoming kinked by the cannula of the nail, and of being driven in ahead of the nail. Final anteroposterior and lateral roent-

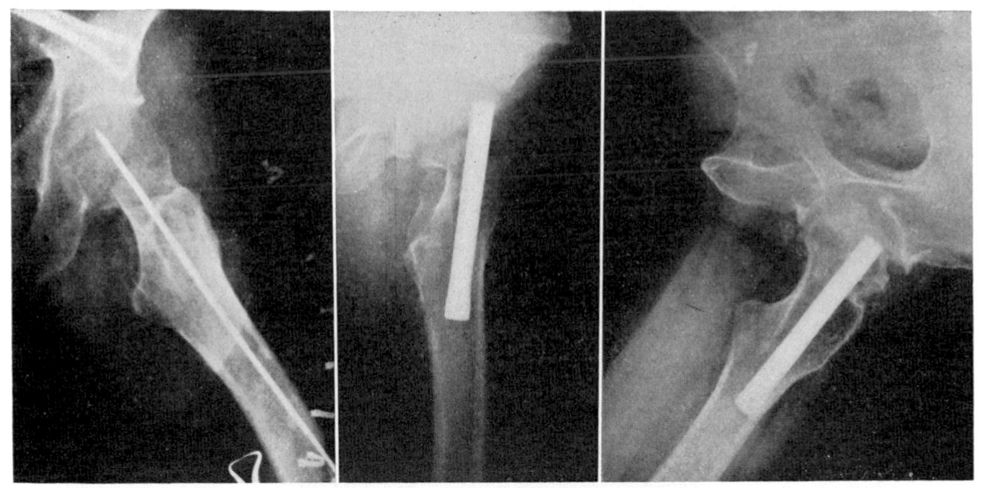

Figure 15–15. Impacted valgus fracture seen in lateral view.
Left. Guide wire in position, but failing to transfix the head to the acetabulum.
Center. Displacement of the head and disimpaction produced by the impact of the nail.
Right. Segmental necrosis 18 months later. This complication was preventable.

genograms are taken after removal of the guide wire. The wound is closed loosely, obliterating dead space but permitting escape of accumulated blood. Final roentgen confirmation of the length and position of the nail is essential.

Postoperative Treatment. The patient starts knee-bending and leg-raising exercises, and is gotten out of bed (Fig. 15–*11*) to the wheelchair within 24 hours after operation. Moderate discomfort in the thigh is usual, and accentuates the patient's natural fear. It is the surgeon's task to reassure the patient until confidence has been regained. As soon as muscular control has been re-established, instruction in crutch walking is begun. This usually starts in the walker on about the fourth day after operation. Repeated, step-by-step, painstaking guidance converts the majority of these patients into expert crutch walkers. If, after an adequate trial of instruction, it becomes apparent that the subject will not be safe on crutches, time is spent in teaching the use of the wheelchair. The wheelchair patient should also be able to use the bathroom, dress, and live relatively independently. The average patient leaves the hospital between the second and third week after operation. Weight bearing is allowed about four months after injury.

Treatment of type II (mid-neck). The displaced fragments must be repositioned before nailing. Accurate reduction is necessary, and a stable position is usually obtainable because the type II fracture is relatively horizontal (Fig. 15–*16*). The angle is 35 to 70 degrees from the horizontal (Pauwels), so that impacting force offsets shearing stress if reduction is proper. Roentgen criteria for the completeness of reduction are often misleading. The writer and his associates are unwilling to rely upon roentgenographic evidence alone, and, for this reason, during recent years

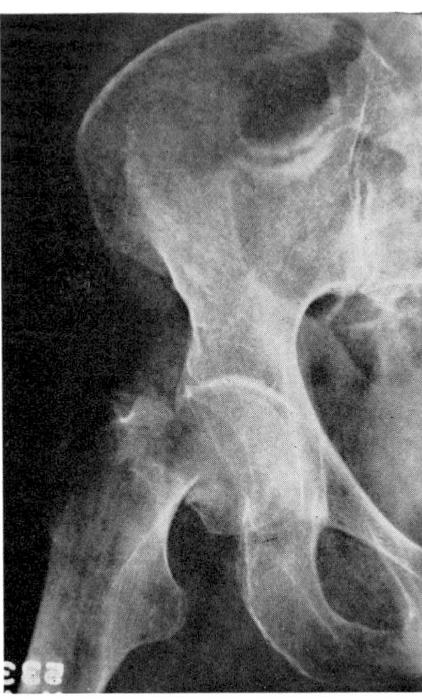

Figure 15–16. Type II intracapsular fracture. Angle of inclination is less than 70 degrees. A stable reduction should be possible.

have performed open reduction of all type II fractures. Reduction is more certain when performed under direct vision. The head of the femur should be balanced securely on the neck before the nail is inserted. Recent studies show that accurate stable reductions by the open method have reduced the incidence of nonunion. These studies indicate that, contrary to previous belief, avascular necrosis of the head fragment occurs no more frequently after technically adequate open reduction than after closed reduction and "blind" nailing.

TECHNIQUE OF OPEN REDUCTION. A lateral approach seems preferable to an anterior or posterior route. The anterior (Smith-Petersen) incision gives a good view of the fracture, but offers little room for nail insertion, and it is difficult to maintain reduction of the fragments during the nailing procedure, if the patient is positioned for a posterior exposure. It is preferable to have the limb free, and the patient supine on an ordinary operating table. Lateral exposure (Fig. 15–*17*) begins 1 inch behind the anterosuperior iliac spine, and passes downward over the greater trochanter, extending the same distance in line with the shaft of the femur. The sheath of the tensor fascia lata is opened along the anterior margin of the muscular portion and the muscle is pushed forward. As the fascia lata is opened, the vastus lateralis and the insertion of the gluteus medius come into view. The precapsular fat is found just anterior and medial to the gluteus medius tendon, and through this the capsule can be opened from the acetabulum to the intertrochanteric line. The vastus lateralis is

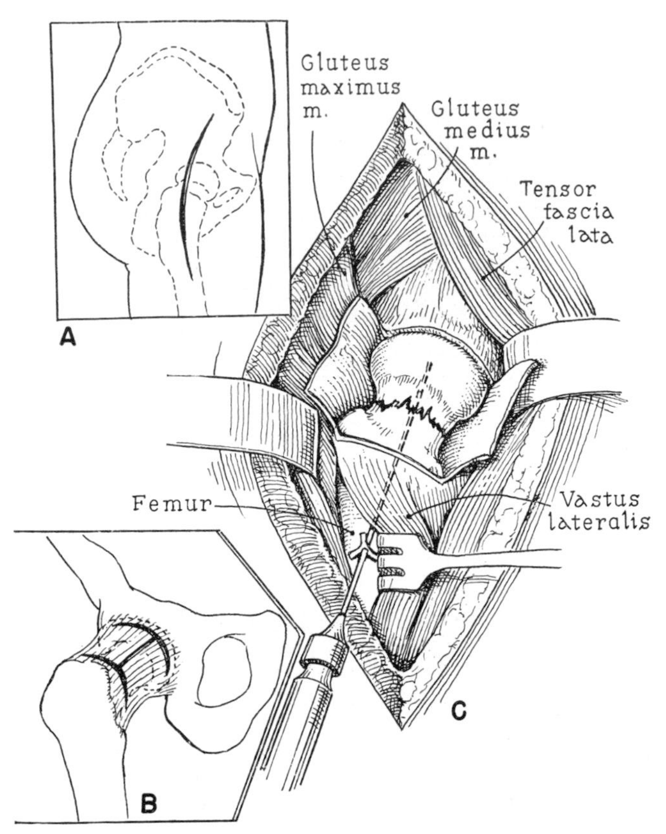

Figure 15–17. Technique of open reduction.

A. The incision begins 1 inch behind the anteroposterior spine and passes downward over the trochanter.

B. The anterior capsule is opened by an H incision.

C. The tensor fascia muscle is retracted forward.

incised, care being taken to clamp and ligate the large transverse branches of the lateral circumflex femoral artery contained within it. The capsule should be opened sufficiently to permit good visualization of the fracture. The limb is rotated inward, and abducted, and the neck is pushed medially under the head. Following complete reduction of type II fractures, there should be sufficient stability so that the head moves with the neck as one piece when the limb is gently rotated. *The nail should not be inserted until a completely stable reduction has been obtained.* Internal fixation with guide wire and nail follows the same steps as in "blind" nailing. However, a plate often must be attached to the base of the nail to prevent motion of the nail within the neck of the femur (Fig. 15–*18*). The fragments may be impacted before wound closure.

AFTERCARE. Treatment in the hospital and during the first few months after operation differs in no way from that following "blind" nailing. Early, intensive, detailed instruction soon makes crutch walking possible for most of these patients. The others are accommodated to a wheelchair existence. Local reparative processes demand abstinence from weight bearing

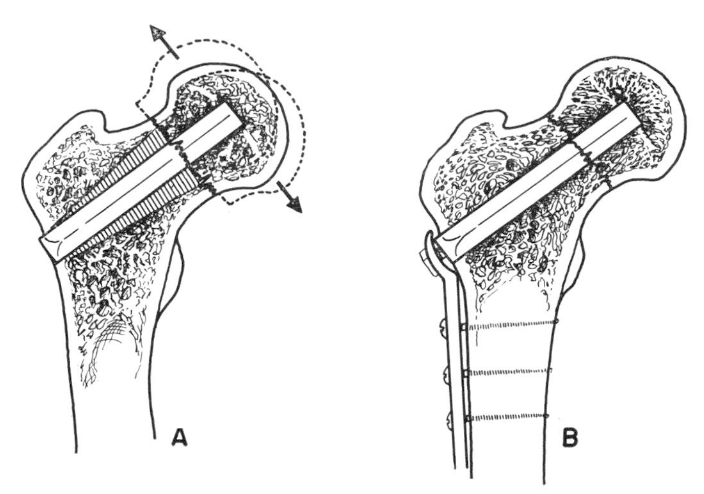

Figure 15–18. The wobble of the nail in the neck of the femur (A) may be eliminated by addition of a plate at the base of the nail (B). The proximal portion of the neck does not grasp the nail securely.

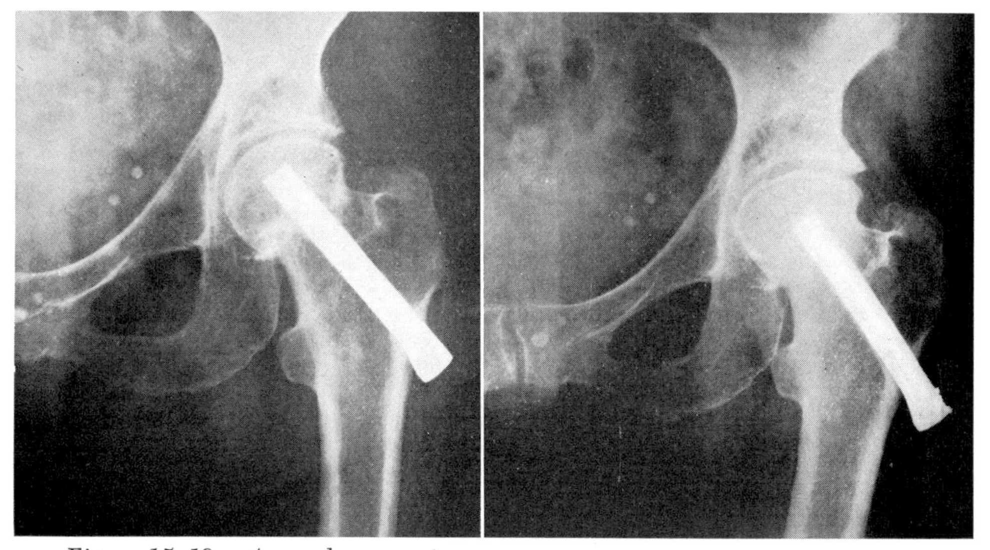

Figure 15–19. Avascular necrosis.

Left. Well healed fracture and normal contour of the head one year after injury, at which time weight bearing was begun.

Right. Ten months later showing collapse of the head. The second nine month period is critical!

until the fracture has united and the head fragment becomes revascularized. Other than the more nearly horizontal direction to the fracture line, type II lesions present the same problems as type III fractures. Although there is a higher incidence of nonunion following type III lesions, vascular damage is essentially the same in both situations. Where there are massive areas of bone necrosis, 18 to 24 months will be required for revascularization and replacement. If weight bearing is begun before this process is complete, the head will collapse (Fig. 15–*19*). To date there is no accurate method for determining the state of the blood supply to the femoral head, nor any measure for gauging termination of the non–weight-bearing period. Union of type II fractures generally is complete within six months. Sherman and Phemister suggested that crutch walking for an additional period of a year or so after union has occurred would eliminate late collapse of the femoral head. Unfortunately, the age of these patients makes it impossible to enforce such a program, and the average patient will bear weight after the sixth month, regardless of instructions.

Treatment of type III (vertical subcapital). There is no more difficult problem in fracture surgery than that presented by this injury. Even if the most thorough reduction is carried out, the head still has a tendency to slip downward. The head lacks purchase on the neck (Fig. 15–*20*), and motion often occurs at these unstable fracture lines, despite internal fixation. Bone absorption and nonunion are common (Fig. 15–*21*). Type III intracapsular lesions accounted for 75 per cent of the nonunions in a series of 500 hip fractures reviewed.

There is a way to eliminate the mechanical problem presented by these vertical fractures. The contour of the bone can be changed to produce a more horizontal fracture and minimize the shearing force. This should be done at the initial operation by a primary osteotomy upon all type III fractures. The osteotomy should convert shearing strain to impacting pressure by shifting the fracture line to a more horizontal direction, and should not preclude internal fixation.

TECHNIQUE OF PRIMARY OSTEOTOMY. The osteotomy may be made at

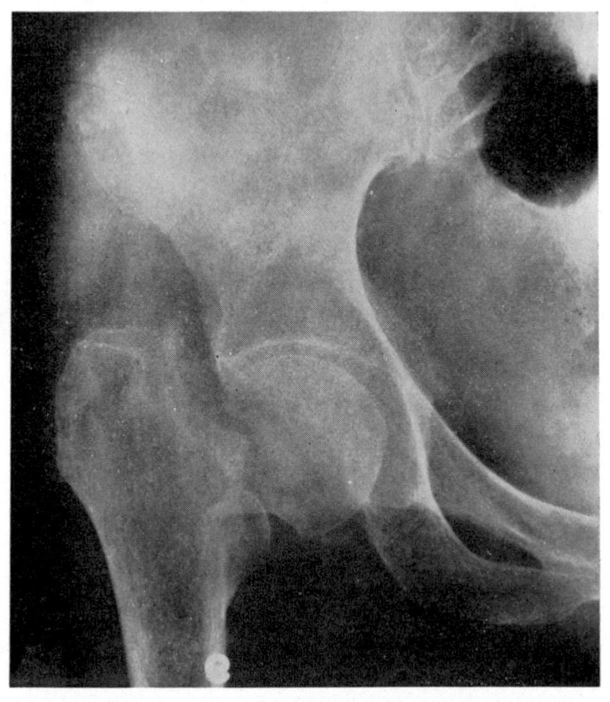

Figure 15–20. Type III fracture of the femoral neck. Note the shape of the head fragment.

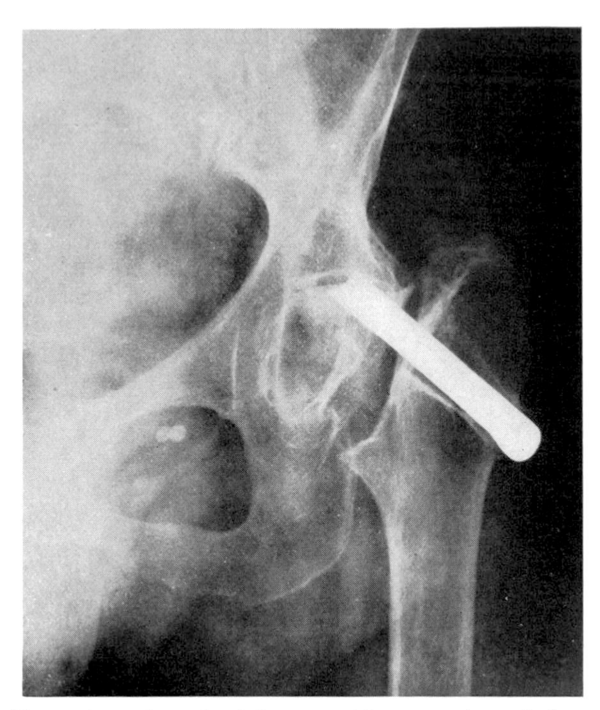

Figure 15–21. Nonunion of neck of femur with resorption of the neck. The pseudoarthrosis interferes with revascularization of the head.

one of two levels: (1) intracapsular (cervical osteotomy), and (2) intertrochanteric. It is most desirable to avoid the need for postoperative plaster casts because elderly subjects tolerate immobilization poorly. The hospital stay and the incidence of medical complications are minimized by internal fixation. Most surgeons prefer the intertrochanteric level because it presents a broader surface for healing, and the cancellous bone at this level unites more rapidly. In general, the displacement osteotomies (McMurray, Lorenz) have been supplanted by angulation osteotomies because of the greater ease of internal fixation and improved range of hip motion. The wedge type of angulation osteotomy is recommended. At times, however, inspection of the fracture makes it apparent that cervical osteotomy offers the simplest and most direct solution.

The fracture is exposed by a lateral approach (Fig. 15–*17*). The lesion is inspected, and, if removal of a spike of neck fragment permits a stable reduction, it is removed (cervical osteotomy). Internal fixation with a Smith-Petersen nail and femoral side plate (Fig. 15–*18*) follows in the usual manner. If the neck is short, one must resort to a more distal osteotomy lest shortening of the neck produce an impingement of the trochanter against the acetabulum. If the osteotomy is to be performed at the intertrochanteric level, the fracture is reduced and an assistant continues traction until the head has been fixed to the neck with a Smith-Petersen nail. The point of entrance of the nail should be near the ridge of origin of the vastus lateralis (about 1 inch proximal to the usual level). Next, a wedge is removed distal to the nail and above the lesser trochanter (see

Fig. 15–27, *B*). This wedge should comprise an angle of about 30 to 45 degrees. It is undesirable to place the hip in greater degree of valgus because of the loss of the abductor lever and the altered weight-bearing surface of the femoral head. If possible, the inner cortex is left intact at this time. The nail driver is then applied to the nail for control of the short upper fragments and the shaft is abducted until the osteotomy is closed. The shaft is rigidly attached to the nail with a femoral side plate and screws.

AFTERCARE IN PRIMARY OSTEOTOMY. The postoperative treatment of these patients differs in no way from that outlined for type II fractures. Early osteotomy does not increase morbidity; it has reduced the incidence of nonunion, but has not reduced the incidence of late avascular changes in the femoral head. Indeed, a superficial appraisal of the results would suggest that this procedure has contributed to vascular damage. Late collapse of the head occurs less frequently in type III fractures treated with internal fixation without osteotomy. However, the difference can be accounted for by the fact that there are fewer nonunions in the osteotomy group. The head rarely collapses so long as the fracture remains ununited. There is usually inadequate weight-bearing thrust to collapse the head in ununited fractures. Nevertheless, the alarming incidence of head changes demonstrates the need for precautions when discussing the prognosis after even the most mechanically perfect osteotomy.

Complications Following Intracapsular Fractures

"The three causes of failure are: (1) failure of reduction, (2) failure of fixation, (3) failure of the blood supply to the femoral head," said Kellogg Speed. Most of the bad results are the consequence of bad nailing. Accuracy is essential. The surgeon cannot be satisfied until a nail of the proper length lies in the center of the head and is properly attached to the shaft. Painstaking care, skill, and patience will determine the result. Hastily performed operations too often end in disaster, and the few minutes saved serves no purpose other than to inflate the ego of the misguided surgeon. Time spent in precise roentgen control does not harm the patient. The clock should be forgotten. The operator must have the courage to continue until he has obtained a stable reduction of the fragments and has fixed them with a well-placed nail. We will consider the complications in two groups: (1) complications associated with the operation, and (2) complications unassociated with the operation. The majority of complications are avoidable.

Complications and pitfalls of the operation. INACCURATE REDUCTION. When a stable reduction has been obtained, the fragments will move together as one piece while the limb is gently rotated. The accuracy of reduction can best be determined by arthrotomy and direct visualization of the fracture. Roentgen views are often misleading. Malalignment in the lateral plane makes central placement of the nail impossible, and is a precursor to "cutting out" of the nail with loss of fixation. In considering the anteroposterior view, one strives to place the neck well under the

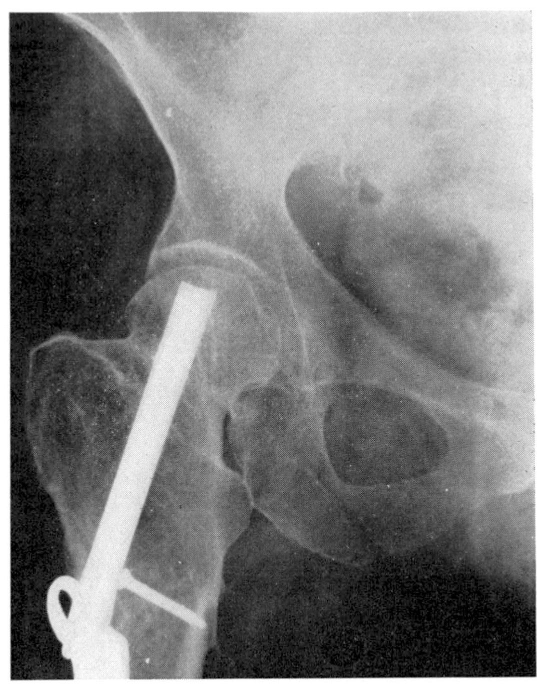

Figure 15–22. Two years after primary trochanteric osteotomy for a vertical unstable fracture. Union followed when shearing force had been eliminated. This particular osteotomy was done at a level lower than ideal.

head. Varus deformity is completely eliminated. It is often desirable to obtain a slight coxa valga because this changes shearing force to an impacting influence. If motion and instability are present at the time of nailing, bone resorption and nonunion often follow despite internal fixation. Vertical type III fractures often require stabilization by osteotomy at the time of nailing (Fig. 15–22).

INACCURATE INSERTION OF THE GUIDE WIRE. The position of the guide wire must be checked with *clear* anteroposterior and lateral roentgenograms before the nail is driven. The position of this wire can be changed without damaging the bone. However, once the nail has been inserted, its position cannot be changed without weakening its grasp upon the bone. The nail must pass through the center of the head. This is important. The two most common causes of the nail "cutting out" through the head are: (1) marginal placement (Fig. 15–23), and (2) second insertion of the nail. The nail can penetrate deepest when inserted dead center. If the nail is directed toward the articular margin it cannot be inserted as far without penetrating into the joint and, therefore, must have a weaker hold on the head (Fig. 15–24). Reinsertion of the nail crushes the head and enlarges the tract so that its grasp is loosened (see Loss of Fixation, infra).

ROLLING OF THE HEAD AS THE NAIL IS DRIVEN. The end of the nail may spin the head as it first strikes it. The reduction is lost, and the bent guide wire fouls the nail. The nail and wire must be extracted. This can

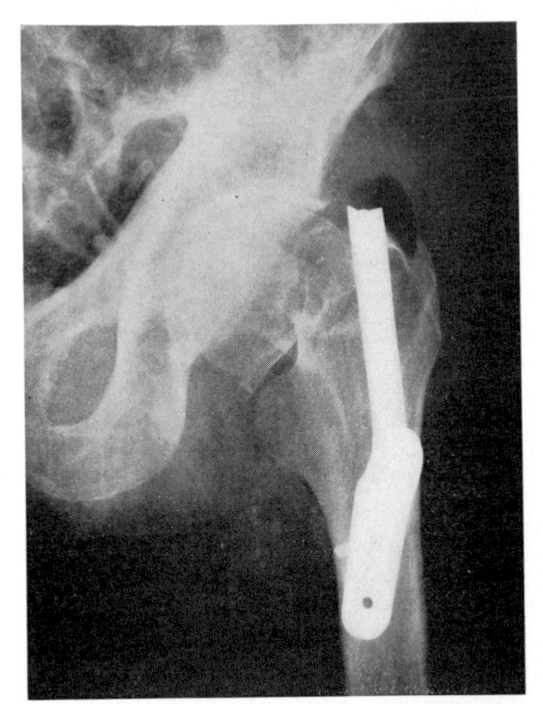

Figure 15–23. A nail which cut out of the head following marginal placement.

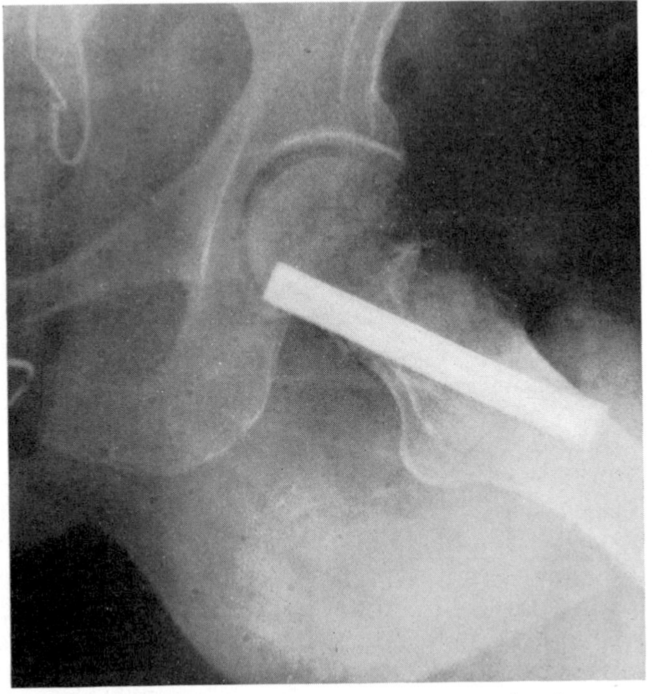

Figure 15–24. Lateral view in the operating room showing marginal position of the nail with damage to the head and neck. This tragedy could have been avoided by guide wire localization prior to nail insertion.

be difficult and traumatic. The fracture must be rereduced and each step in the nailing procedure repeated. Impacted valgus fractures can be displaced by the impact of the nail, and in this instance the blood supply to the head is damaged as the reflected capsule is torn (Fig. 15–*15*). Rolling of the head can be avoided if a *stiff guide wire is used and inserted through the neck and head and into the acetabulum.* The largest wire that can be inserted through the cannula of the nail should be selected. A thin limber wire may bend, especially if it fails to transfix the head.

PUSHING GUIDE WIRE INTO PELVIS AHEAD OF NAIL. The wire may be caught by the nail and carried inward as the nail is driven. Large bowel and bladder perforation has resulted, and on occasion removal of the wire has required an abdominal approach. These complications can be avoided if precautions are observed in starting the nail. The point of the nail may skid if driven directly into the hard outer femoral cortex. It is here that the wire may be indented by the cannula and caught. This is the danger point. Skidding is prevented by making an opening into the lateral femoral cortex sufficiently large to engage the tip of the nail before it is driven.

SHORT NAIL. The nail must penetrate a sufficient distance or it will break out of the head. In subcapital fractures the greatest possible depth short of joint penetration is desirable. If the nail is not long enough to extend 1.5 cm. within the head fragment, it should be extracted and exchanged for one of the proper length. Recent adjustable nails eliminate the need for these extractions and their adverse effects upon the fixation finally obtained.

LONG NAIL. Intrusion of the nail into the joint can be prevented only if extreme care and accuracy are exercised in measuring the length of the femoral neck. If final roentgenograms indicate penetration into the joint, the nail should be withdrawn a sufficient distance to correct this error. If this is not done, the intruding nail will damage the acetabulum. "Scratching" of the acetabulum is not necessarily accompanied by pain because articular cartilage has no sensory innervation; however, it is undesirable because of the articular injury it produces. Partial extraction of the nail weakens its grasp, and further "backing out" of the nail or extrusion may occur later (see Loss of Fixation, infra). Spontaneous extrusion can be prevented by fixing the base of the nail to the shaft with a short plate.

POSTOPERATIVE HEMATOMA. Complete hemostasis is usually impossible when working with fractured bone and injured soft tissue. "Watertight" closure of the skin and subcutaneous tissue often prevents the escape of blood, and a hematoma forms. A deep collection of blood may produce systemic effects and a febrile reaction, but, more important, it constitutes an ideal culture medium devoid of resistance to bacterial growth. Such a hematoma is the precursor of the great majority of postoperative hip-joint infections. The insertion of a drain, widely practiced in the early days of internal fixation, has now been generally discarded because of the danger of a persistent sinus tract and low-grade infection in tissues around the drain. Escape of blood is permitted if the wound is closed in such a way as to obliterate dead space, with widely separated (1.5–2 cm.) fascial and dermal sutures.

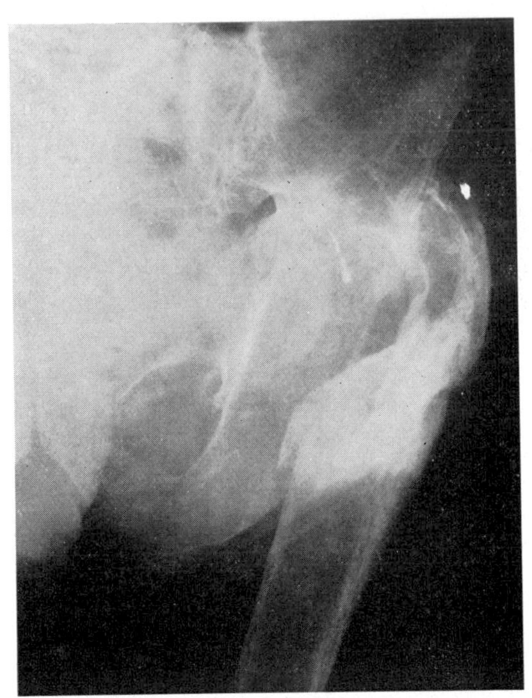

Figure 15–25. Three years after an infected fracture of the femoral neck. The bone had become extensively involved before the presence of the infection had been recognized, because of the masking effect of "prophylactic antibiotics." Adequate early drainage might have averted this problem.

INFECTION. Bacteria seeded in deep hematomas may smolder under the suppression of antibiotics and blossom forth weeks after surgery. In this situation much damage can occur before the infection is recognized (Fig. 15–25). Modern surgeons are becoming increasingly skeptical of "prophylactic antibiotics" in hip surgery, and feel that when infection occurs their masking effect interferes with early recognition of the infection and delays adequate drainage and proper selection of the appropriate antibiotic by determination of bacterial sensitivity.

LOSS OF FIXATION. Late extrusion or "cutting out" of the nail from the head occurs as a result of:

(1) loose nail tract, following reinsertion or partial extraction of the nail;

(2) marginal insertion of the nail in the head;

(3) use of a nail that is too short;

(4) fracture of inadequate metal;

(5) loosening of the nail by motion associated with an unstable reduction;

(6) failure to eliminate "wobble" of the nail in the neck by failing to attach a plate to the base of the nail (Fig. 15–26);

(7) unauthorized weight bearing by the patient.

When loss of fixation occurs, the choice lies between accepting a nonunion or undertaking reconstructive surgery. The treatment must be

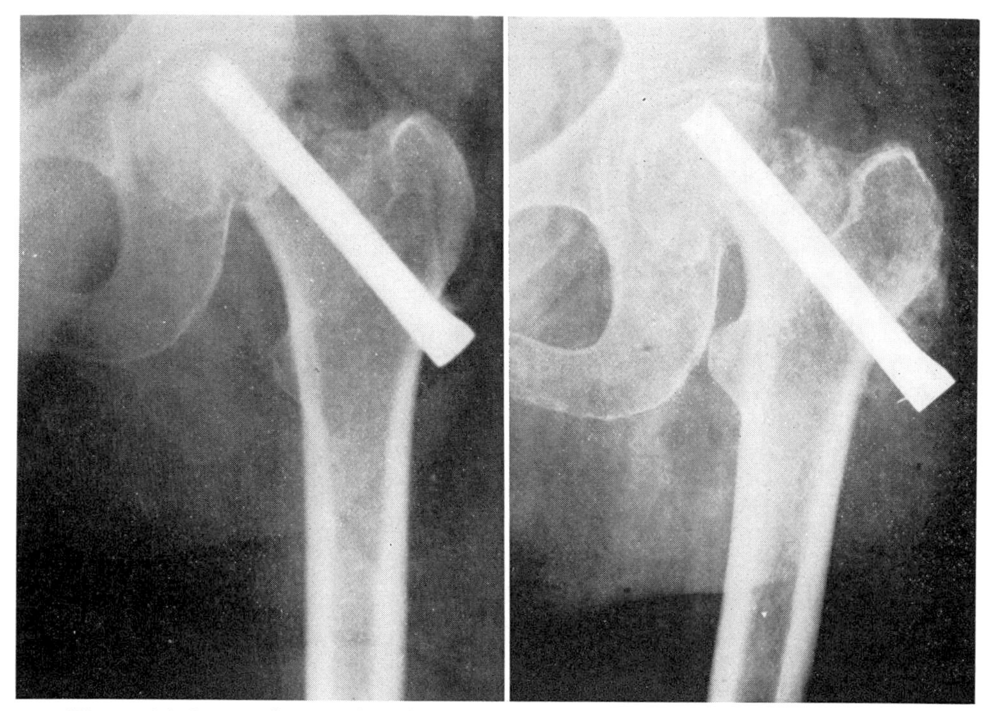

Figure 15–26. Tilt of nail within the neck.
Left. Postoperative position.
Right. Four months later, showing maintenance of nail-head relationship, but a shift of the nail in the distal segment.

individualized, and depends upon the patient's general physical status, the viability of the head fragment, the status of the neck of the femur, and the duration of the injury. In most recent fractures complicated in this way the tissues are vascular and osteogenic, and a simple abduction osteotomy at the time of refixation suffices.

NONUNION FOLLOWING FEMORAL NECK FRACTURE. Unstable reduction and inadequate fixation are the chief causes of nonunion. Loss of blood supply is a less important factor. On the other hand, the presence of the nonunion makes revascularization of the head impossible. Motion at the fracture line causes absorption of the neck (Fig. 15–*21*). Eventually a false joint is formed. These conditions prevent revascularization of the head. The fulcrum of support at the hip is lost, resulting in a telescoping instability, and the opposite hip falls rather than rises when weight is borne upon the affected limb (Trendelenburg's sign). The hip abductors are rendered ineffectual, causing a "gluteal lurch" type of gait. This telescopic instability accounts for the pain and fatigue often present because the abductor muscles are contused and become edematous and tender.

Surgical treatment is directed at: (1) creating a fulcrum for the abductors, (2) redirecting weight-bearing thrust through the acetabulum, (3) preserving or forming an articulation, and (4) eliminating instability. The types of operations and their indications are summarized in Table 15–2. The degree of absorption of the femoral neck, the viability of the

TABLE 15–2. SURGERY FOR NONUNION OF FEMORAL NECK FRACTURE

Indications	*Indicated Procedure*
Good head, adequate neck, young patient	Bone graft, osteotomy, and internal fixation
Good head, short neck, young patient	Brackett vs. intramedullary prosthesis
Dead head, old patient	Intramedullary prosthesis

femoral head, and the general condition of the patient influence the choice of procedure. It should be emphasized that many patients with established nonunions have satisfactory, although not perfect, function, and perform their usual activities with little discomfort. In this situation surgical treatment is neither necessary nor justifiable.

If the *head is viable* and the age and general condition of the patient permits, one of the operations in which the head fragment can be preserved is selected (Table 15–2). The condition of the head is often best appraised at operation because roentgen evidences of avascularity (spotty increased density, fragmentation, or resorption) are not always definite. If the nonunion has existed for a short period of time and there is *minimal absorption of the neck*, the outlook is more favorable. In this situation the best results have been obtained from bone graft combined with an angulation osteotomy (Figs. 15–27, 28) which creates a valgus position of the head and

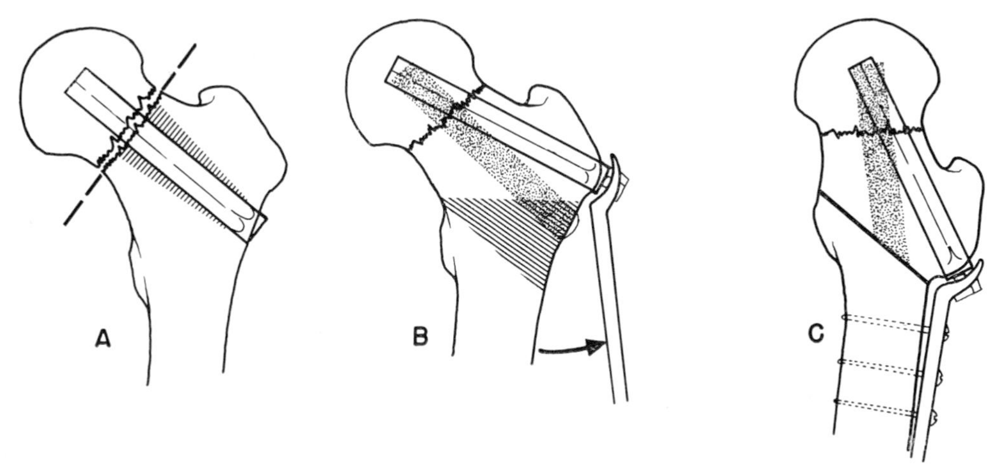

Figure 15–27. Trochanteric osteotomy and bone graft used for ununited fracture.

A. Preoperative problem showing moderate resorption at the neck and wobble of the nail.

B. New nail inserted above the previous one, bone grafts filling the old nail tract, and a 35 to 45 degree wedge resected at a level just above the lesser trochanter.

C. Final position showing elimination of shearing motion; bone grafts crossing area of fibrous union and serving as a framework for revascularization.

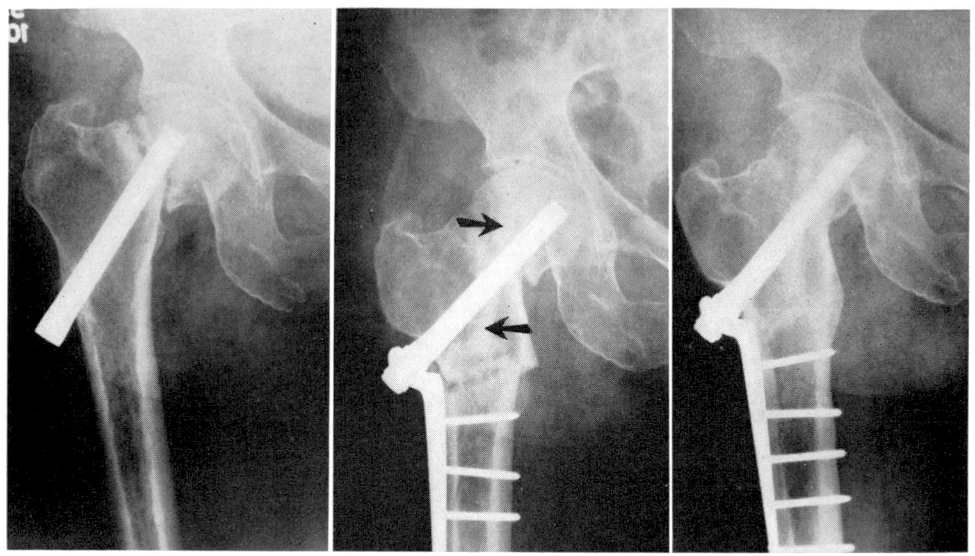

Figure 15–28. Nonunion of the femoral neck treated by trochanteric osteotomy and bone grafting.

Left. Preoperative problem 1½ years after injury.

Center. Postoperative roentgenogram. Note bone graft (arrows) in original nail tract.

Right. One year later. Union had occurred within four months.

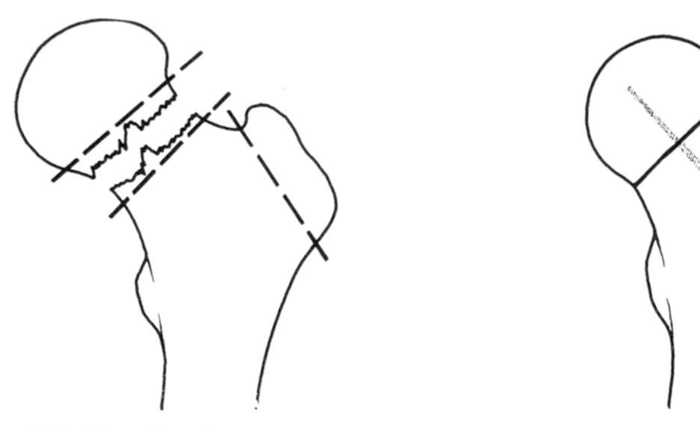

Figure 15–29. Brackett operation for nonunion when neck resorption is excessive. The indications for this procedure are few, since its use is limited to young patients in whom the head fragment appears viable.

converts shearing to impacting pressure. When the neck is short, the Brackett operation may be used (Fig. 15–29). An ununited fracture should be crossed with bone grafts which will serve to maintain a pathway through the scar tissues for circulation to enter the head and for repair. It is desirable to appose broad surfaces of cancellous bone at the osteotomy site, and for this reason the intertrochanteric level is preferable. Drilling and renailing and insertion of an intramedullary graft of fibula, and other types of osteosynthesis procedures which fail to eliminate shearing force by osteotomy, have been less successful. Internal fixation ensures better contact and shortens bed stay and, therefore, displacement osteotomies have become less popular because they are more difficult to fix internally. The

Dickson geometric or the intertrochanteric wedge osteotomies are preferable. Following wedge resections at the intertrochanteric level, interval fixation can be accomplished with a Smith-Petersen nail and plate attachment (Thornton-McLaughlin). With secure internal fixation these patients may be out of bed within a day or two after operation. Gooseneck blade plates (Moore, Blount) have a tendency to "cut out" of the head. A spline (Bosworth) creates excessive valgus which is undesirable. Severe valgus produces weakening of the abductor muscle, and increases the pressure on the femoral head. *If maximal absorption of the neck* is present, it may be necessary to modify the osteotomy so as to restore length of the neck by including transposition of the greater trochanter (Brackett).

If the head fragment is necrotic and adherent, it should be removed. Head resection alone is sometimes utilized for infected nonunions and poor-risk patients. When the general condition of the patient permits, reconstruction should accompany head removal. Medullary replacement prosthesis has supplanted operations of Whitman, Colonna, and short-stem replacement prosthesis for the head (Judet). Medullary prosthesis is now widely used for nonunion in older patients, or in any patient in whom the femoral head is necrotic (Fig. 15–*30*). The stem prosthesis (Judet) has essentially no place in the treatment of fracture or its complications because the neck of the femur is shortened. The medullary prosthesis offers the advantages of preservation of the length of the neck, and more diffuse pressure on the bone in an area where the blood supply is superior. When replacement arthroplasty has failed, recourse may be had to trochanteric arthroplasty, resection, or arthrodesis (Fig. 15–*31*). Arthrodesis (Fig. 15–*31, C*) is of value in an occasional young, active, laboring man with nonunion. However, replacement of the head and neck offers a quick result with minimal convalescence for older patients. A number of pros-

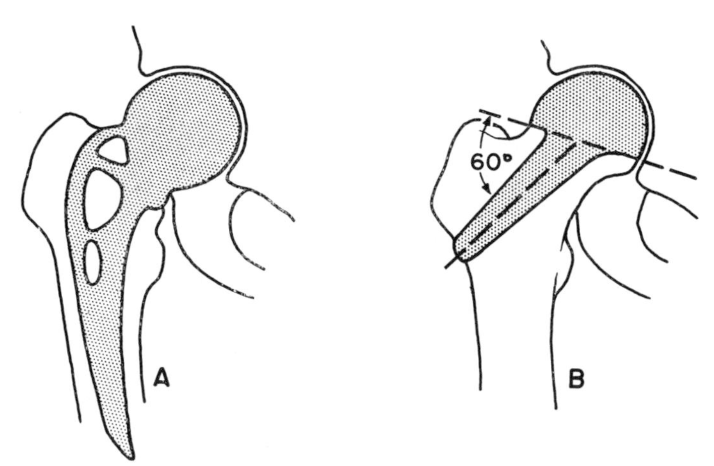

Figure 15–30. The two types of replacement prosthesis for the femoral head.
A. Intramedullary prosthesis.
B. Stem prosthesis.

The intramedullary prosthesis has supplanted the stem type because of better diffusion of strain on the supporting bone, superior blood supply of the trochanteric region as apposed to that of the neck, and better preservation of length of the neck.

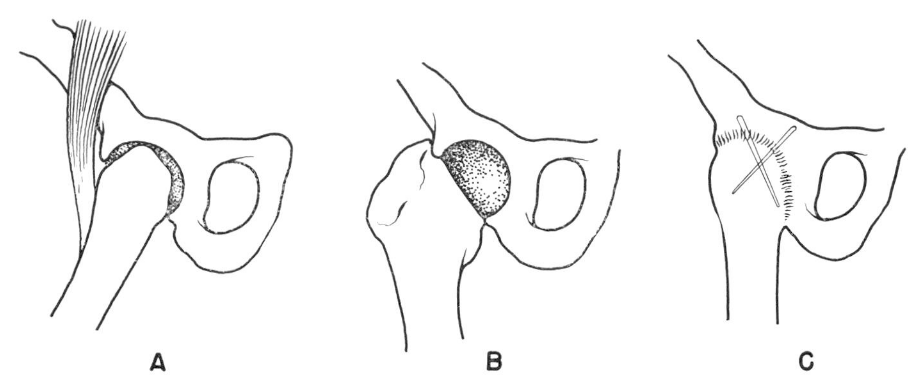

Figure 15–31. Procedures available when replacement arthroplasty has failed.
A. Trochanteric arthroplasty.
B. Resection.
C. Arthrodesis.

thetic appliances have been developed during recent years. Vitallium or stainless steel may be used. Acrylic is not strong enough and has shown breakage and wear. Nylon is to be condemned because of lack of inertness and sensitiveness to the material which have been reported. The durability of the prosthesis is dependent upon: (1) material that is strong and inert, (2) a design which diffuses pressure, and (3) a secure seat in healthy bone with good blood supply.

LATE COMPLICATIONS OF THE NAIL. Should the nail be removed after union of the fracture? It poses a theoretical barrier to complete revascularization of the head, and a painful bursa may form over its protruding base in the trochanteric region. Furthermore, fractures may occur adjacent to the rigid metal. The normal elasticity of the bone in the neck of the femur is reduced, and this accounts for the subtrochanteric or subcapital fractures that may result if re-injury should occur. For these reasons, the nail should be removed in all young patients when union is complete. In older persons it is not necessary to remove the nail unless bursal pain or other complication arises.

Complications not associated with the operation. AVASCULAR NECROSIS OF FEMORAL HEAD. The fate of the head is sealed at the moment of injury. Closed reduction with lateral nailing is followed by avascular necrosis as frequently as is properly performed open reduction. No form of treatment yet devised will prevent the development of bone necrosis. Careful follow-up studies indicate roentgen changes after union in 40 per cent of displaced femoral neck fractures. The reflected capsular vessels are usually spared in impacted valgus lesions (Fig. 15–*13*), and yet 10 per cent of these fractures display late alterations in density and contour of the femoral head. Changes are often not visualized until the second nine months after injury, at which time the fracture has united and the hip is subjected to weight-bearing stress (Fig. 15–*19*). Alterations in the contour of the articular surface of the femoral head are associated with excessive wear and hypertrophic osteoarthritis follows. If the hip becomes painful, further treatment is necessary. The age, general health, and activities of the patient are major considerations in planning therapy.

Nonoperative treatment consists of restriction of activities within the limits of pain and fatigue, weight reduction where indicated, physical therapy to eliminate contracture, salicylates during acute exacerbations, and intra-articular instillation of Hydrocortone. This is the therapy for any osteoarthritic joint. It is indicated when symptoms are mild, or when the patient is a poor risk for operation.

Operative treatment may be classified in three categories: (1) arthroplasty, (2) arthrodesis, and (3) interruption of sensory innervation. The *Smith-Petersen cup arthroplasty* (Fig. 15–32) utilizes sound physiological principles. The fibrous repair at the articular surfaces of the femur and acetabulum is converted to fibrocartilage and "molded" by motion of the metallic cup. After several months it resembles normal articular cartilage, although it can be distinguished from hyaline cartilage microscopically. The concept of remolding the joint to normal contour is appealing. Unfortunately, however, it is a difficult operation technically, and few surgeons claim relief of pain in more than 60 per cent of their patients. It is the procedure of choice, however, in young patients who are unsuitable for or refuse arthrodesis.

Arthrodesis is a more certain method of stopping pain. If the hip is fused with 25 degrees of flexion, neutral rotation, and neutral abduction-adduction, the gait is excellent and there is minimal handicap. The function of a fused hip is dependent upon increased pelvic excursion in walking

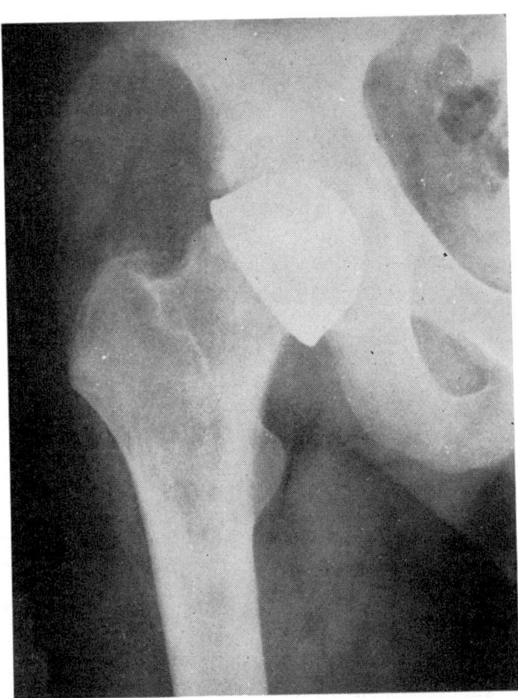

Figure 15–32. Smith-Petersen cup arthroplasty is useful in young patients with avascular necrosis of the femoral head, provided the area of collapse is limited.

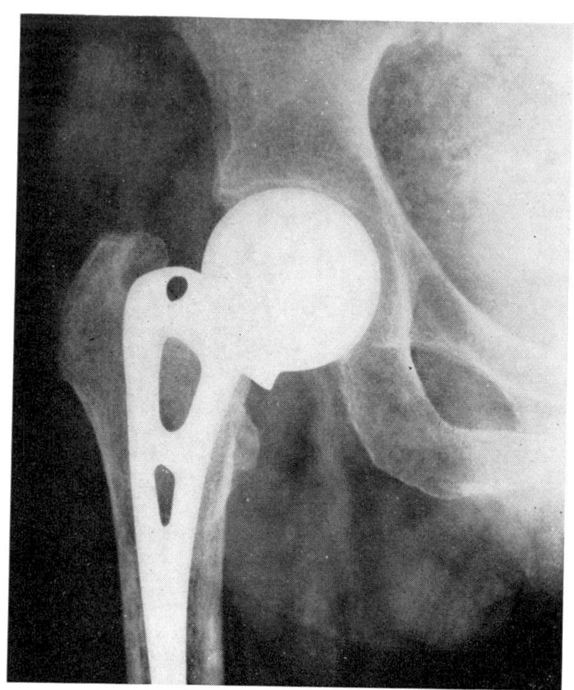

Figure 15–33. Medullary replacement prosthesis preserves good surface contact against acetabulum by correct head size, maintains normal neck length for abductor power, and diffuses strain over a broad area of calcar and shaft.

and sitting and, therefore, low back difficulties are a consideration. Likewise, bilateral hip disease causes one to favor arthroplasty over arthrodesis. In general, fusion is the procedure of choice in young active patients. In older patients *replacement arthroplasty* is preferred, because it is a less shocking operation and requires a minimal recovery period.

Neurectomy of the obturator, femoral, and sciatic branches has so often failed to relieve pain that it has been generally abandoned.

Chordotomy, or division of the contralateral spinothalamic tracts at the upper thoracic level, has been tried in certain poor-risk patients, but without consistent success.

EXTRACAPSULAR FRACTURES

Basal fractures of the neck of the femur, intertrochanteric fractures, and subtrochanteric fractures occur through or outside the ligamentous attachments of the hip joint and, therefore, have a good blood supply. Union is the rule, provided the fracture is immobilized. Immobilization can be accomplished by means of traction, plaster immobilization, the Roger Anderson "well-leg" traction device, and internal fixation. There is no fear of necrosis of the femoral head. Nevertheless, the treatment of patients with extracapsular fractures is often most difficult. Soft callus bends, and coxa vara with shortening of the limb develops in comminuted fractures (type III—see Fig. 15–9), unless they are immobilized for five or six months. Furthermore, displaced trochanteric fractures more frequently cause severe systemic effects and are associated with a much greater mortality than are intracapsular fractures. Intertrochanteric and subtrochanteric fractures lack ligamentous and capsular support, and are associated with soft tissue injury and hemorrhage equaling that of fractures of the femoral shaft. Most surgeons agree that internal fixation has reduced mortality by 50 per cent. However, 20 per cent of patients with a displaced extracapsular fracture die within six months from causes related to the injury (Table 15–*1*). Therefore, these fractures must be respected as the serious injuries they are.

Diagnosis

The mechanism of fracture, history, and physical findings correspond to those of the intracapsular group; however, if an external rotation deformity greater than 45 degrees is present, one is dealing with an extracapsular rather than an intracapsular lesion. The splinting effect of the capsule limits displacement in the intracapsular lesion so that external rotation deformity is less than 45 degrees. Nondisplaced or incomplete lesions produce minimal signs and pose a diagnostic pitfall. Clear anteroposterior and lateral roentgenograms must be obtained promptly in any injured individual complaining of hip or knee pain.

Treatment

Most extracapsular fractures unite with treatment by traction or plaster, but these methods have been replaced by internal fixation since the hospital stay and mortality have been greatly reduced by early mobilization of the patient. Internal fixation by means of a Smith-Petersen nail which is rigidly fastened to the femoral shaft with a plate permits the patient to be out of bed within a day or two following operation. The nail must be fixed to the shaft because the cancellous bone in the trochanter is too soft to hold the base of the nail securely. This applies to basal neck and subtrochanteric fractures, as well as to intertrochanteric lesions.

Fractures of base of femoral neck. Treatment by traction is definitely inadequate for this group. Nonunion may result from incomplete immobilization. Internal fixation is required. These fractures respond well to proper internal fixation, however, and union within three or four months is the rule.

Intertrochanteric, type I. Nondisplaced or incomplete fractures are accompanied by minimal soft tissue injury. They produce little pain. For these reasons the systemic effects are minimal. No reduction is necessary. The healing time is shorter than in any other "hip fracture." Roentgen evidences of consolidation are present within two months after injury (Fig. 15–*34*). The aim of treatment is protection from further injury throughout the healing period. Most surgeons prefer internal fixation and early crutch ambulation because they feel the elderly patient should be up and about during the healing period, but they are afraid to trust the patient on crutches without added internal support for the fragments. In any case,

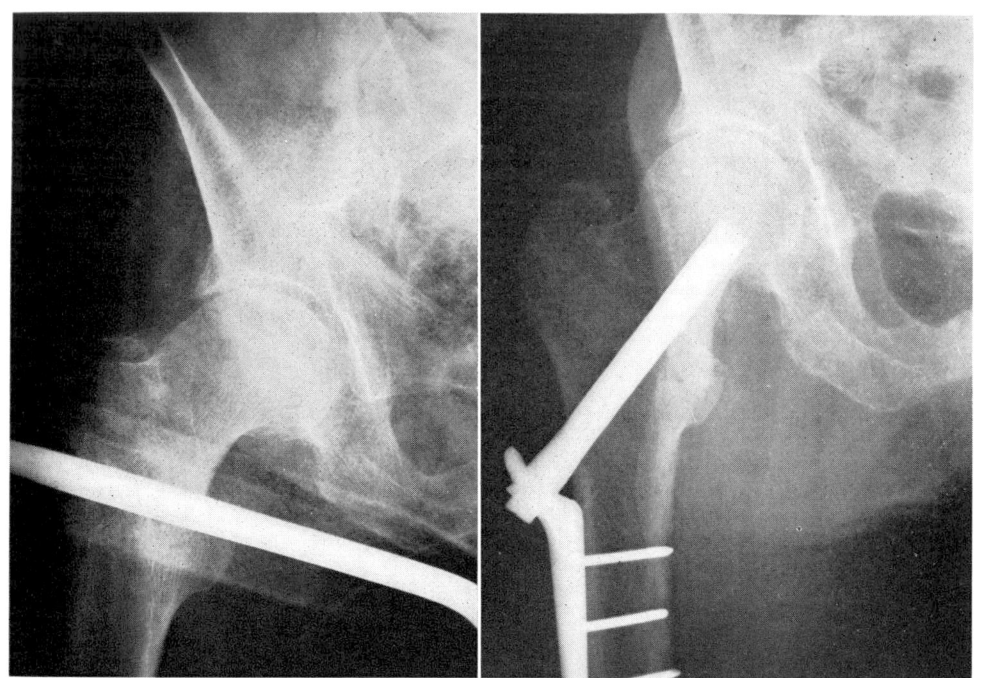

Figure 15–34. Type I, nondisplaced, intertrochanteric fracture.
Left. At time of injury.
Right. Solid union two months later.

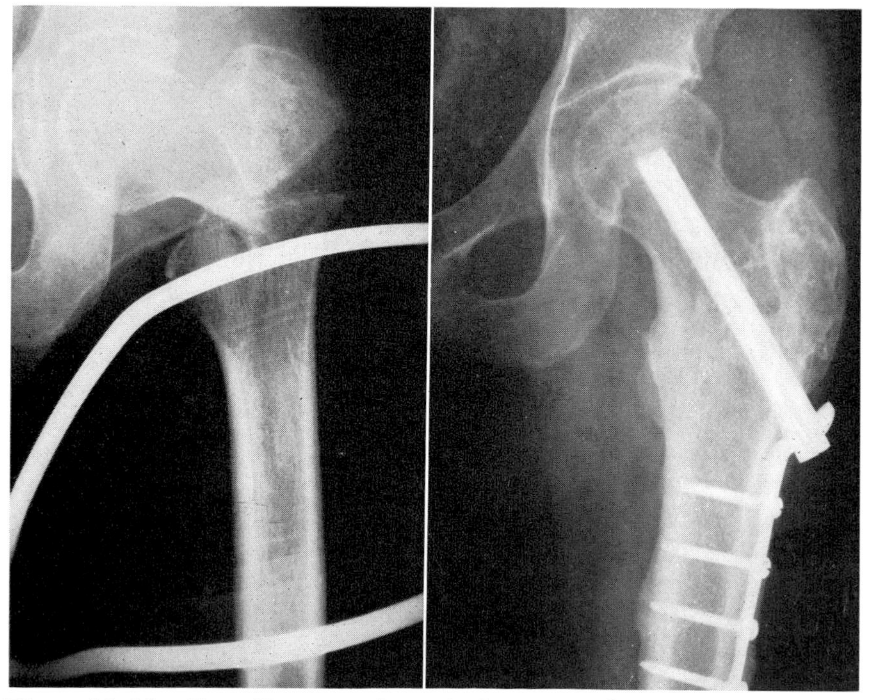

Figure 15–35. Type II intertrochanteric fracture with intact medial buttress.
Left. At time of injury.
Right. Accurate reduction was maintained until union occurred.

the prognosis is excellent, provided the good position of the fragments is maintained until they have united.

Intertrochanteric, type II. These displaced fractures lack the comminution of the "unstable" group. There is firm bone on each side of the fracture line. Good anatomical results can be obtained because the bone does not tend to collapse into varus and shorten, as occurs so frequently after comminuted fractures. If an accurate reduction is obtained, it is possible to maintain anatomical position with internal fixation (Fig. 15–35). A good reduction is essential. Inaccurate initial replacement of the fragments accounts for most of the shortening that follows type II fractures. Mortality following these lesions is comparable to that of the comminuted group, type III, and indicates extensive local tissue injury and blood loss.

Intertrochanteric, type III. When the buttress of cortex along the medial side of the fractured bone is lacking (Fig. 15–36) there is no fulcrum for the maintenance of length. The angulated femoral neck acts as a lever. Following reduction there is an overwhelming tendency toward varus rotation and shortening of the extremity. Alignment can be maintained by traction, but the soft callus bends when this is discontinued. Few patients can tolerate traction for the five- or six-month period required for firm consolidation. Furthermore, shortening occurs in four out of five patients treated by internal fixation. To date no infallible method of pre-

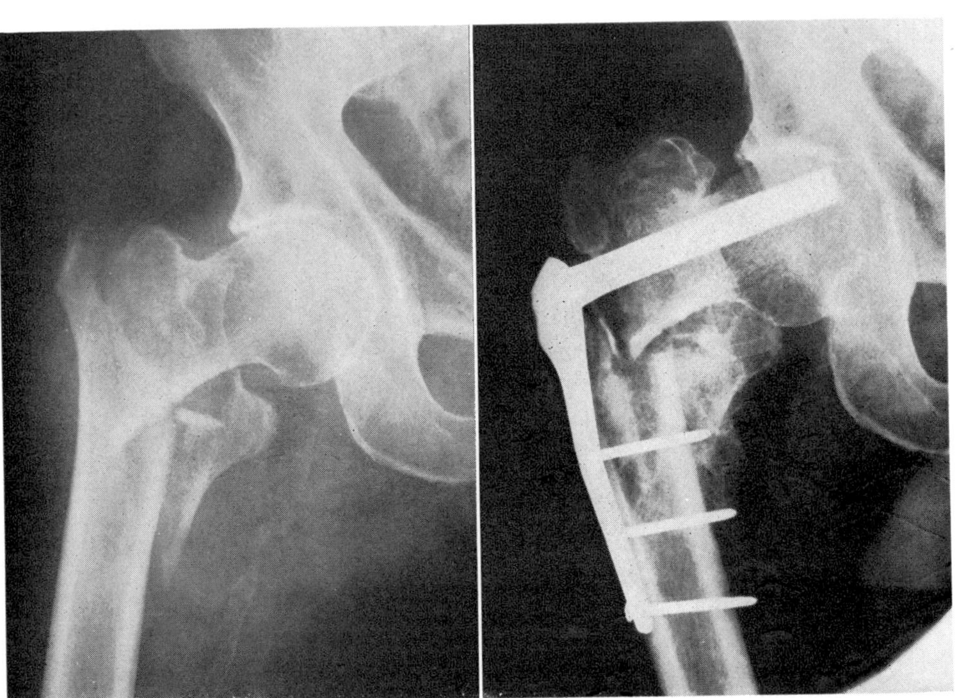

Figure 15–36. Type III intertrochanteric fracture. The medial buttress has been destroyed.

Left. At time of injury.

Right. Anatomic reduction was followed by collapse and varus rotation of the proximal segment.

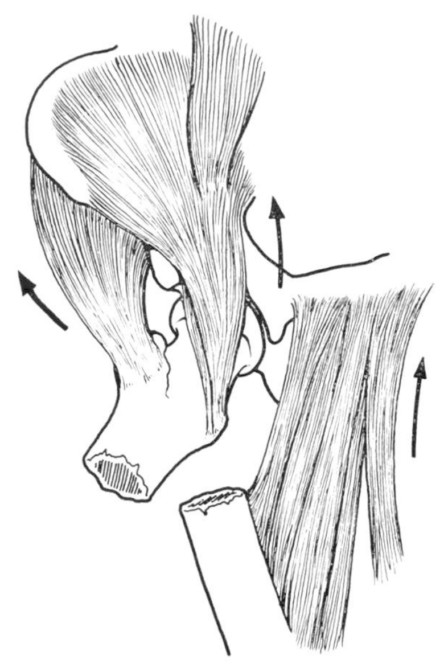

Figure 15–37. *Subtrochanteric fracture. The proximal fragment is flexed by the iliopsoas, abducted by the lesser glutei, and externally rotated. The distal fragment is adducted and pulled proximally.*

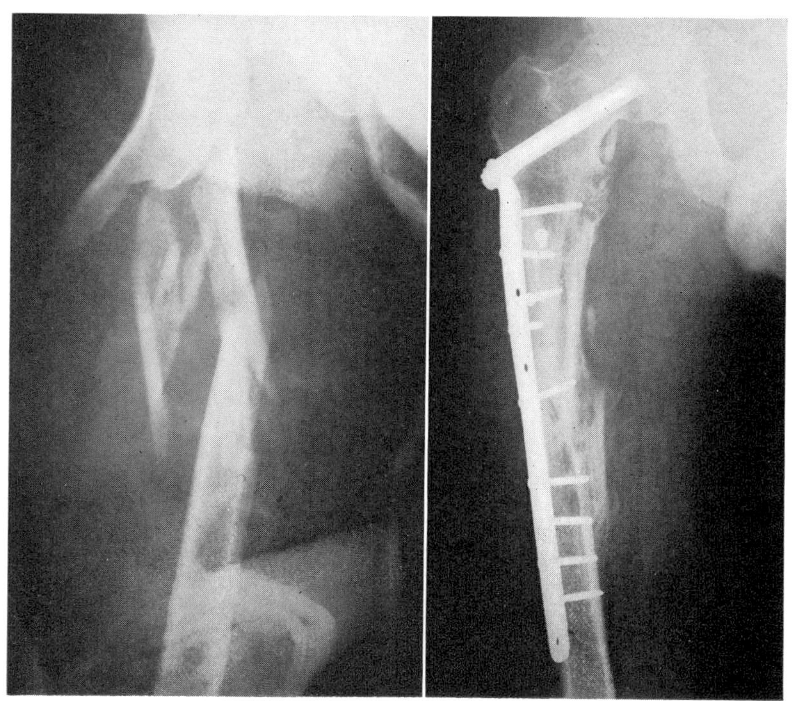

Figure 15–38. *Comminuted subtrochanteric fracture.*

Left. *Original treatment in plaster spica inadequate because of flexion of proximal fragment and interposition of muscle.*

Right. *Open reduction and internal fixation produced excellent result.*

venting collapse of these unstable lesions is available. Often it is advisable to nail the fracture in varus position for the sake of faster union. Patients with the better results survive long enough to suffer the crippling effects of a shortened extremity. The mortality has been reduced by internal fixation. This is the treatment of choice. But, even so, the prognosis must be guarded.

Subtrochanteric fractures. These fractures comprise approximately 10 per cent of the trochanteric lesions and result from severe trauma. The patients are often active individuals from a younger age group. The fracture is usually comminuted. The abductors, flexors, and external rotators of the hip act upon the proximal fragment while the shaft is displaced upward and inward by the adductors (Fig. 15–37). Interposition of soft parts is not uncommon and, if present, demands open reduction. Nonunion occurs if the fragments are improperly aligned or poorly immobilized. Internal fixation is the favored method in adults. At times it is not possible to obtain secure internal fixation because of comminution. In this situation supplemental traction or plaster should be used postoperatively. Open reduction with internal fixation is essential if interposition of soft tissue is present (Fig. 15–38). The presence of interposed muscle can be determined by persistent posterior displacement of the shaft as seen in the lateral view and the absence of bony crepitus.

Technique of Internal Fixation of Trochanteric Fractures (McLaughlin)

A lateral incision is made from the level of the trochanter downward. The tensor fascia tendon and vastus lateralis muscle are incised longitudinally. Care is taken to find and ligate the large branch of the lateral circumflex femoral artery found within the muscle about 3 inches below the trochanteric ridge. If the fracture is markedly displaced, it is exposed and reduction is carried out under direct vision. However, good position often can be obtained by merely abducting the limb and rotating it inward. *The amount of internal rotation required is generally less than enough to bring the limb to the neutral position.* Unlike the reduction of intracapsular fractures, intertrochanteric lesions usually should be nailed with the limb in moderate *external rotation.* Fixation is made easier by a preliminary tri-flange window in the lateral cortex, and the use of a guide wire. A modified Smith-Petersen nail, with a bolt extending from the base, is inserted to the level of the junction of the head and neck. The length of the nail should be such that about ½ inch protrudes from the lateral cortex at this time. The plate then is attached to the base of nail and held parallel to (but not in contact with) the femoral shaft, as the lock bolt is tightened. Only in this way can the plate be locked securely to the nail. The nail is then driven inward until the plate is in contact with the femoral shaft. The plate is held to the shaft with a bone clamp and a second set of anteroposterior and lateral roentgenograms is taken to ensure proper position. The tip of the nail should not penetrate deeper than ½ inch from the articular surface to allow for subsequent collapse of comminuted fragments. The plate is secured with screws only after satisfactory final roentgenograms have been seen.

Complications of Intertrochanteric Fractures

Realization that the three types of intertrochanteric fractures produce different systemic and local effects is essential to a discussion of this problem (Fig. 15–9). Nondisplaced fractures (type I) can be treated by any method with uniformly good results. Displaced fractures cause an impressive mortality and may produce shortening of the extremity. Of 266 intertrochanteric lesions studied, only one failed to unite, and this was due to interposition of muscle in a fracture treated by traction. There was no instance of avascular necrosis of the head.

Mortality. Most surgeons agree that internal fixation has reduced mortality. Nevertheless, the prognosis must be guarded. Of 235 intracapsular fractures treated on the Fracture Service of the New York Orthopaedic–Presbyterian Hospitals only nine deaths (4 per cent) were related to the injury. Of 266 intertrochanteric fractures, treated during the same period, 49 deaths (19 per cent) were from related causes. This emphasizes the serious effect of extracapsular lesions upon aged patients.

Shortening of the extremity. To date there is no method that ensures a good anatomical result when the fracture is comminuted (type III). Traction with internal fixation has been followed by collapse and varus rotation (Fig. 15–*36*) in 75 per cent of these fractures. On the other hand, anatomical restoration should be the rule in type II lesions, provided there is an accurate reduction. Operative treatment has improved the results in these stable lesions (Fig. 15–*33*).

ATYPICAL FRACTURES OF THE HIP

Childhood Fractures

Trochanteric fractures in immature bone present few problems. As a rule, these can be reduced by manipulation and held with plaster. These fractures are usually healed within eight weeks (Fig. 15–*39*).

Intracapsular fractures of the femoral neck, however, are especially unfortunate in children. The incidence of avascular necrosis and nonunion is generally greater than that following similar lesions in adults. This is thought to be due to the fact that the ligamentum teres artery is less well formed before the epiphysis closes, and often the sole source of blood supply to the caput is the retinaculum, which may be damaged. In the writer's experience, childhood hip fractures have invariably occurred at one of two levels: (1) trochanteric, and (2) epiphyseal separation of the capital epiphysis (Fig. 15–*40*). Congenital coxa vara has been confused with nonunion of fractured femoral neck. A true intracapsular fracture through the neck of the femur (other than basal neck) has not been seen, and must be extremely rare if it does occur. Epiphyseal fractures usually require internal fixation; plaster immobilization is uncertain and often inadequate (Fig. 15–*41*).

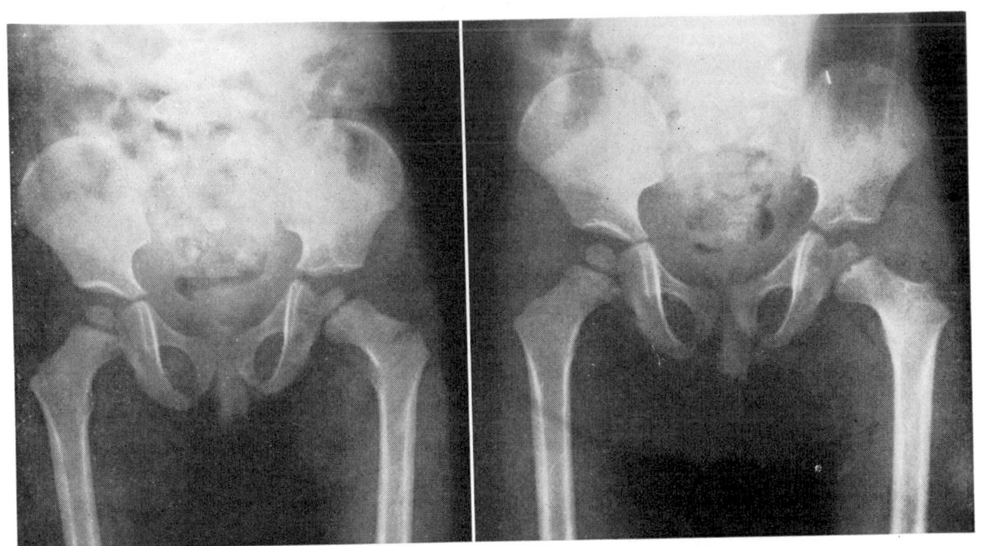

Figure 15–39. Intertrochanteric fracture in a six-year-old child.
Left. Original injury.
Right. Union was complete after eight weeks in a plaster spica.

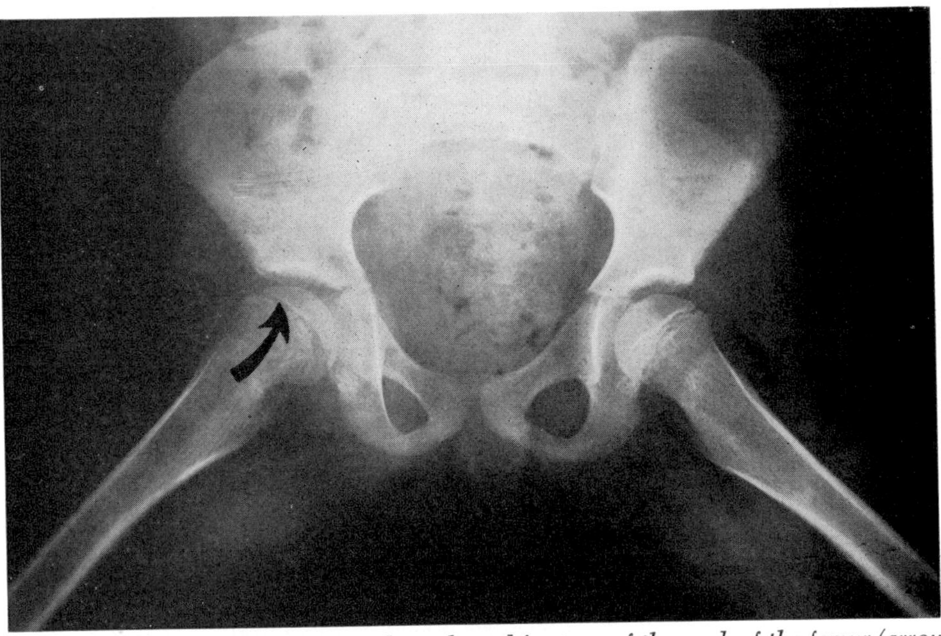

Figure 15–40. Minimally displaced epiphyseal fracture of the neck of the femur (arrow) in a six-year-old girl, which was successfully treated by plaster immobilization.

Irradiation Fractures

Spontaneous fracture of the femoral neck following irradiation of the pelvis for malignancy is not rare. The blood supply to the neck of the femur is damaged by heavy irradiation and this, coupled with local tissue necrosis, predisposes to fatigue-fracture. With continued use, the deformity increases

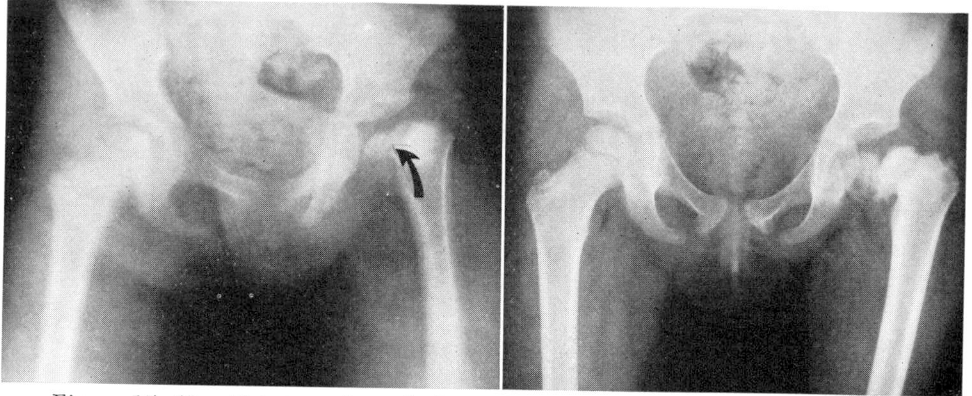

Figure 15–41. Fracture through the neck of the femur zone in a five-year-old girl. Left. The epiphyseal zone was involved (arrow).

Right. The result six months after plaster immobilization, showing marked varus deformity following this inadequate treatment. The osteotomy now required could have been avoided by proper initial internal fixation.

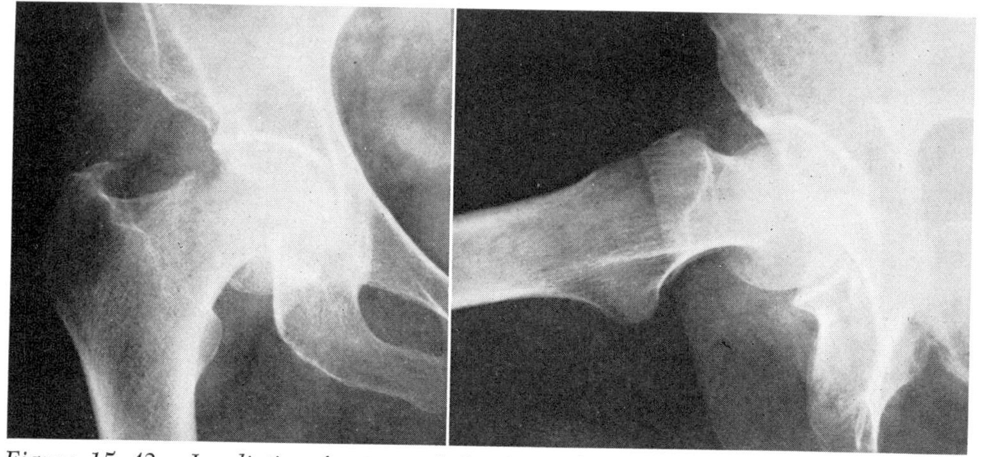

Figure 15–42. Irradiation fracture of the femoral neck. Note the lack of rotatory deformity in the lateral view (right).

(Fig. 15–42). The results in patients treated early are superior to those in patients with marked deformity created by continued weight bearing. This condition should be suspected in any female patient having hip pain subsequent to radiotherapy to the pelvis. Repeated roentgenograms may be necessary to establish the diagnosis. Later, the characteristic displacement is one of varus without lateral rotation deformity. Internal fixation without correction of the displacement has given good results in a high percentage of patients treated early. The prognosis is less hopeful when softening and severe displacement are present.

Fracture Due to Metastasis

The presence of metastatic bone destruction does not preclude surgical intervention. Internal fixation of the fracture often is possible (Fig.

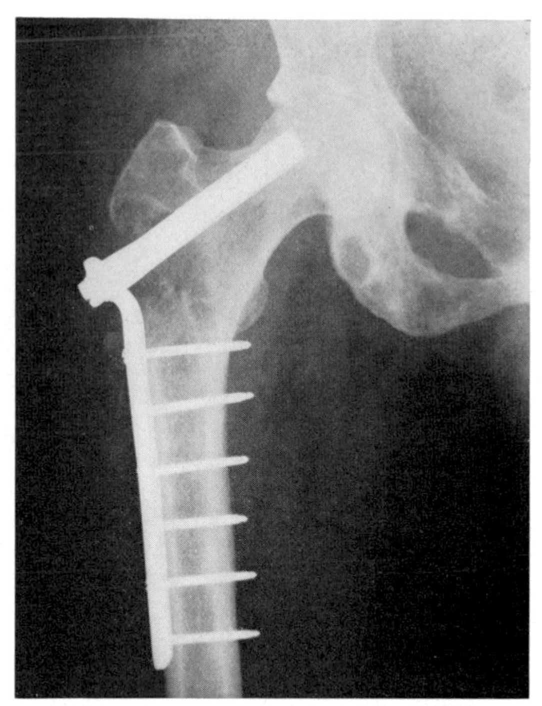

Figure 15–43. Pathological fracture due to metastatic carcinoma from the breast. Internal fixation stopped the pain. Irradiation was given, and the fracture subsequently united.

15–43). Pain is alleviated, and union may occur. At times replacement prosthesis is indicated, however, because this permits early weight bearing and gives a more rapid result in these patients whose life expectancy is limited.

TRAUMATIC DISLOCATION OF THE HIP

Fractures are usually encountered in immature and aged femurs. Dislocations are seen almost exclusively in young adults or individuals in middle years of life. In this age group the bone is so strong that a powerful force may push the head of the femur through the capsule or into the acetabulum, rather than break the femur. Three varieties of dislocation occur: (1) posterior—the head of the femur rests behind the acetabulum ("sciatic" dislocation); (2) anterior—the head of the femur rests in front of the acetabulum ("obturator" dislocation); and (3) central—the femoral head is forced through the floor of the acetabulum ("intrapelvic" dislocation). Automobile accidents have greatly increased the frequency of traumatic dislocation, particularly of dislocation with posterior displacement.

POSTERIOR DISLOCATION

The anterior capsule is reinforced by the powerful Y ligament of Bigelow (iliofemoral ligament) and the oblique head of the rectus femoris muscle.

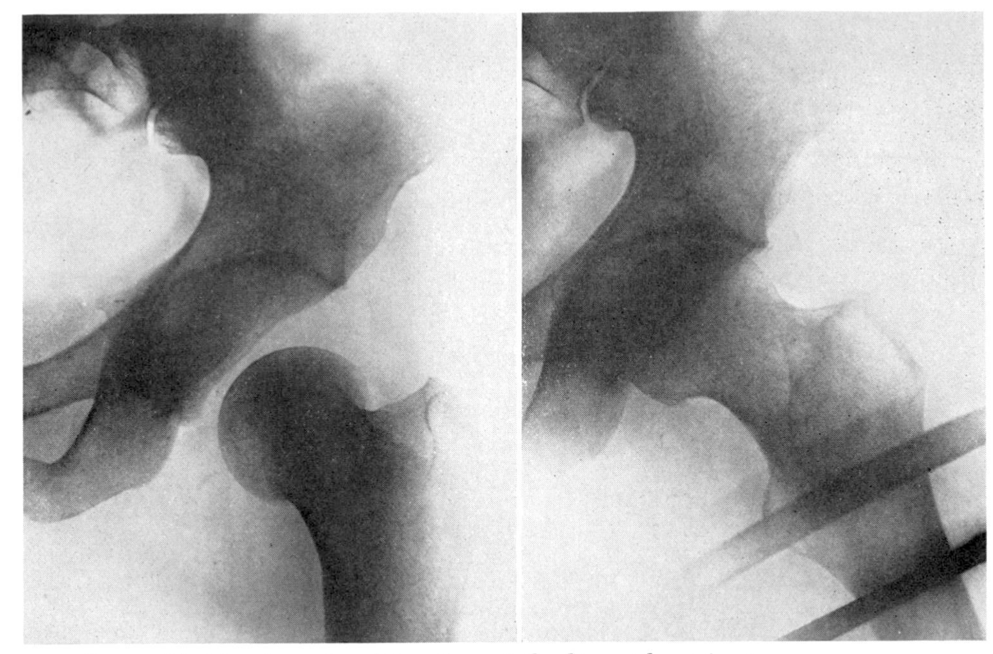

Figure 15–44. Posterior dislocation of the hip without fracture.
Left. Typical deformity with marked internal rotation.
Right. Closed reduction is followed by satisfactory result, provided damage to the blood supply of the femoral head has not been significant.

The posterior capsule is weaker. The joint is particularly vulnerable when flexed and adducted. A passenger in the front seat of an automobile with legs crossed may be thrown against the instrument panel. The impact can push the head of the femur out of the back of the socket (Fig. 15–*44*). This type of dislocation occurs more frequently than any other.

Pathology

The impact often displaces the posterior rim of the acetabulum and may produce segmental fractures of the femoral head. The sciatic nerve may be injured. The ligamentum teres and posterior capsule are torn. The important vessels within these structures are damaged. Late avascular necrosis of the femoral head occurs in approximately 30 to 40 per cent (Fig. 15–*45*). There are no completely accurate statistics on this. Furthermore, it is probable that some idiopathic necroses of the upper femur are based upon spontaneously reduced luxations of the hip (Fig. 15–*46*).

Diagnosis

The most striking physical sign is that the entire limb is held in marked internal rotation. No other condition produces this picture, and the diagnosis of posterior dislocation can be made from across the room. In addition, the limb is moderately flexed and adducted. There is an exception to the

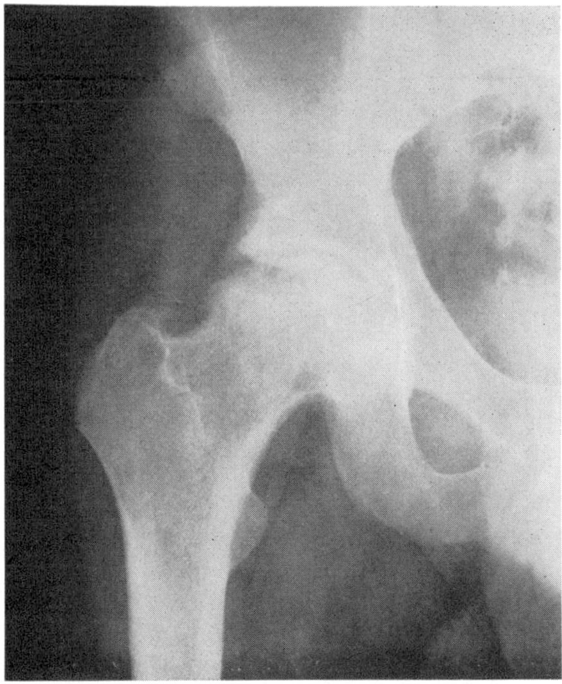

Figure 15–45. Avascular necrosis of the femoral head 18 months after traumatic posterior dislocation. The ligamentum teres and posterior capsular vessels are injured.

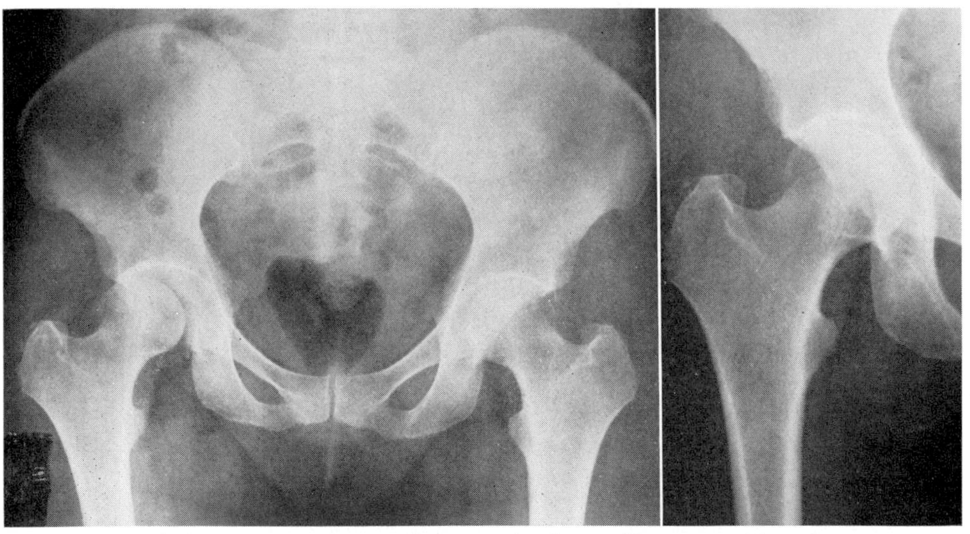

Figure 15–46. Spontaneous reduction of a hip subluxation. After the roentgenogram at the left was taken, the patient felt a click as the technician lifted the limb. Evidence of avascularity of the femoral head was seen sixteen months later.

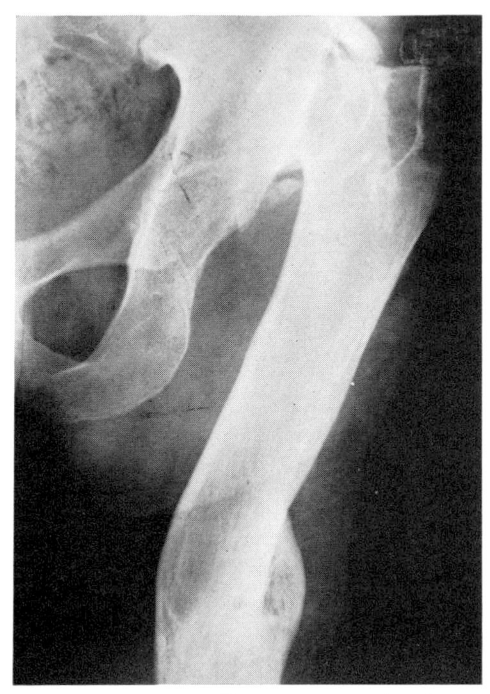

Figure 15–47. Roentgenogram made two years after fracture of the femoral shaft with concomitant posterior dislocation of the hip. The dislocation had not been recognized, and the femoral fracture had healed with 90 degrees rotatory deformity.

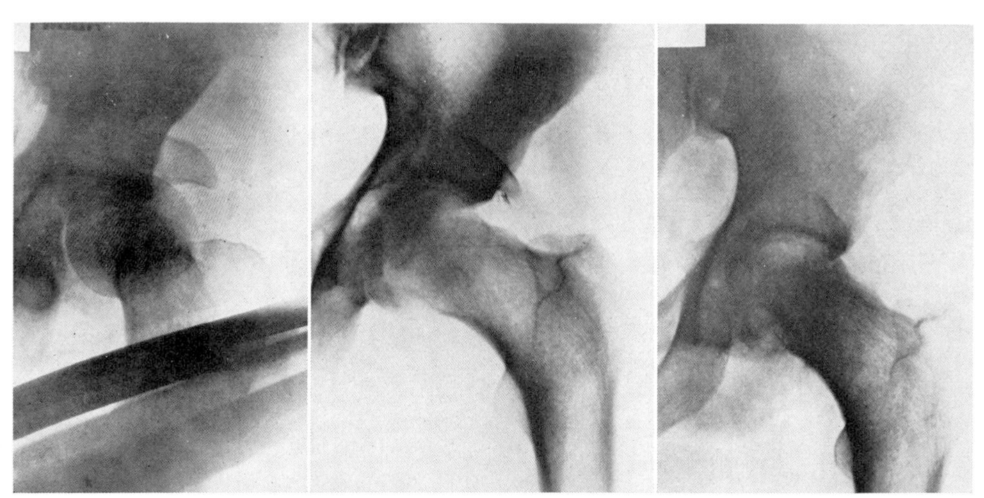

Figure 15–48. Posterior dislocation associated with fracture of the acetabular rim.
Left. Prereduction roentgenogram.
Center. After closed manipulative reduction.
Right. Late arthritic changes due to instability caused by incomplete reposition of the large rim fragment. Open reduction and internal fixation should have been done for the elimination of instability.

rule. When the dislocation is combined with a fracture of the shaft of the femur (Fig. 15–47), the typical attitude of internal rotation is lacking and, if attention is limited to the shaft fracture, the dislocation may be overlooked.

Treatment

Small fragments of acetabular rim may be ignored, but when the segment is so large that it renders reduction unstable, internal fixation is advisable (Fig. 15–48). Two major therapeutic categories exist: dislocation (1) with significant fracture, and (2) without significant fracture. In the latter instance, manipulative reduction is adequate; in the former, accurate open reduction with internal fixation of the rim segment is mandatory. In borderline cases it is well to remember that a good percentage of these patients develop necrosis of the femoral head whether operated upon or not. This thought may sway the decision against operation in questionable situations.

Among the methods of manipulative reduction perhaps the best known is that of Bigelow. The patient is anesthetized supine upon the floor and the limb is flexed as upward traction is applied, bringing the femoral head opposite the acetabulum. The limb is then externally rotated to beyond neutral, and brought out in abduction as the hip is extended. Following reduction, the limb is suspended in balanced suspension and motion is

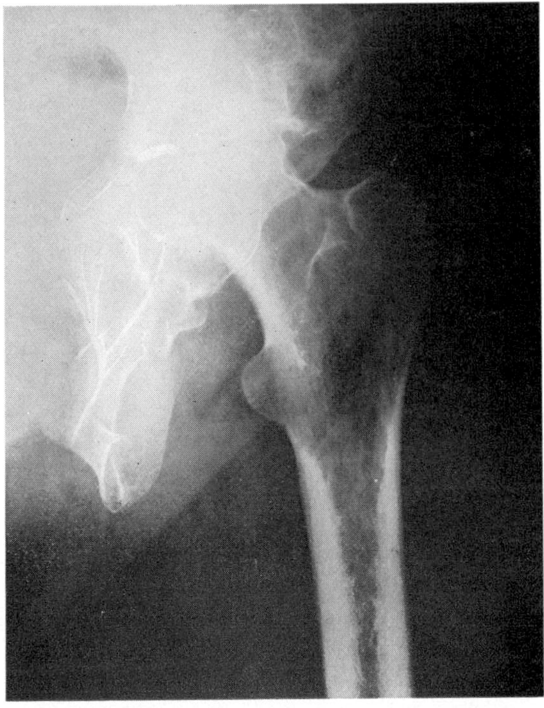

Figure 15–49. One year after posterior dislocation with acetabular rim fracture. In attaching the acetabular lip, a screw had been inclined too far anteriorly and entered the head of the femur.

progressed within the limits of pain. The average patient is allowed up on crutches without weight bearing about two weeks after reduction.

When open reduction is necessary because of a large acetabular rim fracture, the approach passes along the superior and lateral borders of the gluteus maximus. The fragment should be retracted and the joint inspected for loose pieces of bone. Care is taken to avoid injury to the sciatic nerve. After the femoral head is replaced in the acetabulum, the rim fragment is accurately reduced and fixed in place with one or more screws. Care must be taken lest the screws penetrate the acetabulum (Fig. 15–*49*). After operation, the unstable hip should be immobilized in a plaster spica for four to six weeks, until union of the fracture has occurred.

In any case, the problem of *when to begin weight bearing arises.* There are two schools of thought. One group advises non–weight-bearing crutch walking for 12 to 24 months. They believe that this permits revascularization by creeping replacement of any areas of avascular bone in the femoral head, and gives these young patients the best chance to avoid late joint changes. The other school emphasizes that to date the previously described concept is merely theoretical, and that the true value of a prolonged non–weight-bearing régime has not been established. They believe that joint changes occur in spite of this program and, therefore, permit weight bearing within two or three months after injury. Most textbooks suggest starting ambulation six months after injury. This lacks the logic of either school of thought.

Complications of Posterior Dislocation of the Hip

Sciatic nerve damage. Associated sciatic symptoms are usually transitory and disappear progressively. When symptoms of complete paralysis below the knee and wide sensory disturbances persist, the prospects for recovery are poor. The results of surgery upon the sciatic nerve have not been encouraging.

Avascular necrosis of the femoral head. This is the most important complication (Fig. 15–*45*). If pain and disability result, surgical intervention is required. Inasmuch as these patients are usually young, arthrodesis of the hip is often indicated. Arthroplasty lacks the certainty of a lasting result, but is preferable in certain individuals with sedentary occupations, and in older patients.

Fracture of Femur Associated with Dislocation

When fracture of the femoral head is associated with dislocation of the hip, segmental fragments, if small, should be excised after the dislocation is reduced. If a fragment is large and attached to the ligamentum teres (Fig. 15–*50*) it should be reduced and internally fixed. Femoral neck fractures and femoral shaft fractures accompanying dislocations are seen on occasion, and these should be internally fixed after the dislocation has been reduced. If concomitant femoral shaft fracture is present, open reduction of the fracture usually is necessary, at which time the hip can be

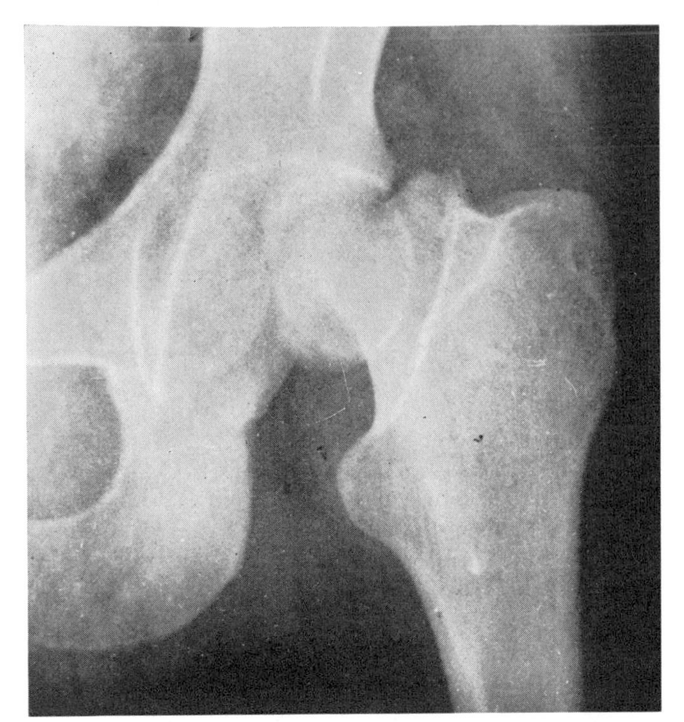

Figure 15–50. Fracture of the femoral head with dislocation. Large fragments attached to ligamentum teres should be reduced and internally fixed.

reduced and the fracture internally fixed with an intramedullary nail. In patients where the hip dislocation is overlooked because of its association with a shaft fracture (Fig. 15–47), the femoral fracture unites in 90 degrees malrotation. In this situation little can be done other than arthrodesis of the distorted hip joint.

ANTERIOR DISLOCATION

Anterior displacement of the femoral head is produced by forced abduction. The stevedore standing with one foot on the boat and the other on the dock as the boat moves away from shore, or a dancer doing the "splits," may sustain this lesion. The femoral head may produce pressure upon the femoral vessels.

Diagnosis

Upon inspection the limb is abducted and externally rotated. There is palpable fullness in the groin due to the displaced femoral head. Roentgenograms complete the differentiation from a fracture of the femoral neck.

Treatment

Reduction can be accomplished by traction and internal rotation. It is necessary to remember that anterior displacement may embarrass the

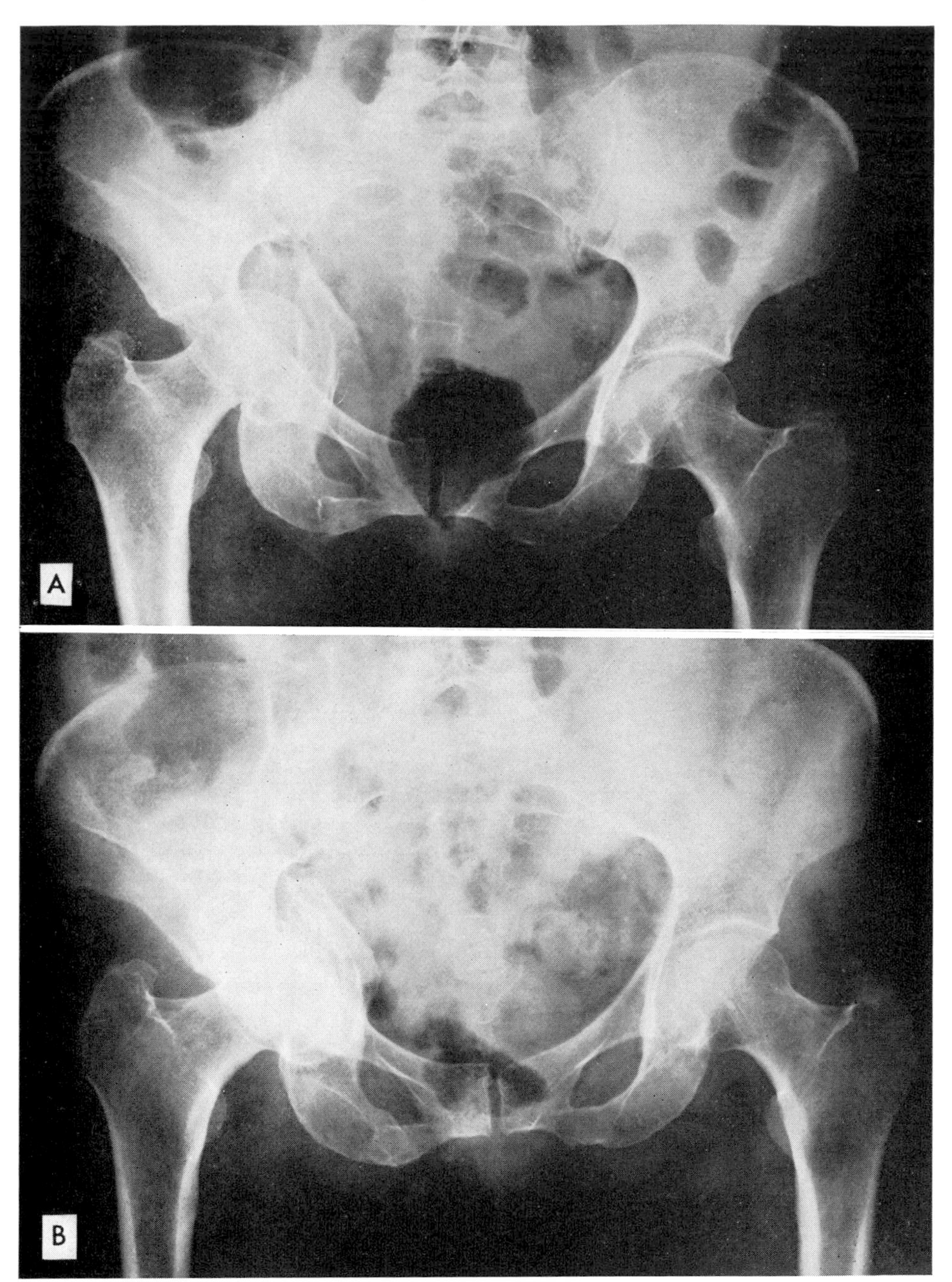

Figure 15–51. Central dislocation of the hip in an elderly patient.

A. Traction failed to improve the position.

B. Three and a half years later the patient was walking without significant disability. In a younger patient open reduction with internal fixation would have been preferable.

femoral vein and that massive pulmonary infarction with sudden death has followed manipulation. This dramatic complication has occurred, as a rule, when reduction was delayed more than 12 hours. For this reason, vein ligation should precede reduction in neglected cases. Aftercare is as discussed for posterior dislocations. As in posterior displacements, late avascular necrosis is a frequent complication.

CENTRAL DISLOCATION

A blow upon the trochanter may drive the femoral head medially against the floor of the acetabulum. The ischiopubic rami are rotated inward. There may be extensive comminution. Muscle spasm exaggerates the displacement.

Treatment

When displacement is minimal, early motion is begun and progressed within pain limits. Weight bearing is deferred until a firm fibrocartilage repair has minimized discrepancies in the articular surface (four to six months). Displaced lesions may be reduced by skeletal traction combined with a lateral swathe. Often certain fragments fail to follow the head of the femur (Fig. 15–*51*). In this case open reduction with internal fixation of certain major segments may be advisable. The fractures are exposed by a posterior approach or by reflecting the origin of the iliacus muscle from the inner aspect of the bone. Internal fixation is accomplished with screws and is supplemented by skeletal traction postoperatively. Weight bearing is begun four to six months after injury. If pain exists after a year or two, arthrodesis or arthroplasty may be necessary. However, the functional result in these patients is generally far better than the roentgenograms suggest.

Part IV

THE TRUNK

CHAPTER 16

INJURIES OF THE PELVIS

By HARRISON L. McLAUGHLIN, M.D.

THE INNOMINATE BONES and the sacrum form a circle of bone that is virtually rigid. The sacroiliac and interpubic ligaments allow no measurable motion at the symphysis pubis or sacroiliac joints, but provide for sufficient resilience in these areas to absorb some of the impact of direct or indirect trauma to the pelvic girdle. The strength and self-sufficiency of the sacro-iliac ligaments are well illustrated by a preservation of pelvic stability and an absence of locomotor difficulty even after removal of the entire anterior segment of the pelvic girdle (Fig. 16–*1*). The abdominal contents are supported on the saucer formed by the iliac wings, and the pelvic viscera are contained and protected by the cup formed by the pubic and ischial bones. Body weight is borne by the ischial tuberosities in the seated position, and is transmitted through the innominate bones to the femora when the body is erect.

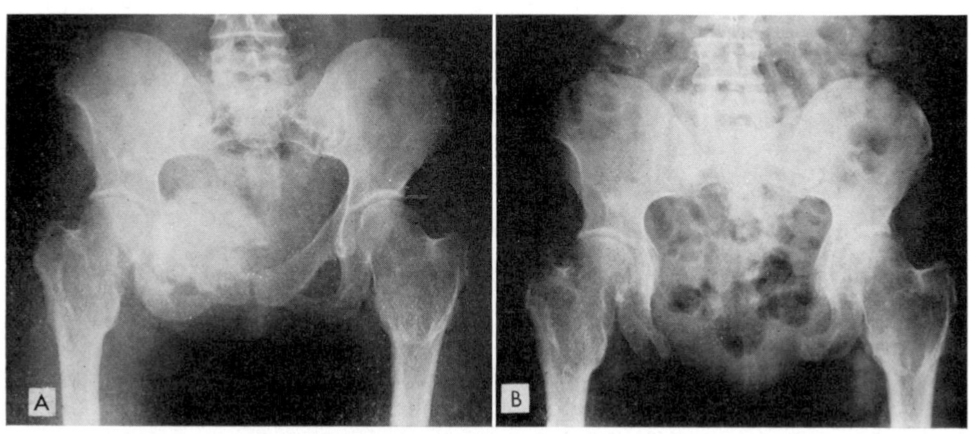

Figure 16–1. Intact sacroiliac ligaments are sufficient for locomotion.

A chondrosarcoma (A) which, 17 years after local excision, recurred and obliterated the pelvic cavity. Radical excision required ablation of both pubic segments of the pelvis (B). Ambulation remained undisturbed, adductor muscle function remained intact with reduced power, and the sacroiliac joints remained stable and free from discomfort.

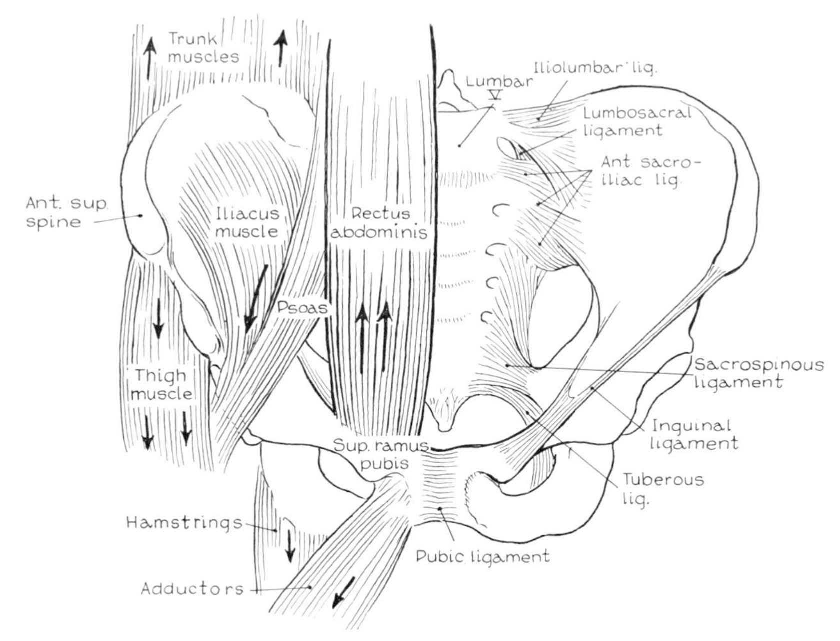

Figure 16–2. The motor-skeletal anatomy of the normal pelvis.

AVULSION FRACTURES OF THE PELVIS

The pelvis skeleton is common anchorage for both trunk and locomotor muscles. It is suspended between these two powerful muscle groups (Fig. 16–2) and serves as a fulcrum over which the upright position is maintained and the lower extremities are propelled. A violent contraction against resistance may avulse the bony attachment of a muscle from the pelvis skeleton, but, despite the great power of the muscles attached to the pelvis, this type of injury is seldom encountered, except in youthful patients, and at the ischial tuberosity or anterior superior iliac spine. The cause is consistently some ultimate athletic exertion of adolescence or young adult life. Strong fascial connections prevent gross displacement of the avulsed bone fragment. Spontaneous sound healing is the rule. Recovery is complete, except for the frequent repair of an avulsed ischial tuberosity by exuberant callus, which may cause some inconvenience when the patient sits on a hard surface.

Avulsion of Ischial Tuberosity (by Hamstring Muscles)

The buttock is tender, swollen, and painful. The thigh cannot be flexed. Extension of the knee produces buttock pain. Maximum displacement occurs at the time of injury, seldom exceeds 2 cm., and does not increase (Fig. 16–3). Operative repair, which does little except make it necessary for the patient subsequently to sit on a scar, as well as an over-sized tuberosity, is contraindicated. Bed rest and control of pain should be provided until ambulation with the aid of crutches is tolerated, usually a

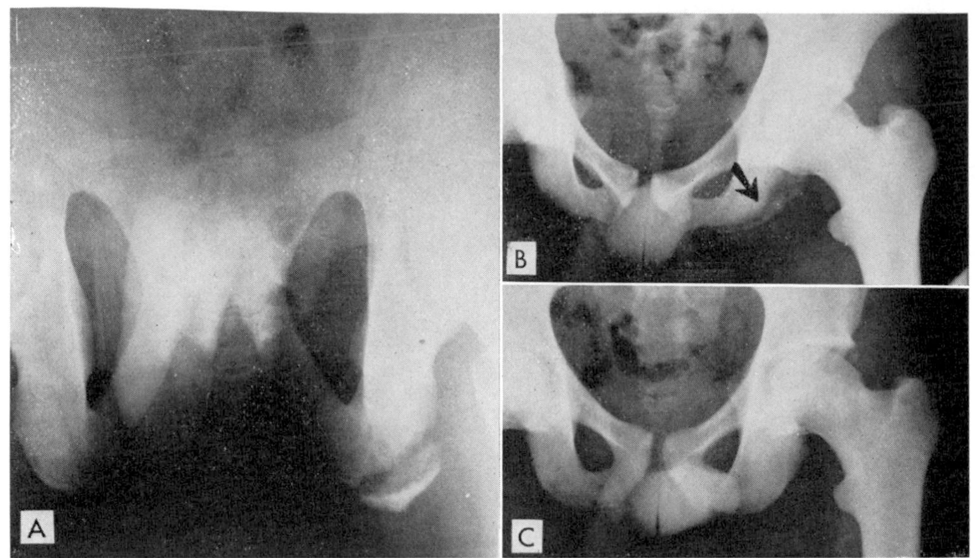

Figure 16–3. Avulsion of the ischial tuberosity by the hamstring muscles.

Maximum displacement of the avulsed apophysis occurs immediately and does not increase. Attempts at suture fail to maintain reduction, owing to the strength of the displacing muscles, and the patient is forced to sit on an operative scar.

A. Tangential view of avulsed ischial tuberosity.

B. This is less apparent (arrow) in ordinary anteroposterior films.

C. Note the over-sized tuberosity present after healing of the fracture.

period of two to three weeks. The patient should be warned that the injured region may remain sensitive for several months, and that healing may produce a slightly over-sized tuberosity.

Avulsion of Anterior Iliac Spines

Displacement of a fragment of anterior superior iliac spine avulsed by the sartorius muscle usually is limited to less than 3 cm. by surrounding fascial connections (Fig. 16–4). When the anterior inferior iliac spine is avulsed by the rectus femoris, gross displacement is prevented by the reflected head of this muscle, which remains intact (Fig. 16–5). With either injury, bed rest with the thighs flexed for one or two weeks, after which ambulation may be resumed progressively, is followed by complete recovery. Operative repair is unnecessary, and has produced functional results no better than those in which the avulsed fragment was allowed to heal in a slightly displaced position.

Avulsion of Ilium by External Violence ("Motorcycle Injury")

This injury is limited almost exclusively to motorcyclists. At the impact of a collision the motorcyclist throws himself sideways from his seat, but his forward momentum drives him against one rubber-shod steering handle, which sinks into the lower quadrant of the abdomen and hooks against the abdominal surface of the iliac wing. Variable amounts of ilium are

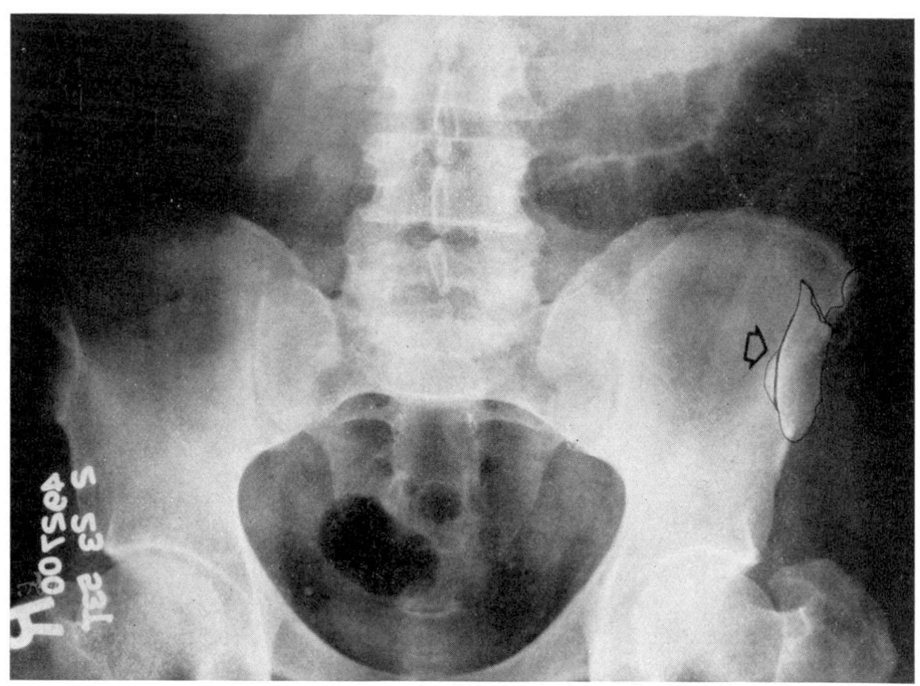

Figure 16–4. *Avulsion of anterior superior iliac spine by sartorius muscle.*
The fascial investments of the sartorius muscle prevent its contraction sufficiently to prevent gross displacement of the bone fragment.

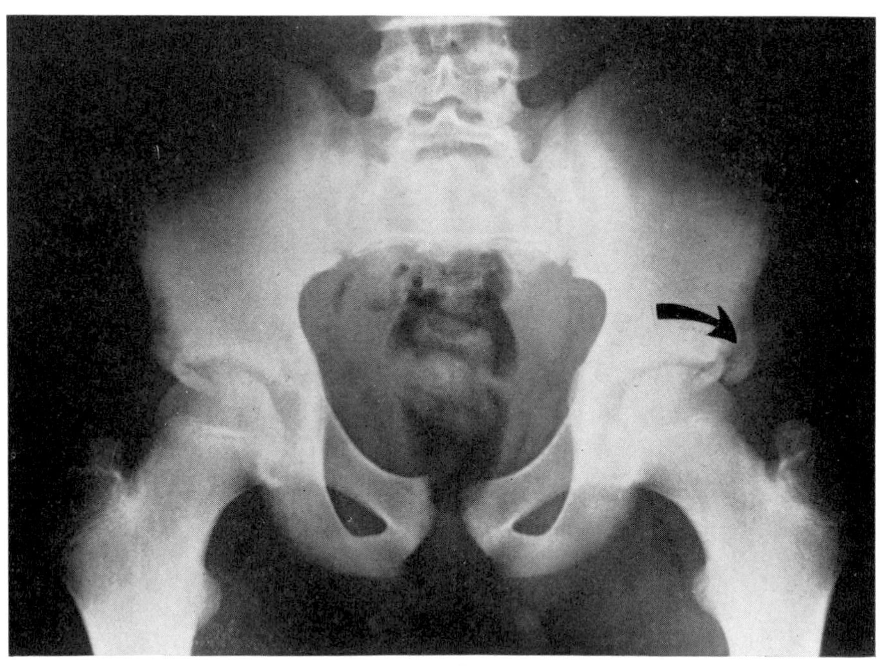

Figure 16–5. *Avulsion of anterior inferior iliac spine by rectus femoris.*
The intact reflected origin of the muscle prevents gross displacement of the bone fragment. Note bilateral separate centers of ossification in the rim of the acetabulum, which should not be confused with this injury.

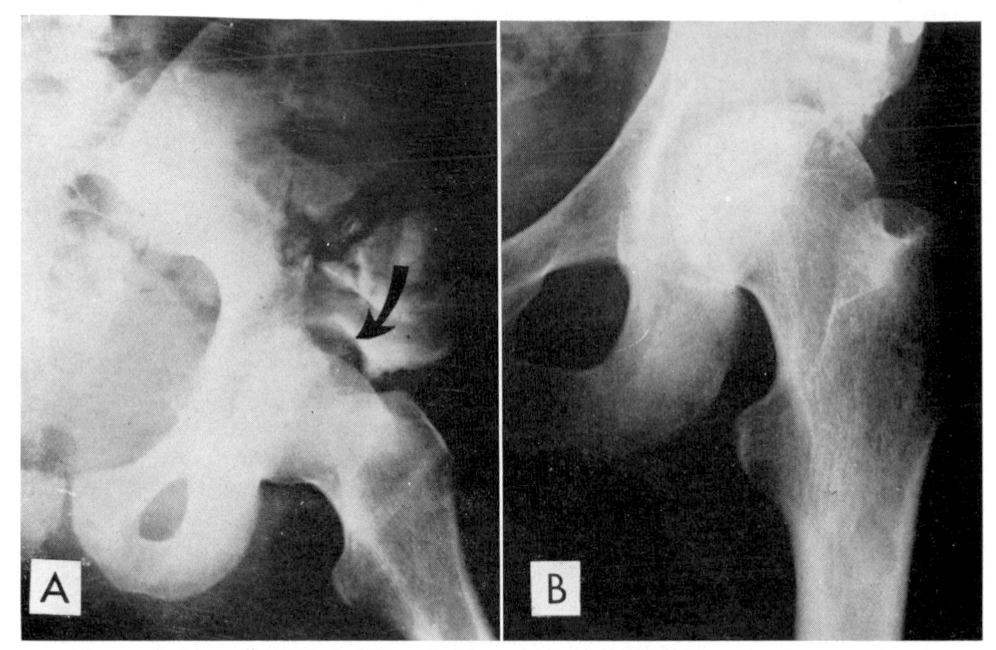

Figure 16–6. "Motorcycle" fracture of anterior ilium.

The iliac wing was shattered, and the acetabular roof disorganized (A). There was a contused laceration of the abdominal wall, but the peritoneum and viscera were intact. The largest iliac fragment, including the roof of the acetabulum (arrow), was reduced at the time of wound excision and fixed in place by plates and screws (B). Transfixion pins may also serve as internal fixation devices (see Figure 16–15, C).

shattered and gouged toward the surface, but, more important, the cecum or descending colon may also be damaged (Fig. 16–6). A contused wound of the belly wall often contaminates the fracture, and, if the peritoneum has been lacerated, the danger of infection may be increased by the presence of intestinal contents in the wound. A prompt surgical toilet should be carried out. If the peritoneal cavity is open, the abdominal and pelvic viscera must be examined and, when necessary, repaired. If the peritoneum is intact, exploratory laparotomy may be deferred pending the development of appropriate indications, as outlined in Chapter 17, on Injuries of the Abdomen.

The shattered ilium, per se, is of minor importance, since the main bony circle of the pelvis is intact. The broken fragments may be removed, reduced, or left undisturbed, as the local circumstances dictate. In the absence of bone infection an excellent result is the rule, unless the acetabulum has been damaged by the injury. If this has occurred (Fig. 16–6), the acetabulum should be reconstructed at the time of wound excision and cleansing. The displacing power of the muscles attached to the anterior ilium usually makes some form of internal fixation necessary to maintenance of acetabular reconstruction. There should be no hesitation in accepting the calculated risk of implanting foreign fixation materials in such a contaminated but cleansed wound, for without internal fixation failure is virtually certain.

STABLE FRACTURES OF THE PELVIS

A single break in the continuity of the essentially rigid pelvic girdle remains undisplaced. When an apparently isolated break in continuity of the pelvic girdle is characterized by displacement, a second injury must be present (see Fig. 16–7, *D*). Frequently this second injury is a small disruption of one sacroiliac joint, which may be difficult or impossible to identify in a roentgenogram.

Fracture of a Single Pubic Ramus

Displacement cannot occur with fracture of a single pubic ramus (Fig. 16–7, *C*, *a*), because the pubic ring is a rigid circle of bone. Sound union and complete recovery are certain. Except for a short period of rest and palliation for one or two weeks following injury, treatment is unnecessary. Weight bearing may be allowed as soon as it can be tolerated.

Unilateral Fractures of Both Pubic Rami

This injury creates a break in the continuity of the main pelvic ring (Fig. 16–7, *C*, *b*), but so long as the pelvic ring is broken in only a single

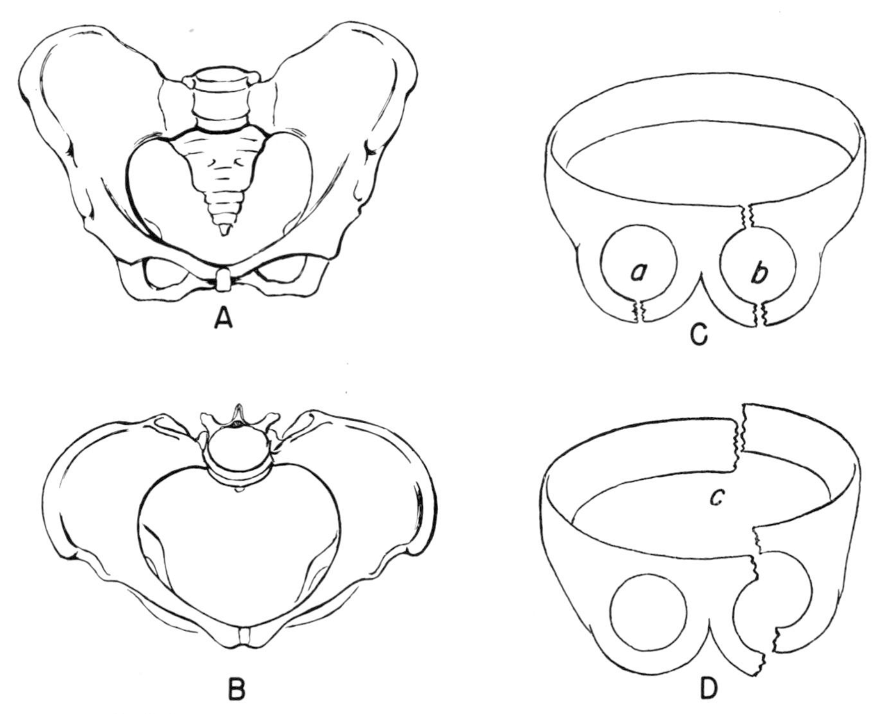

Figure 16–7.

A, B. The pelvis skeleton is the equivalent of a rigid bony circle.

C. Fracture through a single plane of the pubic ring (a) or through a single plane of the pelvic ring (b) cannot displace.

D. Displacement in fracture of the pubic ramus is indicative of simultaneous injury to another segment of the pelvic ring (c).

plane displacement cannot occur. Weight-bearing strain is transmitted to the injured segment via the "give" of the sacroiliac ligaments, and, although this cannot produce displacement of the bone fragments, painful symptoms on weight bearing often are perpetuated for four to eight weeks. Several weeks of bed rest often is required before progressive weight bearing becomes tolerable. Complete recovery occurs within several months.

The "Sprung" Sacroiliac Joint

Unilateral fractures of both pubic rami with a small amount of displacement often are accompanied by some distortion of one sacroiliac joint. Roentgen recognition of the latter injury is possible only with gross displacement, and the clinical signs of a sacroiliac joint injury are seldom present. Such a subluxed or "sprung" sacroiliac joint is an innocuous injury which rarely produces early or late symptoms. Indeed, even gross disruption and prolonged sacroiliac instability (see Fig. 16–*14*) seldom has been observed to be a source of significant pain. This writer has yet to recognize an isolated subluxation of a sacroiliac joint. Such a lesion, in the absence of a fracture elsewhere in the pelvic ring, is usually accompanied by a comparable small distortion of a relaxed symphysis pubis. This may result from infection in the interpubic syndesmosis, but is more commonly encountered following parturition, when all the pelvic ligaments are relaxed, and a painful and palpable separation of the symphysis pubis may temporarily occur.

BLADDER INJURY COMPLICATING MINOR PELVIC FRACTURES

Injury to the genitourinary tract, especially to the bladder, may complicate the simplest and most minor injury to the pelvis. An empty bladder is relatively immune to rupture, and can be lacerated only by gross displacement of fracture fragments, but a distended bladder may be ruptured, even by the impact of force to the pelvis which is insufficient to cause a fracture. Rupture of a distended bladder is not uncommon with relatively undisplaced pubic fractures (Fig. 16–*8, A*), and often is accompanied by some contusion and subsequent edema of the urethra.

Even without direct damage to the genitourinary tract, the hemorrhage from fractures of the pubis extravasates along the urogenital diaphragm to puddle around the neck of the bladder. Sphincter spasm is produced by the consequent local inflammatory reaction. With all pubic fractures extracellular fluid accumulates and partially obliterates the lower pelvic cavity, to lift the bladder cephalad and often to displace it away from the side of the injury (Fig. 16–*8, B*). The common combination of sphincter spasm, contusion, stretch, and external pressure against both urethra and bladder frequently results in an obstinate but temporary retention of urine which requires management by catheterization. *The integrity of the urinary tract should be confirmed in every pelvic injury, no matter how minor it appears.*

Bladder rupture may be extraperitoneal, with extravasation of urine

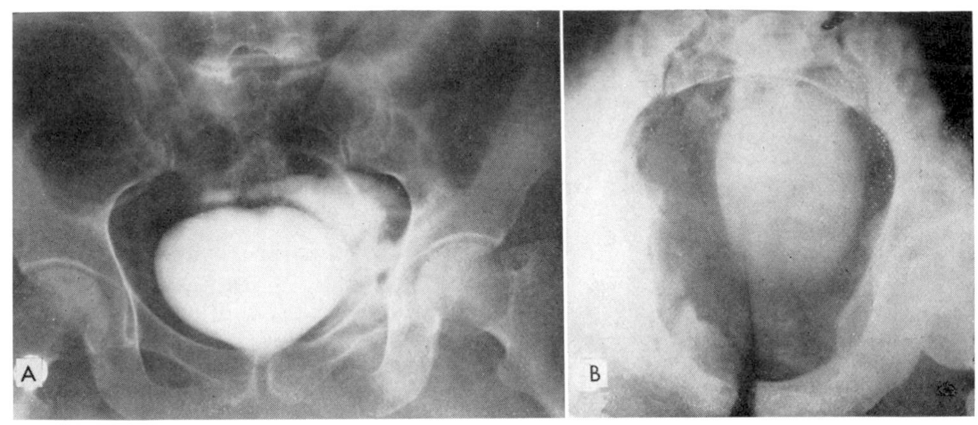

Figure 16–8. Genitourinary tract involvement in fractures of the pelvis.

A. Stable fracture of both rami of pubis without gross displacement. Bladder ruptured, with extravasation of dye.

B. Stable pubic ramus fracture, bladder intact, but intravenous pyelogram shows it to be elevated, flattened by intrapelvic swelling, and displaced away from the side of fracture.

into the regional tissue spaces to produce a severe retroperitoneal reaction, or intraperitoneal, with spillage of urine into the abdominal cavity to produce acute peritonitis. In either event, rapid and profound shock is the rule. All infected areas must be drained widely, and the urine stream must be diverted by suprapubic cystostomy at the earliest possible moment.

Diagnosis of Bladder Rupture

The following procedures are useful in determining if the bladder has been ruptured:

1. Catheterize immediately unless spontaneous voiding occurs:
   (*a*) if clear urine is recovered, bladder rupture is improbable;
   (*b*) if bloody urine is recovered, bladder rupture is probable;
   (*c*) if no urine is recovered, bladder rupture is probable.
2. Confirm the diagnosis by
   (*a*) injection of 200 ml. of sterile water through the catheter—if the full amount is not recovered, bladder rupture of some degree is fairly certain (a negative result does not preclude a small rupture);
   (*b*) injection of radiopaque dye into the catheter, followed by roentgenogram (see Figures 16–8, 16–*10*);
   (*c*) intravenous pyelogram, except in the presence of profound shock, during which the kidneys are unlikely to excrete enough dye to produce adequate visualization of the bladder.

UNSTABLE INJURIES OF THE PELVIS

"Straddle" Injuries

Direct trauma to the pubes or perineum may produce grossly unstable fractures limited to the anterior segment of the pelvic girdle. The pubic bones are shattered and may be torn free from their abdominal- or thigh-muscle attachments. To nurse a patient with such an injury in the supine position is poor treatment, and may result in a silent displacement of the fracture fragments cephalad by the abdominal muscles (Fig. 16–9, *B*), or into the thigh by the adductors (see Figure 16–*14*). Recumbency is mandatory, but patients with these injuries *should be nursed or immobilized in a semi-sitting position.* When the urinary tract is displaced or overstretched by soft-part connections to the displaced bone segment, open reduction and internal fixation of the fracture may be necessary to control of urinary dysfunction. Otherwise, bed rest in a semi-sitting position to maintain relaxation of both abdominal and thigh muscles should be continued until the fracture heals strongly enough to withstand the pull of the displacing musculature.

Rupture of urethra by "straddle" injury. The anterior urethra is most commonly ruptured by a "straddle" injury, whereas the posterior urethra is usually lacerated by a displaced fragment of bone. The diagnosis may be suspected when there are acute urinary retention and inability to void, blood at the urethral meatus, and swelling and ecchymosis in the perineum, scrotum, or lower abdomen. It is confirmed by finding a movable prostate on rectal examination, by inability to pass a urethral catheter, and by roentgen evidence of the rupture (Fig. 16–*10*).

If a catheter can be passed, it should be left in place. So long as the urine stream is diverted and further extravasation prevented by an indwelling catheter, an injured urethra will heal, and, although dilatation of the scarred segment may subsequently be required, the urinary tract remains patent. After the successful passage of a catheter, doubt may remain concerning the presence or absence of a urethral rupture. This may be dispelled by injection of a small quantity of concentrated dye into

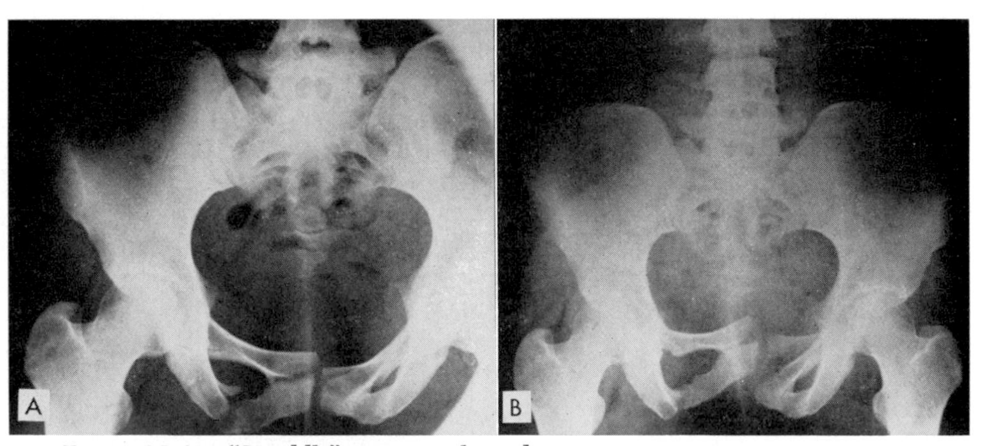

Figure 16–9. *"Straddle" injury to the pubes.*

Multiple fractures of the pubic bones (A) with little or no displacement. The patient was nursed supine rather than in a semi-sitting position. The rectus abdominis muscles produced cephalad displacement of the pubic fragments (B) and secondarily distorted and jeopardized the function of the urinary tract. Patients with unstable pubic fractures should be nursed in a semi-sitting position.

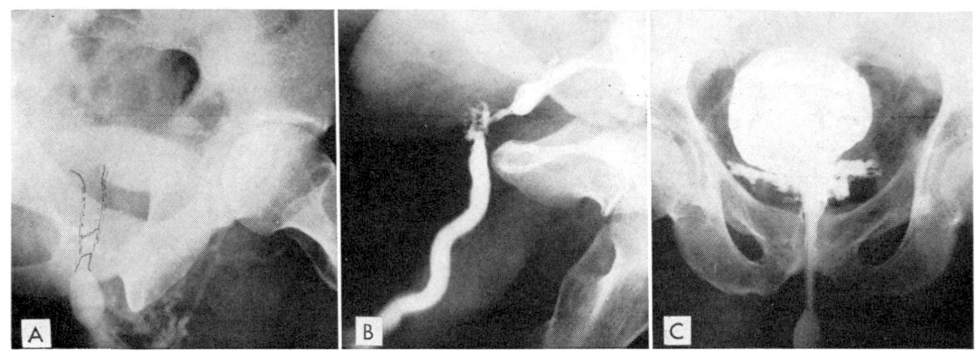

Figure 16–10.

A. Pelvic injury complicated by rupture of the posterior portion of the urethra. Note the extravasation of dye throughout the perineal veins.

B. "Straddle" injury complicated by rupture of the anterior portion of the urethra.

C. The urethra has been incompletely avulsed from the neck of the bladder.

the urethra, following which roentgenograms will confirm the presence or absence of extravasation.

Extravasation warrants suprapubic cystostomy and wide drainage of all involved tissues. Inability to pass a catheter past the rupture, or even to find the torn ends of the urethra, is common. Under these circumstances two metal sounds should be passed, one from the open bladder cavity, and one from the urethral meatus, until their ends meet at the point of urethral rupture. If these ends are maintained in contact, it is then possible to guide the distal sound into the bladder. A catheter then can be locked or tied to the end of this sound, and withdrawn retrograde through the urethra.

DISLOCATIONS OF THE PELVIS

Disruption of the pelvis by rupture of its great supporting ligaments results from rotation of one innominate bone in the sagittal plane while the remainder of the pelvic ring remains fixed. The primary force is leverage by the hyperextended femur (Fig. 16–*11, A*). When the femoral lever is also abducted, the pelvis splits apart at the symphysis, and the two halves swing open like an oyster shell on a posterior hinge made possible by disruption of the sacroiliac ligaments. However, if the hyperextended femoral lever is adducted, the two pelvic segments telescope so that the pubic bones overlap (Fig. 16–*12, A, B*). Associated fractures, except for avulsion of flakes of bone by the ligaments, are rare, but concomitant injuries to the pelvic viscera are common. As a rule, reduction of the displaced pelvic segment greatly facilitates repair of the associated visceral injuries.

The "Burst" Pelvis (Dislocation by Hyperextension and Abduction)

The affected extremity lies in lateral rotation. A palpable hiatus at the symphysis is filled by a massive hematoma. Rupture of the bladder or

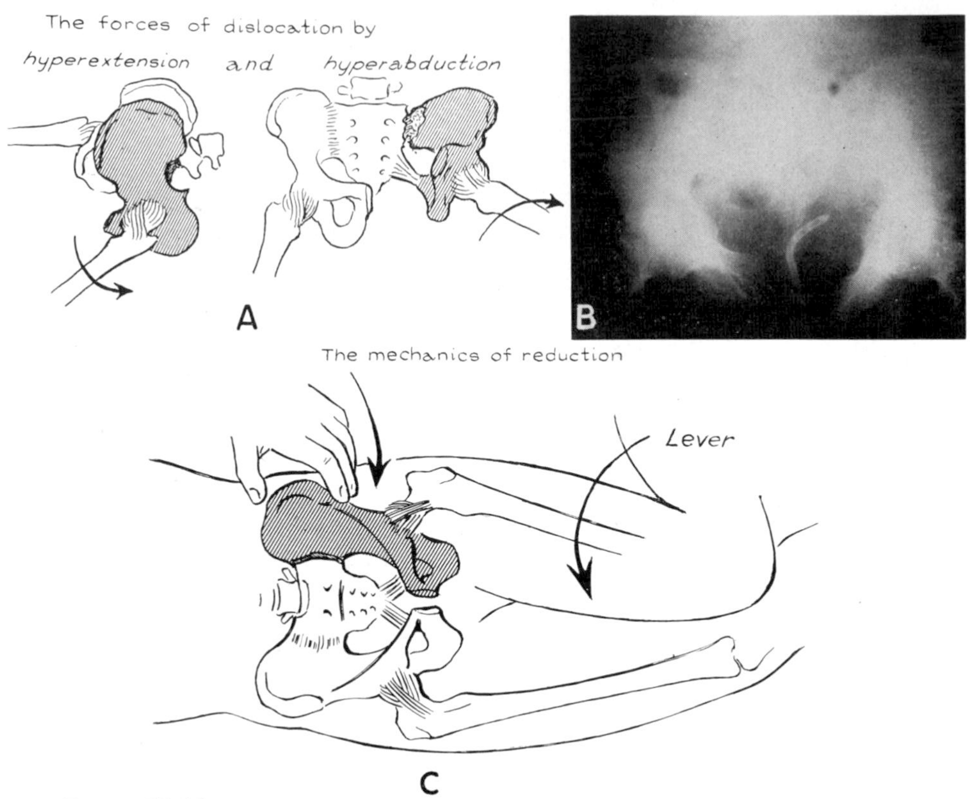

Figure 16–11.

A. Dislocation of the hindquarter results from violent hyperextension of the femoral lever, sufficient to rupture the ligaments bridging the symphysis pubis and the sacroiliac joint. When this force is combined with abduction, the pelvis splits open like an oyster shell.

B. The roentgenogram indicates it is probable that the bladder followed the displaced pelvic segment.

C. Reduction by manipulation should reverse the offending forces. The patient is placed on the intact side. The pelvic segments are compressed manually. The femoral lever is adducted, flexed, and rotated medially.

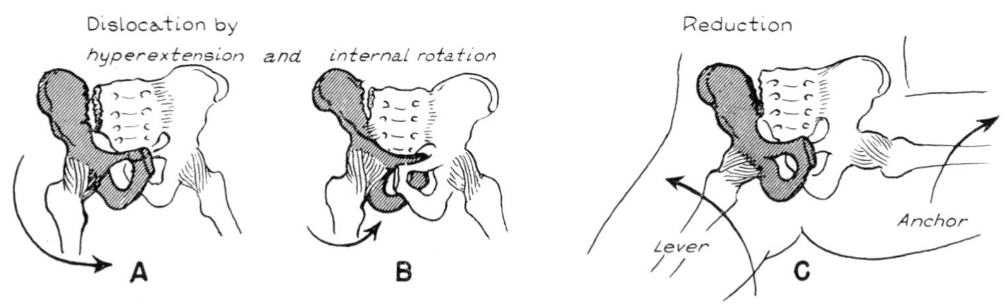

Figure 16–12.

A, B. Following disruption of the ligaments by hyperextension, adduction of the femoral lever produces a scissors dislocation. The displaced pelvic half may come to rest in front of (A) or behind (B) its mate.

C. Reduction requires the intact pelvic segment to be stabilized and anchored by abduction and external rotation of the femur, the other femur then being used as a lever to disengage the locked pubes.

urethra or avulsion of the urethra from the bladder must be suspected. Urine may be spilled into both the extraperitoneal and intraperitoneal spaces. Under any circumstances all the signs of acute peritoneal irritation are present, and profound shock is to be expected.

Reduction should be done as soon as possible, for little else can be accomplished until the bones are replaced. Small separations of the symphysis can be closed by placing the patient in lateral recumbency and compressing the two pelvic segments. Gross disruptions often require utilization of the femoral lever to reverse the forces which created the displacement. The patient is placed recumbent, lying on the intact side so that the weight of the displaced hindquarter will aid in its replacement. The extremity of the affected side is then flexed, adducted, and rotated inward coincident with a strong downward push against the iliac crest of the dislocated segment (Fig. 16–*11, C*). Maintenance of reduction requires a continuous compression force which may be provided by a double plaster spica from rib margins to just above the knees or, when plaster encasement is contraindicated, by balanced suspension of the pelvis in a hammock or sling arranged so that body weight creates a continuous compression force.

The "Telescoped" Pelvis (Dislocation by Hyperextension and Adduction)

The hip is flexed and rotated inward. The thigh and buttock remain off the table. Bladder damage with transection of the urethra is a common result from the scissors-action of the overlapping pubes. Repair of bladder and urethra is difficult or impossible until the pubic bones are disengaged. The displaced pubic arch may rest behind or in front of its mate (Fig. 16–*12, A, B*).

Reduction is not difficult when the displaced pubis lies in front of its counterpart. With the patient supine, pressure is made over the iliac crests sufficient to derotate the displaced segment. When this is not successful, or when the dislocated pubis is jammed behind its mate, femoral leverage is required (Fig. 16–*12, C*). With the patient supine, the intact side of the pelvis is locked in place by full flexion, abduction, and lateral rotation of the extremity. This fixation should be maintained by an assistant. The femur of the affected extremity is similarly locked on its acetabulum, and then gently rocked into hyperabduction. Derotation and reduction may take place with an audible snap. There is little danger of recurrence of such an overlapping displacement, and the patient may be nursed supine.

Aftercare of Dislocated Pelvis

The patient with a reduced dislocation of the pelvis should remain recumbent with the pelvis compressed by a suspension hammock or plaster spica for eight weeks. Similarly, the patient with a grossly telescoped pelvis should remain recumbent for at least six to eight weeks, but pelvic compression is not required. Weight bearing on the affected extremity should

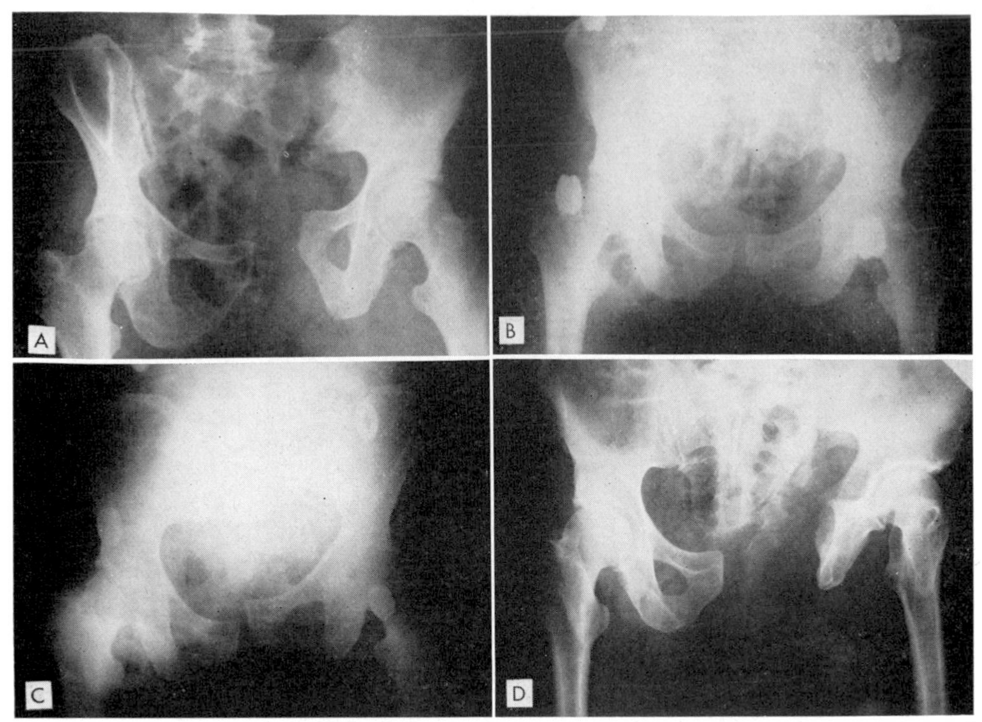

Figure 16–13. Silent cephalad displacement following reduction of dislocated hindquarter, the constant potential penalty of omitting traction from the aftercare of this injury.

A. Roentgenogram before reduction.

B. Roentgenogram after reduction. The patient was nursed in a compression hammock.

C. Two weeks after reduction–beginning loss of reduction completely unaccompanied by symptoms.

D. The end result.

be gradually resumed on crutches, increasing progressively as symptoms subside.

Silent cephalad displacement of the unstable segment is a constant possibility during the first few weeks following reduction of the burst pelvis. Roentgen examination to exclude this complication should be carried out at least once a week for several weeks. When such displacement remains unrecognized for even a short time, correction is precluded by repair of the soft tissues (Fig. 16–*13*). As soon as any tendency toward cephalad migration of the reduced innominate bone is observed, continuous traction should be applied to the affected extremity. Skeletal pin traction through the upper tibia, with the foot of the bed elevated on 6-inch blocks, should be instituted promptly, and continued for several weeks.

FRACTURE-DISLOCATION OF THE PELVIS

Massive crushing injuries may produce gross ligament disruption combined with multiple fractures throughout the pelvic ring. Some visceral

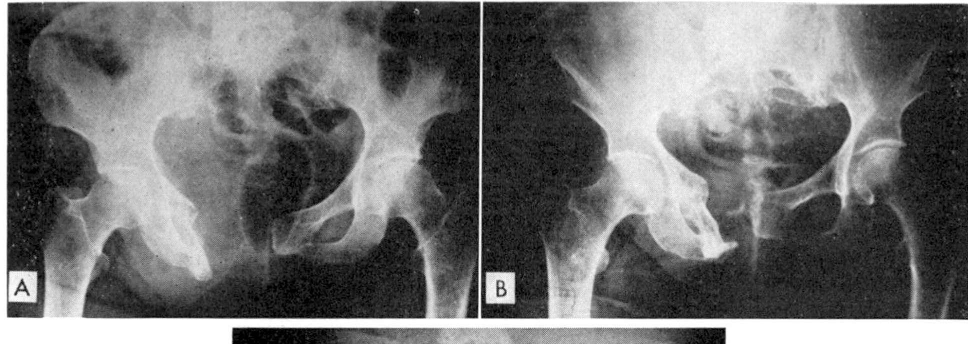

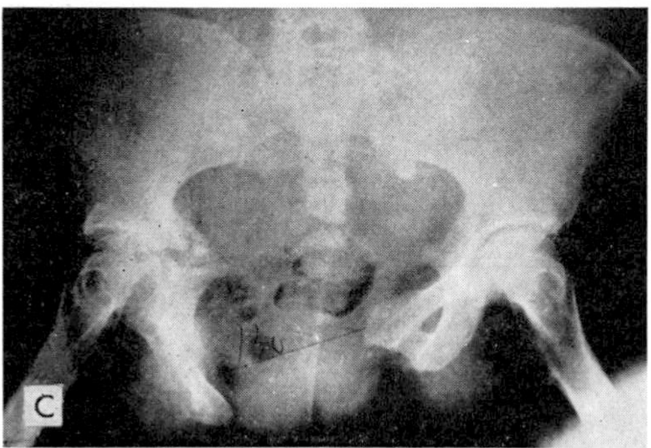

Figure 16–14. Ipsilateral and contralateral fracture-dislocation.

A. Disruption of symphysis, right sacroiliac joint, and right pubic arch. The fracture fragments are avulsed from the abdominal muscles and displaced into the thigh by the adductors.

B. Later film representing the late range of hypermobility persisting in the right sacroiliac joint (difference in distance between the pubic arches in A and B) without symptoms in this region. No significant defect in locomotion.

C. Disruption of symphysis, left sacroiliac joint, and fracture of the right innominate bone at the level of the acetabulum. The pubic arch is again pulled into the thigh by the adductors. No reduction. Considerable interference with locomotion due to the right hip joint deformity, but no symptoms in the left sacroiliac joint.

damage is almost always present. There is no consistent pattern of injury, except that the pelvic girdle usually is disrupted in both anterior and posterior segments. Entire segments may be not only displaced from the remainder of the pelvis, but also torn loose from much of their muscular supports. The remaining attached muscles then produce great displacement (Fig. 16–*14*). Profound shock makes any operative procedure precarious, but visceral damage must be repaired at the earliest possible moment, and at times this requires prior re-assemblage and fixation of the displaced bones. In themselves, displaced pubic segments produce relatively little disability, and acceptance of malunion may prove a lesser risk than an uncertain repair in a patient who is a poor operative risk. As pointed out early in this chapter, the entire anterior wall of the pelvic girdle is functionally unimportant to locomotion (see Fig. 16–*1*), and, if necessary, late excision of a grossly displaced pubic segment can be done. Except when it is necessary to the control of visceral injuries, the only common indication for early open reduction of the damaged pelvis skeleton

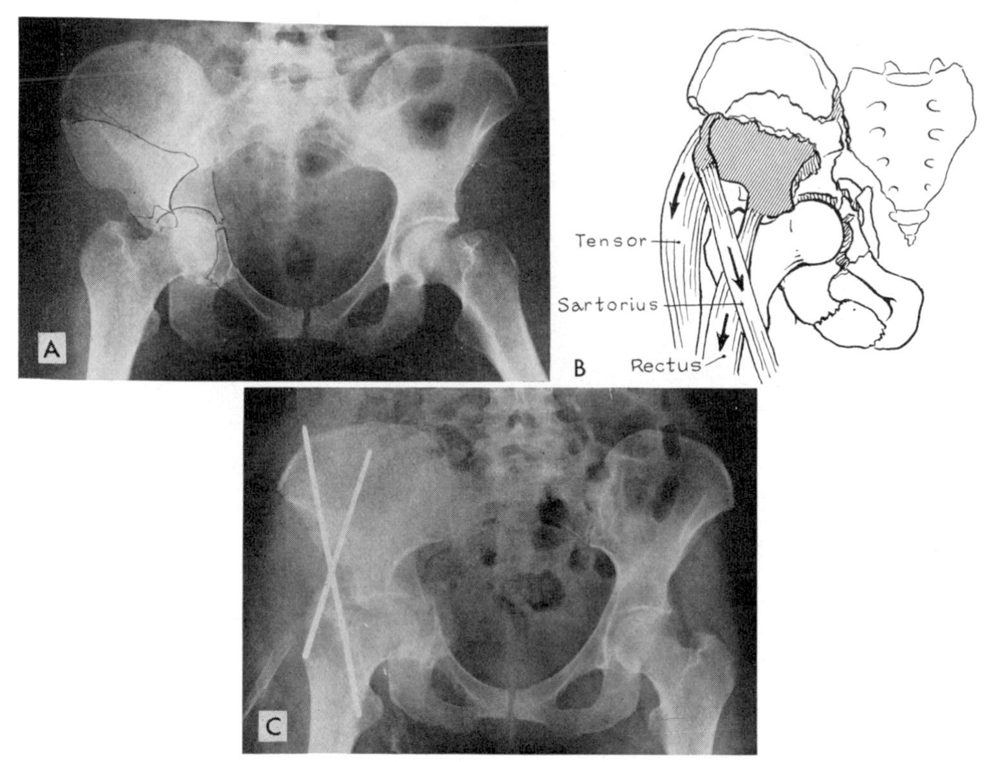

Figure 16–15. The roentgenogram is an incomplete index of bone damage in the pelvis.

A. The main fracture lines as seen in the original roentgenogram are marked.

B. The actual findings at operation. The anterior (shaded) iliac fragment, containing 50 per cent of the acetabular surface, was rotated through 90 degrees by the thigh muscles (arrows).

C. Reconstruction of the acetabulum was maintained by transfixion of the main iliac fragments with heavy pins. Immobilization in a plaster spica for eight weeks was followed by a good result.

is gross disorganization of the roof of the acetabulum (Fig. 16–*15*). Such a lesion requires open reduction and internal fixation as soon as the patient's general condition will permit.

Permanent sacroiliac instability or hypermobility is likely if the symphysis remains separated. It is not usually a cause of significant pain nor, except in the presence of cephalad hindquarter displacement, does it produce much difficulty in locomotion. The involved hindquarter swings like a gate on the massive fibrous-tissue hinge formed by healing of the disrupted sacroiliac joint; the symphysis gap increases or decreases, depending on femoral leverage (Fig. 16–*14, A, B*). However, the trouble likely to be caused by the loose sacroiliac joint is much less serious than are the chronic urinary difficulties attendant upon the disturbed symphysis.

COMBINED PELVIC INJURIES IN CHILDREN

The pelvic bones of a child are more elastic than those in an adult, and they usually give way before their connecting ligaments do. A crushing

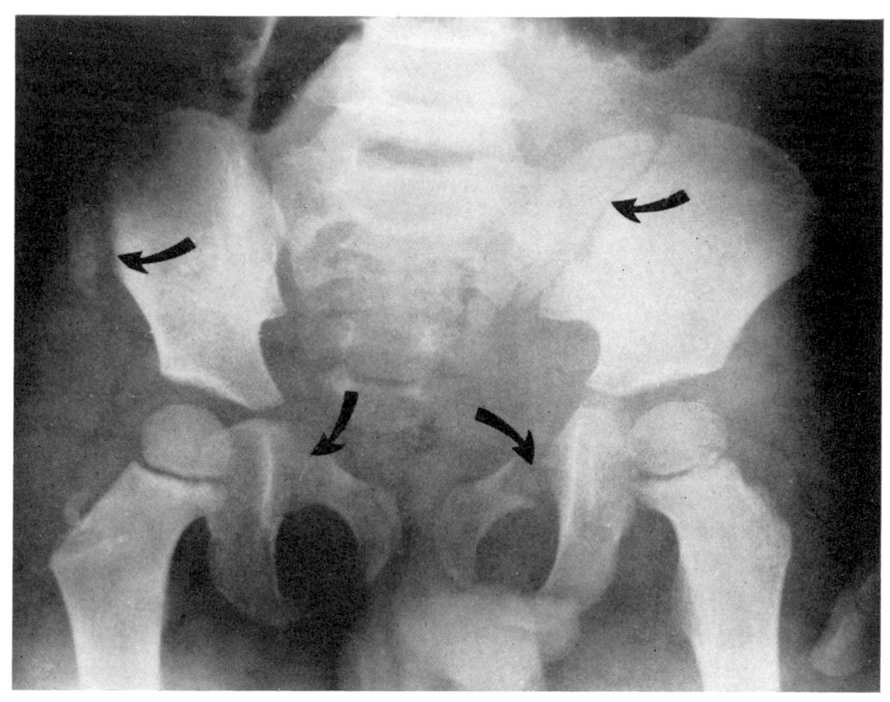

Figure 16–16. "Balloon tire" runover injury in a child.

The tire was soft enough and the pelvic girdle of the child resilient enough so that gross deformity did not occur. All four pelvic quadrants are the seat of multiple fractures (arrows). The sacroiliac and interpubic ligaments remained essentially intact. The patient was nursed supine until the intra-abdominal status was stabilized, and then was dressed in a plaster spica for eight weeks. Recovery was uneventful, with little or no permanent defect.

injury is more apt to produce multiple fractures (Fig. 16–*16*) than joint disruption. Gross displacement is consequently less common than in the adult, since the fracture fragments remain somewhat stabilized by relatively intact soft-part supports, and the displacing power of the muscles is relatively small. Supportive therapy, management of associated visceral injuries, and bed rest until the fragments unite constitute the essentials of treatment.

FRACTURE OF THE SACRUM

The sacrum is fractured by direct trauma, usually the result of a fall against a hard object. The fracture is transverse, and there is seldom any displacement; it is exquisitely tender and painful, but not often of serious import. The upper half of the bone is relatively protected by the posterior iliac spines and securely stabilized by the sacroiliac ligaments. Consequently, fractures which damage the second and third sacral nerves and create serious bladder and rectal complications are uncommon. Injury to the lower and relatively unprotected sacral segments is unlikely to be complicated by more than mild and transient neurological complications.

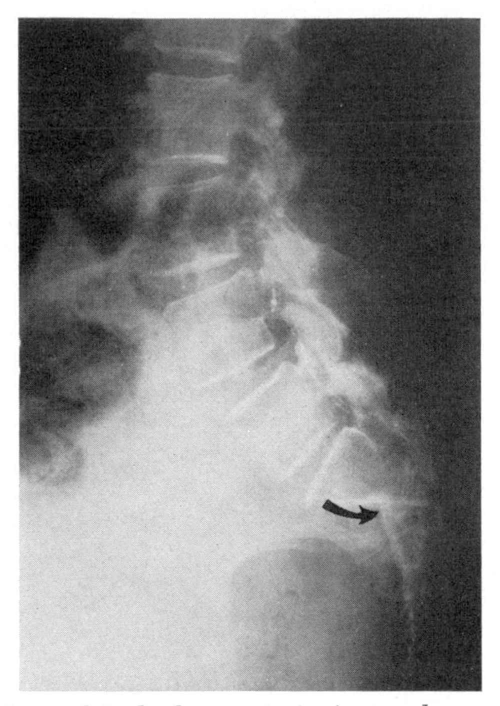

Figure 16–17. Intrapelvic displacement of a fractured sacrum.

Marked cauda equina damage by the fracture at the level of the second and third sacral vertebrae produced intractable bladder and rectum paralysis. The atonic rectum permits a firm grasp upon the distal fracture fragment, and manipulative reduction should be attempted.

Constipation should be prevented, and the fracture area protected from undue external pressure for four to six weeks, after which sound healing is present.

Gross displacement of the lower segment of a fractured sacrum (Fig. 16–*17*) causes injury to the cauda equina and may produce a complete paralysis of bladder and rectum, as well as saddle anesthesia in the gluteal cleft. Through the atonic rectal sphincter two fingers may be inserted easily to permit a firm grasp on the displaced fragment. An attempt to reduce the displacement in this manner should be made in all early cases, but within about two weeks fibrosis precludes manipulative replacement, and neurosurgical decompression of the cauda equina offers the sole but rather forlorn hope for improvement.

INJURIES TO THE COCCYX

Because of the variable shape and axis of the coccyx, many more coccyx fractures are diagnosed roentgenographically than really occur. Contusion of the coccyx is common, and is equally capable of producing the early acute or protracted chronic pain of coccygodynia. Both injuries should receive the same treatment during the phase of acute pain, namely, protection from external pressure by correct sitting posture, protection from the internal irritation of a constipated stool by laxatives, warm baths, and other simple palliative measures. In the absence of some continuing irritation of the injured area, complete recovery is to be expected within a few weeks.

Coccygodynia is caused and perpetuated by improper posture. When an individual sits up straight on a hard surface there is little or no pressure on the coccyx. However, the human is inclined to slouch, get his feet up in the air, and sit in soft chairs, all of which tend to give the coccyx a weight-bearing function for which it is not suited. Such continued mechanical abuse of the coccyx following injury is the most important single factor in perpetuating the discomfort of coccygodynia. Once firmly established, this painful syndrome is persistent, but recovery is virtually certain if, until the symptoms subside completely, the patient adheres to three rules—never to become constipated, never to sit except bolt upright on a hard chair, and always to sleep on a firm bed. Only when a thorough trial of this program has failed to bring relief is coccygectomy justified.

CHAPTER 17

INJURIES OF THE ABDOMEN

By LAWRENCE W. SLOAN, M.D.

Combined Thoraco-abdominal Injuries

GENERAL CONSIDERATIONS

The thorax and abdomen are subject to every type of injury. The effects produced are fundamentally the same as those produced by trauma elsewhere in the body. The factors which are responsible for the seriousness and distinctive nature of these injuries are derived from the variety and complexity of the hidden, vital, contiguous structures involved. These same factors are responsible also for the difficulties of interpreting physical signs. This is unlike trauma of the extremities and periphery, where inspection alone often reveals the essential facts regarding the nature, extent, and seriousness of the injury. The *complications* and *sequelae* of these injuries, particularly of those of the abdomen, are often puzzling for the same reason. They beget their own problems of diagnosis and treatment. These often are as difficult to interpret and manage as the original trauma, and sometimes are even more difficult.

Whether gains have been made in useful knowledge of the pathophysiological mechanisms of injury and repair as the result of war may well be questioned. It cannot be denied, however, that war has been a proving ground for surgical principle and practice. Also, much valuable experience has been gained by a great many physicians in the application of principles of surgery which have been tried and proved or discarded in combat surgery. The use of primary delayed closure of debrided contaminated wounds, which was practiced so extensively and successfully in World War II, was regarded by some as the discovery of new knowledge. Actually, this principle of treatment was well known in civilian practice long before then, but its teaching had been neglected; and its importance and value even today are widely underestimated because of an easily accepted tendency to rely so heavily upon antibiotics and chemotherapeutic agents. In general, significant advances in knowledge are made between wars in everything except how to adapt what has already been learned to uses of war.

Wartime vs. Peacetime Injuries

The significant differences between abdominal injuries inflicted in war and those incurred by civilians in peacetime should be pointed out, for the sake of perspective. In the former, and until the pattern of armed conflict changes substantially, as it seems likely to do, penetrating and open abdominal trauma will greatly exceed closed, blunt, or nonpenetrating injury, whereas in peacetime civilian life, including traffic, occupational, domestic, and rural accidents, the reverse is true. This situation alters importantly the role of diagnosis, but not the principles of treatment. Important as is diagnosis in the handling of open wounds from the standpoint of avoiding unnecessary celiotomy, the number of operative procedures that will have to be carried out perforce and speedily, without exact diagnosis of the extent of the injury, will be far greater for open wounds than in the closed trauma group. In the latter better judgment, based on accurate diagnosis, will be required to decide not only whether visceral injury has occurred but also whether to operate if it has and, lastly, when it should be done. It follows also that in war injuries the hollow viscera will be injured more frequently than the solid viscera, the opposite in general being true of civilian accidents. Direct, nonpenetrating force may produce ruptures of the stomach, duodenum, small and large bowel, and bladder, but this is relatively uncommon. Penetrating wounds entering the abdominal cavity almost invariably produce perforations of one or more of these structures. Intraperitoneal hemorrhage therefore will frequently be associated with blunt trauma of the abdomen, which will be sustained much more frequently in civilian accidents than in war wounds.

In our present peacetime motorized and otherwise mechanized civilization, traffic and industrial accidents constitute the major causes of abdominal and thoraco-abdominal injuries. In peacetime civilian life the general surgeon sees nowhere near the number or the variety of injuries that is encountered in wartime. Many of the mass techniques developed for handling injuries on such a scale would, therefore, not apply in civilian practice. On the other hand, it was only the employment of sound surgical principles, adapted efficiently and with competence to wartime needs during the latter months of World War II and the Korean conflict, that resulted in such great improvement in mortality and morbidity over the performance in World War I.

The use of chemotherapeutic and antibiotic agents certainly modified but did not replace the application of sound surgical principles. This is illustrated by the initial ill-considered use of sulfonamide powder in fresh wounds. Such a measure not only was found to be insufficient to replace early, rational debridement, splinting, and careful transportation of patients with open wounds (supplemented, it is true, by the intelligent use of these new agents) but was often found to be actually harmful. What new techniques will be devised to meet the contingencies of another world conflict is well beyond the scope or intent of the present text. It is safe to say, however, that the basic principles we have learned will not change. Success in saving the civilian and military population from death and incapacitating disability resulting from physical trauma will be in proportion to the degree, intelligence, and organizational efficiency with which these principles are applied to a large number of casualties.

Principles of Management of Multiple Injuries

Abdominal and abdomino-thoracic injuries are among the most serious with which the surgeon has to cope. It must never be forgotten that serious as these injuries may be or may seem to be, other even more serious injuries may also have been incurred. Associated injuries often prove to be more important and their treatment more urgent than the abdominal one. If an associated thoracic injury is present, either separately or as a component of the abdominal injury, treatment of this, generally speaking, will take precedence, and always will if respiratory function is jeopardized.

Disregard of the fundamental precept of examining casualties for multiple injuries was constantly warned against in handling battle injuries. In peacetime injuries, particularly in traffic accidents, it is not so much the pressure of the load (which was frequently the case in handling combat casualties) which is responsible for overlooking important hidden associated injuries. The masking effect of alcohol must be cautioned against particularly in evaluating civilian traffic injuries. Although in research studies on traffic accidents a relatively small number are attributable *directly* to drunkenness,* the number of accidents caused indirectly because of the effects of alcohol undoubtedly is very much higher and would be almost impossible to compute accurately. The signs and symptoms of injury in an intoxicated person are difficult, if not impossible, to interpret. Vomiting is common, and it should be recalled that vomitus which does not contain blood is of little diagnostic significance in thoracic and abdominal trauma. The examiner nevertheless is forced to make important decisions affecting the injured person's welfare or chance of survival on the basis of objective evidence alone, which, in the case of central injuries (as opposed to peripheral ones, which generally are obvious), may be fatal. The great danger is in assuming that the injuries are minor in such cases, and allowing the patient to be removed from observation prematurely during the lag interval between the time of injury and the development of signs of serious damage.

In civilian practice there is seldom the excuse for making this serious mistake. It is a rare injury which requires such urgent treatment that one does not have a chance to think—to size up the situation, and to formulate a plan for doing first things first and then to proceed in an orderly fashion to treat the injured person. Occasionally one must and does act by instinct, which is better if it has been trained. This will occur most frequently in providing an airway and in arresting hemorrhage—more likely in the proper sequence, when the two occur simultaneously, if the instinct has been trained. The treatment of most injuries permits, and under certain circum-

* Nine per cent reported in a panel discussion on Crash Injuries and Their Prevention at the 51st Annual Meeting of the Sixth District Branch of the Medical Society of the State of New York.

stances demands, thoughtful reflection. Under no other circumstances is this more important than in handling abdominal and thoraco-abdominal injuries.

Priority of Treatment of Multiple Injuries

In learning to work out the problems which arise in handling injuries to the thorax and abdomen, a principle of the utmost practical importance is to reduce them to their simplest possible terms: (1) a partially disabled respiratory mechanism, (2) hemorrhage, and (3) infection. Any one of these may, at the time of injury or subsequently, dominate the picture, and alone be responsible for the death of the patient. Death will occur most rapidly from acute failure of respiration which, at times, results from the simplest of causes such as obstruction of the airway by the tongue when the jaw muscles are relaxed with the patient in the supine position, or from more complex causes such as a severe injury producing multiple rib fractures and a flail chest. Respiratory function must be restored and maintained. Therefore, attention to injuries jeopardizing this mechanism must take precedence whenever it is compromised or threatened. Hemorrhage may also prove rapidly fatal either directly as the result of exsanguination, or indirectly, as by cardiac tamponade. Arresting the bleeding or relieving the tamponade may have first priority. Infection develops later, but may be the sole cause of death. Usually, of course, non-lethal components of all three are present in varying proportions. It is the ability to assess these accurately, and to implement treatment based on such an evaluation, which constitutes skill in handling abdominal and thoraco-abdominal injuries.

Frequently these injuries are complex, or seem so when first seen. One is baffled not only in making an accurate diagnosis of injury, especially in nonpenetrating trauma, but also in assessing extent of the injury. Frequently, these days, there are multiple injuries because of the large number of traffic accidents. The priority and manner of going about treating them, as in war injuries, may be puzzling unless one has trained himself to consider the problem in terms of relative urgency with respect to the threats to life and function.

A good working plan for establishing priority of treatment in this group of seriously injured patients has been suggested by Curry and Lyttle. Of first priority are the injuries which interfere with vital physiological function (e.g., flail chest, tension pneumothorax, cardiac tamponade, severe bleeding, obstructions of the respiratory tract). Of second priority are those injuries which do not produce death early but the persistence of which, untreated, adds to the shock and will probably result in death if treatment is unduly delayed (e.g., perforation of a hollow viscus). Of third priority are those injuries which contribute little to the persistence of shock or to the impairment of ultimate function if the injured parts are properly splinted and dressed (e.g., fractures, and superficial, peripheral soft tissue injuries). Let it be emphasized that *the greatest danger lies in failure to recognize the existence of injuries of second priority* either because of the urgency of those in the first group or because those in the third group are so obvious and often dramatic that those in the second group are overlooked. Injuries of second priority are often silent at first, their effects delayed, and symptoms obscured or masked. Many abdominal injuries fall into this group.

Alterations in Physiology Produced by Thoraco-abdominal Injuries

The significant systemic responses of the body to trauma are discussed in Chapter 1. It should be noted that, because of the relatively greater severity and consequently the greater morbidity and high mortality rate of abdominal and thoraco-abdominal injuries, the greater is the need for those undertaking the care of patients who have incurred them to understand what the mechanisms are which produce deleterious systemic responses due to trauma, how to recognize them, what causes them, and how to treat them. The development of perspective in the use of many of the advocated agents and methods of handling abdominal trauma and its complications is a process of slow evolution, as in other fields of medicine.

Primary shock is a constant and familiar concomitant of injury. Its diagnosis and treatment are well understood. The subsequent shifts in body fluids accompanying changes and losses in electrolytes and the relation of these to fluid administration to the injured are now much better understood than before World War II. The mechanism of renal failure associated with an increase in circulating potassium and nitrogen, and the harmful effects of anoxia and other fundamental physiological disturbances associated with severe trauma are still under investigation.

The solution of problems of wound healing and failure to make satisfactory nutritional gains following hepatic damage caused by trauma, which are exceedingly important factors in treating patients suffering from abdominal trauma, are being facilitated by the development of solutions of utilizable protein and fat which can be tolerated when given intravenously. The enzymatic debridement of burns and sloughing wounds and the dissolution of collections of clotted blood within closed cavities are now possible under certain conditions. The value of antibiotics and chemotherapeutic agents used locally and systemically both in the prophylaxis and treatment of infection in abdominal trauma is gradually being evaluated.

CLINICAL AND ANATOMICAL CHARACTERISTICS OF THORACO-ABDOMINAL INJURIES

Clinical and anatomical features relevant to trauma of the abdomen and thorax in particular must be considered by anyone caring for injuries within these compartments.

External Evidence No Index of Extent or Import of Injury

Estimation of the extent of injury, of whatever type, cannot necessarily be based on the external evidence. Serious direct and indirect effects of trauma to the abdomen and chest may result from causes which produce little or no external evidence of violence. These are often overlooked in the presence of multiple, more obvious, external injuries. A relatively slight contusion or small wound may produce a fatal rupture of liver, spleen, pancreas, or hollow viscus (the symptoms of which may be slow in developing), or a sudden, fatal intrathoracic hemorrhage, or collapse of the lung.

Autogenous Potential Sources of Contamination

Within the peritoneal cavity are hollow viscera which contain gas and fluid. Many of the bacteria within these structures, as well as those which are introduced from the outside via penetrating agents, are pathogenic. The enzymatic secretions from some intra-abdominal structures when activated become capable of digesting organic material, either autogenously or synergistically.

Vascular Viscera

The solid viscera within the peritoneal cavity are unusually vascular and relatively fixed. Bleeding from them is hidden, particularly in nonpenetrating injuries. Large vascular trunks lie within or in close proximity to them. Even though serious or fatal hemorrhage may not result directly from injury to these vascular organs or to their blood supply, the nutrition of an organ may be impaired, with consequent serious or fatal effect, particularly in the abdomen, for example, impaired nutrition of a segment of bowel with resulting obstruction, gangrene, perforation, and sepsis.

Primary—Secondary Trauma Sequence

A single type of primary injury, such as a simple contusion, may be responsible for other types of injury by a sort of chain reaction. The primary injury may be relatively trivial, but the secondary trauma may be fatal. Thus a blunt blow which may not even break the skin or cause any external evidence of trauma may result in peritonitis or fatal hemorrhage. Such an injury may also occur from blast, either in air or when the abdomen is submerged under water. Likewise, a severe contusion may be responsible for fracture of a pelvic bone, a fragment from which may lacerate or puncture the bladder, rectum, or other pelvic viscera, such wound in turn leading to bleeding and sepsis.

Single Agent—Multiple Injuries

Multiple injuries may be produced by a single agent in structures which are capable of producing further contamination as well as those which are not. Thus a bullet may produce lacerations of bowel, liver, and major blood vessels. It may pass from one compartment of the abdomen to another, or to adjacent body compartments. A knowledge of anatomy, particularly of the normal and abnormal anatomical relationships within the abdomen, is of first importance. An awareness of what structures probably are involved on the basis of the direction taken by the penetrating object and its probable behavior in passing through these structures will solve most of the problems of diagnosis in dealing with such injuries.

Upper vs. Lower Abdominal Injuries

The concentration of important vascular structures in the upper abdomen, and the great possibility of contamination by highly pathogenic bacteria in the lower abdomen and pelvis, account for the principal characteristics distinguishing acute injuries in these two areas. Injuries of the lower abdomen which disrupt the colon or lower urinary tract are characterized chiefly by the development of infection and sepsis, whereas trauma of comparable type and severity in the upper abdomen will be characterized rather by hemorrhage and immediate or early severe shock. Sepsis and delayed shock, of course, often ensue.

The very acuteness of the symptoms produced by upper abdominal trauma, however, favors early operative intervention. This usually leads to prompt operative interference, early attempts to arrest hemorrhage, and closure of sources of contamination. Nevertheless, a greater number of early fatal injuries are sustained in the upper than in the lower abdomen, owing to the frequently associated injuries to vital blood vessels and extremely vascular solid viscera. Whether there is more rapid absorption from the peritoneal surfaces in the upper abdomen is doubtful. If true, this would predispose also to a rapid and acute response to injury. When a severe infection develops here the degree of acute toxemia generally is greater and the systemic effects more acute than those produced by infection in the lower abdomen. However, many factors besides rapid absorption may influence this.

Natural Defenses of Peritoneum

Tending to neutralize the effects of traumatic, bacterial and chemical insults within the peritoneal cavity is the natural defense which the peritoneum, when intact and undamaged, is known to possess. Hence the importance of gentleness in exploration is evident, as is also that of using non-irritating solutions for irrigation and debridement, and of introducing drains only when clearly indicated.

Influence of Speed of Traumatic Force

As has been pointed out elsewhere, a factor of great importance responsible for abdominal visceral damage and its degree of severity is the speed with which the force is applied. Pressure of considerable force, if exerted slowly, will usually cause little or no damage. A lesser blow delivered swiftly may, however, produce widespread damage from which the fixed solid and hollow viscera and the distended hollow viscera suffer most.

Combinations of Trauma Factors

Trauma frequently produces immediate or late effects resulting from combinations of the above factors in dealing with which speed, but not haste, is of the essence. The net result of severe abdominal trauma will be hemorrhage, inflammation (usually as infection), or both. Diagnosis will be derived from an analysis of history, signs, symptoms, and special examinations aimed at discovering the sites and extent of injury. Treatment will depend upon knowledge of the actual or potential consequences of injury at such sites that it is capable of producing hemorrhage or inflammation (including infection) or both.

THORACO-ABDOMINAL VS. PERIPHERAL TRAUMA

In peripheral trauma the severity and extent of the damage produced, including the degree of shock, are roughly proportional to the severity of the trauma responsible for the injury. There are, of course, exceptions to this general rule, as for example when an insignificant burn or scratch is the portal of entry for a highly pathogenic organism which may result in a lethal septicemia. However, in case of thoracic, and particularly in abdominal, trauma, an injury, either of the penetrating or of the nonpenetrating variety, which would be trivial if sustained at the periphery might very well cause death. This fact has been alluded to already in other connections, but its importance deserves emphasis. The management of peripheral injuries, because they are peripheral, and therefore so frequently obvious, is likely to be more promptly and better handled than most intra-abdominal and intrathoracic injuries. The principal factors which may mask the nature and extent of the latter are their hidden location, shock, and impairment of the sensorium from associated brain injuries or by alcohol.

The integrity and continuity of function of intra-abdominal and intrathoracic structures are *dependent* upon an *absence* of bleeding and/or inflammation. On the other hand, although bleeding always accompanies a fracture of the extremity, interruption of continuity of the bone is the principal cause of loss of function—not the bleeding or infection, unless they are severe. If bleeding or inflammation were not associated with "fracture" of the liver, the body economy would not suffer irreparably so long as enough functioning liver was left to supply it. If not enough functioning hepatic tissue remains, death ensues. In injury to the spleen function is not important at all, whereas loss of blood is critical.

In the cardiovascular, gastrointestinal, and genitourinary tracts, perforations or interruptions of continuity, if unaccompanied by bleeding or infection, would lead to relatively short periods of non-function. When present in such injuries these two factors often cause death, which is seldom true in injuries of the extremities. The emphasis in handling injuries in these areas therefore is vitally different. In injuries of the extremities, restoration of function absorbs the attention of the surgeon from the beginning, except when associated hemorrhage threatens life. In injuries of the cardiovascular, gastrointestinal, and genitourinary tracts, restoration of function is dependent upon the prevention or control of hemorrhage and infection, which therefore takes precedence over everything else at every stage of active treatment.

SYMPTOMS MASKING LOCALIZATION AND EXTENT OF THORACO-ABDOMINAL TRAUMA

In thoraco-abdominal injuries, as in chest injuries alone, there are likely to be symptoms referable to the disturbed physiology of respiration due to possible injury to the diaphragm or even to the fracture of a rib. At first, these symptoms may predominate, but usually the reverse will be true, and the injury to the diaphragm or rib will not be recognized because of the preponderance of *abdominal* signs and symptoms. In crush injuries of the chest, however, there may be associated upper abdominal injuries, particularly of the pancreas, liver, and spleen, and distended hollow viscera. However, if there are multiple rib fractures, paradoxical respiration may occur with inward motion of the chest wall on inspiration, and the resulting respiratory embarrassment and loss of ventilation will most likely mask the abdominal injuries, severe though they may be.

Severity of the abdominal injuries will depend to a large extent upon whether the crush injury is produced suddenly or slowly. The respiratory difficulty may be increased by the associated subdiaphragmatic injury and by bleeding from ruptured or torn upper abdominal viscera. Bleeding from above, if from the lung, is seldom severe or incapacitating, but bleeding from the chest wall itself, as well as from the damaged abdominal viscera, may be so severe as to produce critical respiratory embarrassment, as well as significant blood loss resulting in rapidly developing shock.

Added to this loss of the normal bellows action of the chest wall may be the contusion and possible laceration of the lung itself and possibly the diaphragm, with resulting edema of the lung tissue involved, extravasation of blood into the air passages and peritoneal cavity, and pneumothorax. The effects of these chest wall–lung–bronchial–diaphragmatic injuries are compounded by the ineffectiveness of cough and by the retention of mucous secretion, blood, and edema fluid in the tracheobronchial passages. Bleeding from the chest wall may be so severe that it fills the pleural cavity and enters the abdominal cavity, causing further respiratory embarrassment, as well as significant total blood loss.

IMPORTANCE OF POSTURE IN PENETRATING WOUNDS

Wounds penetrating the lower chest or upper abdomen at right angles to the body, or slanting wounds penetrating either compartment at almost any point, may inflict severe injury to parietes or viscera in either compartment or both. In addition, there may be associated wounds of the spine and spinal cord. Injuries to the retroperitoneal viscera also may result, particularly to the kidneys (and adrenals), duodenum, pancreas, great vessels, cisterna chyli, and thoracic duct. Unless deflected by bone, a high velocity missile will almost always produce a straight track. Bizarre, apparently inexplicable visceral wounds found on exploration are usually *the result of the position of the body* at the time of penetration of the missile.

Injuries Involving Only the Abdomen

DIAGNOSIS

DIAGNOSIS of abdominal injury, particularly of the effects of injury upon intra-abdominal structures, is ideally a synthesis and astute interpretation of the data derived from careful interrogation regarding the manner in which the injury was sustained and from accurate observation of the effects produced. When possible, this is then supplemented by various tests and special examinations based on the interpretation of these clinical data. At times, in emergency situations, the diagnosis must be based solely on clinical observations, perhaps entirely on physical examination. This, when performed with competence and experience, yields more information by far than any other examination or test.

If physical examination is to be the tool of reliability and dependence needed in evaluation of these injuries, it must be stated, at the risk of being trite, that its value depends on the ability of the examiner to know with assurance that the signs elicited are actually there and that others he fails to elicit are absent. There is no room for guesswork or inaccurate observation. The examiner must be a capable and experienced observer. He must *know* when he hears bowel sounds, when shifting dulness is present, when muscle spasm is present, *and when these and other critical signs are changing.* The serious errors in physical examination are usually those of observation rather than of incorrect interpretation of correctly observed physical signs. In order to have this assurance, the examiner will often have to go back and check his findings repeatedly, especially in patients who have sustained injuries such as those under discussion *in which the situation during the critical early phase is never static.*

Exploratory Celiotomy

Open injuries of the abdomen ordinarily do not present the same problems in diagnosis that closed, or nonpenetrating, injuries do, largely because so much is known or can be inferred from the fact that a wound has been produced. Usually, also, one knows the object which produced the wound, as well as the characteristics of the damage inflicted by it in the different types of tissue traversed. One may also surmise what structures will have been injured, with the certainty that the wound will be contaminated from the first. The likelihood of injury to hollow viscera will be far greater in open than in blunt injuries, and therefore speed, but not haste, in closing these wounds is imperative. This means operation at the earliest possible moment in all of these injuries, and celiotomy in the vast majority of them. Much about the diagnosis is already known, and, in these patients in whom the abdomen is opened, diagnosis of the *extent* of the injury is made concurrently with treatment. Important, even critical, injuries which might not have been suspected are likely to be found and corrected.

Current opinion, generally, takes the point of view that these patients are better treated because the diagnosis is established and the extent of the injury can be more accurately evaluated simply by careful inspection. There is such an advantage in being able to do this that, with improved anesthesia, and availability of blood, blood fractions, and plasma substitutes, and antibiotics, the conservative point of view held 30 years ago regarding the handling of both types of injuries, but particularly of the nonpenetrating ones, is giving way to a more aggressive approach in handling patients in whom the diagnosis is in doubt.

Today many surgeons consider operation less hazardous than the delay entailed in dealing with a *possible* but barely suspected injury which cannot be proved to exist by current diagnostic procedures, but which, if it did exist and were not treated promptly by surgery, might well prove fatal. In other words, what might have been taking a desperate chance by operating 30 years ago might today be justifiably considered safe. A rough estimate of the over-all results in terms of lives which might have been saved has been made in some reports by reviewing the case histories of those patients who have died because a critical diagnosis, which would have been made (and the patient's life saved) had operation been performed, was missed.

This in no way lessens the importance of making as accurate a diagnosis as possible. But today there certainly are more patients upon whom an *exploratory celiotomy* may safely be carried out because of an honest doubt than there were 30 years ago. This is no reflection upon the diagnostic acumen of the surgeon then, who as often as not is the same surgeon today; it is rather an acknowledgment of the great progress surgery has been able to make, thanks largely to the contributions of knowledge and skill from allied branches of medicine.

History—Examination—Re-examination

Obtaining as much information as possible about the circumstances associated with production of the injury is an essential first step. It should include, if possible, such pertinent data as the time the injury was sustained; the position of the body at the time; how recently the patient had eaten, voided, and defecated; the nature, direction, and force of the agent or mechanism responsible for the trauma; the exact site of the injury or wounds produced, especially of wounds of entrance and exit in penetrating injuries.

If the patient is conscious, his reaction to the situation will be carefully noted. These observations will include the patient's facies and general physical attitude of pain, alarm, apprehension, excitement, euphoria, delirium, or ominous stillness with barely perceptible respiration and pulse; whether he moves about or lies still and is afraid of being moved, or seeks a more comfortable position; the color, state of hydration, turgor, and temperature of his skin; the quality and rate of his pulse, and his blood pressure and pulse pressure.

DIAGNOSIS OF PENETRATING ABDOMINAL WOUNDS

In addition to thus estimating clinically the patient's general physical status with reference to the peripheral circulation and state of hydration,* one should examine the patient with a penetrating abdominal wound for particular injuries in an effort to decide which one probably has first priority in treatment after resuscitative measures have been taken. If there is only an abdominal wound, or if the abdominal wound is of first priority among a number of wounds, the response to the resuscitative efforts becomes one of the important criteria in deciding whether celiotomy should be performed. It may also give some idea about the patient's chance of survival.

Response to Resuscitative Measures

These early supportive measures often establish or at least strongly suggest the type and severity of intra-abdominal damage sustained. If the response is good and rapid, usually either no injury of the alimentary tract has occurred or the injury is very recent and slight. If the alimentary tract has not been injured, there will be no significant distortion of vital signs, although symptoms simulating shock may be present. Resuscitative measures may even not be required if such a patient is kept under observation and followed closely. If the response is poor, or if the patient's condition actually deteriorates during treatment, there is either *extensive damage to the alimentary tract, severe hemorrhage,* or both, and the severity of the damage (and consequently the prognosis) will be found proportional to the lack of response.

Splinting of Abdomen and Absence of Peristalsis

If there is splinting of the abdomen on respiration with diffuse tenderness, pain, and rigidity, and absence of peristalsis on auscultation, the alimentary tract has been perforated, although severe bleeding may not have occurred. Celiotomy must be performed.

The importance of auscultation, especially, must be emphasized, and of estimating as accurately as possible the course of the missile track

* Rob makes the observation that most of the patients with war wounds of the abdomen were dehydrated when seen. This might be attributed to the state in which they reached the medical installation where definitive surgery was performed following transport and morphine administration. However, unless seen early, the same is true in civilians with intra-abdominal wounds.

in deciding in less obvious cases whether celiotomy should be performed. Rob offers the following dictum with regard to auscultation: "The absence of peristaltic sounds, confirmed and reconfirmed, is a positive indication for laparotomy, but the presence of peristaltic sounds is only a valuable guide toward, and *not a positive indication for, conservative treatment.*" The point is that this sign changes as peritoneal irritation develops. This usually occurs coincidentally with peritoneal insult, but it may not occur until several hours after injury, particularly in vascular accidents which produce slow compromise of a segment of intestine, or in freak accidents, such as one he cites. The wound of entrance should be excised in these cases.

In cases in which doubt exists as to whether the peritoneal cavity was penetrated the question of celiotomy is often decided by this procedure. Taking into consideration the site of wounding and the criteria for celiotomy already discussed, together with the estimate of the patient's condition, decision may be made against celiotomy even if the wound has penetrated the peritoneal cavity and a foreign body or other missile is lodged there or beyond. Many wounds of the liver with deeply situated small missiles, such as rifle bullets, do not require celiotomy, even though hemoperitoneum results. Attempts to expose these sites and control bleeding therefrom frequently results in more and possibly uncontrollable bleeding. Wounds involving only the extraperitoneal or retroperitoneal attachments of the colon may not require celiotomy. Suture of a wound of this aspect of the colon wall may at times be carried out if the external wound is excised and tamponed open. Considerable judgment and experience are needed in deciding these points.

Missile Tracks

The value of determining the probable course of the missile track is of much assistance in planning the site of the abdominal incision as well as in judging the structures probably traversed. The value of roentgenography and fluoroscopy in this connection is inestimable for localizing the site of lodgment of a radiopaque missile. Often the track itself may be identified. If only the missile is apparent, the course of the track may be quite accurately estimated from the point of entrance by a straight line to it if the position of the patient at the time of injury is known and the missile was not deflected by bone.

If roentgen study is not possible but the patient's position and the direction the missile was traveling are known, the probable course of the missile track through soft parts may still be estimated with considerable accuracy. Wounding of bladder, kidney, or ureter in the track of a missile may be established by catheterization. Digital examination of the rectum may reveal injury of the colon or rectum. A missile track which completely traverses the body will be a straight line between the wound of entrance and the wound of exit, taking into consideration the position of the body at the time of wounding and possible deflection of the missile by bone.

Misleading Signs in Diagnosis of Penetrating Wounds

In penetrating wounds it has been pointed out, as the result of experience with large numbers of war injuries, that some of the signs ordinarily relied on in physical diagnosis are either not reliable or are less reliable than usual. The absence of liver dulness may be of no importance in estimating liver injury, owing to the entrance of air along the missile track; abdominal rigidity is frequently absent or diminished in gunshot wounds of the abdomen which produce perforations of the alimentary tract, whereas the "boardlike abdomen" is thought of as the sign par excellence denoting this catastrophe. On the other hand, localized abdominal rigidity may be present as a result of injuries just to the abdominal wall, or to adjacent regions, such as chest, buttocks, loin, and retroperitoneal area. Frequently no pain is referred to the shoulder in injuries to the diaphragm.

DIAGNOSIS OF NONPENETRATING ABDOMINAL WOUNDS

The differential diagnosis of blunt or nonpenetrating or "closed" abdominal trauma can be and frequently is very difficult, especially in the early phase of injury. Various factors responsible for this are the mental state of the injured person if he is conscious and the obvious difficulty if he is unconscious; the frequent association of shock; the difficulty of ascertaining accurately the absence or presence of concealed bleeding, or the rate at which this is occurring. The frequent delay in the development of signs and symptoms of concealed bleeding and in the signs and symptoms associated with contusions of solid viscera and extravasation of secretions therefrom is often misleading. This may result in the premature discharge of a patient whose injury is assumed to be trivial. Not infrequently he will be brought back 6 to 10 hours later in a state of shock. Ruptures of hollow viscera are more likely to produce severe abdominal pain, involuntary spasm, and a quiet abdomen.

Masking Effects of Multiple Injuries

Multiple injuries frequently obscure the presence and nature of abdominal damage. Indeed, such damage may be completely overlooked either because of the urgency of another more obvious injury, because the effects of the abdominal injury are slow in exhibiting the symptoms and signs of the damage sustained, or simply because there may be no external evidence of trauma and the examination of the abdomen is casually performed. Another reason for confusion in diagnosis at times when multiple injuries are incurred is the possibility that signs and symptoms due to another injury may be ascribed mistakenly to the abdomen, when in fact there may have been no abdominal damage.

Vomiting, for example, may be considered abdominal in origin, when it may actually be the result of cerebral concussion. Marked and possibly painful abdominal distention may likewise be thought to be due to an abdominal injury, when in reality it may be the result of spinal cord trauma. A painful, somewhat tender, stiff, left upper abdominal wall may be thought to represent splenic trauma when the injury may be intrathoracic.

Careful, complete, accurate, documented physical examinations must obviously be performed repeatedly in the severely wounded or in those about whom there is the least doubt regarding the nature, extent, and severity of the injuries. This point has been stressed repeatedly in military and civilian reports on the handling of abdominal trauma. In civilian practice, with proficiency in physical diagnosis plus the aids usually available for examining these patients, the number of "unnecessary" celiotomies should be reduced somewhat, but probably to nowhere near the vanishing point in doubtful cases since there is no substitute for sound, experienced clinical judgment in making the decision whether or not to enter the peritoneal cavity. Also, since the aids to operative intervention are much improved now, the number of deaths within this group should be exceedingly small.

Penetrating vs. Nonpenetrating Injuries

Since, ultimately, the effects of penetrating trauma may be the same as those of nonpenetrating injuries, namely, peritoneal irritation produced by interruptions in the continuity of the alimentary tract and hemorrhage, many of the criteria for celiotomy will be the same. The important difference between the two types of injury is the great likelihood that, in the first, the continuity of the alimentary tract has been interrupted and, in the second, that it has not; but always there is the *possibility* (although not the same degree of *probability*) that it has been. Hemorrhage, both primarily and secondarily from the spleen and liver, is more likely to follow blunt trauma. If peritoneal irritation occurs, it will result most likely from the rupture of distended hollow viscera or from injured, fractured, fixed, or ruptured hollow or solid viscera which are crushed against the spine, for example, the pancreas, kidneys, and the duodenum.

Factors of importance, therefore, in determining whether to open the abdomen in this type of abdominal trauma are summarized in the following paragraphs.

Criteria for Celiotomy in Nonpenetrating Injuries

If free bleeding results from blunt trauma, it will be accompanied by diffuse abdominal pain, and this therefore may be sufficient reason for opening the peritoneal cavity even though shock has not supervened. At times, however, there may be considerable difficulty in differentiating between intraperitoneal hemorrhage and simply the contusion of the abdominal wall. Hemorrhage of this extent will usually produce early shock. If the picture of shock and diffuse abdominal pain are absent soon after injury, severe immediate hemorrhage is not likely to have occurred, but the possible occurrence later of secondary hemorrhage, or of peritonitis from a ruptured hollow viscus, or both, must not be forgotten. Widespread abdominal tenderness accompanying the hemorrhage would suggest superimposed infection, presumably from a ruptured hollow viscus, and this would occur some hours later. The spleen would be the most likely source of secondary hemorrhage from the rupture of a subcapsular splenic laceration or fracture.

Early, deepening shock. Early shock, in the *absence* of other trauma which might be expected to produce it (such as a fractured femur), would be justification for opening the abdomen, after carrying out resuscitative measures.

Silent abdomen. Another reason for operation would be a silent abdomen, just as in the case of the penetrating wound. In any event, this finding would suggest rupture of the gastrointestinal tract, which might not produce pain at once, depending on a number of factors, such as the site of perforation, its size, and the amount and type of contents in the ruptured segment.

Severe lower thoracic trauma. Upper abdominal visceral injury must always be thought of in association with any type of injury of the lower thoracic wall. Contusions and crushing injuries may produce ruptures of the kidneys, spleen, liver, pancreas, and duodenum, and occasionally of other viscera.

Severe pelvic trauma. Lower abdominal visceral injuries frequently are associated with pelvic fractures. Hematuria may lead to the discovery of a perforated bladder either into the peritoneal cavity or extraperitoneally, requiring celiotomy in either event.

Hematemesis, hematuria, melena. Blood in vomitus, urine, or stool may constitute a reason for celiotomy. A severe upper abdominal blow might produce rupture of both stomach and colon, with the appearance of fresh blood in both vomitus and stool. Vomiting is not a common feature either of blunt abdominal trauma or of penetrating wounds and the character of the vomitus has little diagnostic value *unless it contains blood.* It usually accompanies the ileus which is associated with the development of peritonitis, a later sequela.

If the patient's urine contains blood, the possibility of a ruptured bladder exists. Catheterization, by the amount and type of fluid obtained, would help in deciding whether operation should be done. Large amounts of fluid may be obtained, and the introduction of a known amount of sterile water, expecting to obtain a smaller amount or none at all if the bladder is ruptured, is fallacious and should not be carried out because of the risk of producing wider extravasation of contaminated fluid. Retrograde gravity cystography via urethra would settle the question of ruptured bladder and whether repair and suprapubic cystostomy would be necessary. The female bladder suffers less than that of the male from blunt trauma because of the protection afforded from its lower position in the broader pelvis. The distended male bladder is quite exposed to such trauma.

If blood is passed or found in the rectum, proctoscopy should be done, with suction and irrigation available if the *site* of bleeding is to be found with facility.

Various combinations of these critical manifestations of injury will, of course, be added reason for celiotomy.

ROENTGEN, LABORATORY, AND SPECIAL TESTS IN DIAGNOSIS OF ABDOMINAL TRAUMA

In general, data supplied from roentgen examinations, laboratory tests, and special procedures are factual and accurate. Unlike evidence gained from physical examination, errors are likely to be those of interpretation rather than of execution. Students learn early that involuntary muscular rigidity means guarding or splinting which protects an injured part. The interpretation of the sign is correct. But in a given case is involuntary muscular spasm actually present? Absence of bowel sounds in conjunction with trauma and disease means grave intraperitoneal damage affecting the gastrointestinal tract. But are bowel sounds actually absent?

Subjective vs. Objective Diagnostic Errors

Inaccurate observations, which ordinarily result from inexperience in performance of these tests, will therefore be responsible for erroneous conclusions, especially since so many subjective factors enter into their performance as well as into their interpretation. Roentgen and laboratory tests, on the other hand, are themselves objective data. It is *faulty interpretation* of these data which will lead to incorrect diagnoses from such ordinarily reliable sources. Then, too, if the objective findings are *negative,* recognition of this may be fully as important in the total evaluation of a critical situation as the recognition of positive findings.

Correct interpretation of these tests, rather than accuracy in their performance, which in this case depends so little upon subjective factors, is essential in reaching a correct diagnosis from this sort of information. An illustration of this is the repeatedly negative survey film taken concomitantly with observation of a patient who has suffered blunt trauma to the thoraco-abdominal region. Severe pain, tenderness, and muscle spasm from such an injury may persist beyond the interval within which one would ordinarily expect that they signified only superficial injury. If a survey film at that time was still negative, and evidence of shock was absent, even though pain, tenderness, and muscle spasm were still present, this would be most reassuring, since it would mean that serious intra-abdominal injury very probably had not been sustained.

On the other hand, negative or normal findings in certain situations *do not preclude* the presence of serious injury and *must not be interpreted or accepted as positive evidence that injury has not been sustained.* A good illustration of this point occurs at times in attempts to utilize the procedure of abdominal tap or some modification of this (such as peritoneoscopy, or taking swab smears of pelvic fluid through small surgical wounds) for the purpose of determining the presence of blood or other types of peritoneal contaminants following trauma. Such procedures are safe when performed properly, and are of incontestable value *when positive.* However, results may be negative even when abnormal fluid is present on account of loculation or concealment of the collection, or when the fluid is retroperitoneal but is the cause of symptoms which simulate intraperitoneal injury. A false sense of security may result, and the patient's chances of recovery are thereby jeopardized.

Roentgen Examination

In addition to the information regarding intrathoracic injury gained from postero-anterior and lateral films taken when intrathoracic injury is suspected, much may also be learned or inferred regarding possible injury of and below the diaphragm. The finding of fractured lower ribs implicates the spleen, liver, or kidney, until it is proved otherwise. The finding of outlines of gas-containing structures or even of solid viscera within the thoracic cavity reveals a rupture of the diaphragm.

Enlargement and, later, obliteration of the splenic shadow, and appearance of a serrated line along the greater curvature of a greatly dilated stomach, possible elevation of the left hemidiaphragm, and displacement downward of the left transverse colon and splenic flexure shadow, would afford further evidence of a ruptured spleen.

In many injuries of this nature, vomiting will occur. The absence of blood in the vomitus practically rules out any break in the integrity of the wall of the esophagus, stomach, duodenum, or upper jejunum. Since gastric aspiration is usually carried out in these cases, aspirated gastrointestinal contents also should be examined for blood. Digital rectal examination should also be done routinely, and the presence or absence of blood noted.

The appearance of free gas in the peritoneal cavity following abdominal trauma which ruptures a segment of the gastrointestinal tract is usually not nearly as clear-cut on x-ray films as that following rupture of an anterior peptic ulcer. The presence of gas *within* tissues should be sought as well, particularly in the retroperitoneal region of the mid and upper abdomen, for this may furnish a clue to retroperitoneal rupture of the duodenum. At operation, roentgenographic visualization of the lower common duct–duodenal area may be obtained by introduction of a radiopaque solution into the duct lumen by catheter or T-tube when a retroperitoneal perforation of the duodenum is suspected.

The x-ray appearance of moderately distended intestine due to simple ileus has quite well known characteristics, and accompanies almost every intraperitoneal insult, large or small, whether originating ventrally or dorsally, from the flanks, from above the diaphragm, or from below the reflection of the pelvic peritoneum, or from within the peritoneal cavity itself. This distention is usually generalized. Occasionally it may be localized in the vicinity of an inflamed viscus. In mesenteric vascular occlusion from any source, the bowel above the involved segment will be dilated but may give rise to few symptoms until the features of obstruction, gangrene, and peritoneal irritation develop. The compromised segment of bowel, even when "strangulation" does not exist, ultimately constitutes a point of obstruction as complete as that produced by structural occlusion.

There is also transudation of considerable fluid through the compromised wall, giving rise to an accumulation of peritoneal fluid, eventually purulent. This is often represented by a hazy appearance of the abdominal film which is *not,* however, diagnostic. Traumatic rupture of bowel also produces the appearance of ileus and extraluminal fluid. By far the majority of these ruptures have occurred through normal bowel wall rather than through diseased areas, such as ulcers. The x-ray appearance of bowel seen in acute upper and lower mechanical intestinal obstruction is seldom seen following acute trauma, except as a complication. Tympanites and meteorism sometimes acompany severe cerebrospinal injuries and retroperitoneal damage, and often follow the application of a plaster body spica.

In penetrating wounds the missile track can sometimes be seen on the x-ray films, outlined by contained air and fluid. Aside from this, the appearance of thoracic structures will resemble that resulting from external blunt trauma associated with penetrating fractured ribs. The thoracoabdominal roentgenograms may show, in addition, abdominal viscera within the thorax. In wounds of the pericardium and heart the cardiac shadow will not be much enlarged, but fluoroscopic examination will show rapid, narrow excursions of the cardiac borders. Occurrence of this serious injury probably will have been ascertained already from the site and directions of the wound, the muffled, faint, rapid heart sounds, the small pulse pressure, the pallid (shock-type) cyanosis, and feeble paradoxical pulse. (Paradoxical pulse: diminution or disappearance of pulse on inspiration, noted best with blood pressure cuff adjusted to level at which systole is first heard.)

In gunshot wounds of the abdomen, roentgen examinations may show the missile itself, which is of great value since, by knowing the location of the wound of entrance, the surgeon may frequently plot the course of the missile, and is thus able to determine the most suitable incision of approach and the viscera which are probably injured. (The track may also be deduced from the wounds of entrance and exit, if the position of the patient at time of injury is known.) Air may be sucked in along the missile track. This may actually outline viscera, but also may be misleading by obliterating liver dulness, which on physical examination may produce the false impression that the gastrointestinal tract has been perforated.

The employment of bedside roentgenography in all severe injuries has been advocated by Orkin, chiefly, he suggests, for the valuable aid given in determining the presence and extent of renal and other urinary tract injuries. With justification, however, he points out that such a procedure provides additional information regarding the presence and extent of other associated injuries. In so far as the urological problems are concerned, he advises a survey film and excretory studies in *all* such patients, and retrograde studies as well, whenever feasible. It is almost always possible, by these means, to determine whether both kidneys are present, and to decide *early* between operative and non-operative treatment for injuries of the urinary tract. Since *associated* injuries account for most of the deaths in urological trauma, this is a point well taken.

Obliteration of psoas margins and of renal outlines is common in retroperitoneal injuries, especially in renal trauma and subsequent infection, flank injuries with hemorrhage, with or without spine fractures, and in dissecting and ruptured abdominal aneurysms. Associated with these disorders, lateral scoliosis will be found on examination of posteroanterior survey films of the abdomen, showing the spine with the convexity of the curve toward the side opposite the injury, because of muscle spasm on the injured side.

In the pelvis, anorectal, urethral, bladder, and ureteral injuries are almost always of the penetrating variety or associated with pelvic fractures. External inspection and digital rectal and vaginal examinations, supplemented by anoscope, proctosigmoidoscope, and vaginal speculum, will reveal the nature and extent of most of the external urethral-rectal-genital damage. Urethral cystograms will show injuries of the urethra and bladder. Extraperitoneal rupture of the bladder results in extravasation of urine into the space of Retzius, upward as far as the umbilicus and downward to the knees, as well as throughout the perivesical and lower retroperitoneal tissue spaces. The appearance by cystography is usually described as "tear-drop," unless the rupture is extensive, in which event the radiopaque medium will radiate out into a wide peripheral zone, or is posterior, when the appearance will simulate a bladder diverticulum. Fractures of the pelvis producing bladder rupture are almost always caused by lateral or anteroposterior compression injuries. Intraperitoneal rupture of the bladder may occur as the result of blunt trauma, although it is not as likely to occur as with penetrating injuries. The same examinations should be carried out as described for extraperitoneal rupture, provided the urgency of the situation does not demand prompt operation, which is likely with missile wounds.

It is well to remember that injury of any degree of severity to the lower urinary tract is likely to produce acute urinary symptoms: urgency without being able to void, and frequently dysuria when voiding *is* possible. Also, grossly bloody urine may be passed after relatively trivial trauma to urethra and bladder, and clear urine may be voided even when the bladder has been ruptured. All of these pelvic injuries should be investigated by the special procedures outlined, no matter how insignificant they may seem to be.

Laboratory Tests

Laboratory tests usually cannot be relied on to make or even to aid in making a diagnosis of specific injury without other, usually clinical, confirmatory evidence. These tests have quite limited usefulness. Blood counts may be helpful in following the progress of an injury with reference to the development of anemia or infection, but are of little value in the early diagnosis of acute hemorrhage. Evidence of rapid, concealed bleeding will be detected *first by looking at the patient* and by carefully assessing his vital signs. Continued severe bleeding usually will be indicated by failure of the vital signs to become stabilized, and by a falling hematocrit. A leukocytosis usually accompanies bleeding of this degree of severity, but is not diagnostic. It will be present also when blood has collected in cavities, spaces, and tissues outside the vascular bed; it will also accompany supervening infection except, at times, in the aged and the debilitated.

Dunphy points out that intractable hypotension accompanied by severe abdominal pain occurring soon after major trauma may be the result of spinal cord injury *which may simulate an acute abdominal injury*. Also that head injuries damaging the basal ganglia, fat embolism, and associated multiple injuries may be responsible for intractable early hypotension.

Devitalization of a segment of intestine usually will be associated with a sharp rise in the white blood cell count, often to a height of 20,000, with 90 per cent polymorphonuclear leukocytes. This will occur quite early, frequently even before any trend toward an elevated pulse rate is apparent, and certainly preceding elevation of the temperature or development of clinical symptoms and signs of impending intestinal gangrene. Inconspicuous distention may be present, but x-ray examination may show a loop or segment of moderately distended bowel out of proportion to the physical signs.

Serum amylase determinations aid in the diagnosis of pancreatic injuries if it is remembered that elevation of the amylase is delayed for about 48 hours and if the diagnosis has not already been established by other means in the interim. It is one of those tests which, when negative, does not necessarily rule out pancreatic injury. The serum amylase will become elevated in case a pseudocyst ruptures. Roentgenograms of the abdomen should be taken at intervals following trauma which might have injured the pancreas, especially when abdominal symptoms persist. The development of a pseudocyst may be discovered, or plaques of saponified fat seen which, when present, albeit uncommon, have a sufficiently characteristic appearance to make the diagnosis of pancreatic injury.

Determinations of electrolytes help greatly in the diagnosis of complications associated with obvious or occult fluid losses from the body which so frequently accompany injury, both in the acute and in the chronic phases. The principal value of electrolyte, protein fraction, and steroid excretion determinations, however, is to provide a precise basis for supplementary support of the injured person, chiefly by parenteral routes.

Numerous other tests and procedures have been devised for the purpose of delineating more clearly the diagnosis of injuries, especially of nonpenetrating injuries of the abdomen. Caution must be emphasized in using (1) those which employ blind instrumentation into already injured structures, cystoscopy and catheterization, for example; (2) those by which fluid or air is introduced into contaminated tissue spaces, both because they may further disseminate contamination and because they require manipulation of a severely injured patient in order to carry out a procedure which may yield information of equivocal value at best; and (3) those which, to delineate injured organs more clearly, utilize harmful radiopaque substances which cannot be recovered, such as Thorotrast.

All things considered, it is understandable that open trauma should be better managed than closed trauma. The facility and accuracy in making a diagnosis and in assessing the extent of open injuries are in no small part responsible for this state of affairs. In essence, the present day ability to *safely* convert a closed injury to an open one by surgical intervention is one of the bases for advocating a more aggressive approach to the management of nonpenetrating abdominal trauma.

TREATMENT OF ABDOMINAL INJURIES

Except for a word of additional caution because of the possible masking effect of narcotics and alcohol on physical signs, symptoms, and patient behavior, as well as their depressive effects on the sensorium, respiration, and blood pressure, the measures employed for the relief of pain in acute thoracic and abdominal trauma, including the parenteral use of morphine, and handling, positioning, splinting, and transporting of injured persons, are similar to those employed in other severe injuries. These are discussed in other chapters.

Treatment of Shock and Hemorrhage

Any severe abdominal injury will at some time produce shock unless prophylactic treatment is given, and even then it may subsequently supervene. In these injuries a very frequent cause and concomitant of shock is hemorrhage. In those patients with internal injuries in which the effects of trauma are developing slowly, shock will not occur until later. Therefore, in every case in which the history suggests the possibility of internal abdominal injury, and in every case in which such injury is even suspected, it is imperative that the patient be observed repeatedly and closely for signs and symptoms of impending shock. Meantime, without delay, equipment and other means of combating it, should it begin to develop, should be assembled.

The treatment of shock in a patient with an acute abdominal injury does not differ, in principle, from the treatment of a patient suffering from shock from any other cause. Hemorrhage is the most frequent cause. If hemorrhage is obvious, it must, if possible, be controlled. If it is not obvious, and this is often the case, fluid must be started. Whole blood is a good fluid to use in case of doubt, although before long it may become obvious whether continued bleeding is actually the cause of the shock. This should be kept in mind because of the hazard of over-transfusion and the possibility of subsequent homologous serum hepatitis. Recovery from primary shock will permit more careful evaluation of the possibility of continued bleeding.

Meanwhile, recovery from shock may occur, and the extent and severity of the injuries may be properly assessed. Until such recovery has occurred, operative interference is fraught with danger. Nevertheless, in doubtful situations accurately evaluated, early operation will save more lives than will watchful waiting. The danger inherent in operative interference *must* be faced in the presence of obvious, active hemorrhage—steps being taken at the same time to make up the blood volume deficit by *intravenous* transfusion of whole blood. If blood is not available, an attempt must be made to control hemorrhage under any circumstance, and without regard to asepsis if need be, as in any other case of acute hemorrhage. The problem at that desperate moment is simply to save life. (Recognition of the shock state ordinarily is not difficult. The gray color, apathy or unconsciousness, cool clammy skin, thready pulse, and low blood pressure and narrow pulse pressure are familiar indices.)

The immediate treatment of the patient is the conservation of body heat rather than application of external heat, which may be injurious; provision for and maintenance of an adequate airway, with administration of oxygen, if available; placing the patient supine or in the lateral decubitus position if there is an airway problem, with head down to forestall aspiration of vomitus or blood, having respect always for the possibility of an associated head or spinal injury; the administration of blood, plasma, plasma expander, glucose in isotonic saline solution, or isotonic saline solution alone, depending upon the situation—whether the shock state is thought to be associated with acute blood loss or not, and what solutions, if any, are available.

Treatment of Abdominal Wounds

Once shock has been controlled, definite treatment may be directed toward the injuries responsible for it. In fact this frequently will already have been started, especially if there is an associated open wound.

The first emergency treatment of an abdominal wound may be simply the application of a sterile or clean dressing. If the wound is extensive, it may be accompanied by prolapse or frank evisceration of the abdominal contents. It may still be possible only, at the initial treatment of such a wound, to cover it with a sterile or clean or sometimes an improvised dressing, meantime treating the patient for shock and hemorrhage.

When definitive treatment becomes possible in such a case, it is to be carried out under general anesthesia, with provision to maintain the blood pressure to prevent the patient from relapsing into shock.

The abdomen is prepared as for any intraperitoneal procedure. Eviscerated bowel may be protected with sterile pads moistened with warm isotonic saline solution while the wound is debrided and the bowel examined for penetrating or lacerated wounds, or for devitalized segments. These might necessitate resection or, if extensive, and the condition of the patient is precarious, exteriorization, especially if the large bowel has been injured; or drainage of the contaminated area with a proximal, completely diverting colostomy may be necessary. Occasionally a vascular injury may be responsible for devitalization of a long segment of bowel. This, too, may require resection or exteriorization, after it has been observed for a sufficient length of time to determine its ability to survive. Resections will depend on whether it is thought that such a procedure will be tolerated.

Examination of the peritoneal cavity must be thorough and complete. The wound may have to be enlarged in order to facilitate this, even though the exploratory incision should be on the liberal side to begin with.

Lacerations of blood vessels in which clot may have formed, but which later may give rise to secondary hemorrhage, should be noted, and the vessels ligated, repaired, or, if essential, replaced by substitutes if feasible. There may be lacerations of the liver and spleen, from which hemorrhage generally is severe and controlled with difficulty. Secondary hemorrhage from these sites may occur as late as three weeks after injury. One of the absolute essentials in the treatment of this type of injury is availability of adequate *suction* apparatus. The importance of this adjuvant can hardly be over-emphasized. It is as important in the handling of abdominal injuries as of cranial and brain injuries, and *must* be part of the operating room equipment available for both the urgent and the definitive treatment of these wounds.

If, in such a severe abdominal wound, the spleen has been lacerated or torn, it should be removed. The risk of delayed or secondary hemorrhage is too great to permit consideration of controlling hemorrhage from this source by suture, ligation, or pack, except under the most dire circumstances.

If, on the other hand, the liver injury is the source of bleeding, it must usually be controlled by ligatures, tapes, and rubber-shod clamps or other devices. Large portions of the liver may have to be removed in order to control the bleeding and prevent subsequent devitalization and necrosis of liver parenchyma. It must be remembered that bile ducts, sometimes major ducts, may be implicated in such an injury, resulting in the extravasation of bile into the peritoneal and thoracic cavities. The bile passages and vascular channels are contiguous, so that direct communication may become established between them. Bleeding may then occur into one of the larger ducts, giving rise to tarry stools and severe or chronic anemia. Such a condition was observed as the result of a sledding accident a few years ago, in which at least half of the right lobe of the liver became necrotic from the loss of its blood supply, the patient becoming anemic owing to an open communication between a major branch of the hepatic artery and a large branch of the right hepatic duct.

Treatment of Wounds of Gastrointestinal Tract

In general, wounds of the stomach, duodenum, and small bowel may be sutured, provided the viability of the structure is assured. If not, a resection should preferably be done or, as a measure of necessity, the injured segment exteriorized if possible or, if not, possibly a sump drain installed or drainage via an incision in the flank to a contaminated retroperitoneal wound of the colon with a diverting colostomy above. Heretofore wounds of the large bowel have usually been exteriorized, especially if the wound is as much as 6 hours old. However, with the present availability of antibiotic solutions for irrigation of contaminated wounds and drugs for oral and parenteral administration, and considering the decreased time factor in rendering definitive surgical treatment, exteriorization of injured large bowel does not occupy the important place it occupied in wartime military surgery. Nevertheless, it is safer to exteriorize a segment of injured large bowel under any circumstances if the injury is more than 6 hours old, or to provide drainage to the exterior, with proximal colostomy, as described above. In repairing wounds of the stomach, duodenum, and small and large bowel, it must be remembered that the more obvious wounds of the antimesenteric surface may be associated with wounds of the mesenteric wall and mesentery opposite, with mesentery-retroperitoneal areas, and with the lesser sac.

Wounds involving the duodenal-pancreatic region are particularly treacherous because of the difficulty of access for exploration, and the possibility of injury to major vascular channels, including those in the mesenteries, and to pancreas, colon, spleen, and liver. Wounds of this region are frequently associated also with injuries to intrathoracic structures. Closing all the wounds in hollow viscera or resecting badly injured or non-viable segments, exteriorizing, or otherwise handling these wounds, as described above, together with controlling hemorrhage, constitute the principal surgical measures in dealing with these severe wounds. Toilet of the peritoneal cavity must be attended to, and is partly accomplished during this phase of the procedure. This is then completed, and the operative sites sprayed or irrigated with an antibiotic solution such as neomycin-bacitracin.

The value of this, in comparison with debridement, which includes the irrigation of contaminated wounds and adjacent areas with sterile isotonic saline solution, is not settled beyond controversy. The danger lies in allowing the local use of antibiotics to be depended on as a substitute for thorough and often time-consuming debridement. After gloves, drapes, and contaminated instruments are changed or discarded, the viscera are replaced within the peritoneal cavity and the peritoneum is closed. The fascial layers of the wound should be closed also, but the subcutaneous and skin wounds should be left open, and the edges of the wound kept apart by strips of sterile petrolatum gauze and perhaps a small tampon of gauze to forestall the development of a serious mural infection. Placing the skin sutures is an acceptable procedure and makes delayed primary closure of many contaminated wounds easily possible three to six days after the operation. Rigidity and fixation of the tissues beyond that time interfere with approximation of the wound edges. After such a procedure the patient is placed on a broad-spectrum antibiotic or a combination of synergistic antibiotics, such as penicillin and streptomycin.

Retained Foreign Bodies

One must be on the lookout for foreign bodies, depending on the agent thought or known to be responsible for the injury. Intra-abdominal foreign bodies may originate from outside the body or from within. Ingested objects which may produce trauma are legion, and are encountered chiefly in psychopathic individuals and children. Whenever the continuity of the gastrointestinal tract is interrupted or the integrity of its wall compromised, as by wounds and ruptures, any of its contents may become a foreign body. Blood itself, free in the peritoneal cavity or extravasated into normal body cavities, such as the bladder, stomach, or intestine, or into cavities traumatically produced, becomes a foreign body. Similarly chyle, lymph, bile, and other body fluids, and particularly activated digestive enzymes, diverted or displaced from their normal sites by any type of trauma, superimpose other types of injury. Other body tissues, especially bone fragments, may become traumatic agents.

The commonest foreign bodies originating outside the body are parts of the individual's clothing and frequently the agents themselves which carry the clothing into the abdomen. Removal or evacuation of these various foreign bodies is essential in order to forestall mural or intra-abdominal infection, and to arrest primary hemorrhage and prevent secondary bleeding. Their removal is necessary also to prevent fistula and sinus formation; intestinal, vascular, urinary, biliary, or thoracic duct obstruction; pressure necrosis of tissue; and the formation of such pathological structures as traumatic cysts of pancreas and liver.

Drainage

The question of drainage of such wounds is one about which there is great difference of opinion. The indications, however, are fairly clear in most instances. If tissue of doubtful viability cannot be removed or exteriorized, but must be left in the peritoneal cavity, drainage should be provided to that area. Also, if closure of a wound in bowel is insecure, drains should be placed to the vicinity of such a site, but not against the suture line. The breakdown of a wound drained in such manner should be expected. A sump drain may even be placed in anticipation of such an eventuality, and intubation of the intestinal tract provided to try to minimize the likelihood of breakdown of the intestinal wound by reduction of pressure from gas and fluid within the lumen at that site. Drainage of the entire peritoneal cavity is impossible, and attempts to do so are undesirable.

If the gastrointestinal closures are thought to be complete and secure, and devitalized tissue is not found on exploration, drains should not be used, even though there has been considerable and widespread contamination. To place a drain down to a good closure of an intestinal wound is an invitation to the formation of a fistula which may prove fatal. Every expedient should be used to avoid the use of a drain. One situation in which use of a drain is justified is insecure and incomplete hemostasis. Packing may be necessary in some instances, and this may so interfere with approximation of the wound margins that the development of a hernia must be considered inevitable. But this is of relatively minor importance. A drain used to permit the exit of serum from a large wound which may be expected to close without infection should be removed early, by which is meant the day after operation or the day following. If it is left longer, the occurrence of a wound infection, usually mild but at times severe, becomes increasingly likely.

Drainage of a liver wound is imperative because of the leakage of bile. This is of even greater importance if hemostatic agents such as Gelfoam and Oxycel gauze are used. These agents prevent the formation of adhesions, thus facilitating the diffusion of bile into the peritoneal cavity if external drainage is not provided.

CHARACTERISTIC FEATURES OF SPECIFIC TYPES OF ABDOMINAL INJURY

GUNSHOT WOUNDS

Probably physicians and lay persons alike have taken more interest in gunshot wounds than in any other type of trauma. One of the reasons for this is the widespread use of firearms in war and peace since their introduction into Europe in the 14th century. The history of the development of these weapons may be traced in medical annals from the very beginning. In the course of these developments something was learned about anatomy, but relatively little progress was made in handling the injuries produced by firearms until the ligature was introduced by Ambroise Paré in the 16th century, and John Hunter (1728–1793) made surgery a science. Really significant advances in the treatment of gunshot wounds of the abdomen had to await the discoveries, and their acceptance, of Semmelweiss, Pasteur, and Lister, and the skill and courage of their convictions of a number of surgeons late in the last century who resolutely stood for "intervention" in treating these injuries, as opposed to "abstention."

Almost all of the significant progress since this transition has occurred within the last half century. The mortality rate for penetrating abdominal wounds at the Charity Hospital of Louisiana in New Orleans from 1890 to 1900 was 68.9 per cent of those operated on, against 53.6 per cent of those who were not. The mortality rate for these wounds in World War I is reported as 56 per cent. The practice of intervening surgically in these cases was not officially adopted in the British Army until 1915. Even in the Spanish Civil War (1939), the highest mortality rate was quoted as 71.8 per cent, the lowest 53.7 per cent. The mortality rate from penetrating missile wounds of the abdomen in World War II was 25 per cent.

Another reason for the general interest in these wounds is the associated human interest or drama; *someone* invariably had to fire the pistol or gun, giving it a personal, human touch, in contrast to the impersonal sort of trauma produced by an automobile, a machine, or that caused by common farm or domestic accidents. Frequently there is considerable human drama* associated with these injuries, as in the assassinations of the three

* An interesting case in the personal experience of the writer during World War II, although it did not involve abdominal injury, illustrates this point. A G.I. infantryman, who had killed an English woman, was cornered by the military police in the flat where he had taken refuge. As they closed in, tossing tear gas through the transom, he turned his carbine on himself, firing a shot upward which entered the neck above the hyoid bone. When taken, the soldier was conscious and seemed little the worse for his self-inflicted wound. He was brought to our nearby military hospital where he arrived conscious, not in shock, and without any neurological findings. A wound leaking sanguineous cerebrospinal fluid was seen high in the posterior pharynx. X-ray showed a bullet lying in the left frontal lobe of the brain. His condition remained good but, because of the probability of meningitis, it was deemed essential to stop the leakage of cerebrospinal fluid. That evening, a bone flap was turned, the left frontal lobe gently lifted, and the

American Presidents, which have been the subject of an article by Miller, and one of which was recently reviewed by Vincent.

If the gunshot wound is through and through, the wound of entrance will usually be small and inconspicuous, unless the shot is fired so close that the heat of the blast produces a burned contusion of the wall, the presence of powder marks depending on the type of propelling charge; the wound of exit, on the other hand, may be ragged and gaping. The track is a straight line unless the missile is deflected by bone or other resistant tissue as it loses velocity in the body. The effect on soft tissues en route is complete disruption and disorganization, both because of the force of impact and because of the positive and negative pressure effects within the hollow viscera and abdominal cavity produced by the speeding missile. This behavior sometimes accounts for perforation of bowel which has not even come directly in contact with the missile. This phenomenon must be taken into account when one is exploring an abdominal wound produced by a rifle bullet, particularly a glancing wound in the flank near the retroperitoneal aspects of gas-containing ascending or descending colon, for perforations of the bowel wall may be produced without penetration of the wall by the missile itself.

The most mutilating variety of gunshot wound seen in civilian practice is that produced by the shotgun. It is not an uncommon injury. When fired at short range (frequent when homicide is the intent), the blast often carries away part of the thoracic or abdominal wall or even drives it into the cavity, destroying deeper structures in its path. Thus these two varieties of penetrating wounds are virtually always associated with very rapidly developing shock, whereas piercing, penetrating wounds of the thorax and abdomen, such as those produced by knives, ice picks, pitch forks, and the like, ordinarily are not associated with rapidly developing shock. Moreover, the intraperitoneal visceral wounds usually produce single injuries, whereas gunshot and shotgun wounds usually produce multiple injuries.

The principles involved in the treatment of gunshot wounds of the abdomen and thorax are set forth in the discussion of penetrating injuries. Other important and more detailed aspects of treatment are discussed in

---

wound, as it entered through the base of the skull, was found to have performed an anterior hypophysectomy en route, passing between the optic nerves just in front of the optic chiasm without traumatizing either these or the major vessels at the base of the brain, entering the left frontal lobe, causing minimal bleeding. A flap of dura was fashioned, elevated, and turned back over the wound of entrance of the bullet. Penicillin (which had become available shortly before) was introduced at the site of injury, the lobe replaced, and the wound closed without any attempt being made to remove the bullet. The patient's immediate postoperative recovery was uneventful. About eight days later he was transferred to a garrison hospital.

Approximately three weeks later he was sent back to our hospital, with symptoms suggestive of an abscess at the bullet site in the left frontal lobe. The flap was again raised, and the bullet was found lying within a small abscess pocket. Its removal was simple. The abscess cavity was swabbed out, penicillin again introduced, and the wound closed. The patient made a rapid and apparently completely satisfactory recovery from this second procedure and was soon returned to the garrison hospital. Follow-up a short time later revealed that soon after his second return to the garrison hospital he was taken out and hanged.

the following sections. (See also the discussion on Retained Foreign Bodies, p. 519, and on other related subjects under Complications and Sequelae of Abdominal Trauma, p. 530.)

INJURIES OF THE COLON AND RECTUM

Various aspects of injuries of the colon and rectum have been discussed previously. In these the diagnosis of intraperitoneal injury as opposed to extraperitoneal injury is obviously of great importance. In most abdominal wounds, particularly in penetrating ones, exploratory celiotomy is considered by far the safest course. Are there ever circumstances in which celiotomy is considered unnecessary? In patients with gunshot and impaling wounds of the perineum and buttocks, there are rarely, if ever, any exceptions. In other mural areas of the abdomen and thorax, when a retained penetrating object is radiopaque and good roentgenograms are available, there undoubtedly are times when exploratory celiotomy will not be necessary. Further confirmation of this fact may be established by *exploration of the wound,* debridement, and establishment of hemostasis, with or without removal of the foreign body. If a large bowel perforation is found extraperitoneally, it may be possible to close the defect in the wall, leaving the debrided wound of access wide open.

Local application of antibiotic solutions and the use of antibiotics parenterally or orally are a matter of judgment, depending largely on length of time since injury, extent of damage, type of injury and object producing it, for example, knife wounds vs. missile wounds and traffic injuries. When defects with loss of segments of contused bowel wall have been produced, whether intraperitoneal or extraperitoneal, a proximal colostomy or exteriorization of the injured segment of bowel or both should be carried out. The colostomy should be a simple loop colostomy (in preference to a Mikulicz procedure), with division of the bowel which shall provide complete diversion of the fecal stream from the site of injury. This is of particular importance when the anal sphincter has been disrupted, in order to permit healing of the plastic repair required to forestall incontinence. Colostomy, by preference, should not be performed through the exploratory incision, but should be made at a distance proximal to the site of injury to the bowel, to permit subsequent procedures to be performed with greater facility and safety.

Primary repair of perforations of the large bowel produced by knife and gunshot wounds of the abdomen in civilian practice is being carried out more frequently and with less morbidity and a lower mortality rate than was considered possible under wartime conditions. Early and prompt treatment of these injuries places them essentially in the category of elective large bowel surgery except when there is obviously extensive contamination by fecal contents or widespread devitalization of tissues. Almost all knife wounds (which usually are small perforations) treated within 6 hours of injury may safely be handled in this manner without proximal colostomy or exteriorization, and the same is true of many perforations by bullets. Shotgun and, in fact, most types of gunshot wounds will be associated with shock, and the former will very likely produce extensive destruction of tissue. Two-stage procedures therefore will usually be necessary in shotgun wounds.

The immediate debridement of these wounds usually cannot be carried out without risk of losing the patient from hemorrhage and shock. The initial surgical procedure is to start resuscitation by intravenous fluids, transfusing blood as soon as possible. The stomach should be emptied and a large nasogastric tube left in place to provide for further aspiration and possibly for inflation of the stomach and duodenum at operation, as described by Pontius and others (see duodenal injuries, p. 528), to facilitate the discovery of perforations or lacerations of the duodenum. An indwelling catheter should be introduced, which will serve the immediate purpose of diagnosis and decompression and later serve as an aid in estimating fluid balance and renal function. Roentgen examination will show the approximate locations of retained radiopaque missiles. If rectal examination shows the presence of blood, proctoscopy should be done, with adequate suction apparatus at hand, to determine whether the source of bleeding is a rectal wound.

In recent sharp, penetrating, and stab wounds, exploration may be done through or by extension of the wound of injury, to determine whether the wound enters the peritoneal cavity, whether wounding of a retro- or extraperitoneal viscus has occurred, and, if it has, to determine the procedure to be carried out, possibly without celiotomy. In older wounds of this type, celiotomy should be done through clean tissues, an incision being used which will give good exposure; a long, midline incision will usually be the best. The intra-abdominal procedure should then be carried out and, as a separate procedure, debridement and usually drainage or tamponade of the skin and subcutaneous wound of entrance. At least the skin and subcutaneous wound should be left open, with or without placing skin sutures for delayed primary closure.

In the wounds produced by firearms, celiotomy may usually be carried out rapidly and with excellent exposure by a long midline incision. Arrest of hemorrhage is of first importance, and should be followed by suture repair of obvious visceral injuries. Intestinal wounds should be closed transversely. Finally, a careful, thorough, and systematic examination of the peritoneal cavity should be made for injuries which may have been overlooked. Of these, the most dangerous are in the retroperitoneal portions of the duodenum and the right and left colon. Therefore these segments of bowel should be mobilized almost routinely. Mesenteric attachments and mesenteries themselves should be inspected with particular thoroughness for evidence of obscure perforating wounds into them and for blood vessel injuries producing slow devitalization of segments of bowel. Recovery of the bullet or other missile will not be worth while and may actually be detrimental if search for it jeopardizes the life of the patient. However, in the case of a bullet, its recovery may be important from the standpoint of ballistic study in criminal cases, and this should be taken into account by the surgeon. The complications and sequelae of retained foreign bodies should also be remembered in reaching a decision on this point.

INSERTED FOREIGN BODIES

Foreign bodies inserted into the rectum for purposes of examination or therapy (such as proctoscopes and bougies or rectal tubes and enema tips) or accidentally or intentionally inserted objects (the number and variety of which are almost beyond belief) constitute serious hazards because of (1) the local irritation produced, (2) the danger of perforating adjacent structures outside of or within the peritoneal cavity, and (3) the danger of either or both of these accidents occurring during extraction of the foreign body, which can, on occasion, thwart the most ingenious efforts. The same situation may prevail following insertion of foreign bodies into the vagina or urethra.

Another injury of somewhat the same type is the accidental or very occasional intentional serious distention of the colon with fluid or gas from below. Caution must be used in giving rectal treatments, particularly colon lavages, to avoid over-distending the bowel. In the conscious patient there will usually be warning of this by the patient's voiced objections, but not so in the case of an unconscious patient. Death has been caused both by unintentional rupture of the large bowel in this manner and by the intentional distention of the rectum and colon by compressed air and by the introduction of fluid into the rectum under pressure.

RUPTURE OF THE SPLEEN

Spontaneous rupture of the normal spleen (i.e., occurring in the absence of both trauma and disease) has been reported, but its undisputed occurrence has been denied by several authors. A recent critical review of the reported cases establishes it as a rare occurrence of unknown etiology.

Traumatic rupture of the spleen is relatively common and not infrequently is the sole critical injury produced by blunt trauma to the left anterior or lateral thoraco-abdominal wall. In the presence of possible masking effects of the contusion, so often characterized by a sharp, catching chest pain on inspiration, signifying pleural irritation due often to a fractured rib, it is highly important to recognize the diagnostic features of a ruptured spleen per se. These are highlighted by the reports of *spontaneous ruptures,* the essential features of which, as summarized from the literature by Orloff and Peskin, are (1) the history of trauma; (2) abdominal pain in all cases reported; (3) tenderness usually confined to the left hypochondrium or generalized over the abdomen; (4) not infrequent aching pain on reclining or coughing referred to the top of the left shoulder (Kehr's sign) or to the axilla or supraclavicular region; (5) left upper quadrant rigidity, maximal in the left hypochondrium but distributed to the same areas generally as the tenderness; (6) shifting abdominal dulness or *occasional non-shifting* but increasing *dulness* in the left upper quadrant (Ballance sign); (7) dizziness or faintness and frequent actual syncope; (8) nausea and vomiting; (9) elevated pulse rate with normal temperature; and (10) usually rapid progression of symptoms. (In a small proportion of cases, after the injury, the onset of left hypochondriac pain and tenderness is followed by a latent period of varying duration—for as long as 3 weeks and occasionally longer, associated with vague abdominal discomfort—and then the acute symptoms signifying resumption of bleeding abruptly develop.)

The immediate blood count almost always shows a leukocytosis but rarely shows anemia. Roentgen examination is of value, as it may show increased density in the left hypochondrium, with obliteration of the splenic outline, the left renal outline, and the psoas shadow; serration along the greater curvature, and displacement of the stomach to the right; elevation and limitation of motion of the left hemidiaphragm; downward displacement of the splenic flexure; gastric and intestinal dilatation (or dynamic ileus), and the suggestion of free peritoneal fluid. If the diagnosis is in doubt, needle aspiration of the left upper quadrant may prove of value, but only if the findings are positive. Negative results are meaningless and should not be taken as evidence *against* splenic rupture, since blood is frequently loculated and may be missed.

The triad of pain, tenderness, and rigidity in the left upper quadrant after direct trauma to the left thoraco-abdominal wall should suggest the possibility of a ruptured spleen, and call for continued observation, repeated physical examinations, and the performance of appropriate tests and examinations as outlined above. Preparations should be made for transfusion, and blood should be started if further evidence of bleeding is elicited. When operation is performed, the incision used is important. A sufficiently long left rectus incision usually gives adequate exposure for splenectomy and should be used, especially if multiple associated abdominal injuries are suspected. A combined left thoraco-abdominal incision may be *planned* when ruptured spleen is considered quite definitely to be the only significant injury, as is often the case in nonpenetrating trauma. The abdominal part of the incision may then be made, the intraperitoneal situation assessed, and the incision carried into the thorax through the 8th or 9th left costal interspace if necessary. The diaphragm should be examined thoroughly for small tears or lacerations, which should then be repaired, and the surgical diaphragmatic wound closed with strong nonabsorbable suture material.

The over-all mortality rate in ruptured spleen in a number of reported series of cases is about 30 per cent. It is lower in children, and higher in adults and in patients who sustain multiple injuries. When the sole injury has been the ruptured spleen, the mortality rate in reported series has been 0.7 to 6 per cent.

Postoperative complications of splenectomy are frequent, the most common being pulmonary atelectasis, pneumonitis, and dynamic ileus. Venous thrombosis may occur as the platelet elevation reaches its peak, usually during the second postoperative week. Prophylactic anticoagulation measures should then be instituted.

The most dangerous aspect of splenic rupture is lack of awareness that it may have occurred, especially in persons sustaining multiple injuries.

INJURIES OF THE LIVER

The over-all mortality rate from *injuries* to the liver has been reduced within the past half century from over 60 per cent to around 15 per cent, owing largely to improvement in the treatment of wounds by the development of methods of blood replacement and control of infection. These same factors have aided in the reduction of mortality from associated injuries. However, there has been very little reduction in the mortality rate from *ruptured liver* during this same interval, the high percentage—78 per cent reported by Edler in 1888—being essentially the same today.

It may be reasonably inferred that ruptures of the liver probably account for many of the deaths in today's crash injuries. The exact proportion of fatalities so produced is not known, because unfortunately so few postmortem examinations are performed on victims of these accidents. When sudden impact occurs, the size and weight of the liver are important predisposing factors in the production of tears along the lines of its attachments due to inertia. It is easy to understand how ensuing hemorrhage can rapidly be fatal, resulting in a relatively low incidence of hepatic injuries observed in hospital series. When death does not occur at the site of accident, the patient may survive even in the presence of massive hemoperitoneum, particularly if replacement therapy is promptly instituted. Thus, Rob can say quite honestly (speaking, however, of liver *wounds*) that under circumstances when liver damage can safely be presumed to be the sole injury to a patient surviving transportation to hospital, operative attempts to control the hemorrhage may themselves prove fatal.

Usually, of course, in today's crash injuries, multiple injuries will be incurred, and indications will be quite clear for entering the peritoneal cavity. At such times, if bleeding occurs from the liver, and the site is accessible, it must be controlled if possible, at least temporarily, by the simplest measures, such as tamponade and packing. Exploration should then be carried out and other necessary intra-abdominal procedures completed, because it is recognized that the mortality rate in patients sustaining liver injuries and surviving long enough to reach hospital is in direct proportion to the number of *associated injuries*. The very fact that the patient has already survived the liver injury indicates that, with further supportive measures and *minimal* operative interference, unless it is urgently required (more than this being capable of precipitating further and fatal bleeding), he will in all likelihood be safe from this immediate hazard at least. Unfortunately, in most accidents producing *rupture* of the liver, control of bleeding from this source leaves very little time or opportunity for other elaborate procedures. If other hazards can be forestalled by prompt surgery and the patient's condition becomes stabilized by the supportive measures employed, the surgeon, relying on judgment and experience, will determine at that time whether it is safe to proceed with resections of probably devitalized liver segments or with other measures of hemostasis to protect against secondary hemorrhage, infection, and bile peritonitis. There is no rule of thumb in such situations. The decision must be the result of individual and collaborative assessment of the patient's condition by the surgeon, anesthesiologist, and frequently the attending physician. *The principal limiting factor is inadequate means of controlling severe bleeding from this organ.*

These wounds must be drained, particularly if Gelfoam or Oxycel gauze has been employed to help control bleeding from the liver wound. As mentioned earlier, these hemostatic agents also inhibit the formation of adhesions, with the result that extravasation of bile may take place into the free peritoneal cavity unless provision has been made for its escape to the exterior through a soft, fenestrated tube drain or drains.

INJURIES OF THE DUODENUM

Fortunately, duodenal injuries are relatively uncommon, for less progress has been made in the past 50 years in terms of reduced morbidity and mortality following these injuries than after any other thoracic or abdominal injury. In fact, the mortality rate for duodenal injuries in the Korean conflict was 41 per cent. By far the majority of such injuries are penetrating wounds, a greater proportion occurring in combat than in civilian practice. The mortality rate is higher for blunt injuries, about one-third of which are retroperitoneal perforations or tears, than for penetrating wounds, the reasons for which are fairly obvious. Stab wounds carry a far lower mortality rate. Among civilians, pistol, shotgun, and stab wounds account for the majority of these injuries. Traffic accidents, direct blows, and falls account for most of the remainder. Since most of the injuries are due to firearms and traffic accidents, they will be associated with other, multiple injuries. This always increases the gravity of the prognosis. As with other serious injuries, an awareness that such an injury may exist is probably the most important single factor on which to place our hope for a lowered mortality rate.

Suggestive findings in the examination of the injured person which should produce awareness of this injury are the site of the injury and type of trauma; the presence of blood in the vomitus; roentgen evidence of free air in the peritoneal cavity or *in the retroperitoneal tissues* in the vicinity of the duodenum. Use of a swallow of Lipiodol has been suggested by Estes et al. for conscious patients. Since a nasogastric tube is almost routinely employed, a small amount of Lipiodol may be introduced by gravity through this and roentgenograms taken, or air inflation of the stomach and upper intestine, as suggested by Pontius after the abdomen has been opened and the duodenum exposed, may be used. At operation, inspection and palpation may reveal edema and crepitation at the base of the transverse mesocolon, and the presence of dark discoloration of these tissues by blood and bile may also be noted. Finally, one should make certain to mobilize the duodenum so that it can be carefully inspected throughout for both actual perforations and tears and for potential perforations, noticeable as small discolored areas in the wall. To expose the third and fourth parts of the duodenum, the ligament of Treitz will have to be divided and the bowel dissected free at the root of the mesentery.

Mobilization of the hepatic flexure will facilitate exposure of the duodenum. The retroperitoneal aspect of the ascending colon should also be exposed in these injuries, as in other cases of multiple abdominal wounds.

Pain referred to the groin or right testis and crepitus in the retroperitoneal tissues on rectal examination have been described when duodenal rupture has occurred, but these signs have not been consistently reported.

Most of the duodenal injuries will be intraperitoneal and will involve the first and second parts of the duodenum. The most dangerous ones, however, are those involving the retroperitoneal wall, and these are the ones most likely to be overlooked. These wounds should be sutured when possible, making the closure across the bowel to avoid constriction of the lumen, which predisposes to breakdown of the closure. Whether these wounds are sutured or the injured area is resected, the suture lines should be protected by a gastroenterostomy, a gastroduodenostomy, or a duodenoenterostomy, the higher in the small bowel the better. Associated injuries to the gallbladder, liver, and pancreas may require suture and/or cholecystectomy. Major bile ducts may require repair over intraluminal tubes, or anastomosis to bowel.

Associated ureteral injuries are not common, but right renal injury often occurs and may necessitate nephrectomy if the damage otherwise sustained is likely to result in extravasations of blood and urine (see Combined Abdominal and Urinary Tract Injuries, p. 538). Drainage should be provided through a stab wound in the flank, the drain accurately placed and held if necessary by a catgut suture close to, but *not against, the suture line or bowel wall.* Draining through the incision invites breakdown of the wound, with possible disruption, should a duodenal fistula with or without infection develop. This complication is one to be most feared because of problems of fluid and electrolyte loss, nutritional depletion, infection, and associated interference with wound healing. Control of the loss of fluid from a duodenal fistula by means of a catheter snugly placed just intramurally and kept on high negative pressure suction is a method worth trying in managing this difficult problem.

MISCELLANEOUS INJURIES

Many injuries to specific structures not discussed here have been reported in the literature, but most of them are uncommon. The normal aorta may be incompletely lacerated by blunt trauma. This occurs much more frequently in the thorax than in the abdomen. In persons sustaining severe blunt thoracic or abdominal injuries this injury must at times be suspected because of vague, persistent, unexplained chest discomfort and respiratory distress or abdominal discomfort. Roentgen evidence of widening of the mediastinal shadow might suggest what is going on. The initial injury involves the subintimal layer, usually as a transverse laceration with bleeding and scar formation, which result in weakening of the wall, the basis for the later development of aneurysm and possible rupture. Acute traumatic rupture of the normal abdominal aorta from blunt trauma has been reported, but is extremely rare. Today these injuries are not necessarily fatal, thanks to the advances which have been made in blood vessel substitution surgery.

Chylous ascites and chylothorax are infrequently caused by penetrating and rarely by nonpenetrating trauma to the thoracic duct and cisterna chyli and to the root of the mesentery. Chyluria may be a rare complication or sequela of injury in this area, resulting from extensive blocking of lacteals by cicatrization at a retroperitoneal site of injury near the receptaculum chyli, with associated renal or ureteral injury.

Rarely spontaneous rupture of one of the gastroepiploic vessels into the lesser peritoneal sac will produce a syndrome called "abdominal apoplexy," simulating acute pancreatitis by the severity, type, and distribution of pain, but with a normal serum amylase and a drop in the hematocrit. Spontaneous ruptures of blood vessels in the abdominal wall, simulating acute intraperitoneal disorders such as acute intestinal obstruction, are more frequent but still are very uncommon. Passage or lodgment of a missile or other foreign body between large arteries and accompanying veins will rarely produce a disabling arteriovenous aneurysm. Such an aneurysm has been produced between the aorta and the inferior vena cava.

Of very serious import is the occasional occurrence of mesenteric thrombosis from severe, blunt abdominal trauma. It is a little surprising that this does not occur more frequently than is reported, considering the relative present-day frequency of severe blunt trauma to that area.

Certain *types* of trauma will produce many other different combinations of associated injuries in addition to those discussed, notably missile wounds and crash injuries. Usually such trauma produces so many complex injuries of such serious proportions that we find ourselves once again considering the immediate individual problem from the point of view of general principles and priority of treatment. Unfortunately, most of today's "dangerous" and "fatal" highway and airplane accidents fall into this category. The principles and many of the methods of handling these injuries are discussed in other chapters of this book.

COMPLICATIONS AND SEQUELAE OF ABDOMINAL TRAUMA

In addition to an intimate familiarity with the immediate anatomical, physiological, and technical problems of survival in dealing with injuries to the thorax and abdomen, the surgeon must have a sound knowledge of the probable and possible *consequences* of injury in these areas when produced by various types of trauma. The variety of complications and sequelae of injuries to thoracic and abdominal viscera is larger by far than the variety of primary injuries, and can be more difficult to diagnose and manage than the immediate effects of the injury itself. Intelligent handling of the primary damage will minimize but will never eradicate these early and late consequences of trauma.

When one considers what may be the effects of a single retained foreign body, the complexity of the subject becomes obvious. It is true that many foreign bodies remain silent, in fact, they may not even be known to exist.

For example, a roentgenogram taken because of "arthritis" may reveal the presence of a bullet in the paraspinal muscles, as it did in a man who had sustained what was thought to be an inconsequential wound some 45 years previously, in the Spanish American War. The "arthritis" was treated conservatively, and the bullet was carried to his grave.

On the other hand, consider the mischief which may be produced by just two of the commonest effects of retained foreign bodies, infection and hemorrhage. These two complications, either separately or together, can be exceedingly difficult to treat successfully. Attempting to stop a secondary hemorrhage resulting from necrosis of the wall of a large vessel, most likely inaccessible, in the middle of the night, can be one of the most frustrating and distressing episodes that a surgeon experiences. The subsequent development of fistulas of various types may not be dramatic, yet they will inevitably tax the skill and resourcefulness of every surgeon who does abdominal and thoracic surgery in this century of armed conflict and automobiles, with hydrogen bombs, rockets, and space travel in the immediate offing.

As with primary injury, a classification more or less arbitrary and overlapping, but based on knowledge of the early effects and late results of trauma, is invaluable in systematizing one's thinking and planning in the management of the consequences of thoracic and abdominal injuries. To do this, and to organize and execute an intelligent plan of treatment, takes a good *working knowledge* in particular of anatomy, physiology, pathology, and bacteriology.

The consequences of trauma may be divided into: (1) immediate, (2) proximate, and (3) late complications, and (4) sequelae. The immediate complications merge with the injury itself. They constitute, essentially, the anatomical and physiological derangements which are the immediate and direct results of the primary trauma which, when severe, often threaten life, such as compromise of the airway, cardiac tamponade, cardiac arrest, exsanguination, and the like.

The proximate complications may be thought of as those closely related to the *early phase of injury*, or as secondary injuries which follow and result from the initial injury. These also may threaten life, as, for example, secondary hemorrhage and shock and the development of infection of many different types. Extravasation of blood and of body fluids other than blood, including urine, lymph, gastrointestinal contents, activated or inactivated enzymes of pancreatic fluid, bile, cerebrospinal fluid, and chyle, may occur.

Late complications which may be associated with or may result from these include secondary shock associated with fluid and electrolyte loss and imbalance; or generalized, spreading, dissecting, necrotizing, or circumscribed infection, the effects of which, coupled with nutritional depletion, delay and interfere with wound healing. These factors in turn predispose to dehiscence of suture lines and of other surgical wounds, causing disruption and evisceration. Anemia often is also associated with this unfortunate train of events.

Within this same phase of continuing or secondary injury, many of the fistulas will develop. These will include internal and external fistulas communicating with or connecting hollow viscera, principally of the gastrointestinal and urinary tracts. Probably the most serious of these is a duodenal fistula (see Injuries of the Duodenum, p. 528). Arteriovenous fistulas also may develop. Developing somewhat later, and usually associated with infection, are the fistulas associated with retained foreign bodies, whether autogenous in origin, such as bone fragments, tendon, fascia, and cartilage sloughs, or heterogenous, such as the traumatic agent itself or clothing and other non-metallic objects carried into the body cavities and tissues with it.

Ingested foreign bodies or objects inserted into body orifices constitute a form of primary trauma which also may lead to the above-mentioned complications. Oftener they require merely conservative treatment during a period of careful observation, as will frequently occur following the ingestion of non-absorbable objects by children and psychopathic persons. They may, however, require early surgical intervention at some point, depending on the location, size, and type of object ingested or inserted. (See under Characteristic Features of Specific Types of Abdominal Injury, Injuries of the Colon and Rectum, p. 523, and Inserted Foreign Bodies, p. 525.)

Of some interest among the late complications of abdominal trauma is the development of pseudocysts of the pancreas. These are relatively common following pancreatic trauma. Usually they present between the stomach and the transverse colon. They cannot be easily removed because of hemorrhage and because there are no normal anatomical cleavage planes. Usually they are marsupialized or, on occasion, anastomosed to a contiguous segment of small bowel.

Bile cysts, splenic cysts, liver cysts, and chyle and lymphatic cysts have resulted from trauma to corresponding structures. Peritoneal implantations of splenic tissue have been found after traumatic rupture of the spleen.

Late complications may develop into permanent sequelae, or sequelae may result from permanent primary or secondary injury, for example, sphincter incontinence, partial or complete cord bladder, and other neurologic residua associated with loss or devitalization of important nerve pathways which affect abdominal structures and their functions. Diaphragmatic hernias are frequently produced early, owing to small perforating wounds or tears overlooked at the time of injury and operation. It must again be recalled that over 50 per cent of strangulated diaphragmatic hernias are traumatic in origin.

The surgical treatment of most late complications and sequelae of thoracic and abdominal trauma falls into the groups of elective procedures handled by surgeons in whose field they lie. Details of their management are to be found in appropriate texts and articles, and are not within the scope of this work.

MANAGEMENT OF THORACO-ABDOMINAL INJURIES

Thoraco-abdominal injuries from the point of view of the chest surgeon are considered in Chapter 18, to which the reader is referred. From the point of view of the abdominal surgeon certain particularly pertinent features are discussed here, at the risk of repetition.

These injuries are usually of the penetrating type, comparatively seldom the result of blunt injury. Occasionally, crushing injuries and other indirect trauma sustained in automobile accidents will produce rupture of the diaphragm. The majority of war missile wounds passed from the thorax into the abdomen rather than in the reverse direction (about 12 to 1), and the same is probably true of civilian injuries of this type. In either event, interference with the dynamics of respiration usually calls attention to the intrathoracic component which requires priority of treatment even though much more time will usually be spent subsequently in dealing with the abdominal component of the injury, whether through the thoracotomy incision or through a *second* abdominal incision. To embark upon a long abdominal procedure in the presence of a damaged respiratory mechanism is to court disaster. Rarely, a bullet or knife wound of the abdomen will perforate the diaphragm without producing any signs or symptoms of intrathoracic injury.

The chief area of vulnerability to thoraco-abdominal wounds is that section of the body between planes transecting the level of the costal margin and the 12th rib below, and the nipple (male) and angle of the scapula above. A knowledge of the anatomy of and approaches to this section of the body is therefore of the greatest importance. Rarely injury to the abdomen may be caused by agents entering through wounds in the neck, axilla, buttocks, and thighs. The value of posteroanterior and lateral roentgenograms in localizing radiopaque foreign bodies within this zone is obvious.

Not infrequently the abdominal damage sustained in thoraco-abdominal injury may be dealt with adequately through thoracotomy incisions used to repair the intrathoracic damage sustained. This is not only feasible, but far safer, in early operation, than an abdominal approach, especially on the left side, if the diaphragm has been opened widely and the pleural surfaces are contaminated. It offers an opportunity to debride the pleura thoroughly and to close the diaphragm accurately and securely. In a series reported by Wylie et al. the entire abdominal procedure was performed through the thoracotomy approach in 362 out of 903 patients. Wounds involving the superior surface of the liver, the right kidney, and the hepatic flexure could be dealt with usually through a thoracotomy incision on the right side. Injuries caused by missiles entering the lower zone of the diaphragm on that side, however, were explored through the abdomen, after the diaphragm and wounds of entry in the chest wall were debrided and closed.

Most small wounds of the diaphragm on the left side should be approached through the abdomen because of the danger, otherwise, of contaminating the pleura should it be necessary to open the diaphragm widely from above in attempting exploration of the abdomen through a chest wall incision. However, this is a debatable point, and each situation must be considered as an individual problem. The wound in the diaphragm should be closed with non-absorbable suture material.

In those who survive thoraco-abdominal injuries, the abdominal injuries sustained are frequently complex and the mortality rate is high. Among World War II casualties, the over-all mortality rate in those who sustained thoraco-abdominal wounds was roughly 25 per cent. In analyzing the case records of 903 such casualties, Wylie stated that the most lethal part of the injury was the abdominal component, depending on the type and number of organs below the diaphragm which were involved. Wounds involving five or more organs were fatal.

In civilians penetrating thoraco-abdominal wounds are produced chiefly by knives and other penetrating objects, intentionally or accidentally, and by firearms. Damage produced by the first type of agent is far less serious than that produced by the second.

The most difficult and serious injuries occurring in this area, from the standpoint of detection and treatment, are severe traffic and crushing injuries which almost always are multiple. Frequently there will be injuries of both chest and abdomen, but seldom do abdominal injuries extend into the thorax. Ruptures of the spleen, liver, pancreas, and distended hollow viscera are commonly associated with injuries inside the thorax and of the thoracic wall. Additional data regarding these injuries will be found in Chapter 18.

Rupture of the Diaphragm

Rupture of the diaphragm does occur, but it may be masked by shock or be overlooked because of the severity of associated injuries. The left hemidiaphragm is usually affected, because of the protection given the right side by the liver. Pain may be present in the left chest or referred to the left shoulder. Usually there will be dyspnea and cyanosis. Dulness or tympany may be present over the left lower chest, and the mediastinum may be shifted to the right. Roentgenographic and fluoroscopic examination may reveal the presence of hollow abdominal viscera within the thoracic cavity, and by that time, if the associated injuries are not too severe, there may be complaints of indigestion and abdominal pain.

Symptoms may even suggest a coronary occlusion. The onset of crampy pains, sounds of hyperactive peristalsis, nausea, and vomiting herald the onset of acute intestinal obstruction which urgently demands surgical intervention. In this event the approach should be through the chest wall because of the facility with which the obstruction can be relieved and even a segment of nonviable bowel resected by enlarging the opening in the diaphragm. It should be added that repair of the diaphragm from above gives greater assurance against recurrence of a hernia than inexact repair of a defect from below. This is particularly true when the defect in the diaphragm is small and peripheral. Such defects are frequently overlooked from below. It is to be remembered that *the majority of strangulated diaphragmatic hernias are traumatic in origin.*

Crush injuries may occasionally cause fracture of ribs, which may perforate the diaphragm and the viscera beneath. Such injuries are rare.

Blast injuries do not produce rupture of the diaphragm, the mechanism of damage in such trauma being dependent on the presence of gas within the tissues or lumens of hollow viscera affected, which may lead to hemorrhages within the lungs and perforations in the walls of hollow abdominal viscera but no damage to solid viscera. In such injuries the lungs suffer most.

ABDOMINAL INJURIES ASSOCIATED WITH FRACTURES

The regions in which abdominal injuries are associated with fractures are the spine, the sternum, and lower ribs, the pelvis, and the upper femurs. Both penetrating and nonpenetrating injuries of the lower thoracic cage may result in fractures of the ribs and sternum, which in turn may produce intra-abdominal damage. The most frequent injuries are diaphragmatic tears; splenic, liver, and renal lacerations resulting in intra- and extraperitoneal bleeding or hemorrhage, and possible perforation of the splenic flexure or stomach, depending on the direction and force of the traumatic agent and the state of distention of the viscera. Damage to hollow viscera is uncommon in nonpenetrating injuries. In such a situation, injury to the spleen, with hemorrhage, is the most serious, though frequently overlooked, associated injury, and should always be considered. In fact, celiotomy is indicated in severe contusions and crushing injuries involving the lower thorax, not only because of the possibility of secondary damage associated with fractured ribs, but also because of associated trauma to viscera other than those injured by the fractured fragments of bone, notably the duodenum, pancreas, and small intestine.

The major problem resulting from fractured ribs, however, is not intraperitoneal injury, but rather associated intrathoracic injury to soft parts, and, when multiple, flail chest and vasculorespiratory embarrassment, which may be rapidly fatal.

Fracture of the Spine and Retroperitoneal Hemorrhage

The retroperitoneal effects of these direct blunt-trauma spine fractures and other injuries to the thoracolumbar regions, however, often give rise to difficulty in differentiating between retroperitoneal and intraperitoneal damage due to contusion and hemorrhage contiguous with and adjacent to the posterior and lateral peritoneum. Intraperitoneal injury of course may also occur with these injuries, the most likely being rupture of the spleen, liver, or kidneys. If ribs also are fractured, other structures may be damaged, including diaphragm, pleura, lung, and colon. The confusing abdominal symptoms and signs produced by these flank injuries are tenderness, pain, and, not infrequently, spasm of the lateral abdominal muscles and psoas, and, somewhat later, abdominal distention. Often the distention becomes marked and extraordinarily difficult to alleviate, but it is a diffuse type of paralytic ileus not difficult to differentiate from intraperitoneal irritation or mechanical intestinal obstruction.

The problem of differentiation between intraperitoneal and extraperitoneal damage becomes more difficult when injury to the *anterior* abdominal wall has occurred, producing rupture of relatively large vessels, such as the inferior epigastric artery. Such rupture, of course, may rarely occur "spontaneously" when the vessel is diseased. In either event, the effect may so closely simulate acute intestinal obstruction or compromise of a segment of bowel as to warrant emergency celiotomy. Usually, in the course of making the incision, the nature of the pathology is revealed.

Fractures of Pelvis and/or Skull

Fractures of the pelvis and skull are not infrequently associated with abdominal injuries. Of particular interest in this connection are symptoms and signs incorrectly attributed to intracranial pressure, and misconstrued as evidence of skull fracture when actually none has occurred. Usually, of course, this is not a difficult problem in differential diagnosis. Nausea and vomiting without hematemesis are not uncommon in severe cerebral concussion, and occasionally there is also abdominal pain, but the absence of other critical evidence of intra-abdominal injury will be quite obvious to a perceptive observer. (The same may be said for a patient with congestive heart disease or one who is on an excessive dose of digitalis.)

Pelvic fractures, particularly fracture of the pubic rami in the male by lateral or anteroposterior compression of the pelvis, may produce rupture of the bladder, with extravasation of blood and urine throughout the pelvic tissues; perforation of the rectum and pelvic viscera and small bowel may also occur in the female. These are serious injuries and require prompt closure of the perforations and removal of the penetrating bone fragments. Examination of the voided urine for blood, roentgen examination, digital and proctoscopic examinations, and visualization of the urethra and bladder areas by retrograde gravity urography via urethra are the most revealing and safest diagnostic procedures to carry out. The use of a catheter may be dangerous and misleading when a urethral tear has been produced, or when intraperitoneal extravasation has occurred and is drained per catheter. The constant desire to void, with inability to do so, is characteristic of bladder and urethral injuries.

Fractures of the pelvic bones by *penetrating* missiles or other agents, combined with associated injuries to pelvic and peritoneal viscera, are particularly dangerous and will be discussed together. These include impaling injuries which may or may not be associated with fractures. The fractures may or may not be important, depending on whether the *missile* or the *resulting bone fragments* are responsible for the injuries to adjacent structures—the urethra, bladder, or ureters, genital viscera, pelvic colon and sphincters, large and small intestines lying within the pelvis, major blood vessels, or the cauda equina and sacral nerves. Missile wounds and impaling injuries of the perineum, buttocks, and upper thighs may also produce intraperitoneal injuries. In treating these, the soft parts leading to the damaged viscera must be opened widely, debrided, and drained; the visceral tears and lacerations should be repaired when possible, with protection to the closures by a proximal colostomy, a suprapubic cystostomy, or both; and antibiotics used locally and parenterally, combined with an exploratory celiotomy performed coincidentally, by another operating team, if possible, or as a separate, proximate procedure.

The morbidity and mortality resulting from these injuries, owing to frequent anaerobic infections, notably gas, were very high prior to World War II. When such injuries were treated early and adequately, as outlined above, the mortality was reduced from 70–80 per cent to about 15 per cent.

ABDOMINAL INJURIES ASSOCIATED WITH INJURY TO THE SPINAL CORD

Injuries to the spinal cord are not infrequently associated with intrathoracic, thoraco-abdominal, and abdominal injuries. The usual type of trauma responsible for such a combination of injuries is a gunshot or missile wound. However, injury to any part of the spinal cord alone may produce alterations in the function of thoracic and abdominal viscera and parietes, as well as peripheral muscular and sensory changes. Thus, a fall from a height may produce a fracture of the cervical spine with cord compression and resulting quadriplegia. At the same time, there will be serious disturbances of bladder and colon functions involving both sensory and motor components of the walls of these structures and their sphincters. The innervation of the small bowel may be affected, resulting in distention amounting even to tympanites or meteorism. If, in addition, there has been an associated contusion of the lower thoracic wall or abdomen, intrathoracic and intra-abdominal injuries must also be considered. If the injury has also produced extraperitoneal damage, signs and symptoms of *intra*-peritoneal injury may be present although intraperitoneal damage actually may not have been sustained.

For the abdominal surgeon, the problem is primarily one of diagnosis. Wounds penetrating the abdomen and injuring the spine and spinal cord will have to be explored intraperitoneally. Whether to follow this with decompression of the cord will depend on a number of circumstances, not the least important of which is the general condition of the patient. If the cord itself has been disrupted by a missile, by the bony fragment of a fractured spine, or by other direct disruptive trauma, decompression seldom helps. If, however, the trauma is indirect, producing simple contusion or hemorrhage, restoration of function may depend on prompt decompression of the cord. Laminectomy should be carried out as soon as the condition of the patient permits. In such circumstances the importance of accurate roentgen diagnosis is obvious.

Usually penetrating injuries producing spinal cord damage will be associated with spine fractures. On the other hand, most fractures of the dorsolumbar spine produced by indirect trauma, and many direct blows producing fractures of transverse processes and lumbar ribs, will produce no cord damage and will infrequently cause spinal root compression.

COMBINED ABDOMINAL AND URINARY TRACT INJURIES

Injuries of the external and internal genital and lower urinary tract are not infrequently associated with perineal, buttock, and thigh wounds. These are practically never isolated visceral injuries. Injury of the lower ureter is uncommon but may be suggested by the presence of urine in the wound or in the rectum, even on digital examination. If divided, torn, or perforated, the ureter should be repaired, if possible, at the time, over a ureteral catheter which is left in place, implanted into the bladder; if the ureter is avulsed with loss of substance, the proximal end may be implanted in the large bowel or the excretion of urine be otherwise temporarily exteriorized, as by nephrostomy.

Excretory urography usually is of little value in the diagnosis of these *lower* urinary tract injuries, because of associated suppression of renal excretion of urine which persists for several hours after injury and insufficient concentration of the opaque medium, resulting in absence of outlines of ureters and bladder. Retrograde cystoscopy is not without danger from the instrumentation and is time consuming. Retrograde gravity urography via urethra probably provides the safest and surest means of defining lacerations and perforations of these structures in doubtful cases. These injuries nearly always require celiotomy because of the great likelihood of intra-abdominal damage, and this is preferable to prolonged observation. Exploration must include the ureteral and bladder regions for evidence of injuries, and these should be repaired at the time, with vesical drainage by suprapubic cystostomy.

Upper urinary tract injuries, particularly penetrating injuries, are often associated with intraperitoneal damage. It should be pointed out that, although kidney injury is quite frequent, a minority of renal injuries require nephrectomy. Most renal injuries associated with nonpenetrating trauma are contusions. Early suture of a small laceration with drainage to the site of closure is usually all that is required in minor wounds and lacerations. Greater damage is most safely and conservatively treated by nephrectomy. This point of view presupposes the demonstration of a normally functioning opposite kidney and takes into account the known high incidence of morbidity and mortality following conservative treatment for renal injuries in which there has been extravasation of blood and urine outside of the capsule.

Many contusions will produce gross hematuria, as illustrated by the effects produced in boxers and prizefighters by infighting. The amount of hematuria may seem out of all proportion to the extent of demonstrable damage. Repeated damage of this type may ultimately result in impaired renal function.

Thus, although rupture of the spleen requiring splenectomy is a common sequel to severe blunt trauma to the left lateral thoraco-abdominal region, sufficient injury to the kidney to necessitate nephrectomy will seldom occur. Most single renal injuries are contusions without extravasation which heal in about two weeks with bed rest, and are not usually associated with impaired renal function.

BIBLIOGRAPHY

Curry, G. J., and Lyttle, S. N.: Treatment of multiple severe complex injuries, Am. J. Surg. 83:703, 1952.
Dunphy, J. E., and Botsford, T. W.: Physical Examination of the Surgical Patient, ed. 2. Philadelphia, W. B. Saunders Co., 1958, p. 304.
Estes, W. L., Jr., Bowman, T. L., and Meilicke, F. F.: Non-penetrating abdominal trauma with special reference to lesions of the duodenum and pancreas, Am. J. Surg. 83:434, 1952.
Miller, J. M.: The death of James Abram Garfield, Surg., Gynec. & Obst., 107:113, 1958.
Orkin, L. A.: Bedside urological x-ray examination of the severely injured patient, Surg., Gynec. & Obst. 94:693, 1952.
Orloff, M. J., and Peskin, G. W.: Spontaneous rupture of the normal spleen, a surgical enigma, Internat. Abstr. Surg. 106:1, 1958, in Surg., Gynec. & Obst., January, 1958.
Pontius, R. G., Creech, O., Jr., and DeBakey, M. E.: Management of large bowel injuries in civilian practice, Ann. Surg. 146:291, 1957.
Rob, C. G.: Diagnosis of abdominal trauma in warfare, Surg., Gynec. & Obst. 85:147, 1947.
Vincent, E. H.: Presidential gunshot wounds; three case reports, Surg., Gynec. & Obst. 91:115, 1950.
Wylie, R. H., Hoffman, H. L., Williams, D. B., and Rose, W. F.: The thoraco-abdominal casualty, Ann. Surg. 124:463, 1946.

CHAPTER 18

CHEST INJURIES

By ROBERT H. WYLIE, M.D., and
NORMAN B. THOMSON, Jr., M.D.

GENERAL CONSIDERATIONS

RECOGNITION OF INJURY

In consideration of thoracic trauma, certain general points require emphasis before specific types of injury are dealt with. The first of these is the recognition that an injury of the thorax exists. If there is respiratory difficulty or obvious external evidence of trauma over the thorax, this recognition is usually easy. However, when severe multiple injuries are present, serious damage within the thorax may go unnoticed because of concentration upon a more obvious injury. Thus, in a serious automobile injury with multiple compound fractures of the extremities, a rupture of the diaphragm may escape detection or a large hemothorax may, on occasion, be unrecognized. The obvious answer is found in the dictum that in every case of severe injury there is no substitute for immediate and complete physical examination, which should include an x-ray examination in the posterior, anterior, and lateral positions if injury involving the thorax is suspected.

RECOGNITION OF ALTERED PHYSIOLOGY

In planning the treatment of chest injuries certain changes in respiratory physiology must be given weight even in the most minor of injuries. Thus, in simple fracture of a rib, there will be a disturbance of respiration due to the limitation of normal ventilation by chest pain. When the integrity of the chest wall has actually been destroyed, as in the open sucking wound with collapse of the underlying lung and pendulum swing of the mediastinum, ventilation becomes markedly inhibited and life is threatened. Also, in severe crush injury of the chest, when multiple fractures of the ribs cause the chest wall to lose its rigidity and paradoxical respiration is produced with inward motion of the chest wall in inspiration, the effectiveness of ventilation becomes markedly hampered.

Added to this loss of the normal bellows action of the chest wall are the contusion and laceration of the lung itself, with resulting edema and hemorrhage of pulmonary tissue with extravasation of blood into the bronchial air passages, in addition to pneumothorax and hemothorax. These changes in the lung are compounded by the ineffectiveness of cough and the retention of mucous secretion, hemorrhagic extravasation, and edema fluid in the tracheobronchial passages. Hemorrhage itself, although rarely extensive from the lungs, may be so severe from the chest wall as to fill the pleural cavity, compressing the lung and threatening life with exsanguination.

With these general considerations in view, certain principles of treatment are evident. These comprise (1) early recognition of chest injury and its extent; (2) re-establishment of the integrity of the chest wall and its bellows action; (3) exhaustion of air and blood from the pleural cavity to re-expand the lung; (4) clearance of secretions and blood from the tracheobronchial tree to further facilitate expansion of all lung tissue; and (5) treatment of shock. The methods used to accomplish these general principles in various types of chest injuries will be discussed.

TYPE OF INJURY AND TREATMENT

SIMPLE CHEST WALL INJURY

Simple fracture of a rib is the most minor injury of the chest to require comment as to its management. Commonly this injury is of no consequence except for the incapacity resulting from respiratory pain. However, careful examination of the lungs to detect the presence of pneumothorax or hemothorax is imperative. In most instances roentgenographic or fluoroscopic investigation is indicated. It must be borne in mind that a small pneumothorax or hemothorax, undisclosed by physical examination immediately after injury, may increase markedly in the subsequent 12 to 24 hours. The treatment of pneumothorax and hemothorax is described in later paragraphs.

Respiratory pain may sometimes be minimized by simple strapping of the costal margin to splint chest motion on the side of fracture. Probably the most effective type of strapping is done with elastic adhesive, since this has little tendency to blister the skin. Strapping is often of little help, however, and the resulting denudation of epithelium beneath the adhesive may be of more concern to the patient than the original pain of fracture. When the pain is severe and incapacitating, and particularly when the patient is an elderly person with heart disease, or has emphysema with a marginal respiratory reserve, *intercostal nerve block* with 1 per cent procaine covering an area two interspaces above and below the site of fracture may be indicated; 4–5 ml. of the solution should be used in each interspace. The only serious difficulty encountered with a simple fracture may occur in those patients with greatly diminished cardiac or respiratory reserve. Occasionally such a patient will require bed rest and repeated intercostal nerve block to overcome splinting due to pain and to permit coughing and clearing of the tracheobronchial tree. Oxygen also may be necessary to tide such a patient through the period of acute pain and limitation of respiratory motion attendant upon a simple fracture of a rib.

INTRATHORACIC INJURY WITH CHEST WALL TRAUMA

Single or multiple fractures of ribs may be accompanied by laceration and contusion of the lung, with various degrees of pneumothorax, hemopneumothorax, or hemothorax.

Pneumothorax

In cases of minimal pneumothorax, as evidenced by a 1–2 cm. rim of air at the periphery of the lung, it is usually not necessary to do anything in the way of active removal, but it is wiser to follow such a situation with serial roentgenograms or repeated fluoroscopic examination to be certain that reabsorption is progressing and that no further air leakage has occurred. Similarly, if the amount of blood shed merely fills the costophrenic sinus, serial observation is in order to make sure that it is being absorbed.

When the pneumothorax is more extensive, the best policy is to *re-expand the lung* immediately. This is most effectively done by the insertion of a fenestrated catheter through an intercostal space. Under local procaine infiltration, a trocar and sheath (Fig. 18–*1*, *B*) are inserted through the desired interspace and, upon withdrawal of the trocar, the fenestrated catheter (Fig. 18–*1*, *D*) is inserted into the chest to a depth calculated

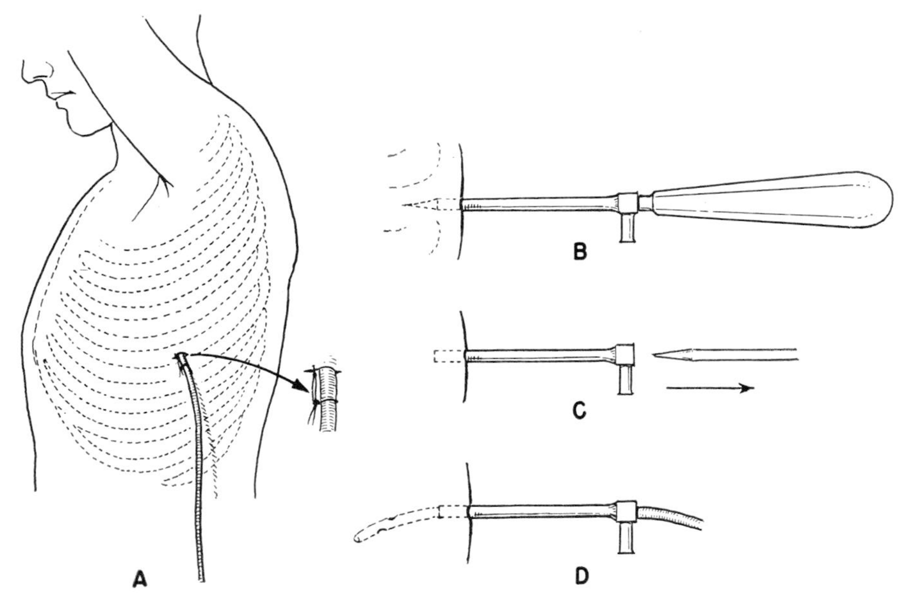

Figure 18–1. Introduction of intercostal tube for drainage of pleural cavity.
A. Intercostal catheter in situ, anchored by suture.
B. Introduction of trocar and sheath.
C. Removal of trocar.
D. Insertion of catheter through sheath.

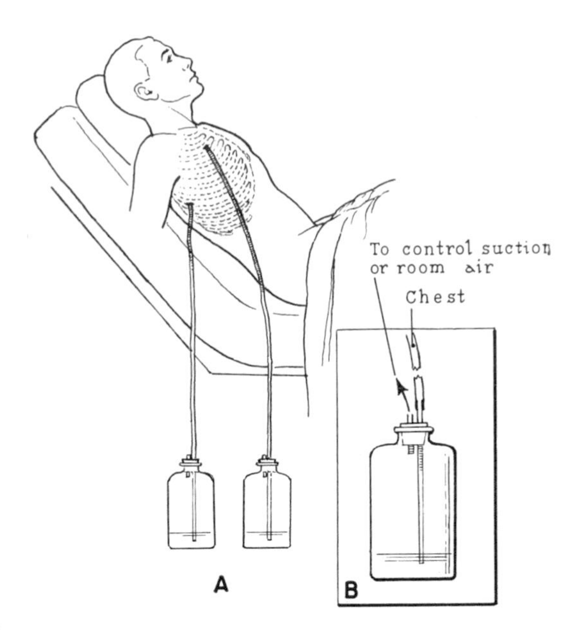

Figure 18–2.
A. Intercostal tubes to water-trap through second interspace anteriorly and seventh interspace in posterior axillary line.
B. Water-trap bottle in more detail.

before insertion so that the most proximal fenestration will be 2–3 cm. within the pleural cavity. Since blood is almost certainly associated with a pneumothorax of this degree, it is wiser to introduce the catheter through the sixth or seventh interspace just posterior to the axillary line, rather than in the second interspace anteriorly in the midclavicular line, which is the favored site when the pneumothorax is not associated with a hemothorax. By placing the tube in a lower space, air may often be exhausted and fluid blood removed with only the one tube. If air is trapped above and the lower tube does not function to remove it properly, an additional tube may be inserted in the superior position (Fig. 18–2, *A*). The use of an underwater trap (Figs. 18–2, *B*, 18–3), rather than suction, is desirable in these cases since suction occasionally tends to isolate the tube by local co-apposition of the pleurae about it. The introduction of a catheter into the chest could be accompanied by the institution of antibiotic coverage.

The presence of a tension pneumothorax should always be suspected in any patient with a chest injury who has shortness of breath. If, on percussion and auscultation and palpation of the position of the trachea, the presence of a pneumothorax is confirmed, a needle of sufficient length to penetrate the chest wall should be introduced through it and *air aspirated.* This is most easily performed through the second or third interspace anteriorly. Such a maneuver is only a temporary expedient for dealing with an acute situation. The needle should be replaced as soon as possible by an intercostal catheter as described above. When the needle cannot be replaced for some time it may be attached by tubing to an underwater trap (Fig. 18–3).

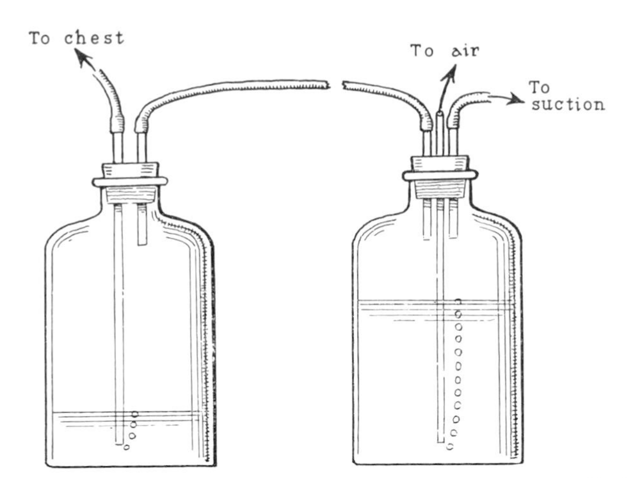

Figure 18–3. Detail of water-trap bottle with intermediate controlled suction bottle.

Hemothorax

Hemorrhage from the lung is self-limiting except when the wound involves the large vessels at the hilus of the lung, as may occur with a penetrating wound of the chest or, rarely, in the most violent types of crush injuries. Laceration of the large vessels is almost always fatal. Persistent hemorrhage, if it occurs, is usually a result of laceration of the intercostal or internal mammary vessels of the chest wall.

The treatment of hemothorax, except for the minimal amount as described previously, is by *needle aspiration.* If a massive hemothorax is present within the first hours of injury, there may be embarrassment of respiration due to collapse of the lung and shift of the mediastinum. Various degrees of circulatory failure will accompany this and the actual blood loss. Transfusion should be started and the hemothorax aspirated. If blood for transfusion is not immediately available the blood thus aspirated from the chest in the first hours following injury may be collected in a sterile manner in a bottle containing citrate and then used for transfusion. A practical method of collection is to attach the aspirating needle in the chest directly to a donor vacuum bottle.

Persistent hemorrhage as evidenced by increasing hemothorax and persistent or recurrent signs of blood loss should be treated as any other hemorrhage, that is, with exploration by thoracotomy and ligature of the bleeding vessels, plus transfusion. In the rare instance in which a pulmonary vessel at the hilus is the cause of bleeding, ligation or even pulmonary resection may be indicated.

A hemothorax should be aspirated immediately if the hemorrhage is massive and encroaches on the respiratory reserve. If it does not encroach on the respiratory function there can be temporization of hours' but not of days' duration. The consideration of postponing aspiration because of the possibility of recurrent hemorrhage is theoretical. No evidence has been offered that hemorrhage is more persistent because of early aspiration.

Certainly when there is a hemothorax of any size a primary aspiration should be performed within the first six hours. It is a common occurrence that hemothorax cannot be dissipated by a single aspiration. Aspiration should be continued daily, at sites determined by physical signs or by the changing x-ray appearance.

Loculation and partial thrombus formation are not uncommon. In most instances the hemothorax can be readily eliminated if aspiration is performed early and repeated daily, but in some cases, particularly if aspiration has been delayed and the chest wall damage is severe, there may be extensive thrombus formation and aspiration will not suffice to remove it. When the remnant of hemothorax, or, more accurately, clotted hemothorax after aspiration, is minimal, showing up as a shadow at the base, obliterating the costophrenic angle and ascending the lateral chest wall a short distance, the wisest decision is to leave it alone. The surgeon should encourage respiratory exercises of the chest wall and diaphragm. At worst, the ensuing deformity and limitation will result only in lateral tenting and fixation of the diaphragm.

If, at the end of a week or ten days, the resultant x-ray shadow is still considerable, denoting a moderate- to large-sized thrombus within the pleural cavity, *streptokinase* should be employed to lyse the fibrin clot and allow it to be evacuated. In preparation for using the fibrinolytic material a fenestrated catheter is introduced through an intercostal space into the clotted hemothorax. One ampule of Varidase is then diluted with 20 ml. of saline solution, to give an adequate volume for injection through the catheter into the thrombus. Antihistamines and aspirin are given to minimize the febrile reaction to the enzymes. After injection of the Varidase, the tube is clamped off and connected to a water-seal trap. The clamp should be left on the catheter for 8 to 12 hours and then released. This procedure may be repeated after an interval of at least 24 hours following release of the catheter. When drainage through the catheter stops, it is withdrawn.

Caution must be exercised in the use of Varidase too early in hemorrhage as its use in the first days after bleeding has been known to start hemorrhage again. Furthermore, when lung tissue has been lacerated, with creation of a bronchopleural fistula, use of the enzyme even in a late period after injury may open up an already sealed fistula.

When a clotted hemothorax has been neglected for four or more weeks, the above methods may not be successful in eliminating the already organizing thrombus. If this thrombus is large, and particularly if it extends along the lateral chest wall, thoracotomy and decortication of the lung will be needed. If aspiration is started early and continued daily, the use of Varidase will rarely be required, and, when both these methods have been employed in a timely fashion, the need for thoracotomy and decortication will be extremely rare.

In addition to neglect of a large clotted hemothorax for four weeks or more, there are two other instances in which decortication may be advisable at an earlier date. The first of these is when a hemothorax has become infected but localization into empyema has not occurred. Here there may be extensive low-grade infection with loculation. When this occurs decortication is indicated for removal of the infected thrombus and re-expansion of the lung. Occasionally, also, when there has been a massive hemothorax with thrombus formation, it may be wisest to operate in the first week to evacuate the clot and re-expand the lung rather than rely on the use of enzymes.

Removal of Tracheobronchial Accumulations

The normal cough mechanism with deep inspiration followed by a phase of increased intratracheal and bronchial pressure with sudden release of air outward in exhalation is the most effective method of evacuation of contents of the bronchi. The preliminary inspiration forces air distal to the bolus, which is then suddenly expelled by explosive exhalation. In trauma this mechanism is crippled to various degrees or rendered entirely ineffectual by the limitations imposed by pain, abnormal mobility of chest wall, or cushioning effects of fluid and air in the pleural cavity. When pain is the prime limiting factor, encouragement to cough after injection of an *opiate* may be all that is necessary. Any opiate used should be given in relatively small doses and repeated every three hours if necessary; 10 mg. of morphine or 75 mg. of Demerol is usually sufficient. If this does not control pain adequately, intercostal nerve block as described previously may be used to abolish pain and allow the patient to cough, or an endotracheal aspiration may be performed. The latter maneuver usually acts to stimulate cough in spite of pain.

Technique of tracheal aspiration. A moderately rigid, open-tipped catheter, about 18-gauge, is best. The catheter is most easily introduced into the trachea with the head extended, tongue out, and during a deep inspiration. At intervals, suction is applied to the catheter for 10–15 seconds

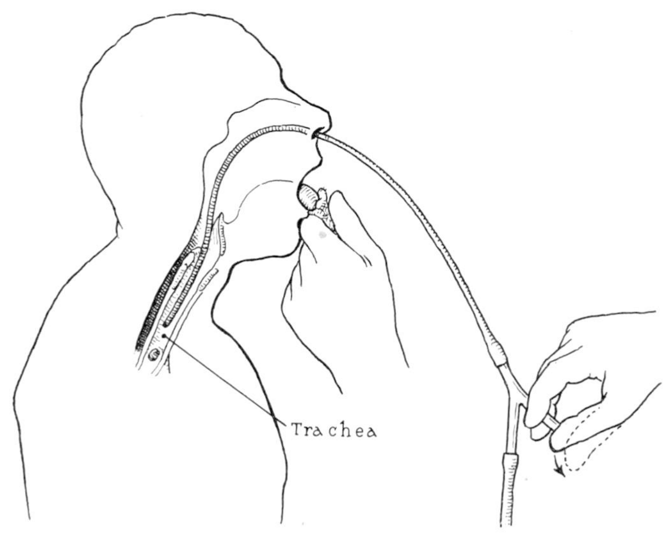

Figure 18–4. Endotracheal aspiration using catheter with Y-tube for intermittent suction.

to prevent anoxia. With the catheter in the trachea it is important not to use prolonged periods of suction, since this may produce a real degree of anoxia. The introduction of a Y-connection to the catheter suction apparatus (Fig. 18–4) will facilitate intermittent use of suction in this procedure. Oxygen may be given through the catheter in the brief intervals between suctioning.

If none of the above methods is successful in removing accumulated secretions to allow lung expansion, *bronchoscopy* must be used. In the severely injured patient this procedure can be performed over the end of a Gatch bed by raising the head piece. When the chest wall has been crushed, or when cough is ineffectual and aspiration unsatisfactory, tracheostomy is indicated and may be life saving.

It is of utmost importance that the post-tracheostomy care be diligently and intelligently applied. It is not enough merely to perform the operation. The nursing care is of even greater importance. Frequent adequate suctioning via a large soft-rubber catheter utilizing the previously described Y-connector is necessary. Humidified air or oxygen should be introduced into the opening of the tracheostomy via a bent 18-gauge needle so that

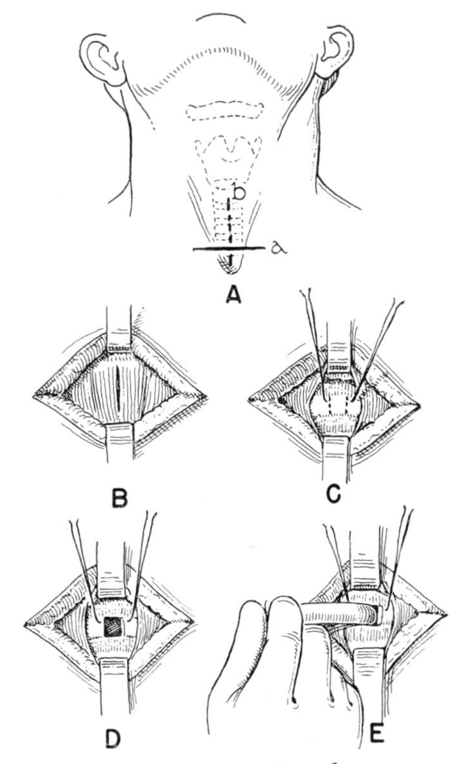

Figure 18–5. Steps in the performance of tracheostomy.

A. Transverse incision (a) with alternate vertical incision (b) to be used in dire emergency.

B. Midline opening of strap muscles.

C. Mobilization of tracheal ring with nerve hooks.

D. Segment of tracheal cartilage excised.

E. Insertion of tracheostomy tube.

a jet of high flow oxygen is not forced into the trachea. Occasionally agents which reduce surface tension or liquefy tenacious mucus, such as Alevaire or sodium lauryl sulfate 0.1 per cent solution, will aid considerably in helping the patient to raise secretions. These agents may be added to the water jar used to humidify the oxygen or may be applied by a nasal spray directly into the tracheal stoma.

A patient with an open tracheostomy tube is unable to produce an effective cough since he cannot raise intrabronchial pressure to initiate the cough. As soon as the acute phase of the injury is over and the chest wall is stabilized, the tracheostomy tube should be plugged off. If the patient demonstrates the ability to raise secretions by himself with the tube plugged for 24 hours, it may be removed. The tracheal stoma will close in a few days.

Technique of tracheostomy (Fig. 18–5). If the patient's condition is precarious, he is kept supine in bed. However, it is easier to perform the tracheostomy if the patient is placed on a stretcher. A sand bag or rolled sheet is placed between the shoulder blades to elevate the upper chest and hyperextend the neck. The neck is prepared and the skin infiltrated with local anesthesia.

If the situation is not urgent, a low transverse skin incision can be used (Fig. 18–5, *A*, *a*). Since exposure is adequate and the resulting scar is less noticeable, this incision is preferred. On the other hand, if the tracheostomy is urgently needed, the vertical incision (Fig. 18–5, *A*, *b*) allows more rapid performance. The strap muscles are exposed and divided in the midline. The thyroid isthmus is retracted upward with a small blunt retractor. If the isthmus is large and covers several rings, it should be divided. A curved clamp is placed behind the isthmus, separating it from the trachea. The isthmus is then clamped on both sides and divided. The cut ends are suture ligated. The strap muscles are retracted with narrow, deep retractors. and the trachea is well exposed. The midline is identified, and a site in a low ring is selected for tracheostomy. This is usually the third or fourth ring. This ring is fixed on either side of the midline by two small skin or dura hooks, and a small segment of the ring is removed. An alternate technique is to make a transverse incision in the soft tissues between two rings, insert the blade of an Allis clamp and grasp the ring. This segment is then excised, and the tube with its obturator is inserted. It is wise to use the largest tube that will fit easily. It is sometimes easier to insert the tube by directing it cephalad. Once it has slipped into the lumen of the trachea it is turned downward and easily falls into place. Several small sutures are taken to loosely approximate the skin edges. The tube is held in place by tying tapes behind the neck.

Treatment of Shock

In treatment of shock in severe injury of the chest, certain important factors should be observed. The usual Trendelenburg position favored in other forms of injury is usually poorly tolerated in patients with respiratory difficulty caused by chest injury. These patients are more comfortable, and are better treated during the period of resuscitation, in a semi-sitting position.

The replacement of blood and the use of oxygen by means of nasal catheter are procedures which should go hand in hand with the measures outlined above to restore respiration equilibrium—stabilization of the chest wall, removal of blood and air from the pleural cavity, and re-expansion of the lung by clearing the tracheobronchial airway.

Blood replacement should be prompt and adequate, but particular care should be taken that the patient does not receive too much fluid or blood. Over-transfusion and/or -hydration may lead to pulmonary edema and death in the person with serious chest injury. Morphine must be used in relatively small doses, and repeated with great caution in the presence of shock, for with restoration of circulation the delayed absorption of the drug given subcutaneously during the period of circulatory collapse may result in serious respiratory depression. The use of oxygen is indicated in the emergency care of chest injury when there is any degree of respiratory difficulty, and when circulatory collapse is present its use is particularly urgent.

CRUSH INJURY OF CHEST

The most serious closed type of chest injury, the so-called crush injury, is of increasing importance because of the accident rate in high speed transportation. Here the chest wall is "stove in" so that it loses its rigidity and becomes a "flail chest." If the crushing force is directed laterally, the pathology of the injury consists in fractures, in two places at least, of multiple adjacent ribs. This results in a central portion of chest wall which is floating, since the ribs are fractured on both extremities of the area. This floating section moves in and out with respiration in a reverse or paradoxical direction to the rest of the chest wall. This paradoxical movement markedly decreases the efficiency of ventilation, is accompanied by severe pain, and renders the coughing mechanism ineffectual. Hemothorax or hemopneumothorax of considerable degree is a frequent accompaniment, together with marked contusion and often laceration of the lung, and with extravasation of blood, edema, and retention of secretions in the bronchial tree.

This type of injury requires immediate measures to relieve a markedly disturbed respiratory physiology. Fixation of the chest wall, removal of blood and/or air from the pleural cavity, and clearing of retained secretions from the tracheobronchial tree are often life saving. When the paradoxical motion of the chest wall is marked, most often anterolaterally where the rib cage is not covered by the scapula or latissimus dorsi, *fixation of a rib is* imperative. A rib should be selected in the central portion of the "floating" section as the pivotal point of fixation. Under local anesthesia an incision is made into the subcutaneous tissues and a medium-sized towel clip is used to grasp about the circumference of the rib. If, on pulling up on this

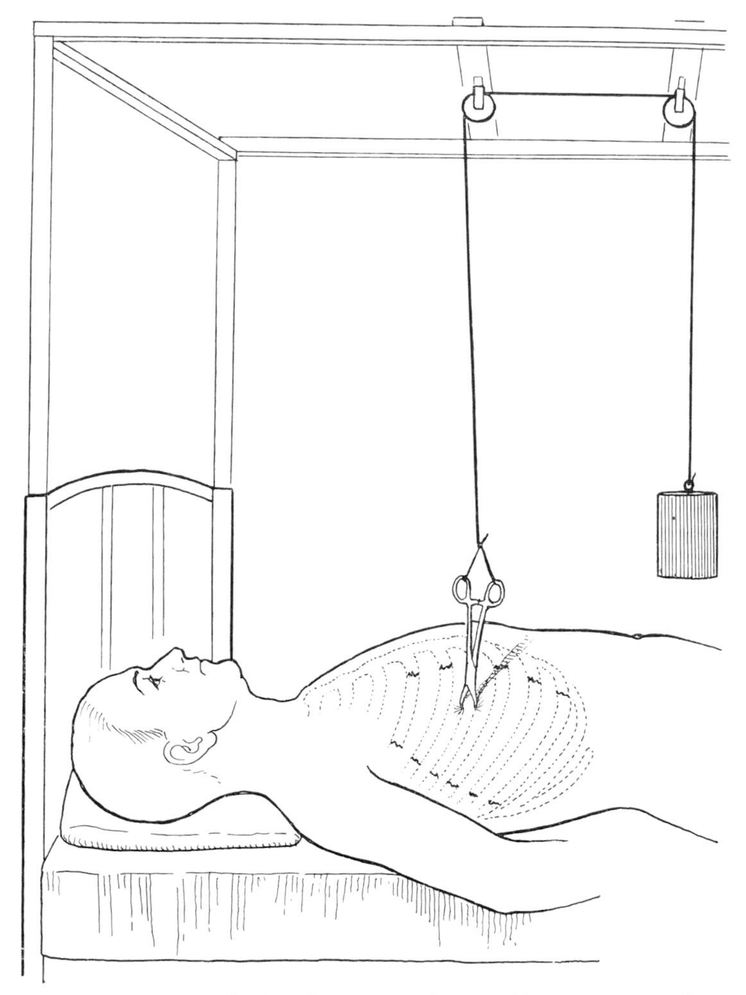

Figure 18–6. One method of fixation of chest wall in severe crush injury.

rib, the chest wall is not stabilized, another rib in the most mobile remaining portion of this section is selected and another towel clip is used to secure it in a similar fashion. Traction is then applied constantly in the desired direction, using a Balkan frame and just enough weight to stabilize the chest (Fig. 18–6). This does not usually have to be more than 3 to 5 pounds.

Direction of the crushing force from front to back rather than laterally produces the so-called "steering-wheel injury," in which the sternum may be fractured transversely, often associated with bilateral fractures of multiple anterior ribs or cartilages. Such a severe anterior crushing injury with a mobile sternum requires fixation immediately. Satisfactory upward traction can be obtained by use of a uterine tenaculum. Under local anesthesia, small incisions are made in the skin on either side of the mobile portion of the sternum. Through these incisions the arms of the tenaculum are inserted to grasp the borders of the sternum. Upward traction is then effected, using a Balkan frame with pulley and just enough weight to overcome the severe mobility. Various other methods of procuring upward traction and fixation have been devised, employing screws, specially constructed tongs, or wire leaders for fixation of the chest wall.

Open reduction of the sternum and fixation by means of wire sutures, under general anesthesia, is rarely indicated, since satisfactory immobilization is most often attained by other methods, as outlined above.

Of greatest importance in the treatment of this most severe type of "crushing injury" is the employment of *tracheostomy.* This procedure has a twofold utility. In the first place, these patients cannot cough effectively because of pain and mobility of the chest wall. Therefore, tracheostomy affords a method by which the tracheobronchial tree may be kept clear of mucous secretions, edema fluids, and extravasated blood. It must be remembered in doing a tracheostomy that cough has been abolished, therefore strict attention must be paid to frequent catheter aspirations of the trachea. Secondly, the tracheostomy by-passes the narrowed area of the larynx and, by permitting freer entrance and egress of air, reduces the effort required by the bellows action of the chest wall and paradoxical motion is minimized. Following tracheostomy the replacement of labored, grunting respirations by quiet, even ventilation may be striking. Also, because tracheostomy by-passes the column of tidal air from the site of the tracheostomy to the mouth, less dead air must be carried back and forth and respiration becomes more efficient.

In some patients with severe bilateral multiple rib fractures with marked paradoxical motion, the above measures may not be enough to allow for adequate ventilation. Under these circumstances use of a mechanical respirator may be indicated. Since the performance of a tracheostomy will be one of the first steps in treating such a patient, the machine will be connected to the tracheostomy tube. If this technique is to be utilized the prolonged use of a cuffed endotracheal tube must be avoided because of the potential danger of damage to tracheal mucosa by pressure and motion of the cuff. It is therefore desirable that a non-cuffed tube be used and ventilation be provided for by high flow. The air which will escape around the tube and into the mouth during inspiration will help expel the secretions which tend to puddle in the pharynx. The information gained through use of mechanical respiratory machines following cardiac surgery indicates that metal or nylon tubes are better tolerated than some of the other types of tracheostomy tubes. The use of a negative phase machine is to be condemned since it increases the paradoxical motion of the chest. In order to adequately ventilate a patient with a machine it is necessary to take over the ventilation rather than to assist it, because most patients with crush injuries are incapable of the respiratory effort necessary to trip the machine.

Since crush injury is indeed serious and often lethal, the importance of the early employment of the above measures in the severely crushed patient cannot be overemphasized.

OPEN WOUNDS OF THE CHEST

In this type of wound, which is associated with an open, "sucking" communication with the pleural cavity, there is a marked disturbance of the respiratory physiology. The lung on the side of the injury is rapidly collapsed. The contralateral lung is seriously compromised in respiratory efficiency, and the cardiac output is diminished by reduction in filling of the heart.

In open sucking wounds of the chest there is a pendulum swing of the mediastinum during respiration. In inspiration the collapsed lung on the side of the open injury moves toward the good lung because of the relative negative pressure on this side. The air entering the contralateral lung is diminished in quantity and becomes a mixture of stagnant air from the collapsed lung and of fresh tracheal air. In expiration there is a swing of the mediastinum toward the injured side, with an increase in intrapleural pressure as the glottis closes in the creation of a grunt, thus the uninjured lung fails to expire efficiently and some of the outgoing air will fill the injured lung. During this phase also, with increased pressure within the thorax, filling of the heart is diminished. These alterations in the physiology necessitate immediate closure of the wound in the chest wall as the first means of resuscitation.

Thus, all open sucking wounds of the chest should be closed immediately by an occlusive dressing, using, if possible, petrolatum gauze next to the skin and a bulky outer gauze dressing held in place by adhesive strips. It is often best, if possible, to apply the closure dressing as the patient makes a forced expiration.

Following the initial and often life-saving procedure of immediate closure of the wound in the manner described, further resuscitation should be carried out before the necessity for operation is evaluated. This resuscitation may require (1) administration of oxygen by nasal catheter; (2) aspiration of blood and air from the chest, usually accomplished by introduction of intercostal catheter–water-trap drainage; (3) blood replacement by transfusion; and, often, (4) the re-establishment of bronchial drainage by intercostal procaine injection with the return of cough or by tracheal aspiration. As soon as resuscitation has been accomplished, the sucking wound of the chest is closed by definitive suture under endotracheal anesthesia.

In choosing the proper time for surgical intervention during resuscitation it must be remembered that the urgency of possible abdominal injury through the diaphragm and/or continued hemorrhage may force the issue and that the act of operation itself under endotracheal anesthesia is a continuation of resuscitation. Control of respiration under endotracheal anesthesia with adequate aspiration of accumulated secretions and blood from the trachea, re-expansion of the lung with removal of blood and air from the pleural cavity, and, finally, control of hemorrhage and firm closure of the chest wall defect, will contribute to the patient's improvement.

THORACO-ABDOMINAL INJURY

Of great importance in the emergency treatment of thoracic injury is an acute awareness that injury to an abdominal viscus may co-exist. Thoraco-abdominal injuries that may be overlooked are of two types. First, there is injury of the lower chest, usually with fracture of the eighth, ninth, or tenth rib in the posterior axillary line, in which there has been rupture of the spleen or liver. In these cases the abdominal signs of tenderness and spasm in the corresponding upper quadrant may be hard to evaluate. The presence of shock and evidence, by hematocrit, of blood loss disproportionate to the chest injury usually give the clues necessary for diagnosis.

Second, the importance of thorough examination of the chest in any serious accident can never be discounted, even when no outward evidence of injury is present. Only by this means can rupture of the diaphragm and migration of the abdominal contents into the chest be detected. X-ray confirmation by revelation of an air-filled viscus in the thoracic cavity above the diaphragm should always be sought. The lateral projection is particularly valuable in this respect. Barium swallow or enema may be used to obtain evidence for more definitive diagnosis.

In penetrating or perforating injuries of the chest, all wounds below the plane of the angle of the scapula posteriorly and the nipple anteriorly should be suspected of having penetrated the abdomen, because of the variable level of the diaphragm and direction of the penetrating agent. Thoracotomy is indicated to rule out perforation of the diaphragm and injury of an intra-abdominal viscus. Conversely, in penetrating wounds of the upper abdomen, the possibility of penetration through the diaphragm into the thorax must always be considered.

The most frequent mistake in dealing with penetrating thoraco-abdominal wounds occurs in failure to suspect penetration through the diaphragm when the external wounds are confined to the chest, and failure to recognize the wound in the diaphragm at the time of abdominal exploration for an external wound of the abdomen.

Various approaches are available for the exploratory operation, i.e., through the chest alone, through the abdomen alone, through the chest and then through the abdomen, and by thoraco-abdominal incision. Whichever approach is employed, measures should first be taken to correct respiratory embarrassment. If thoracotomy is required to accomplish this purpose, it should always precede the laparotomy. The thoraco-abdominal incision should not be elected if the time lag between injury and operation is more than six hours, and if the expected amount of contamination from bowel or stomach is likely to be great. The breakdown of these wounds secondary to infection is more difficult to contend with than a similar complication in the thoracotomy or laparotomy wound because of the division of the costal arch, which is a critical point in the integrity of the abdominal and thoracic parietes of the diaphragm.

Closure of all wounds in either the right or left diaphragm must be accomplished. It is true that small perforating wounds through the chest

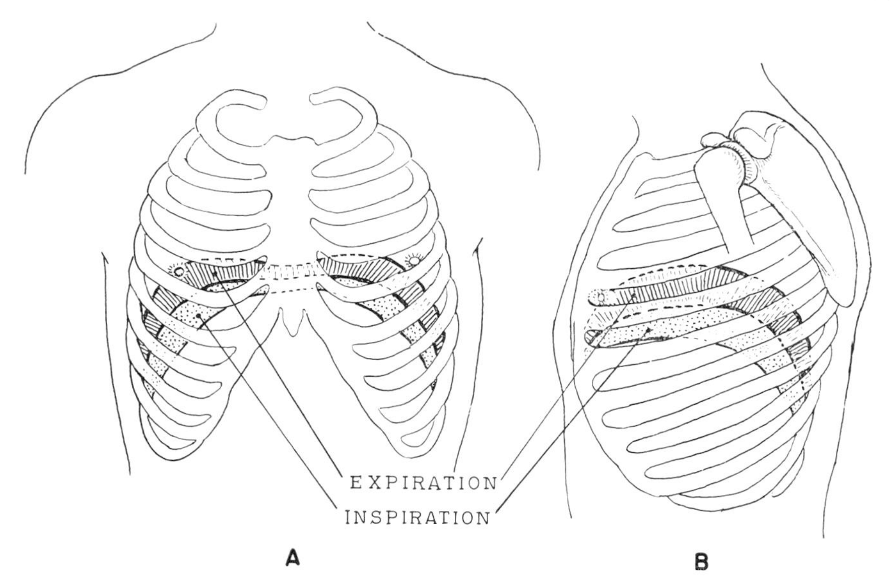

Figure 18–7. Levels of the diaphragm at expiration and inspiration to emphasize the height of abdominal viscera within thorax.

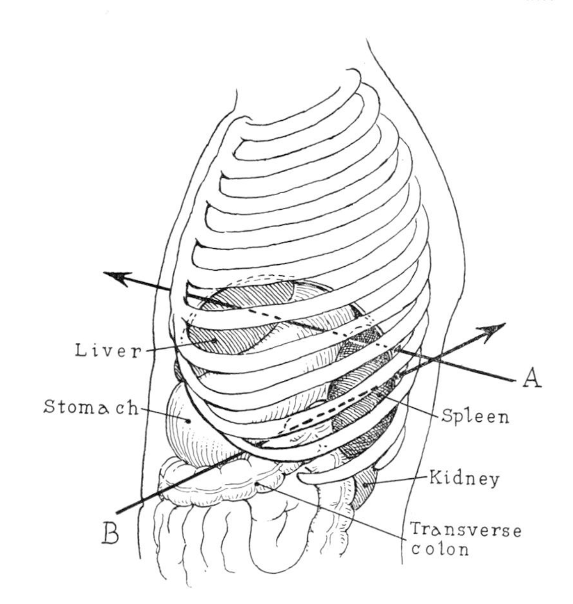

Figure 18–8. Perforating thoraco-abdominal wounds on left side showing viscera. A. Through-and-through chest wound with injury to spleen, stomach, and liver. B. Abdominal wound with exit through chest posteriorly with injury to stomach, colon, and spleen.

and diaphragm and into the liver will sometimes heal spontaneously after drainage of the liver wound below the diaphragm. However, one can never be certain, without adequate exposure, of the extent of diaphragmatic and liver damage or of the amount of retained foreign material. It is always safer to close all wounds of the right diaphragm to protect against bile pleuritis which may on occasion be a serious complication.

Failure to recognize and treat wounds of the diaphragm often results in hernias if the patient survives the injury. In those hernias following indirect trauma associated with rupture of the diaphragm there will be an eventration with, usually, large portions of the stomach and often colon on the left side and liver, occasionally, on the right side entering the chest cavity. When there has been a perforating wound of the diaphragm the resulting hernia may be small, with a small aperture or neck through the diaphragm, and the colon, and sometimes the stomach, may be found within the hernia. Intestinal obstruction may lead to discovery of this type of injury. The diagnosis may be suspected from posterior and lateral x-ray films, disclosing evidence of viscera above the diaphragm. Ultimate diagnosis is made when films following barium enema or barium swallow reveal the presence of the diaphragmatic hernia.

RUPTURE OF THE BRONCHUS

In severe injury, such as occurs in automobile accidents and falls, there may be actual rupture of the bronchus. The diagnosis of this injury may be difficult, but the presence of a large bronchial fistula should make one suspicious of the presence of the lesion. On the other hand, the complete collapse of one lung associated with continuous hemoptysis may also give warning that the bronchus has been lacerated or possibly divided. Diagnosis can be confirmed by bronchoscopy.

When the diagnosis has been confirmed, operation may be successful in re-suturing the bronchial tear and re-establishing drainage of the distal lung. If the bronchus cannot be sutured satisfactorily, pneumonectomy may be necessary.

Patients who have survived undetected bronchial rupture often require surgery later because of bronchial stenosis with distal suppuration and bronchiectasis.

WOUNDS OF THE HEART AND PERICARDIUM

In the severe crushing wounds of the chest, particularly of the anterior or "steering-wheel" type, one must be on the lookout for contusion of the heart or hemopericardium. Injury to the heart will be suggested by transient or persistent tachycardia. Confirmation by electrocardiography should be obtained so that proper treatment with prolonged bed rest is not neglected. Hemopericardium is suggested by muffled cardiac sounds and an enlarged cardiac silhouette on x-ray examination. The presence of tamponade is confirmed in these patients by the finding of a small pulse pressure, paradoxical pulse, and an elevated venous pressure. Immediate aspiration is required, either from below upward on the left at the angle between the costal cartilage and the xiphoid, or directly through the fourth or fifth intercostal space just to the left of the sternum.

The perforating wound of pericardium and heart is more dramatic, presenting almost always an acute tamponade with varying degrees of shock. The treatment of these wounds will vary. Some unquestionably can be managed by aspiration of the pericardium alone, whereas others require thoracotomy and control of hemorrhage. These patients should immediately be given oxygen by nasal tube or mask, made ready for transfusion, and removed to the operating room where, if acute tamponade exists, aspiration of the pericardium may be carried out. If removal of blood from the pericardium relieves the tamponade, further observation in the operating room may demonstrate that massive bleeding is controlled and that judicious subsequent aspirations may be the best course to follow. If, on the other hand, the condition of the patient deteriorates or is not improved following aspiration of enough blood to relieve the acute tamponade, thoracotomy must be performed in the hope of controlling the bleeding. Important, of course, in these patients is the judicious replacement of blood and treatment of the wound of the thorax as outlined previously. Although constrictive calcified pericarditis may follow hemopericardium associated with injury, this is not a common occurrence.

WOUNDS OF THE ESOPHAGUS

Injury of the esophagus may occur (1) by perforation of the thorax by a missile, (2) by instrumentation within the esophagus, or (3) by so-called spontaneous rupture. The last almost always occurs as a result of excessive vomiting or retching (frequently in beer drinkers) and may be associated with esophagitis or ulceration of the lower end of the organ.

Perforating wounds of the chest in which the mediastinum has been entered or traversed require thoracotomy for exploration of the esophagus, and suture if such an injury is present. This type of injury is rarely seen, since a missile traveling in this course will usually penetrate the heart or aorta as well, causing immediate death.

Rupture of the esophagus following esophagoscopy or gastroscopy may occur in the cervical esophagus at the level of the seventh cervical vertebra or just above the cardia at its lowest extremity. In this instance, the emergency treatment is conservative treatment. Nothing is given by mouth. A wide-spectrum antibiotic is administered parenterally, and chewing upon lozenges containing sulfadiazine or neomycin may be of some value. Careful observation is maintained in the immediate period and also during the week following discontinuance of the antibiotic, since paraesophageal abscess may form in the lower neck or upper mediastinum and require drainage by incision in the lower neck. Persistent or recurrent fever is suggestive of abscess, and a lateral roentgenogram of the neck showing a widening of the retrotracheal space often confirms the diagnosis. Paraesophageal mediastinal abscess in the lower mediastinum is less common. Here the x-ray film will show a paramediastinal shadow and often associated effusion in the pleural cavity. Persistent fever is characteristic, and posterior mediastinotomy and drainage of abscess become urgent. Obviously, if pleural fluid or fluid and air are revealed by x-ray within the first six hours following an instrumental accident, it means that the perforation of the esophagus has carried through the parietal pleura and immediate thoracotomy with suture of the perforation is in order. Such extensive perforation, however, is rare.

So-called "spontaneous perforation" of the esophagus most often follows the trauma of vomiting. Sudden pain is most often felt in the epigastrium, but may also be present in the lower sternum and over the lower left chest. The onset of shock and the appearance of subcutaneous emphysema in the neck characterize this injury. X-ray examination may reveal emphysema in the mediastinum, a widened shadow in the lower mediastinum, and often frank fluid in either pleural cavity since very frequently the rupture of the esophagus involves the parietal pleura.

In doubtful cases a swallow of barium may demonstrate leakage outside the main esophageal stream. It has been demonstrated that immediate thoracotomy with suture of the esophageal wound and drainage of the pleural cavity is the treatment of choice. When these patients are seen late, or the diagnosis is not made until after 12 hours has elapsed, catheter drainage of the fluid in the left chest may be undertaken and a few of these patients salvaged. A gastrostomy is employed for subsequent feeding. Since the mortality is excessively high with this form of treatment, early recognition and immediate thoracotomy is the goal to be sought.

CHAPTER 19

INJURIES OF THE VERTEBRAL COLUMN

By FREDERICK M. SMITH, M.D.

GENERAL CONSIDERATIONS

SPINAL INJURIES are common, and are not limited predominantly to industrial accidents, as is often supposed. Fractures may be sustained in such sports as football, diving, polo, and the like; in the home from slipping and landing heavily in a "sit-down" position or falling from a ladder or chair, the impact on a hard surface causing the spine suddenly to flex, or "jack-knife"; or in traffic or highway accidents, many of which may at first seem trivial. Being jounced suddenly in the back seat of a car and striking one's head on the roof is enough to cause a compression fracture or, what is more serious, a fracture-dislocation. In elderly persons with osteoporotic spines it is unnecessary for the head even to hit the roof of a car when jounced. This writer has seen compression of thoracic or lumbar vertebrae occur in these individuals when seized with a sudden attack of coughing or sneezing while bending over to brush the teeth or while merely stooping over to lift a heavy object. Convulsions produced by Metrazol or electric shock therapy are very common causes of compression fractures of the vertebral bodies in young adults.

A spine injury connotes to the layman something serious, and, in his haste to render first-aid treatment or to get the patient to the hospital, he may cause irreparable damage to the spinal cord if the injured person has a fracture-dislocation and is not protected from further damage and transported in a proper fashion. The commonest and least serious type of spine fracture, that is, fracture of a transverse process, is often not well understood by hospital interns or general practitioners with little surgical experience, and may be over-treated and made to assume a seriousness out of all proportion to its actual significance. It is extremely important to understand the differences in spine injuries so that the differences in treatment may likewise be understood, and also that the prognosis may be appreciated and stated with reasonable accuracy.

ANATOMY OF THE VERTEBRAL COLUMN

The vertebral column (Fig. 19–*1*) consists of seven cervical, twelve thoracic, five lumbar, five sacral, and three or four coccygeal vertebrae.

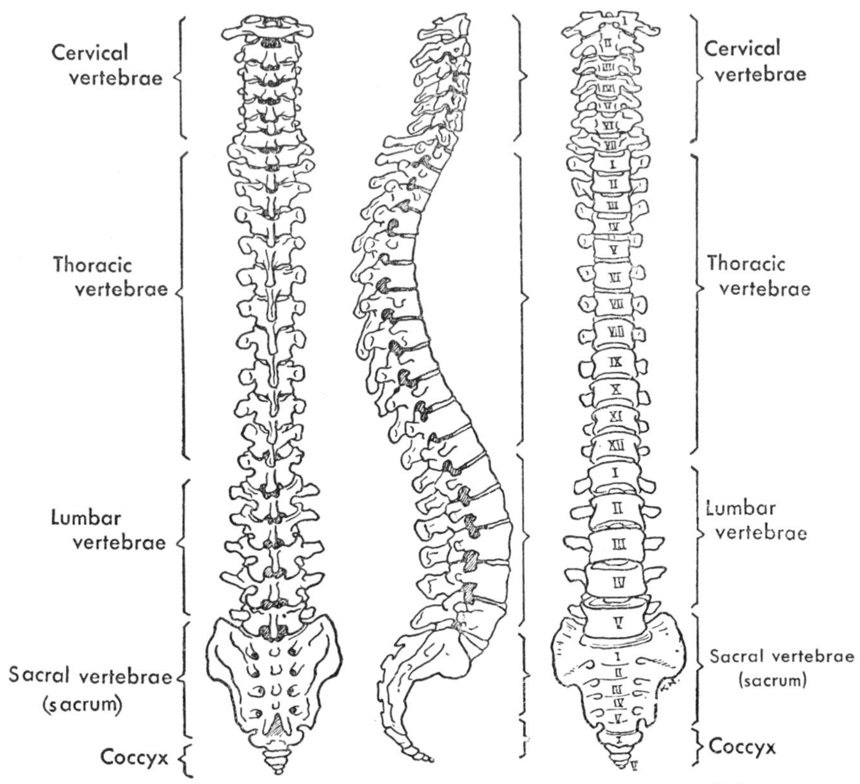

Figure 19–1. Posterior, lateral, and anterior views of the adult spine.

The cervical, thoracic, and lumbar vertebrae are movable upon each other. The vertebrae constituting the sacrum and coccyx are fused to each other, with, however, a joint between the sacrum and coccyx. Each region has its own characteristic features, but, in general, a single vertebra in the movable portion of the spine (cervical, thoracic, or lumbar) has a body which serves the main weight-bearing function of the column, and a neural arch (pedicles, laminae, and spinous processes) to which are attached strong ligaments and muscles and on which are the facets by which the respective adjacent vertebrae articulate, to furnish motion above and below. The neural arch serves also to protect the spinal cord and the nerve roots emerging from the cord. It should be emphasized that the transverse processes projecting laterally from the pedicles are primarily for attachment of muscles, and their displacement by fracture (due to muscular avulsion) can in no way damage the spinal cord. The same applies to isolated fractures of the spinous processes. The vertebrae in general become progressively larger from the upper to the lower region of the spine, to support the increased weight of head and trunk on the lower segments.

Cervical Vertebrae

The cervical vertebrae are small in size and seven in number. The first cervical vertebra (C1, or atlas) has no body or spinous process (Fig.

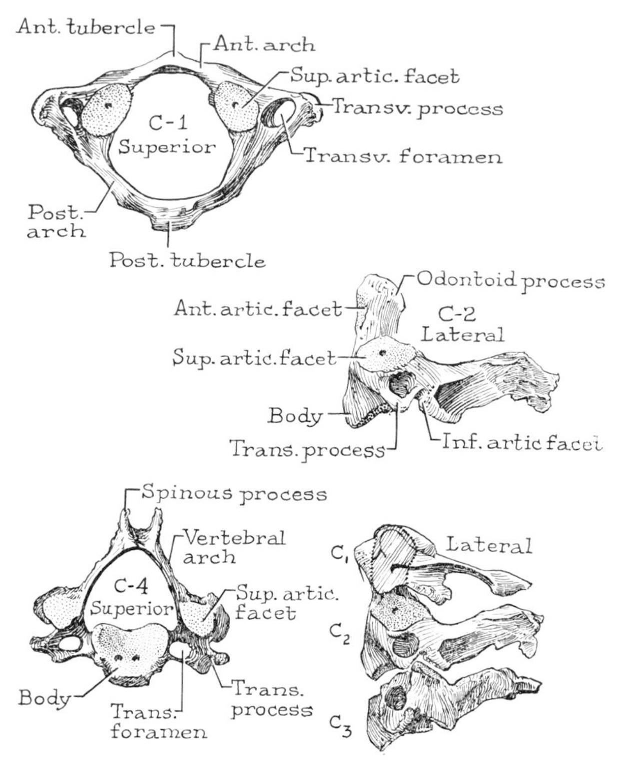

Figure 19–2. Superior views of first and fourth cervical vertebrae; lateral views of first, second, and third cervical vertebrae. (After Spalteholtz.)

19–2). It is formed by an anterior and a posterior arch, which join to form a lateral mass on each side, on the superior aspect of which is a concave, ovoid surface for articulation with the condyles of the occiput, and on the inferior aspect of which is a flat, rounded surface for articulation with the second cervical vertebra (C2, or axis). Its transverse processes are relatively large and contain transverse foramina for transmission of the vertebral arteries. The second cervical vertebra differs from the remaining by the presence of a special structure, the odontoid process, which projects upward from the body. This projecting structure has an anterior process for articulation with the anterior arch of the first cervical vertebra, and a posterior process for attachment of the transverse ligament of the atlas. Lateral to the odontoid process on either side of the body are the slightly convex articular facets for articulation with the inferior facets of the atlas. The third to seventh cervical vertebrae (and the inferior aspect of the second) have their articular facets located lateral to the body at the junction of the pedicles and laminae.

Each cervical vertebra has a transverse foramen in each of its transverse processes for passage of the vertebral artery. The tips of the spinous processes of C2 to C7, inclusive, are bifid. Those of C2 and C7 are longer than the others, and are readily palpable. Connecting the tips of the spinous processes is the supraspinous ligament, and connecting the spinous processes between the tips and the laminae are the interspinous ligaments. The ligamentum nuchae is a midline sheet of ligamentous tissue extending from the external occipital protuberance to the spine of the seventh cervical vertebra, separating the paraspinal muscles on each side.

Thoracic Vertebrae

The thoracic vertebrae are characterized by having facets on the upper posterior parts of their bodies for articulation with the heads of the ribs, and most of them also have facets on the transverse processes for articulation with the tubercles of the ribs (Fig. 19–3). The bodies increase in size

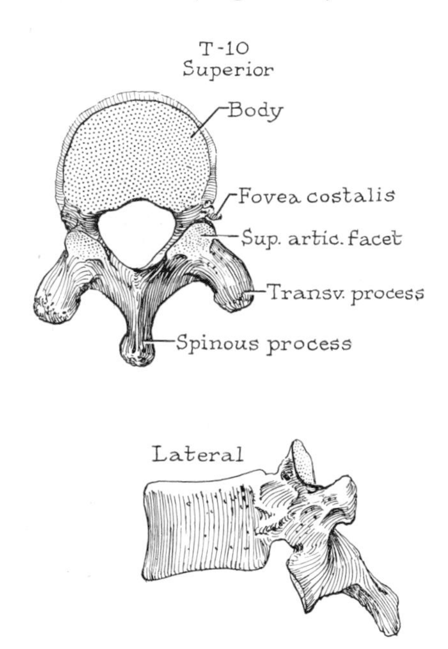

Figure 19–3. Superior and lateral views of the tenth thoracic vertebra. (After Spalteholz.)

from above downward; the laminae are broad, and each overlaps the one below; the spinous processes are long and slender, and slant downward. The articular processes are situated at the junction of the pedicles and laminae on each side, above and below. The superior articular facets are nearly flat and face in a posterior direction, whereas the inferior facets face anteriorly.

Lumbar Vertebrae

The lumbar vertebrae have large bodies, and short and thick pedicles and laminae, and their spinous processes are thick and project almost straight backward (Fig. 19–4). The transverse processes are longer than those of the cervical or thoracic vertebrae. The articular facets are concave superiorly and convex inferiorly, and tend to face inward and outward more than anteroposteriorly. There is, however, considerable variation

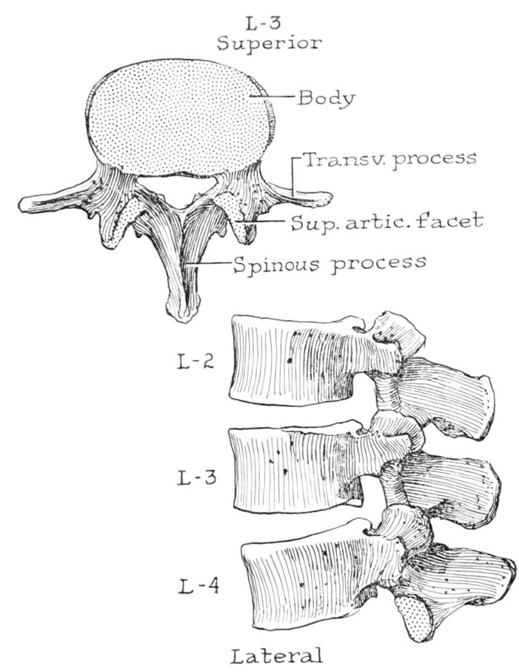

Figure 19–4. Superior view of third lumbar vertebra; lateral views of second, third, and fourth lumbar vertebrae. (After Spalteholz.)

in the arrangement of these facets as seen on roentgenograms of normal vertebral columns.

Sacrum

The five sacral vertebrae are fused into a triangular-shaped bone, the sacrum, with its base directed upward and forward to form an anterior promontory upon which rests the body of the fifth lumbar vertebra. The lateral masses are fused to form the wings of the sacrum, which articulate with the ilia, forming the sacroiliac joints. The anterior surface of the sacrum is concave, and its posterior surface convex. Although the sacral bodies are fused, the sacrum is perforated in front and back by four anterior and four posterior sacral foramina, which connect with the sacral canal and in turn transmit the anterior and posterior divisions of the sacral nerves, respectively.

Coccyx

The coccyx, formed by fusion of the four or five coccygeal segments, is a triangular bone with its base proximal, articulating with the sacrum. It ends distally in a small rudimentary, nondescript nubbin of bone.

MOVEMENTS OF THE VERTEBRAL COLUMN

The vertebral column may be divided into movable and non-movable portions, the former being in the cervical, thoracic, and lumbar regions.

The articular facets between any two vertebrae form true joints, lined by synovial membrane and held together by ligaments. In addition, the vertebral bodies are held together by fibrocartilaginous discs attached to the adjacent body surfaces. The periphery of each disc is composed of a dense fibrocartilage (annulus fibrosus), which is firmly attached to the margins of the bodies, and the center is soft and semigelatinous (the nucleus pulposus).

Extending along the entire vertebral column from C1 to the sacrum is a thick, strong, anterior longitudinal ligament which is attached to the anterior portions of each vertebral disc. *This ligament must be kept in mind always, because it is the chief anatomical structure that makes possible the reduction of a compression fracture of a vertebral body* (see Figure 19–*4*). Extending along the posterior surfaces of the vertebral bodies and attached to these and to the discs is the posterior longitudinal ligament. This extends from C2 to the sacrum and lies in the anterior wall of the spinal canal. Other ligaments uniting the vertebral arches consist of the supraspinous, interspinous, and intertransverse ligaments, and the ligamenta flava. The latter are strong sheets of ligamentous tissue containing elastic fibers, connecting the laminae of adjacent vertebrae and blending with the articular capsules on each side.

Motion in the spine is carried out by a gliding action of the synovial-lined joints plus compressibility and recoil of the intervertebral discs. In the cervical spine anteroposterior motion (flexion-extension) is free. Lateral tilting is possible only by a combination of rotation and torsion. In the thoracic spine lateral movement is freer than flexion-extension because of the vertical arrangement of the articulations. In the lumbar spine flexion-extension is free, but lateral tilting and rotation are limited because of the internal-external arrangement of the articular facets.

SUPPORT OF THE VERTEBRAL COLUMN

Because of the size of the vertebral bodies and the connections of the vertebral arches by a complex arrangement of ligaments and powerful muscles, the vertebral column gives very adequate support to the body. When viewed from behind, the spine forms practically a straight line from occiput to sacrum. Any appreciable curve to either side is known as a scoliosis. When viewed from the lateral aspect any child old enough to walk, and any adult, should show four normal curves in the spine—the thoracic and sacral regions being convex posteriorly, and the cervical and lumbar regions being concave posteriorly (see Fig. 19–*1*). These curves are in general smooth. An abrupt or sharp increase in convexity is known as a kyphosis, or a *kyphotic* deformity, and a similar increase in concavity is called a *lordosis.* It will be noted later that a moderate compression fracture of the body of a thoracic vertebra is more readily detected clinically because the kyphosis is seen or felt early, whereas in the lumbar region a similar degree of body compression will first result in loss of the normal lordosis before one can detect an actual kyphotic deformity.

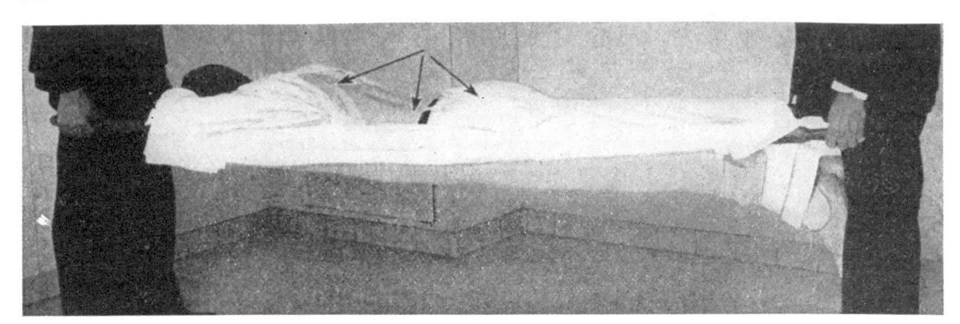

Figure 19–5. Correct prone position for transportation of patient with fracture of thoracic or lumbar spine. (Bancroft and Marble: Surgical Treatment of the Motor-Skeletal System, 2nd ed. Philadelphia, J. B. Lippincott Co., 1951.)

EMERGENCY TREATMENT AND TRANSPORTATION OF PATIENT WITH INJURED SPINE

Whenever injury to the spine is suspected, the patient must be protected against further injury, especially to the spinal cord and nerve roots. Under no circumstance should an injured person with a suspected spine injury be picked up hurriedly with "helping hands" under his knees and shoulders. This method causes further spine flexion and may be the worst procedure that can be carried out. In great haste "to do something" lay persons or even persons presumably trained in first aid may pick up an injured person in this fashion and lift him into the back of a car or truck in order to rush him to the hospital, little realizing that they may, in their haste, cause far greater harm than good.

Emergency treatment for suspected spine injuries and transportation of the injured patient should go hand-in-hand. The best and safest principle to follow is to **prevent** flexion of the injured portion of the spine. Should the injury be in the upper, middle, or lower back (thoracic or lumbar region), the patient must be turned on to his abdomen upon the stretcher, board, shutter, blanket, or whatever else is employed for his transportation (Fig. 19–5). This *prevents* further flexion, and, if anything, allows some extension of the thoracic and lumbar spine which is the very safest position for such transportation. If, on the other hand, the suspected injury is in the neck (cervical region), the same principle is to be carried out, i.e., **prevent** flexion. With an injury in this region, however, it is necessary to roll the patient upon his back, with neck extended, upon the stretcher. This will very effectively guard against flexion of the cervical spine by virtue of gravity alone acting upon the head.

In order to prevent the head from rolling or tilting from side to side during transportation, rolls of clothing, bundles, books, boxes, or the like, may be placed along either side. Better still (if nothing else is available) is another person who can hold the head in slight extension with mild manual traction. Under no circumstances should a pillow or rolled up clothing be used to prop up a patient's head, since this will flex the cervical spine and possibly cause damage to the spinal cord. In event the patient is intoxicated, delirious, or otherwise difficult to control, any attempt to sit up will cause his neck to extend further and added injury will be prevented.

One might ask, "How does one suspect a spine injury?" Soon after an injury the patient may complain of pain in his back or in his neck. This is enough warning even for a layman to suspect a spine injury. If, on the other hand, the patient is unable to move his legs or his attempt to do so is very weak, damage to the spinal nerves (cord or cauda equina) must be suspected. This is a serious injury and all care should be taken to prevent further injury which very likely would make the damage complete and result in permanent paralysis. In a patient with neck fracture or fracture-dislocation, the complaint may be of pain in the arms or hands, and it may be impossible for him to move either his arms or his legs, or weakness may be noted on the attempt. The same extreme care must be followed since partial and remediable damage may be transformed into a complete and permanent paralysis.

Unconscious patients in whom spine injury is suspected naturally do not voluntarily complain of pain or indicate its site, but an examining physician or surgeon may be able to detect considerable information as to the possible level of such injury by firm palpation with thumb and index finger along the entire length of the spine; occasionally percussion by the clenched fist is necessary. In either event the patient, if not too deeply comatose, may "register" pain resulting from this type of examination by groaning, squirming, or moving a leg, and this should be enough to dispel all doubt as to a possible spine fracture.

Associated Injuries

It should be unnecessary to warn of other injuries (chest, intra-abdominal, and of the extremities), and if any are noted, such as extremity fractures, these should be splinted for protection. If an open (compound) fracture is present, the wound must be covered with a sterile dressing (or the cleanest possible dressing if no sterile one is available) before the extremity is splinted. This injury may be more serious than a simple compression fracture of the spine, and its protection against further contamination and further bony or soft part injury is a "must."

FRACTURES OF TRANSVERSE PROCESSES AND SPINOUS PROCESSES

The transverse and spinous processes of the vertebrae furnish prominences for muscular attachments but in no way carry the weight of the body. The spinous processes may furnish some protection for the spinal cord. Having muscular attachments, these processes become fractured almost invariably by muscular violence.

Fractures of Transverse Processes

Etiology. Fractures of the transverse process occur chiefly in the region of the lumbar spine, where the quadratus lumborum muscle arising from the posterior crest of the ilium inserts in turn into each of the transverse processes of L1 to L5 and into the twelfth rib. Any extreme, unguarded, sudden muscular contracture will create a direct pull on the transverse processes and may fracture one or more of these. On the other hand, attempts to resist falling to one side may cause strong enough contraction to avulse one or more transverse processes. On rare occasions a person may fall backward and fracture a transverse process by striking the sharp edge or corner of a bench, chair, or log.

Symptoms. The patient with a fracture of the transverse process suffers immediate pain, which is more severe than that usually encountered in compression fracture of a vertebral body. This is because of extensive hemorrhage and exudation due to soft part injury, with tearing of muscles, fascia, aponeurosis, nerves, and blood vessels. The greater the tear, the greater the damage and concomitant hemorrhage, and hence the increased severity of the pain. Spasm is the greatest factor in causing pain. Attempts to bend to the opposite side or to rotate the trunk with hips fixed will cause severe pain.

Physical examination. The patient moves with extreme caution or refuses to move at all. Attempts to move the patient may cause him to scream with pain. Tenderness is acute just lateral to the paraspinal muscles, and swelling and spasm are often readily detected in this area. There is absence of tenderness over the spinous processes.

Roentgen examination. The *anteroposterior view* is the one most

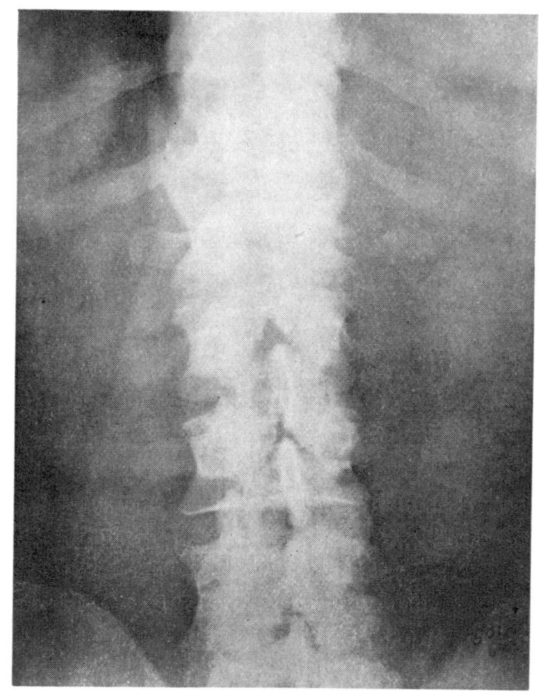

Figure 19–6. Anteroposterior roentgenogram, showing fractures of the transverse processes of the first, second, and third lumbar vertebrae.

likely to show fractures of the transverse processes (Fig. 19–6). These may appear as narrow, jagged fracture lines with little or no displacement or the transverse process of one or more vertebrae may be displaced outward and downward by the muscular pull.

One must not be misled into making an x-ray diagnosis of a fracture of the transverse process in the presence of a congenital separation. This condition shows a smooth rather than a jagged line of separation, and is more apt to be bilateral.

Importance of the injury. It is easy to overrate the importance of this injury and to permit the patient to get the false impression, from the early severe pain and disability, that he is going to be permanently disabled or paralyzed. If one will remember that the injury is essentially a soft part tear, and, because of this, the symptoms are severe, and that the displaced bony fragments are muscular attachments only, play no part in supporting body weight, and are in no way connected with the spinal cord or nerves, he will not make the mistake of treating this injury as a fracture, but will treat it simply as a muscle tear. It is extremely important also to ignore whether the bone fragments subsequently unite by bony union or fibrous union. Function will not be interfered with in the latter event, nor will there be any decrease in strength.

It is probably no more important to keep the transverse process fragments and quadratus lumborum muscle at complete rest during the healing period, nor any more possible to do so, than to keep the abdominal muscles at rest following laparotomy. Despite this, the ease with which the latter heal is well known.

Treatment. The treatment should be directed first toward the local lesion, and second toward rehabilitation of the patient.

The local lesion should be treated in such fashion as to keep the patient comfortable, to hasten disappearance of swelling, tenderness, and muscle spasm, and to permit limited activity in order to prevent the occurrence of severe muscular atrophy from prolonged disuse.

Reduction of the fragment(s) is *impossible and definitely not indicated.* The patient should be kept recumbent in bed with a board beneath the mattress, and physiotherapy in the form of dry heat and gentle massage should be given twice a day for the purpose of hastening dispersal of the hemorrhage and the products of inflammatory exudation. Fairly heavy sedation may be necessary for the first four or five days after injury. The patient may be permitted to turn from side to side when he feels equal to it. No plaster cast is indicated unless this program fails completely in affording relief from pain.

After seven to ten days of the above régime the patient's lower back, ribs, and pelvis may be strapped (Fig. 19–7), and he may be allowed up. Once the patient becomes ambulatory, he may be permitted moderate physical activities, avoiding those motions that put particular stress on the torn quadratus lumborum muscle. After three weeks the patient must be started on regular exercises to improve the strength of his spinal musculature.

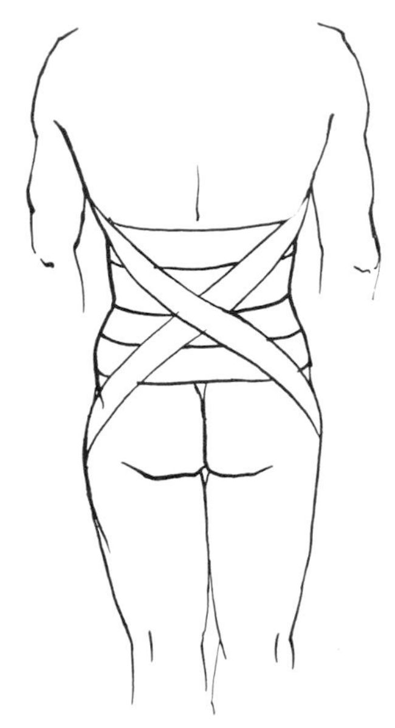

Figure 19–7. Type of strapping used in treatment of fractures of transverse processes of vertebrae of lower back.

Rehabilitation. General rehabilitation of the patient with this injury should start *immediately* with the explanation that his back is not "broken," but that muscles are torn and a few chips that are of no particular importance have been pulled off. The severe pain is best explained on the basis of the muscle tear and not because of the bone injury. The injury *cannot* possibly paralyze him. It should be explained that the sooner he can get up and start using his muscles, the quicker and more complete will be his recovery.

Altogether too many patients are made chronic invalids because they are overtreated for this injury, which treatment (cast, prolonged bed rest, and the like) impresses them with the seriousness of the injury. Many are told that they must not move without assistance, and this in itself creates fear that to do so may cause paralysis or other grave complication.

Spinal braces are not indicated for transverse process fractures. Neither is operation ever indicated for nonunion of any of these fractures.

Fractures of Spinous Processes

Etiology. Spinous processes may be fractured by direct trauma, as with an object falling from a height and striking the patient's flexed spine, or from indirect violence by muscular pull, as in "clay shovellers' fracture," when the injury occurs most commonly in the last cervical or first thoracic vertebra. Such a fracture may also occur in "whip lash" injuries affecting the sixth or seventh cervical vertebra.

Diagnosis. The diagnosis is made on the basis of exquisite pain, local tenderness directly over the fractured spinous process, swelling, and adjacent muscle spasm. Lateral x-ray films show the fracture, but there is rarely much displacement because of anchorage by the interspinous ligaments.

Treatment. Simple fracture of a spinous process requires rest for one or two weeks, physiotherapy (heat and massage) to hasten absorption of exudate, and a Taylor spine brace for the lower thoracic or lumbar region if pain persists for longer than two weeks. Such patients should be put on a program of exercises and mild physical activities as soon as possible, but it may be necessary to keep them out of work that necessitates bending or heavy lifting for six to eight weeks.

Fractures of spinous processes with extension into the laminae require more conservative and prolonged treatment. (See the following section on Neural Arch Injuries.)

NEURAL ARCH INJURIES

Fractures of Laminae

Etiology. An isolated fracture of a lamina or laminae is usually caused by direct trauma, the patient falling against an object or, more rarely, receiving a blow. These fractures are not common, but most of them occur in the neck region. No displacement occurs if a single lamina is fractured. However, if there is a bilateral fracture of the laminae, this portion of the posterior neural arch with attached spinous process may be displaced. If the displacement is in an anterior direction and causes pressure on the spinal cord associated with cord symptoms, the condition is serious and operative decompression is imperative.

Diagnosis. The diagnosis is suspected on the basis of acute pain, local tenderness, muscle spasm, and limited motion, but lateral or oblique roentgenograms are usually necessary to establish a definite diagnosis.

Treatment. An isolated fracture of a single lamina is usually well splinted by the attached muscles and ligaments. If the patient is very uncomfortable he should be treated with physiotherapy in the form of heat and massage, plus analgesics and a felt and cardboard collar for partial immobilization (Fig. 19–8). If symptoms continue severe for more than three or four weeks, it may be advisable to rest the neck in a four-poster type of brace (Fig. 19–9).

In bilateral fractures without anterior displacement and without cord pressure, the treatment may be the same as above, but rest and collar protection may have to be carried out for a much longer period, i.e., for two or three months. Should pain persist in spite of this, and following a long period of exercises in an attempt to strengthen the neck muscles, the surgeon may have to consider operative fusion of the area as a last resort.

Laminal fractures with displacement and cord compression should be operated upon as soon as the diagnosis is made, in order that no permanent damage may result if it has not already occurred. The displaced portion of the neural arch should be drawn posteriorly (away from the spinal cord) and, if redisplacement tends to occur, it should be removed *in toto* and the spinal muscles allowed to fall back into place. Following this the treatment should be identical to that described above.

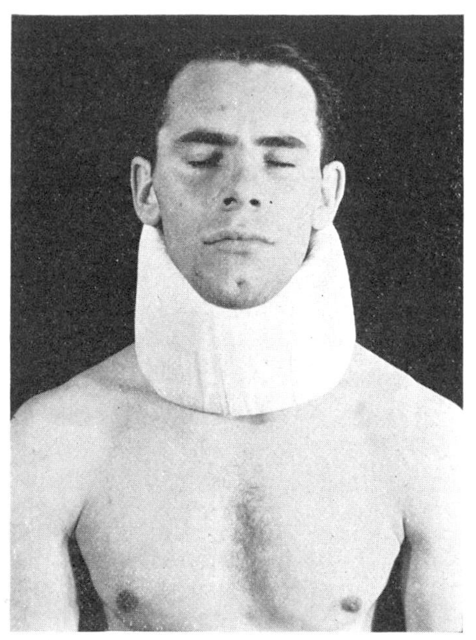

Figure 19–8. *Thomas collar. (Scudder: The Treatment of Fractures, 11th ed., 1938.)*

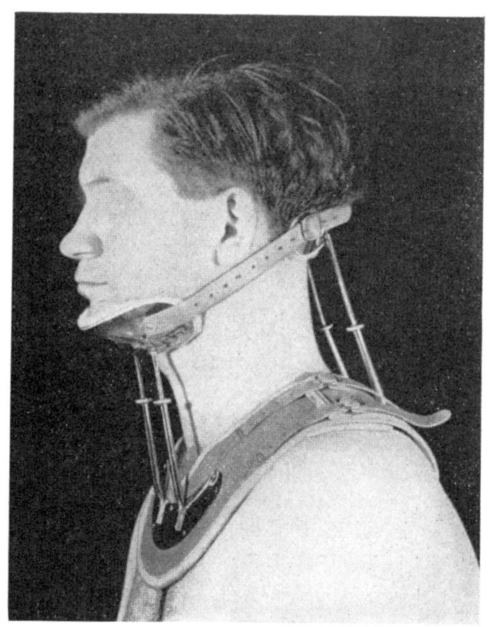

Figure 19–9. *Four-poster neck brace. (Rogers, J. Bone & Joint Surg., 24:245, 1942.)*

Fractures of Pedicles and Articular Processes

Pedicle fractures may result from a direct blow or a severe fall upon the edge of some object. Although fractures of the articular processes may occur from the same cause, they may also occur as the result of severe strain of the lumbar spine. If fracture of either sort is suspected and cannot be demonstrated on the usual anteroposterior or lateral roentgenogram, one should take oblique views as well. Pain may be extremely severe, and disability often is complete. In bilateral pedicle fractures there is frequent displacement. Any cord symptoms make operation and release of pressure from a displaced fragment imperative. It is usually wise to fuse the spine in either type of fracture, since they show poor healing properties and persistent symptoms unless the affected vertebra is stabilized to that above and below. (See Fracture-Dislocation of Thoracolumbar Spine.)

COMPRESSION FRACTURES OF THORACIC AND LUMBAR VERTEBRAE

Etiology. The commonest fracture of the thoracic, thoracolumbar, or lumbar spine is that of the compression type (wedging) of the vertebral body (Figs. 19–*10*, 19–*11*). Such a fracture may be sustained in a fall from a height, but this is by no means the only cause. A patient falling from a ladder or scaffolding, or with a scaffolding, and landing on his feet may fracture one or both ossa calcis and secondarily transmit the force to his spine, flexing it so violently that one or more vertebral bodies are compressed. The flexion force may be a general one, giving a gradual compression, and the spongy bone of the vertebral body is compressed between the superior and inferior plates. Falls from great heights may, with sudden flexion of the spine, be accompanied by tilts or torsion, which in addition may contribute fractures of the posterior vertebral elements (pedicles, laminae, etc.).

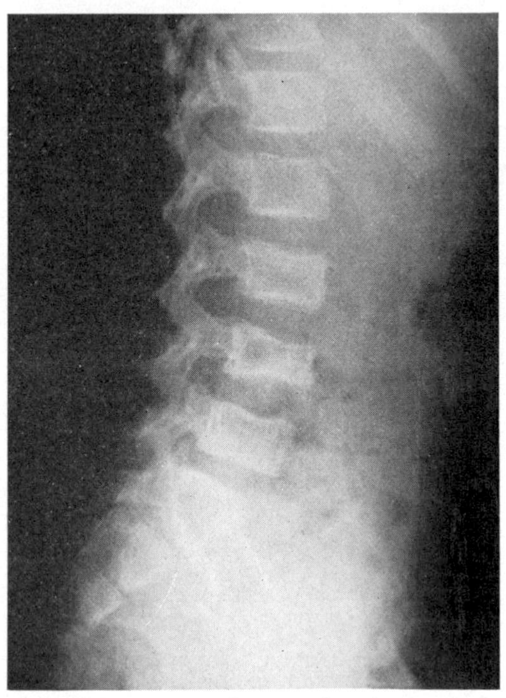

Figure 19–10. Lateral roentgenogram, showing fracture of fourth lumbar vertebra in a child aged 7 years.

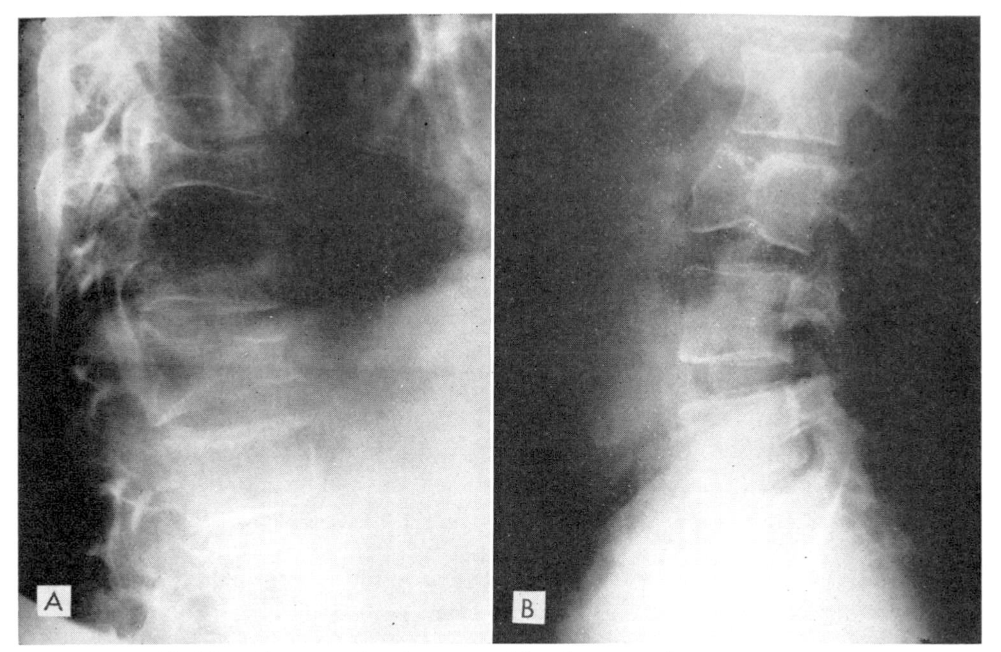

Figure 19–11. *Compression fracture of lumbar vertebra.*

A. Compression fracture of body of first lumbar vertebra in a patient with marked osteoarthritis of the lumbar spine.

B. Lateral roentgenogram made six months after severe compression fracture of third lumbar vertebra, reduced by extension of the spine.

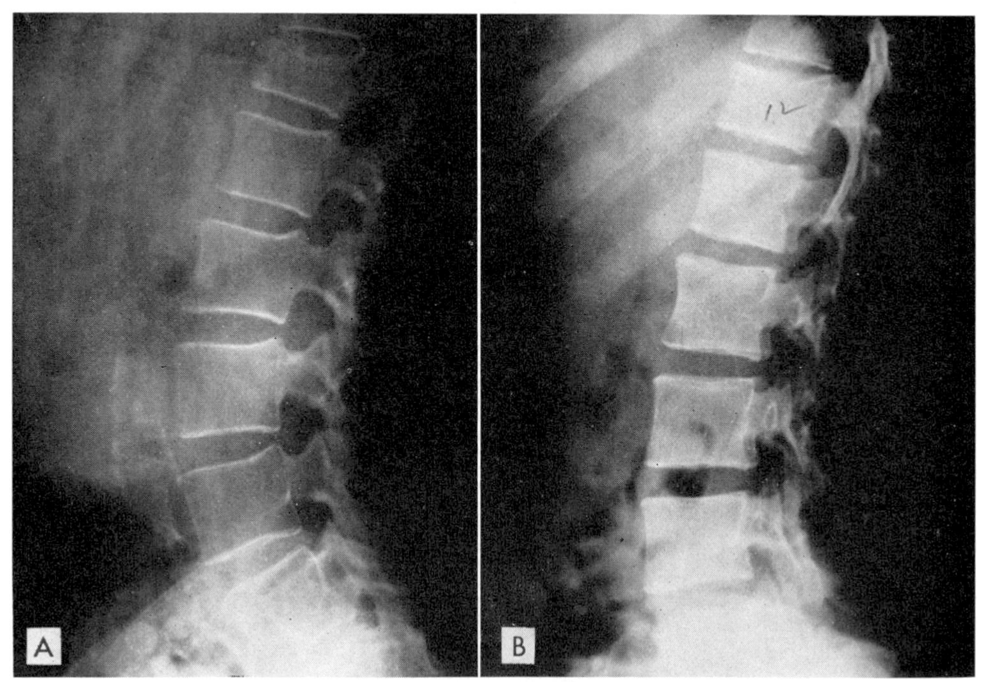

Figure 19–12. *Compression fracture of thoracic vertebra.*

A. Compression fracture of twelfth thoracic vertebra in an osteoporotic spine in a woman aged 60 years. (Note calcification in abdominal aorta.)

B. Lateral roentgenogram showing minimal compression fracture of body of twelfth thoracic vertebra.

Instead of the patient falling and striking a solid surface, the mechanism may be reversed, i.e., a solid surface (deck of a ship, or floor of a tank) may suddenly come up and strike him from below, as has been noted frequently in mined or torpedoed vessels in wartime. With this mechanism fractures of the os calcis have been reported and also fractures of the spine (compression type).

Falling objects (beams, etc.) in construction jobs occasionally strike a workman on the shoulders, thus causing acute flexion of the spine and a compression fracture commonly of the thoracic spine. Mine cave-ins or falling rocks may cause compression fractures, which, owing to the sudden, unexpected impact, may cause more violent acute flexion of the spine and therefore more comminution of the vertebral body. Such lesions are more severe owing to driving of the anterior margin of the body above down into the vertebral body below, not only causing greater comminution and displacement but sometimes driving portions of the displaced body fragment(s) posteriorly where they may impinge directly upon the spinal cord or cauda equina. Even without nerve damage, immobilization after reduction of the fracture must be continued in a hyperextension plaster of paris jacket for perhaps as long as four to six months, to permit bony healing to become firm and strong and to avoid subsequent secondary collapse of soft bony callus.

Predisposing etiologic factors. Certain pathologic conditions of the skeleton, such as multiple myeloma, metastatic tumors, senile(?) osteoporosis (Fig. 19–*12*, *A*), or hyperparathyroidism, predispose to easy compressibility of vertebral bodies with a minimum of external force, as in coughing, sneezing, lifting, being jounced while riding in an automobile, and occasionally in getting out of a chair.

DEFINITIVE TREATMENT

In general the principle of treatment for a compression fracture of a vertebral body is: (1) reduction of the fracture, (2) maintenance of the reduction, and (3) rehabilitation, i.e., restoration of muscle strength, restoration of joint function, and return of the patient to his pre-injury status and occupation. At this point, many exceptions naturally come to the reader's mind, for it is quite obvious that no matter how much one wishes to reduce and immobilize a spine fracture, the age or general condition of the patient may interfere with accomplishment of that aim.

Not only is it difficult to reduce compression fractures in elderly persons, but these patients frequently cannot stand the immobilization given by a plaster of paris jacket because of discomfort, because of interference with respiration when asthma or emphysema is present, or because of senile psychosis. Obesity is another reason why properly fitting casts cannot be applied and expected to maintain reduction. Many of these patients are so uncomfortable and unhappy in a plaster jacket that they beg to be taken out of it, and no amount of reasoning will make them continue with it. Some will remove the plaster themselves by soaking in a bathtub and then unwinding it layer by layer, or will get members of their family or friends to remove it. In such cases it is the better part of wisdom to ignore the fracture treatment per se and to concentrate one's efforts on the handling of the patient. His spine may be given partial protection by fitting him with a Taylor spine brace, provided he will wear it 24 hours a day, but if he wears it only when up out of bed or, at best, only half a day, he is fooling not only himself, but his doctor as well.

Perhaps the best method of handling some of these difficult-to-treat patients is to concentrate upon their spinal musculature, i.e., put them on a regular routine of frequent and graduated exercises to improve the tone and strength of their muscles. The very best physiotherapy for the muscles is *active* exercise, yet many patients still labor under the delusion that treatment of any kind given by someone else is better than anything they can do for themselves.

Methods of Obtaining Reduction

In general, there are three methods of bringing about reduction of a compression fracture:

(1) by hyperextension in bed, using (*a*) a reverse knee gatch, or (*b*) a building jack;
(2) suspension technique (Davis; Rogers);
(3) two-table technique (Watson-Jones).

Preparatory to reducing the compression fracture by any of these methods the patient's body—the entire trunk and upper thighs—is clothed with stockinet, which must be rolled on over his head, and pinned above his shoulders on either side and below the perineum to keep it tight, smooth, and wrinkle-free.

Hyperextension in bed. Use of the reverse knee gatch is an effective method of reducing a compression fracture. It is carried out by placing the patient "wrong-end-to" in the bed, i.e., his head should be at the foot of the bed so that the area of spine to be hyperextended will lie directly over the apex of the knee gatch (Fig. 19–*13*). A hinged fracture board is placed between the mattress and the gatch. The knee gatch is then ele-

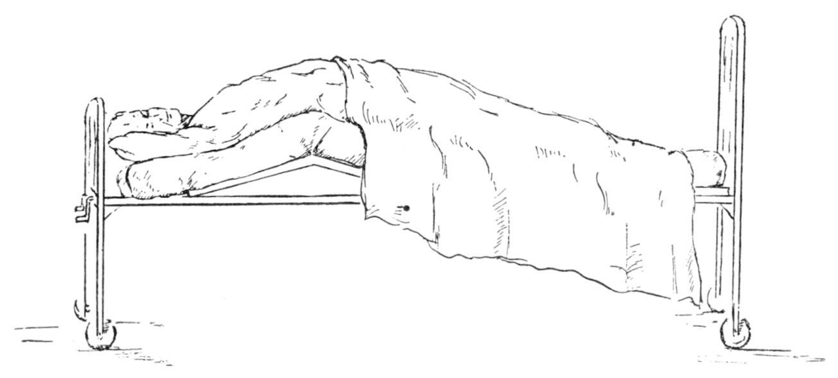

Figure 19–13. Knee-gatch method for obtaining gradual hyperextension of the spine with patient in bed. (An Outline of the Treatment of Fractures by the Committee on Trauma, 6th ed. Chicago, American College of Surgeons, 1956.)

vated at the rate of one full turn of the crank each hour until 10 or 12 such turns have been made, or until it is believed that sufficient extension of the spine has been obtained to bring about reduction of the compression fracture (by tension upon the anterior longitudinal ligament).

The patient of course must remain supine, and enough sedation must be given to overcome severe discomfort, if his cooperation is to be obtained. At the end of 12 hours, or whenever extension is considered sufficient, a lateral roentgenogram centered over the involved vertebra should be made with the portable machine. A careful study of this view will disclose whether or not reduction of the compression fracture is adequate. If it is not sufficient, additional hyperextension is carried out until subsequent check-up shows that the reduction is complete.

Reduction of a compression fracture by means of a jack is carried out as follows: The patient is placed supine in bed in the usual fashion. A narrow board (4 inches wide) is placed transversely beneath the mattress and directly beneath the level of the vertebral body to be reduced. A sturdy car or building jack is so placed on blocks that it lifts the board upward and thus produces hyperextension of the spine at the site desired (Fig. 19–*14*). As with the knee-gatch method of reduction, one or two complete turns of the jack (or raising it one or two notches) per hour is continued until sufficient spine extension has been obtained. A lateral roentgenogram is made with the portable machine, as described for the gatch method of reduction. If reduction is inadequate, further hyperextension is carried out.

When reduction is found to be adequate, by whichever procedure is used, the patient is transferred from his bed (in hyperextended position) to the Goldthwaite frame for application of the plaster jacket (see Maintenance of Reduction, below).

Suspension technique (Davis; Rogers). The suspension method of reduction of a compression fracture as described by Davis or Rogers is carried out by placing the patient prone upon a canvas sling. The chest,

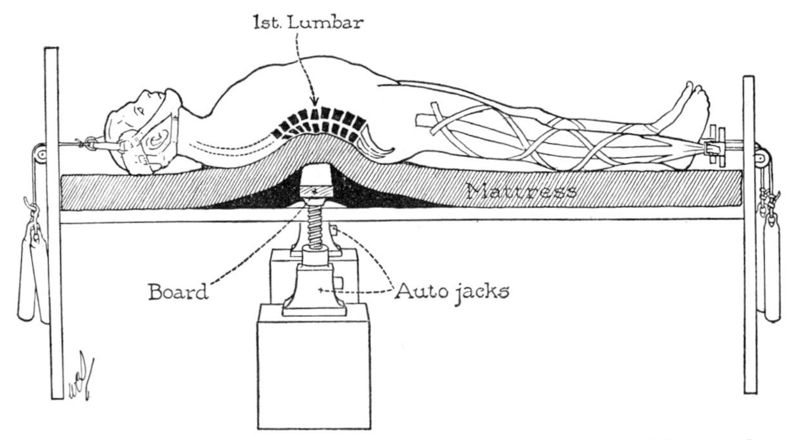

Figure 19–14. Extension of spine in bed by means of building jack method to reduce compression fracture of vertebral body. (Magnuson and Stack: Fractures, 5th ed. Philadelphia, J. B. Lippincott Co., 1949.)

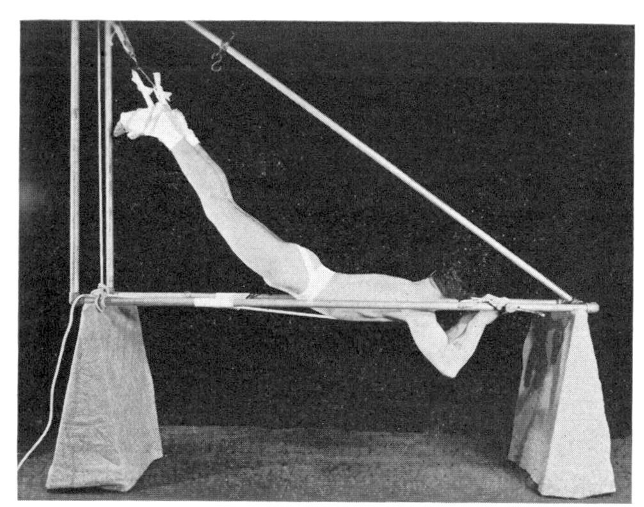

Figure 19–15. Suspension technique of Davis for reducing compression fractures. (Scudder: The Treatment of Fractures, 11th ed., 1938.)

abdomen, and pubis must rest upon the canvas strip, which can be slackened and lowered to bring about further hyperextension of the spine. Traction is applied to the patient's legs by means of padded anklets. The point of exerting traction and suspension upon the legs must be not only well above the patient but at least 12 inches distal to his feet, so that a horizontal as well as a vertical pull is obtained in order to help protect the neural arch of the vertebra (Fig. 19–*15*). In this position the patient is allowed to *sag* into hyperextension. No anesthesia is required, and the whole procedure may be carried out with no more sedation than ⅙ gr. (10 mg.) of morphine. This method of reduction usually gives a very satisfactory and adequate restoration of body height to the crushed vertebra.

By the time the patient has been permitted to sag into hyperextension and the felt pads are properly placed over the bony prominences, as described under Maintenance of Reduction, below, anywhere from 8 to 10 minutes will have elapsed. The compressed vertebra is usually reduced by that time, as may be verified by a lateral roentgenogram with the portable machine. If reduction is adequate, the plaster of paris jacket is applied as described below (see Maintenance of Reduction).

Two-table technique (Watson-Jones). The mechanism by which reduction of an uncomplicated compression fracture is brought about by the two-table technique of Watson-Jones is very similar to that of the suspension method of Davis. Actually, the spine is permitted to sag into hyperextension while the patient is resting in the prone position with his arms on one table and his thighs resting on another which is 12 inches lower (Fig. 19–*16*). His trunk in its entirety (pubis to the sternal notch) **must** remain between the table edges, otherwise adequate hyperextension will not be obtained, and, secondly, unless the trunk is completely free, it will be impossible to apply a plaster jacket of adequate length well-molded to upper sternum, pubis, and spine.

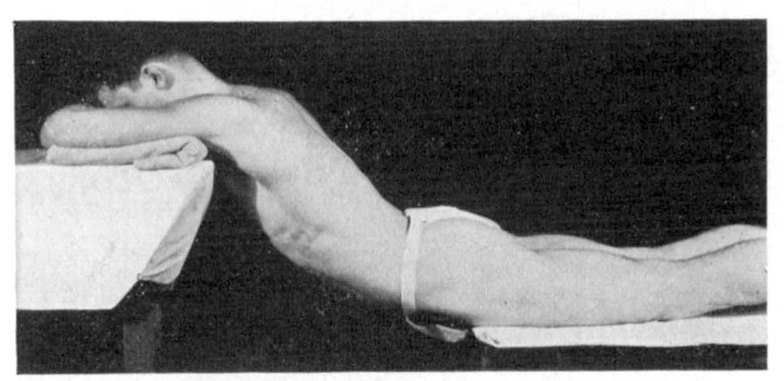

Figure 19–16. The two-table technique of Watson-Jones for reducing compression fractures and for application of plaster jacket. (Scudder: The Treatment of Fractures, 11th ed., 1938.)

X-ray check-up is made after 5 to 8 minutes of sagging (hyperextension) between the tables, and while the film is being developed the bony prominences are properly padded to make ready for application of the plaster. As soon as reduction is found to be satisfactory by x-ray examination, the jacket is applied (see Maintenance of Reduction, below).

Maintenance of Reduction

Application of plaster hyperextension jacket. A plaster jacket, to be effective in maintaining reduction of a vertebral body after compression fracture, *must* keep the spine hyperextended. To accomplish this it must maintain pressure over three bony points: (1) the upper sternum and anterior chest, (2) the pubis, and (3) the spine directly overlying the level of the fractured vertebra. Pressure relying for its purchase on soft parts such as the abdomen, and failing to grasp the pubis or upper sternum, will not prevent flexion of the spine and thus will not maintain reduction of the fracture. Any attempt to curtail this **three-point** bony fixation for the comfort of the patient is a complete waste of effort, time, and material.

While the fracture is being reduced by the suspension or two-table technique, or after it has been achieved by hyperextension in bed, felt pads are placed over the iliac crests and anterior superior spines, rib margins, pubis, upper sternum, and in the region of pectoral muscle margins at the anterior borders of the axillae. These pads are strapped in position with adhesive plaster to prevent their displacement.

When the Goldthwaite frame is used, after the compression fracture has been reduced by hyperextension in bed, a large felt pad is placed on the frame for the patient's sacrum and along the frame for the length of the spine. The patient is then lifted by four persons and his spine is kept hyperextended while he is thus transferred to the Goldthwaite frame and held on this in the same position (Fig. 19–*17*). Several layers of 6-inch strips of plaster bandages, well molded and rubbed, are applied around the body. Heavy reinforcements are added anteriorly from pubis to upper sternum, around the pelvis, around the upper chest, and along the spine, and these are in turn further incorporated and reinforced with additional plaster, smoothly applied and thoroughly rubbed to get rid of air bubbles

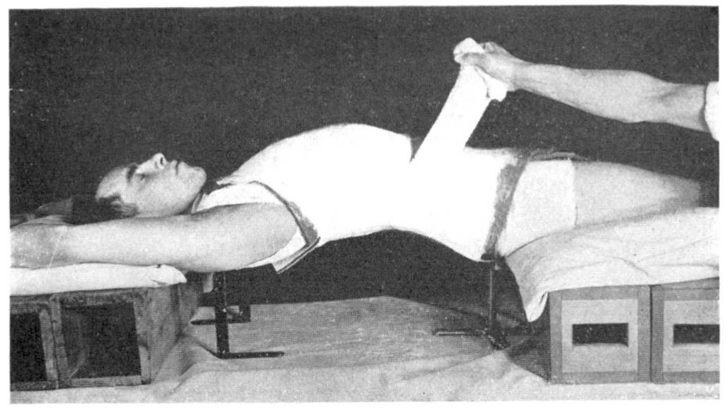

Figure 19–17. Goldthwaite frame (irons) for securing hyperextension of spine and for application of plaster jacket. (Scudder: The Treatment of Fractures, 11th ed., 1938.)

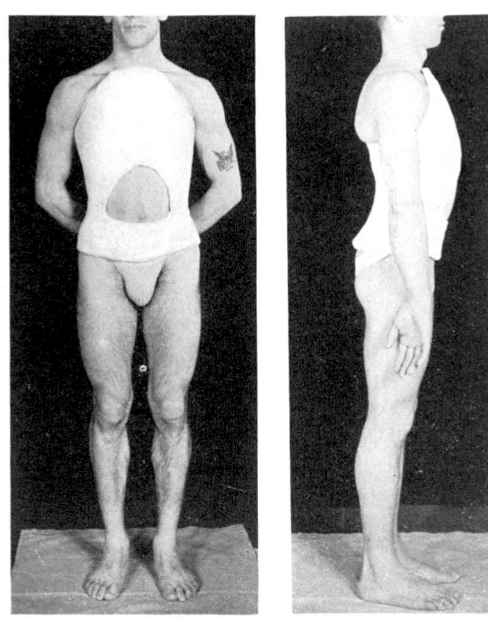

Figure 19–18. Properly fitted and trimmed plaster jacket to allow ambulation. (Scudder: The Treatment of Fractures, 11th ed., 1938.)

and to bring each layer in intimate contact with adjacent layers to prevent lamination.

When the Goldthwaite frame is used, after the plaster has "set" the extension bars of the frame are loosened and the patient with these bars is lifted off the frame and turned prone on the mattress of his bed (now flattened). The extension bars are pulled out from beneath the jacket.

When the suspension method of reducing the fracture is used, reinforcement should be added as described above. As soon as the plaster has hardened, the patient may be taken down from his traction-suspension and the canvas sling pulled out from beneath the plaster.

The jacket should be trimmed at the groins to permit flexion of the hips to 90 degrees, but in no way to release its purchase upon the pubis. It must also be trimmed above, but not lower than the upper border of the sternum. The jacket must be trimmed sufficiently under the arms to permit the patient to bring his arms to his side without the edge of the plaster rubbing the margins of the pectoral muscles. In back the upper border may be trimmed to just below the lower angles of the scapulae to permit free motion of these without local pressure or restriction. Lower down, the plaster must grasp the upper half of the sacrum and not extend distally over the buttocks (Fig. 19–*18*). If the plaster jacket is trimmed correctly, the patient is held hyperextended by having his pubis and sternum held backward while the lumbar and lumbodorsal spine is held forward. He should be able to sit up straight in a hard chair. If the plaster causes pressure in his groins (over femoral vessels and nerves), it will be uncomfortable, and the patient will sit backward in a semireclining position for comfort.

VISCERAL COMPLICATIONS OF COMPRESSION FRACTURES

Abdominal complications, principally distention due to paralytic ileus, result from bleeding into the retroperitoneal tissues from the fracture of a vertebral body. The ileus may be so mild as to warrant no concern and require no particular treatment. At times, however, it may be so severe as to be virtually complete, and the abdominal distention may become extremely marked. Not only may it cause the patient great discomfort, but it may be particularly stubborn and resistant to all forms of treatment employed to combat it. The surgeon cannot apply an effective plaster jacket to a distended patient and expect it to maintain reduction of a vertebral compression fracture. Thus, the abdominal distention must be overcome *before* attempt is made to apply such a cast.

Treatment

The treatment of abdominal distention in these patients is mainly of two types: (1) prophylactic, and (2) definitive.

At this point it would seem advisable to offer a word of caution in embarking upon a specific form of therapy to prevent or correct abdominal distention. It must *never* be assumed that abdominal pain or distention, or both, is the result of a compression fracture only. It is not impossible for the patient, if he has been knocked down by a car, to have a ruptured viscus (e.g., spleen, liver) with intraperitoneal bleeding, or a ruptured intestine with beginning peritonitis plus ileus, or a ruptured bladder or kidney. Early records of the temperature, pulse, blood count, hematocrit, and the like are invaluable for comparison later if the clinical picture worsens. Space does not permit a complete description of the differential diagnosis of the acute traumatic abdomen, but suffice it to say that the surgeon in charge must be ready to suspect almost any type of complication. He must also remember that acute alcoholism may very completely mask all intra-abdominal pain and may likewise make it impossible to elicit tenderness or abdominal rigidity in the early stages, or until the effects of the alcohol have worn off.

Prophylactic treatment. As soon as it has been definitely determined that no intra-abdominal injury or peritonitis exists, the patient is placed on a regular program of medication with 1.0 ml. of neostigmine given intramuscularly every four hours, along with judicious use of a rectal tube. The purpose of this is to stimulate the parasympathetic nerves and thereby keep peristalsis active. If such can be accomplished, intestinal stasis is prevented and no gas or fluid can accumulate to create abdominal distention. This medication, along with sufficient sedation to keep the patient comfortable, is employed until after reduction and plaster immobilization is carried out, if such is to be used. Morphine and codeine should be only sparingly employed except when great pain requires their use, since each tends to depress peristalsis.

Definitive treatment. Many patients with compression fractures are already partially distended when first examined on admission to the hospital. If the distention is at all severe, it will do little good to administer neostigmine hypodermically since paralytic ileus is already present and the drug cannot stimulate paralyzed parasympathetic nerves. Such measures as hot abdominal stupes or poultices with coincident use of the rectal tube may help to relieve the distention. If all of the usual measures, including enemas, high colon lavages, and cathartics, afford the patient no relief, it may be necessary to pass a Miller-Abbott tube into the stomach and through into the intestine, while intermittent suction is applied. All of these measures are difficult to employ, time consuming, and a nuisance. Therefore, the wisest procedure is to try to prevent abdominal distention from becoming a problem by the early prophylactic use of neostigmine and a rectal tube.

AFTERCARE OF COMPRESSION FRACTURES

The principles of treatment of a compression fracture are the same as those of treatment of other fractures, namely, protection from further injury, reduction of the fracture *when necessary,* immobilization of the reduced fracture as long as necessary for firm healing, and restoration of the patient to his pre-injury status and occupation (when feasible) as soon as possible. It may require much time and effort, both for the surgeon and the patient, to accomplish this latter part of the program. As a matter of fact, the initial definitive treatment of the fracture and its possible complications may take but a few hours to a few days, whereas the late treatment must be reckoned in months. One may call it what he prefers (aftercare, late treatment, or rehabilitation), but it must progress *concomitantly* with the actual treatment of the fracture. It is so easy to look upon a fractured vertebra as an injury to the skeleton only. One must never lose sight of the fact that muscle strength, fatigue, slowed circulation, and gastrointestinal physiology are all important factors in the recovery. Besides this, we must remember that we are dealing with a patient with an injury and with altered physiology, and that his well-being and emotions must also be reckoned with.

If a compression fracture is adequately reduced and adequately immobilized in a snug-fitting plaster of paris jacket, the patient should be made ambulatory within one or two weeks and exercises to increase the strength and tone of his spinal musculature must be insisted upon. As a matter of fact, by the time the patient is ready to discard his plaster jacket, his spinal musculature should be so improved that it is better than when he sustained his injury. It is usually necessary for the jacket to remain in place for a period of two or sometimes three months. Some surgeons prefer to follow the jacket with a protective spinal brace (Taylor type—Fig. 19–*19*) for a period of three or four additional months. Watson-Jones strongly advises against the use of a brace following the cast, saying that it accomplishes no real fixation and creates the impression in the patient that it is protecting him when actually he should be relying upon his spinal muscles as the best means of protection. Whatever school of thought is to be followed, the most important part of the patient's aftercare and rehabilitation is for him to practice frequent exercises and follow recreational procedures that will *positively* improve his musculature (see below).

Probably the greatest and most frequent mistake made in treating compression fractures of the spine is to overlook the necessity for improvement of the muscles until it is time to discard whatever apparatus the patient is wearing. This may be as unforgivable as forgetting to advise a patient with an immobilized Colles fracture to exercise his shoulder. Muscles that lack their proper size, tone, and strength tire more readily than strong muscles. When a muscle undergoes fatigue, it aches. When a jacket is no longer worn, weak muscles fatigue early, the patient's back aches, and he lies down for relief. To repeat this frequently is discouraging, and it soon reaches a vicious circle where the patient cannot be on his feet for more than an hour or two at a time, and, when he lies down to relieve his backache or tries to exercise the fatigued muscles, he either promotes

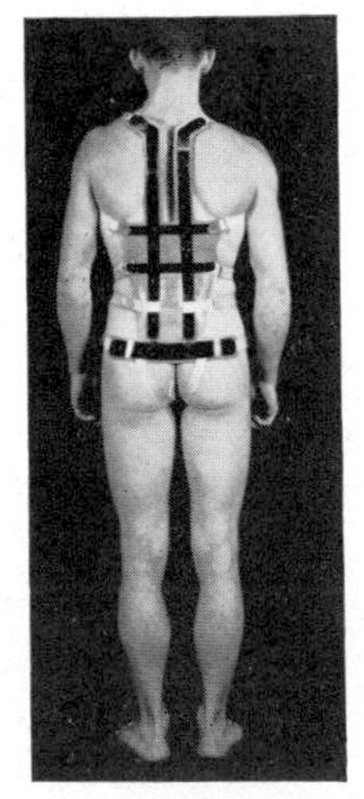

Figure 19–19. Taylor spinal brace. (Scudder: The Treatment of Fractures, 11th Ed., 1938.)

their atrophy or is unable to exercise and strengthen them properly. Disability is thus greatly aggravated owing to the prolonged symptoms of aching and fatigability.

Conversely, the patient who from the beginning of his spine immobilization is compelled to exercise and improve his back muscles will find that he scarcely notices any "let-down" when his cast is discarded. Such a patient will make an excellent and early recovery and be anxious to return to work rather than be constantly offering one excuse after another to postpone starting to work.

Exercises

The general well-being of the patient recovering from a spinal injury will be improved if he can be ambulatory, be out in fresh air daily, and be made to carry out a certain amount of recreational activity. Besides this, however, it is particularly important to strengthen the spinal muscles and the gluteus maximus muscles which help him stand erect. The principal exercises to accomplish this are performed with the patient lying prone upon a floor, mat, padded table, or firm bed (Fig. 19–*20*). While thus placed, and without using his hands or arms to assist himself, he raises his head and shoulders, i.e., extends his spine and holds it thus extended

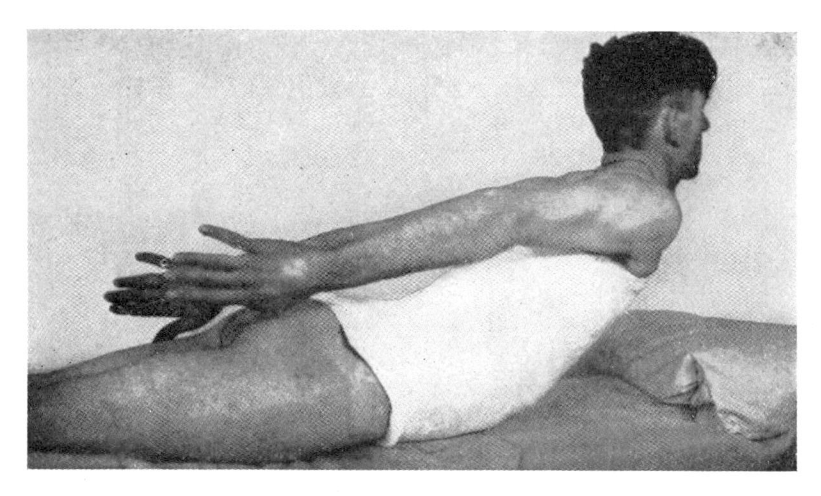

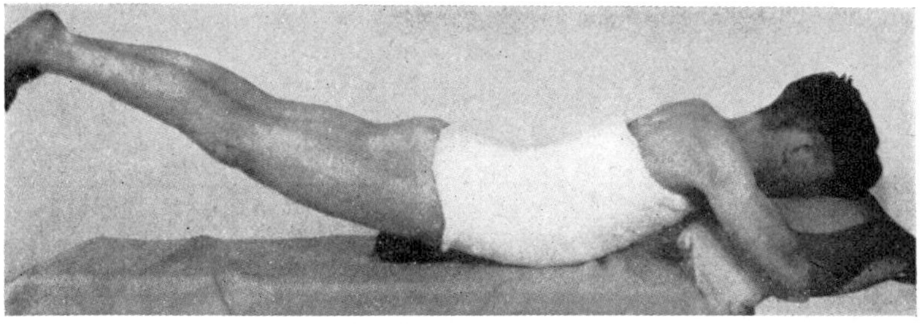

Figure 19–20. Exercises for spinal and abdominal muscles while patient is still immobilized in plaster jacket. (Watson-Jones: Fractures and Joint Injuries, 4th ed., vol. II. Baltimore, Williams & Wilkins, 1955.)

for a period of a few seconds. He then relaxes into his cast for a moment and again repeats the extension. This is performed five times. He then must extend first one hip and then the other (alternately) and hold each in extension for two or three seconds.

This "swim-kick" exercise is repeated until the maneuver (including lifting the leg off the table) has been performed five times on each side. He then relaxes for one half minute and starts again on the spine extension exercise for five more times, to be followed in turn by five more hip extension exercises. In the beginning these exercises are performed at least four times a day, with ten of each exercise done each time. After the first week these may be increased to fifteen each for each exercise period, and after three weeks the patient should do each exercise twenty times each period in divided doses of five.

In addition to back-strengthening exercises the patient may practice straight-leg-raising (while supine), alternating one leg with the other, to help strengthen the hip flexors and also the abdominal muscles. Plenty of walking, stair climbing, and mild recreation, such as tennis or volley ball, may help to keep the patient more interested in his long period of rehabilitation. The patient must be made to understand that massage, heat, and similar modalities can in no way improve his musculature. He must work at this himself, and, if an early start is accomplished, it will help him to realize early how much better he already is beginning to feel.

As for elderly patients or those too feeble to be put on a strenuous program of rehabilitation, it must be remembered that their spinal musculature is the most important bit of anatomy they have. Many elderly patients with osteoporosis who need no reduction of the fracture or in whom reduction is inadvisable may be given temporary corset or brace support for comfort only, but they must also be instructed in an exercise program and compelled to carry this out frequently and regularly, although perhaps not as strenuously as younger individuals should. Improvement of their muscles will pay them high dividends; neglect of their musculature will make them cripples.

Disability Time

The duration of disability will depend upon many factors, such as age, sex, severity of the compression fracture, the level of the spine involved, the patient's occupation, compensation, or litigation status, and the presence of other injuries. According to Davis and Bellinger, 75 per cent of all compression fractures of the spine occur in the thoracolumbar region, i.e., from T10 to L5. Patients who have fractures of moderate severity which are reduced early by one of the methods already described and adequately held in a plaster jacket, and who are put on a program of muscle-strengthening exercises, should have not more than four to six months of disability. Fractures with greater comminution and displacement of fragments may require immobilization in plaster for nearly six months, and therefore the patient's disability will be considerably increased.

Prognosis

It is debatable whether compression fractures occurring in the mid-thoracic and high thoracic region, i.e., above T9, should be reduced at all if they show only a mild to moderate amount of deformity. The vertebrae here are more fixed because of support from the rib cage and rarely collapse as much as those in the lumbar region. Not only is it difficult to reduce these high thoracic fractures, but it is also equally hard to maintain reduction. It is the writer's opinion that a patient with a mild compression fracture between T4 and T9 should be put in a hyperextension jacket even though real reduction cannot be obtained. This will offer some protection and possibly add to the patient's comfort. The after-treatment is the same as that described previously.

It is often unnecessary to immobilize compression fractures in the region of T1 to T4 in a plaster jacket. Very probably a Taylor spine brace for mild protection and prevention of postural slumping is all that is indicated. Watson-Jones believes that it is possible to maintain reduction of a compressed thoracic or thoracolumbar vertebral body by means of a snug-fitting plaster of paris jacket properly applied. It has, however, been shown by Baab and Howorth not only that it is impossible to maintain reduction and that some re-collapse occurs, but also that this makes no ultimate difference in the patient's anatomical, symptomatic, and functional recovery.

Formerly, when Metrazol and later electric shock therapy were employed in certain psychiatric disorders, it was very common to find compression fractures of the thoracic vertebrae. These were usually of a mild degree, and the patients got better with essentially no treatment at all directed to the injured spine. Surprisingly enough, there likewise developed no late sequelae.

HYPEREXTENSION FRACTURES OF THE SPINE

Fractures of the lumbar or dorsolumbar junction caused by *hyperextension* are rare indeed. The mechanism of hyperextension brings about a comminution of the anterior portion of the vertebral body by avulsion of the upper from the lower half through the pull of the anterior longitudinal ligament attachment to its rim (Fig. 19–*21*).

Treatment. It is obvious that treatment of such a fracture by further hyperextension as emphasized in compression fractures would increase the deformity. The fractured vertebra must be immobilized by an adequate plaster jacket, but the jacket should be applied with the patient sitting on a stool or standing erect, with traction upon his head. The erect posture keeps the vertebrae in alignment while the head traction steadies the patient, prevents his swaying or slumping, and makes application of the jacket an easier procedure. The jacket should be worn for three months, and exercises should be instituted for rehabilitation of the spinal musculature, as stressed in the discussion of aftercare of compression fractures.

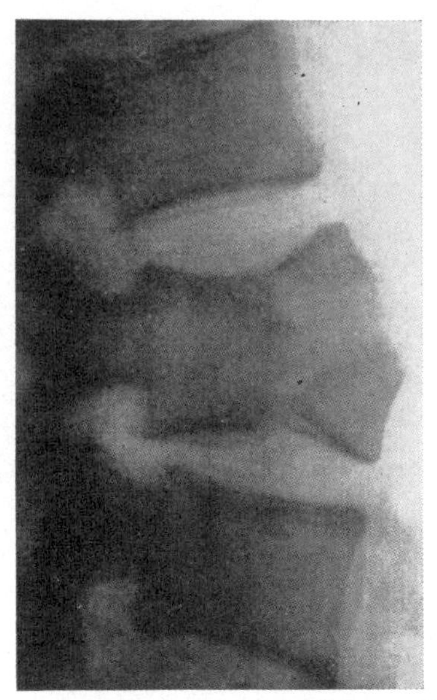

Figure 19–21. Comminuted fracture of body vertebra due to hyperextension. Anterior fragments are avulsed by anterior longitudinal ligament. (Watson-Jones: Fractures and Joint Injuries, 4th ed., vol. II. Baltimore, Williams & Wilkins, 1955.)

FRACTURE-DISLOCATION OF THORACOLUMBAR SPINE

More dangerous than simple compression fracture of the body of a thoracic or lumbar vertebra is the fracture-dislocation (Figs. 19–22, 19–23). This results from a more violent force, as sustained by a passenger who is thrown out of a car which collides with another object or turns over. The great danger, of course, is damage to the spinal cord, with resulting paraplegia.

There are, in general, two types of such injury. One may be a pure anterior dislocation of one vertebra upon the one below. This occurs from a jump type of lesion where the lower facets of the dislocated vertebra lie anterior to the superior facets of the underlying vertebra. Hyperextension is dangerous, and if straight traction with gentle extension fails to reduce the dislocation an open operation is indicated. At operation it may be necessary to excise the upper articular facet on the side preventing reduction and thus allow the upper vertebra to slip back into position.

The second type involves fracture of the pedicles and forward or backward displacement of the body of this vertebra upon the one beneath. Injury to the cord or cauda equina may be present, depending on the extent of displacement.

Treatment. Reduction, when no cord injury is present, is accomplished by gentle traction and mild hyperextension, and usually occurs readily. The patient is then immobilized in a plaster jacket, and a week later spine fusion is performed through a window cut in the jacket. The fusion should include one normal vertebra above and one below the vertebra with fractured pedicles.

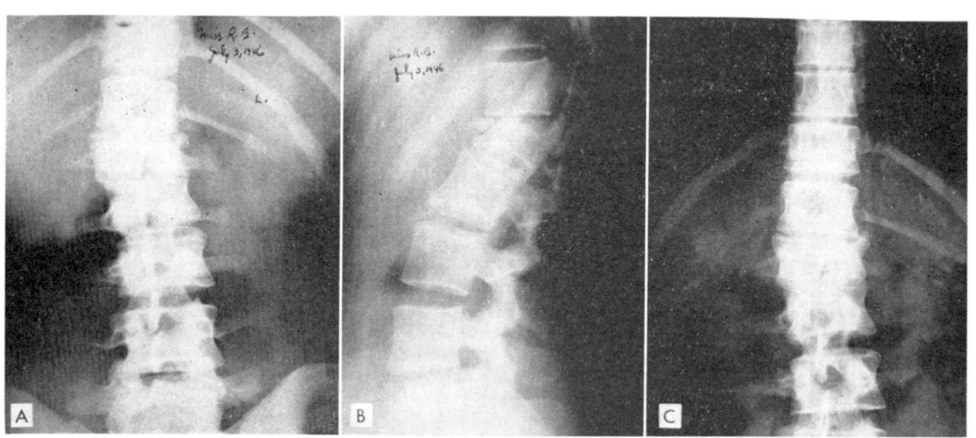

Figure 19–22. Fracture-dislocation of twelfth thoracic vertebra forward upon the first lumbar vertebra.

A. Anteroposterior view.

B. Lateral view.

C. Anteroposterior view, six months after reduction and fusion from eleventh thoracic to second lumbar vertebra.

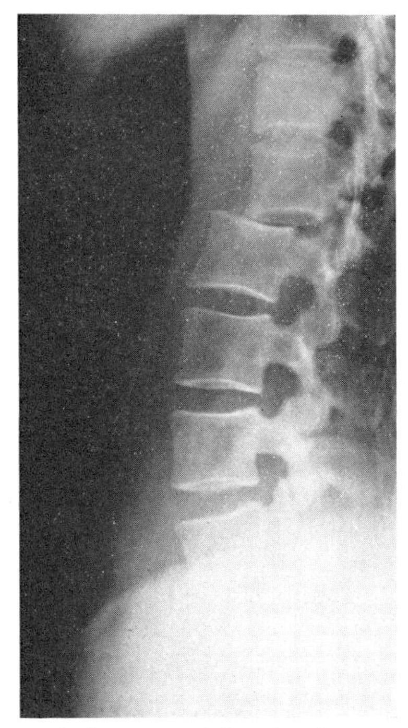

Figure 19–23. Fracture-dislocation of first lumbar upon second lumbar vertebra. Note the unusual posterior displacement of the upper vertebra upon the lower. Reduction by extension and plaster fixation and spine fusion through window in plaster, twelfth thoracic to third lumbar vertebra, gave excellent result.

The patient should be kept in the jacket for two months and subsequently fitted with a Taylor brace; he should also be put on a program of rehabilitation exercises for his spinal musculature.

INJURIES OF CERVICAL VERTEBRAE

Protection of the Cord

The first consideration in a suspected fracture of the cervical spine is protection of the spinal cord or the prevention of further insult if it is already partly damaged. This entails very careful handling of the injured person from the first, as discussed in earlier sections, in lifting him on to a stretcher, transportation, and early examination and management in the hospital. Davis and Bellinger state that the medical profession should assume responsibility for the handling of cervical spine fractures and dislocations from the moment of arrival of the ambulance until the patient is fully rehabilitated. They also believe that house officers and ambulance surgeons or attendants should receive special instruction in the diagnosis and first-aid treatment of these serious injuries.

The surgeon or attendant in charge should apply traction to the patient's head in extension by means of one hand beneath the occiput and one under his chin. The manual traction thus instituted must remain constant while the patient is lifted *by others* and placed upon a stretcher in the **supine** position. (This is in contradistinction to transportation of patients with injuries to the thoracic or lumbar spine, who should be transported in the prone position, but the principle is the same, i.e., to keep the spine in *extension* and prevent flexion which might harm the cord.) A pillow, or rolled or folded clothing or blanket should be put under the patient's shoulders to permit the head and neck to sag into extension. Manual traction in the meantime is continued. Upon arrival at the hospital the patient should be placed directly in his bed in the same position, and manual traction should be replaced by a head halter with approximately 4 or 5 pounds of weight. To afford countertraction the head of the bed must be elevated on high (12-inch) shock-blocks.

Examination and Diagnosis

With emergency transportation completed and all possible steps employed to prevent additional damage, the patient's general condition and neurological status should be investigated. A complete neurological examination must be carried out in order to establish a baseline for future reference. This may be performed just prior to application of the temporary traction by head halter or *immediately* afterward if the patient is having considerable pain in his neck. It is important in addition to examine thoroughly the patient's chest, abdomen, genitourinary tract, and the remainder of the musculoskeletal system for additional soft part or bone injuries. Urine is obtained for analysis, and blood for cell counts, hematocrit, grouping and cross-matching, and the like, if needed.

Roentgenograms should now be made, and these should consist of general survey films in anteroposterior and lateral projection taken with the *portable* x-ray machine. If no fracture is found in the lower cervical spine but a fracture in the region of C1 or C2 or of the odontoid process is suspected, additional films are taken high up, including an anteroposterior view through the open mouth better to outline the odontoid process.

In order to demonstrate C6 and C7 well on lateral x-ray films, it may be necessary for an assistant to pull downward on the patient's arms, to depress the shoulders and prevent their obstructing the view on the film.

One must remember that the x-ray film at this stage may show little bony deformity, and it may be difficult to reconcile the amount of cord damage with these x-ray findings. A certain amount of tissue recoil follows such an injury, and one must suspect and look for real neurologic defects.

Simple Sprains and Subluxations of Cervical Vertebrae

Minor lesions are common and are rarely severe. Sprains result from having the head twisted or snapped but show no characteristic deformity. The symptoms consist of mild pain on motion, partial limitation of motion, and tenderness. No referred neurological symptoms or signs are present. Heat, massage, acetylsalicylic acid, and use of a Thomas collar for the purpose of rest are often indicated.

Subluxations, on the other hand, give more pain, are usually unilateral, and in addition to this may show limited motion to the affected side, and spasm of the sternocleidomastoid muscle on this (the long) side; the head is tilted to the opposite side, and the chin toward the affected side. Such injury may occur without marked trauma and merely from twisting the head as in shaving or being awakened suddenly by an alarm clock. As time goes on the protective spasm increases and in turn causes an increase in the pain.

Treatment of a subluxation consists in overcoming the spasm which can best be accomplished by halter traction with the patient sitting, followed by the application of a Shanz collar. It is sometimes possible (if no traction-halter apparatus is available) to bring about the same result by placing the patient in the supine position with his head hanging in extension over the end of the examining table or stretcher. Gravity thus helps to relax the neck muscles and permits the subluxation to become reduced over a period of 15 to 30 minutes. This treatment should likewise be followed by use of a protective collar. Should either of these methods fail, the patient may be admitted to the hospital for bed rest, head traction, and sedation. Four to eight pounds of traction may be necessary. For longstanding cases, heat, massage, and intermittent traction are often necessary. A Thomas collar should be worn for a fortnight or more after successful reduction (see Fig. 19–8).

Dislocations of Cervical Vertebrae

True dislocation of a cervical vertebra may be a serious injury from the standpoint of cord compression, as well as from the standpoint of treatment.

Unilateral dislocation. In this lesion the head is rotated to the side away from the dislocation. Stereolateral x-ray views from both sides show the dislocation. The chin is also tilted to the opposite side, in contradistinction to the position of simple subluxation. Unilateral dislocation should be treated by the Walton method of reduction.

METHOD OF WALTON. The patient is anesthetized and lies supine with his head hanging over the end of the table. The surgeon supports the patient's head and applies mild traction, while his assistant furnishes countertraction on the patient's arms (and shoulders). The head is then lifted and the cervical spine is slightly flexed. The deformity is now increased while traction is maintained, and the dislocated articular facets become unlocked. The head should now be tilted away from the lesion and the chin rotated toward the lesion. The neck must now be hyperextended to maintain reduction. Reduction is complete if this latter movement (hyperextension) can be obtained freely.

Following reduction the cervical spine should be protected by a four-poster brace or (until such is available) by a snug-fitting Thomas collar (see Figs. 19–9, 19–8).

Bilateral dislocation. This is a serious injury. Even when it is not associated with a fracture, there may be accompanying cord damage, since these dislocations are nearly always complete. The patient's head is displaced forward, with his chin fixed in the midline. He is unable to rotate his head to either side. Weakness, paralysis, or pain is usually present on both sides of the neck in the distribution of the anterior root of the spinal nerve at the level of the dislocated vertebra. Immediate reduction is necessary and is brought about by the method of Taylor (see below). In the meantime, emergency treatment is directed at protecting the spinal cord from any (or further) damage until the diagnosis is clearly established. The patient is kept supine on a firm bed or stretcher with nothing under his head and with sandbags on either side. X-ray examination is made without moving the patient, and traction is applied to the arms so that the relations of the lower cervical vertebrae can be adequately studied.

METHOD OF TAYLOR. The patient is anesthetized in the supine position. Slow, steady traction combined with countertraction is instituted. The surgeon brings about the traction by means of a halter under the patient's chin and occiput and with a band around his own pelvis. The traction is applied initially in the axis of the cervical spine above the level of the dislocation. Such traction may be required for as long as 5 to 10 minutes, and is followed by mild flexion. The head is then rotated from side to side in a mild degree, allowing the dislocated facets to unlock and slide back into place. At this point the neck can be felt to elongate and it is then allowed to drop slowly *backward* into extension while traction is continued. If all goes well, reduction should be complete, and may be confirmed by lateral roentgenograms.

Following confirmation of the reduction the patient's neck should be immobilized by use of a Minerva jacket (Fig. 19–*24*) for a period of two months. This in turn should be followed by a period of protection by a Thomas collar.

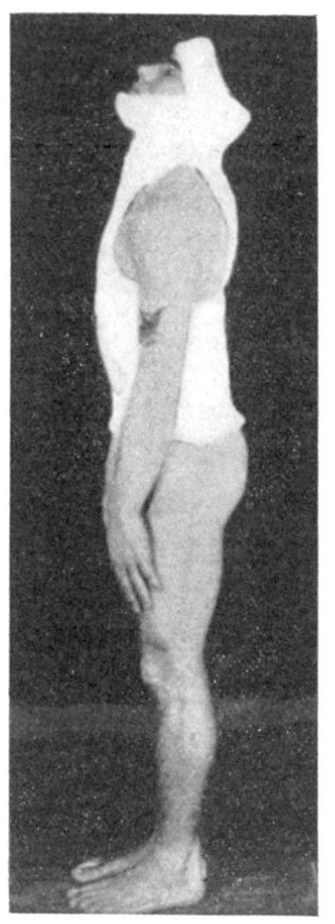

Figure 19-24. *Minerva jacket. (Scudder: The treatment of Fractures, 11th ed., 1938.)*

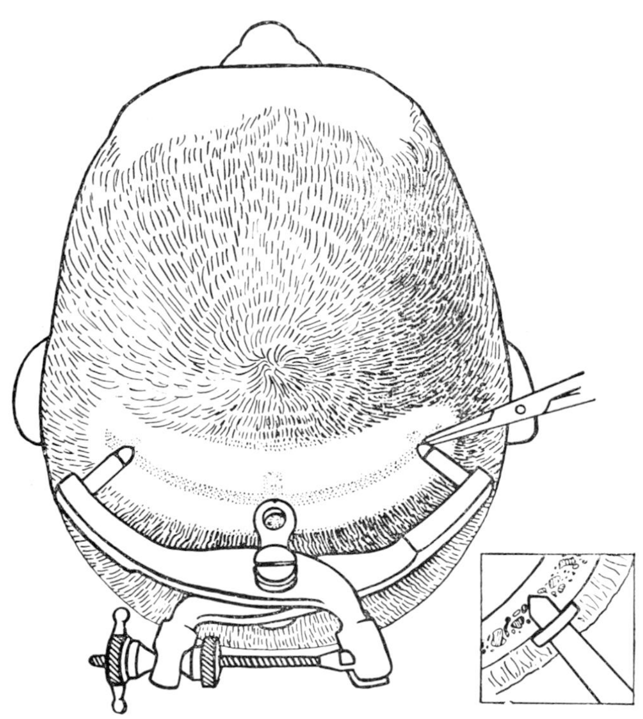

Figure 19–25. *Crutchfield tongs. (Crutchfield, J.A.M.A. 155:29, 1954.)*

Fractures of the Third to Seventh Cervical Vertebrae

Treatment. Definitive treatment for the fractured third to seventh cervical vertebrae is best carried out by application of skeletal traction via Crutchfield (Fig. 19–25) or Barton's tongs (Fig. 19–26) placed in the outer table of the skull. Once tongs have been applied properly they cause no pain, and the patient may have his head raised or lowered or his whole body turned. Five pounds of skeletal traction is usually adequate to reduce a compression fracture, but, if dislocation is present as well, considerably more weight may be required on the tongs, even up to 30 to 40 pounds. Elevation of the head of the bed on high shock-blocks must be continued, as described earlier, for countertraction (Fig. 19–27).

Subsequent treatment may be of a conservative nature, but this requires a long period of bed rest, plaster immobilization, and prolonged disability. Operative treatment, with internal wire-loop fixation and implantation of bone grafts or chips in order to obtain fusion, may be employed. This usually necessitates the wearing of a brace or collar rather than a plaster cast.

CONSERVATIVE TREATMENT. The patient remains in bed with tongs traction for a period of four or five weeks, *flat on his back* on a sponge-rubber or air mattress. At the end of this period, enough healing has occurred so that the tongs may be discontinued, and the patient may be placed in a Minerva jacket or plaster collar to maintain position while bony healing becomes stronger. If other skeletal injuries preclude the

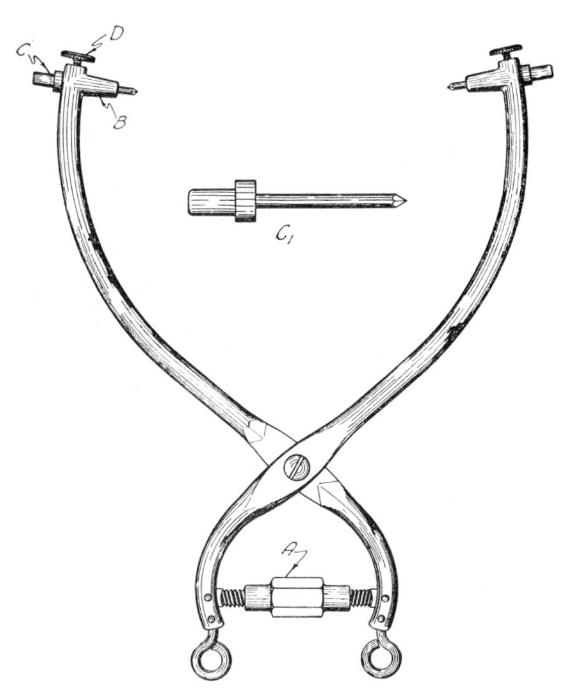

Figure 19–26. Barton's tongs. (Barton, Surg., Gyn. & Obst. 67:94, 1938.)

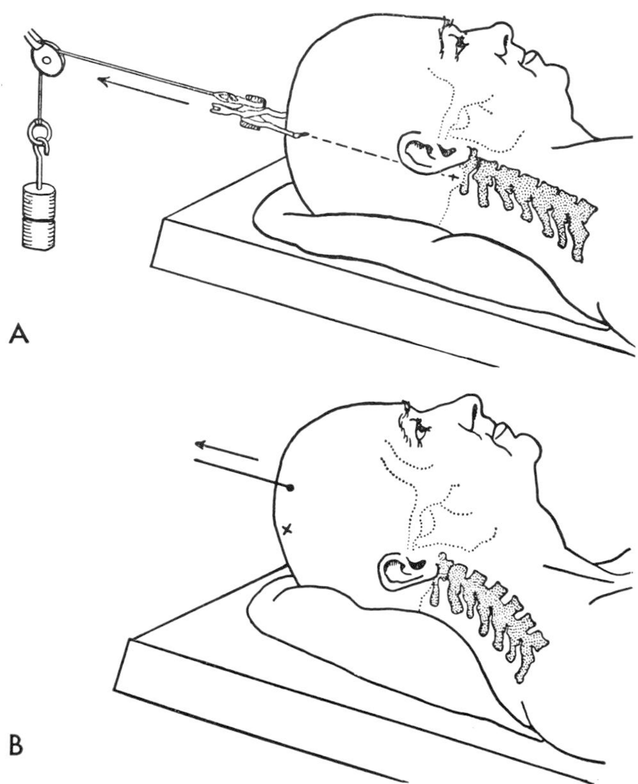

Figure 19–27. Tongs traction employed with countertraction. (Crutchfield, J.A.M.A. 155:29, 1954.)

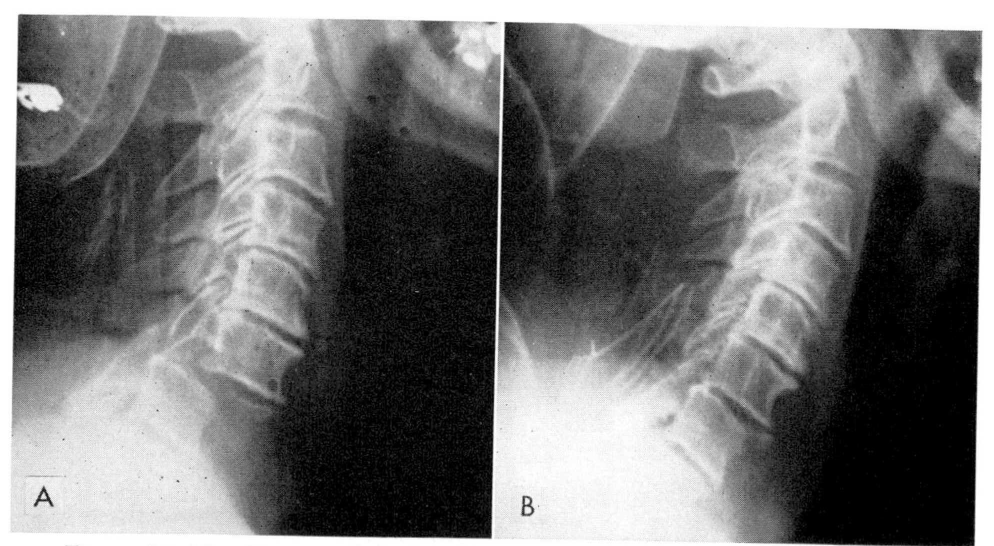

Figure 19–28. Fracture-dislocation of sixth cervical vertebra upon seventh.
A. At time of admission.
B. After fusion from fifth cervical to first thoracic vertebra.

application of a plaster jacket, the tongs traction may be continued while the patient remains in bed.

The average fracture of the third to seventh cervical vertebra should heal sufficiently in three or four months so that use of tongs and plaster fixation need not be continued beyond this time. After removal of the plaster, the patient may be more comfortable wearing a soft Shanz collar for a month while heat, massage, and exercises are employed to loosen the neck muscles and help abolish their soreness.

Operative Treatment. Operation offers a quicker method of securing fixation of the fracture (Fig. 19–28). Rogers, one of its strongest

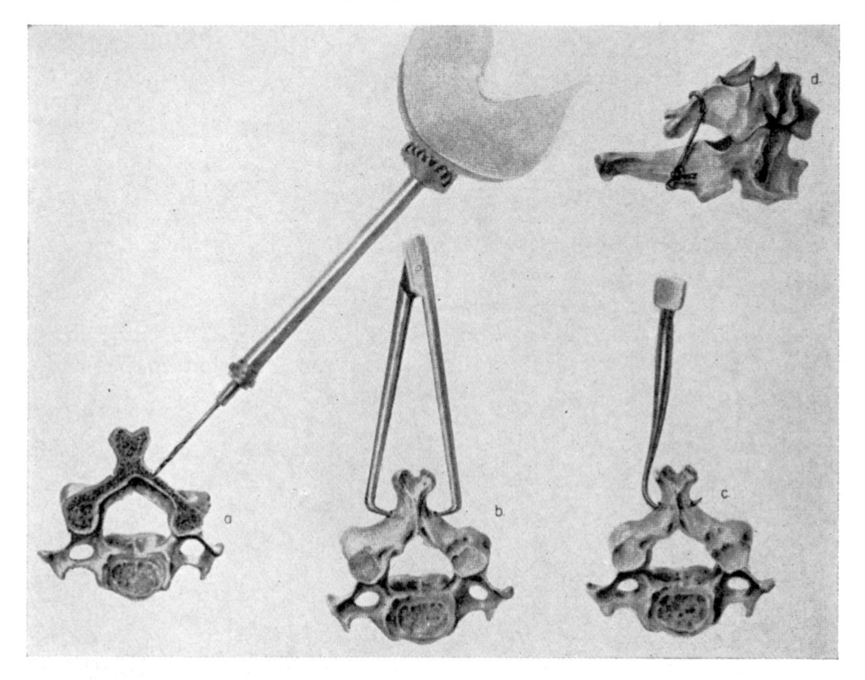

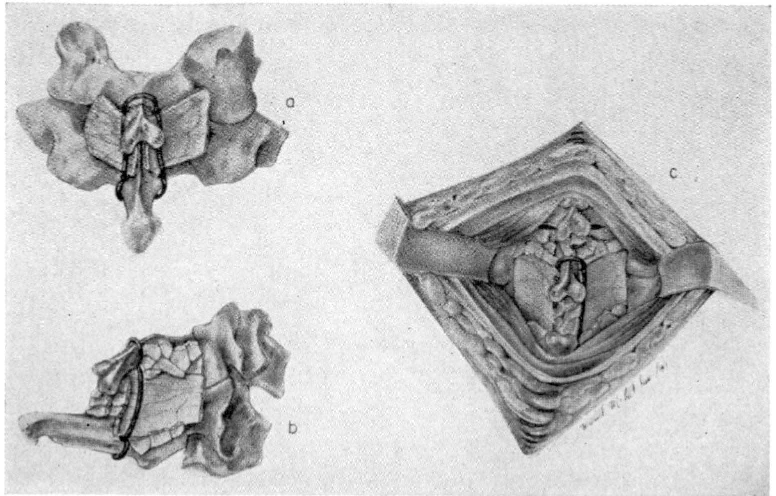

Figure 19–29. Roger's method of wiring and adding bone chips for fusion of cervical spine. (Rogers, J. Bone & Joint Surg. 24:245, 1942.)

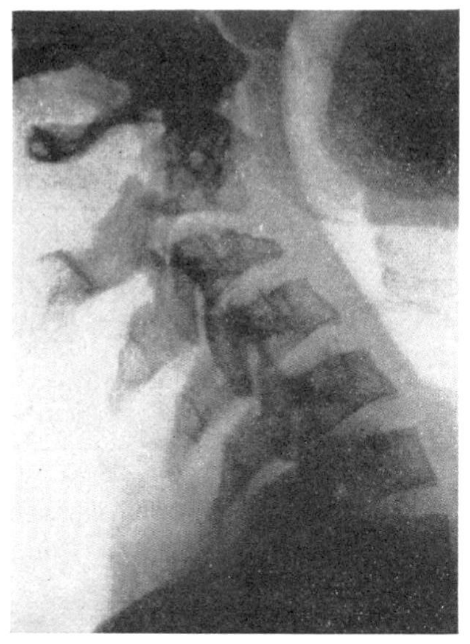

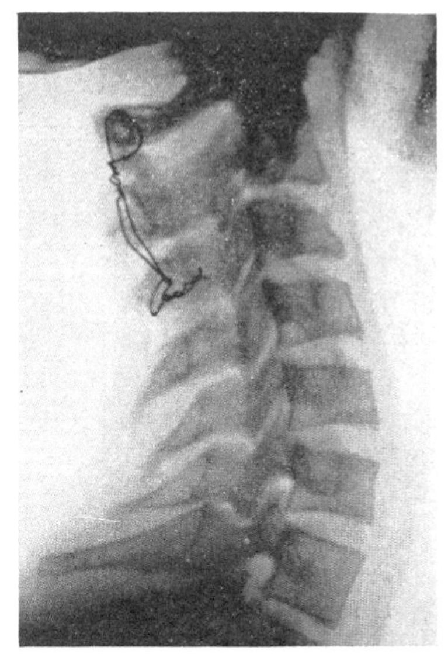

Figure 19–30. Anterior fracture-dislocation of second cervical vertebra on the third; compression fracture of body of third; no cord symptoms.

Left. Roentgenogram on admission.

Right. Complete fusion three months after wire fixation and fusion of first, second, and third cervical vertebrae. Patient returned to work in four months. (Rogers, J. Bone & Joint Surg. 24:245, 1942.)

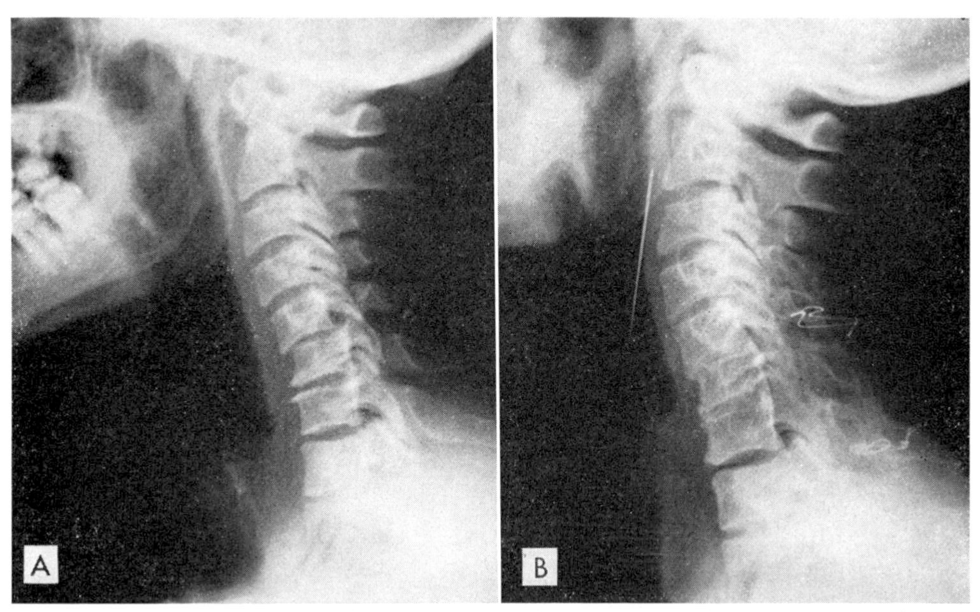

Figure 19–31. Fracture-dislocation of fifth cervical vertebra upon the sixth.

A. At time of admission.

B. After fusion of cervical spine from C4 to C7, utilizing rib grafts held in place with wire loops.

advocates, recommends tongs traction for a week or ten days before operating, to allow the tissues to "jell" a little in cases without cord damage, or, in cases with cord damage, to allow the cord injury to become stabilized. For simple compression fracture he employs 22-gauge stainless steel wire passed through drill holes in the bases of the adjacent spinous processes and packs in iliac bone grafts (Fig. 19–*29*).

Should the pedicles be fractured, the vertebrae above and below the fracture are fused, using the same technique (Figs. 19–*30*, 19–*31*). After operation the patient remains in tongs traction and is permitted to turn at will. After four to five weeks the tongs are removed, a four-poster neck splint attached to a Taylor spine brace is applied, and the patient is made ambulatory. He should wear this brace for three months or slightly longer, at which time good fusion should have occurred.

Fractures and Fracture-Dislocations of First and Second Cervical Vertebrae

Injuries to the atlas and axis (C1 and C2) are more serious than similar lesions in the lower cervical vertebrae because of the higher mortality attendant upon possible paralysis of the respiratory center. For this reason they are dealt with as a special group.

A simple rotatory dislocation of the atlas upon the axis is treated best by Walton's method of manipulation, followed by application of a Shanz collar.

A dislocation of the atlas forward upon the axis without fracture of the odontoid process is usually fatal, because of crushing of the cord at this level against the intact odontoid (Fig. 19–32, *left*). A dislocation of the atlas forward, with fracture and displacement of the odontoid, may be fatal but is less likely to be so because the cord may escape being crushed (Fig. 19–32, *right*). These patients, if not paralyzed, may walk into the emergency ward holding and supporting their heads with their own hands to protect themselves from the sense of insecurity that is always present.

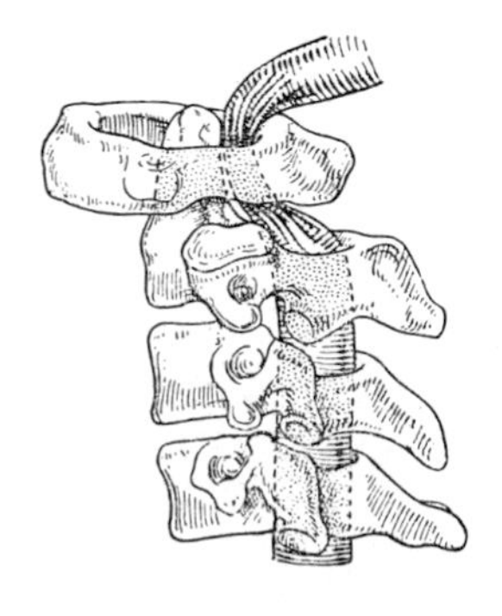

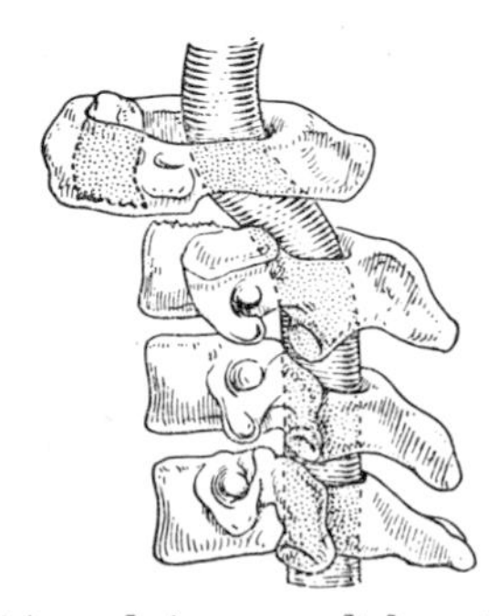

Figure 19–32. Forward dislocation (left) and fracture-dislocation (right) of the atlas (C1) upon the axis (C2). If the odontoid is displaced forward there is less danger of cord compression, and the patient has a better chance of survival. (Watson-Jones: Fractures and Joint Injuries, 4th ed., vol. II. Baltimore, Williams & Wilkins, 1955.)

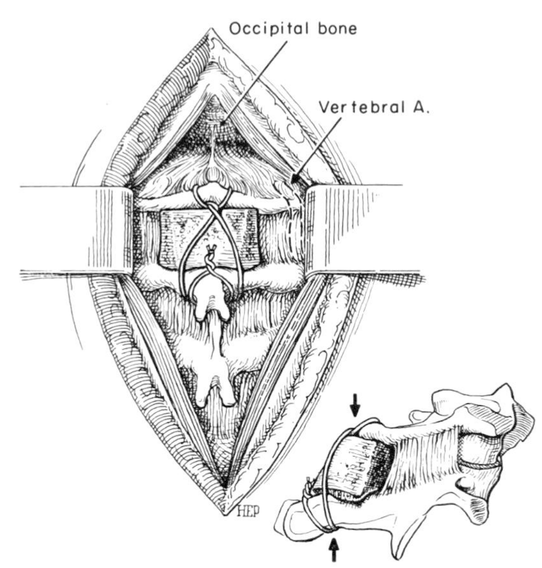

Figure 19–33. Gallie's method of fusion of the first and second cervical vertebrae, with wire loop and iliac bone block.

They should be handled with the utmost care and protection and be x-rayed immediately with special attention being placed on anteroposterior views made through the mouth.

Treatment. In fractures of the first or second cervical vertebra or of the odontoid process, tongs traction should be applied and, if conservative measures are elected, a Minerva jacket must be applied and kept on for four months, followed by use of a high plaster collar for another two or three months, because these fractures are slower to heal than are other fractures lower in the neck. Nonunion of the odontoid may occur if immobilization is inadequate, and this offers some risk of late displacement and subsequent cord damage.

This writer believes that operative treatment of fractures in the region of C1 and C2 is advisable and can be carried out while tongs traction remains in place. Tongs traction may be continued for three, four, or five weeks after operation, and the patient then be allowed up in a collar and brace. The type of operation used for these fractures is similar to that advocated by Rogers, described above, or one may follow the technique of Gallie, who utilizes a bone block cut from the iliac crest and placed between the spinous processes of C1 and C2, with a wire loop snugly holding all three together (Fig. 19–33). This gives a very satisfactory fixation, and the patient is extremely comfortable following the operation.

BIBLIOGRAPHY

Davis, A. G., and Bellinger, M. J.: Injuries to the Spine, in Surgical Treatment of the Motor-Skeletal System, F. W. Bancroft and H. C. Marble, editors. Ed. 2, Vol. 2. Philadelphia, J. B. Lippincott Co., 1951.

Rogers, W. A.: An extension frame for the reduction of fracture of the vertebral body, Surg., Gyn., & Obst. 50:101, 1930.
Rogers, W. A.: Cord injury during reduction of thoracic and lumbar vertebral body fracture and dislocation, J. Bone & Joint Surg. 20:689, 1938.
Rogers, W. A.: Treatment of fracture-dislocation of the cervical spine, J. Bone & Joint Surg. 24:245, 1942.

CHAPTER 20

INJURIES OF THE CERVICAL SPINAL CORD AND ADNEXA

By EDWARD B. SCHLESINGER, M.D.
and JUAN M. TAVERAS, M.D.

ANATOMICAL CONSIDERATIONS

THE ARCHITECTURE of the spinal column is a direct evolutionary response to the demands of function. The large and heavy head, a dynamically changing center of gravity as result of a bipedal gait, and a complex neural apparatus passing to the upper extremities, all play a significant part in the final impress of functional needs on structure. The head must be allowed flexion and extension in the anteroposterior and lateral planes, and in rotation, so that the cervical spine must be designed for wide ranges of motion. The large cervical cord and the roots passing to and from the upper extremities must be buffered against shock and protected against the stresses of wear and tear. All these factors play a part in the ultimate design of the cervical vertebral column and also in the nature of the pathological states which occur there.

At first glance, one notes that the cervical spine differs from the thoracic, particularly in that the intervertebral discs, which convey mobility, are larger, and there is less obliquity to the spinous processes and laminae. The atlas, or first cervical vertebra, upon which the head rests, and upon whose co-joints the head may elevate or depress, forms a unique and ingenious joint for the second cervical vertebra, or axis. By converting the atlas to a mere ring surrounding the odontoid portion of the axis (Fig. 20–*1*), nature has added to the fore-and-aft motion of the head a pivotal motion, allowing rotation. Between the first and second cervical vertebrae there is no true intervertebral disc, but there remains a vestibular remnant of disc where the odontoid attaches to the remainder of the second cervical vertebra below. The lateral joints at these two levels are more horizontal than they are elsewhere, since they are involved in rotation rather than in flexion and extension. Below these levels the structure of the cervical spine is more uniform, with motion based on the intervertebral disc and the lateral joints at each level.

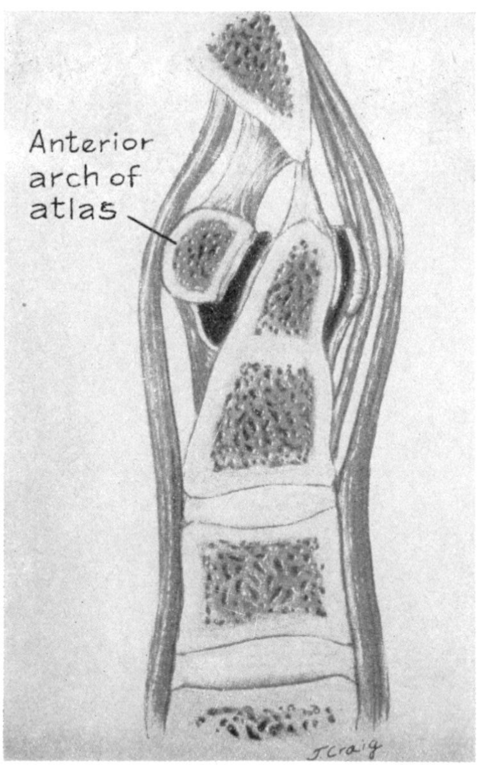

Figure 20–1. *Sagittal cross-section of upper cervical spine according to Testut. Starting at the anterior aspect the ligaments are as follows: anterior longitudinal ligament, atlanto-occipital ligament, apical ligament, transverse ligament, occipito-axial ligament, and posterior longitudinal ligament. Note that the odontoid process is surrounded by a synovial cavity down to its base. There is a small remnant of the disc between the base of the odontoid process and the body of the second cervical vertebra. (Schlesinger, E. B., and Taveras, J. M., Am. J. Surg., 95:641, 1958.)*

SYNDROMES OF THE CERVICAL DISC

Since they bear the brunt of motion, the discs separating the cervical vertebrae, and their limiting ligaments, share the pathology of wear and tear to a marked degree. The center of the disc, or nucleus pulposus, is of semifluid consistency. It is surrounded by the annulus fibrosus or layers of concentric bands of fibrous structure which, with the posterior and anterior longitudinal ligaments, form a unit of structure allowing motion of the vertebral bodies. The semifluid nucleus may be compressed and deformed in various planes to allow range of motion. This hydraulic quality allows the dissipation of stresses to avoid collection of forces at a single point. Pathologic change in the disc consists primarily in degenerative change with loss of fluid. Any unusual focal collection of stresses allows wear and tear on the limiting ligament and annulus so that the hydraulic ram force of the nuclear centrum tends to gradually fray out the limiting layers and the nucleus becomes extruded or protuberant, either posteriorly,

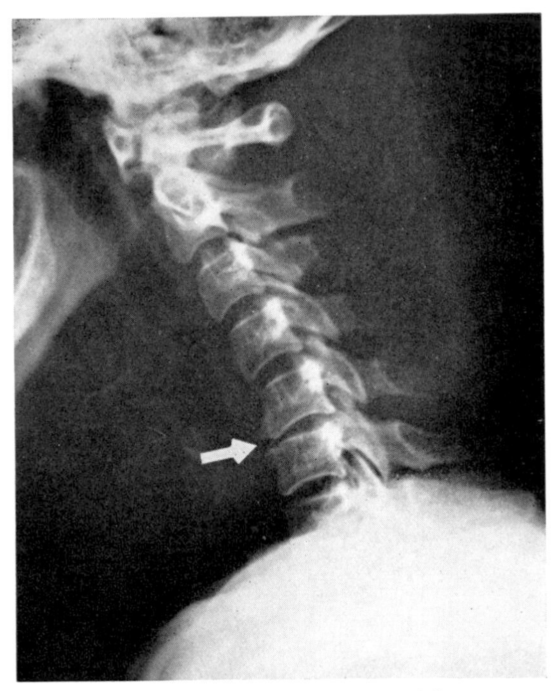

Figure 20–2. Narrowing of the disc space (arrow) between C5 and C6, associated with osteophyte formation along the anterior margin. There is also a sharp angulation of the cervical spine centered at the C5–C6 level, which may indicate that this is the fulcrum of motion. A herniated intervertebral disc was encountered at C5–C6.

in the direction of the spinal canal, or anteriorly, in front of the vertebral bodies.

The limiting ligaments, particularly the posterior longitudinal ligaments, are weaker laterally, and therefore the characteristic lie of the protruded portion of the disc material is lateral, near the site of exit of the nerve roots. If for special reasons the entire posterior longitudinal ligament is weak or weakened, the disc may protrude or extrude uniformly across the canal and come to lie under the spinal cord itself, rather than laterally under the root. Anterior protrusions are of no particular moment or interest here, except as evidence of mechanical abnormality. When the disc material leaves its normal space, a chemical alteration of its contents takes place fairly rapidly. If the protruded portion does not involve the cord or nerve root at a critical point, it may lose fluid rapidly and shrink. It is then covered by fibrous scar tissue and there may be no clinical evidence of its presence. Roentgenography will eventually show characteristic changes of loss of height of the disc space.

Several other related phenomena, however, may take place to alter the eventual course toward the appearance of syndromes of cord or root compression. As soon as disc material protrudes and there is a change in the consistency, volume, and compressibility of the disc, there is a focal collection of stress at this level. Ordinarily motion in the cervical spine is incremental, with very little evidence of a fulcrum at any single joint.

Now, however, as the stress collects, there is pathological wear and tear. The apophyseal joints begin to show arthritic changes. Nature responds to the changes in motion pattern by throwing up arthritic spurs in an attempt to stabilize the area, or merely as a reaction to the abnormal stress. At the same time, at the abutting vertebral margins where the posterior longitudinal ligament and annulus have been disrupted by the nuclear protrusion, a similar reaction takes place. A panniculus of granulation tissue makes its way outward, and spurs begin to form at the vertebral margins (Fig. 20–2). This reaction tends to compromise further the intraspinal space already encroached upon by the disc extrusion.

The stage is now set for compromise of the root as it passes through the foramen, or of the spinal cord, or of both, depending on the size of the disc and whether there is a vigorous arthritic reaction on the posterior aspect of the canal. Where the sequential changes are abrupt and the protrusion is in position to critically compromise the cord or root, the symptoms become apparent early. However, they may not arise until much later in life. With age, there is a change in cervical posture and muscular tone. The spinal canal tends to become gradually narrowed by arthritic changes at various levels. The protruded disc and tissues changed in response to it may then lie closer to the cord, or truly encroach upon it in various positions. In addition, the cord and root may be more vulnerable in that the vessels supplying them blood may have become arteriosclerotic and much more sensitive to trauma. Other variables include anomalies of anteroposterior and lateral diameters of intraspinal space, making the intraspinal space smaller and more vulnerable to any encroachment. Minor or major trauma in a previously well stabilized situation may unfavorably alter the relationships in the intraspinal space by causing edema, further reactive arthritic proliferation, or even further herniation.

Cord Compression by Disc

Cord compression by disc may appear insidiously over a long period of time. Since the anterior aspect of the cord is involved, the syndromes thus created can be very similar to those seen with degenerative diseases of the spinal cord. The compression may be constant or intermittent, depending on posture and on the effect of senescent or pathologic changes in the dynamics of motion. It may chiefly reflect the changes secondary to interference with the anterior blood supply of the cord. In many cases the syndromes are almost indistinguishable from those of ventral tumors or degenerative disease. In early stages the signs may be primarily long-tract in type, with spasticity and sphincteric changes predominating.

There may be focal atrophies at the corresponding segmental levels of the cord, due to compression of the nuclear centers supplying the muscles of the shoulder girdle and upper extremities. When the anterior blood supply is specially vulnerable, the syndromes may be more devastating and the cord involvement more complete. The differential diagnosis of these groups of disorders depends on exhaustive neurological work-up, including myelography. From the standpoint of clinical diagnosis, a careful

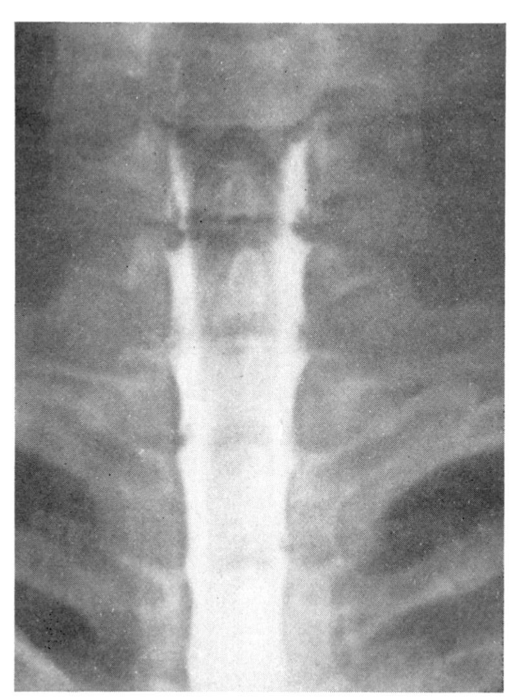

Figure 20–3. Myelogram demonstrating a complete block to the cephalad flow of Pantopaque at the level of the upper margin of C7. Note that the spinal cord (indicated by the radiolucent band in the center of the oil column) suddenly becomes wide just before reaching the point of obstruction. This indicates that the cord is compressed at this point. The cord compression here was due to a large herniation of the C6–C7 intervertebral disc.

history highlighting previous trauma, local discomfort, and lack of other stigmata of demyelinating disease is important. The presence of focal arthritic changes along with alteration in alignment and the fulcrum of motion at a significant vertebral level must throw suspicion on mechanical compression as opposed to degenerative disease.

The ultimate diagnosis must be made by myelography (Fig. 20–3) and spinal fluid studies. Massive, acute extrusion of the disc rarely occurs, except when there has been obvious violent trauma to the vertebral column. This is quite unlike the situation regarding the thoracic region, where previous juvenile disease may leave weakened posterior longitudinal ligaments and allow the occurrence of such extrusions without obvious trauma. Massive extrusion of the disc must be suspected when there is functional evidence of partial or complete transection of the cord despite roentgenographic finding of apparently innocuous fractures or dislocation. In such instances, a deceptive ease of reduction of fracture-dislocations by simple forms of traction may paradoxically denote avulsion of anterior and posterior longitudinal ligaments sufficient to have permitted gross extrusion of the disc into the canal. The so-called recoil injury, implying excursion of the vertebral body against the cervical spinal cord, probably represents in some part disc protrusion against the ventral aspect of the cord rather than slippage of the vertebral body with full and complete return to normal position. It is difficult to comprehend how the latter event could occur without a great deal of evidence of joint injury, at the very least.

The Laterally Placed Disc

When a disc protrudes or extrudes laterally at the most vulnerable point, namely, the site of exit of a nerve root from the canal, the root is caught between the site of its emergence from the cord and its foramen of exit laterally. The course of the root of cervical nerves to the foramen is short, compared with that of the root of lumbar nerves, and there is very little opportunity for the cervical root to slide off of the protuberant mass. If the compression takes place rapidly, the impact on the root may cause edema. This, along with the pressure of the disc on the root, may disturb the blood supply of the nerve, particularly the venous return. The chain of events acts as a vicious cycle in increasing the size of the root and its lack of sufficient space as it passes through the small foramen. The crucial elements in the long-term syndrome lie in the degree of compromise of the root by the actual protrusion versus the part played by edema. Further proliferative change at the vertebral margin in the region of the joints of Luschka and the foramen itself acts to further compromise the root. If the protruding mass is large, the blood supply of the root may be so compromised as to lead to a rapid loss of motor and sensory function in the areas supplied by the root. The adjacent roots may be put on stretch, and the adjacent lateral aspect of the cord may be involved to give an even more florid syndrome.

Symptoms. Although there is a classic picture of lateral cervical disc protrusion, it must be remembered that there are many possible variations, just as there are variations in the patient's appreciation of the symptom complex. Most commonly, the first symptoms are of interference with neck motion, with stiff neck the cardinal feature. Marked tenderness is noted at the paravertebral border of the scapula on the involved side. This always accompanies splinting of the erector capitii muscles, and does not represent a myositic area or so-called trigger point of local muscular pathology. Treatment focused upon it is far removed from the site of the actual lesion.

The head may be held in various fixed positions, depending on the lie of the disc and the opportunity of relieving the pressure on the root by such posturing. This is a clue to the fact that cervical traction, to prove useful, must be exerted in the direction which affords the patient relief of symptoms and not in any classical position of lordosis or extension. Mechanical neck symptoms may ebb or remain severe, or be replaced by vague shoulder cap pain. At this stage there is opportunity for great confusion with local lesions of the shoulder. At times, it is almost impossible to differentiate the two at any early stage. However, there comes to be engrafted upon the vague diffuse pain a truly radicular component, which follows anatomically the course of the involved root and its sensory dermatome. At this juncture, the patient ordinarily notes paresthesias or numbness in the involved dermatome. There may, likewise, be weakness of the muscle group supplied by the nerve root. Actual neuritic tenderness of the peripheral branches supplied by the root may be present when the root compression is severe and protracted.

Sites of Predilection of Disc Protrusion in the Cervical Region

Although motion in the cervical spine is incremental, there is more motion at C5–C6 and C6–C7 than elsewhere. Accordingly, more stress falls in these areas, and disc protrusion and wear and tear of the ligamentous structure occur more frequently here than elsewhere. With advancing age one notes by x-ray increasing narrowing of the disc at the cervicothoracic junction which is unrelated to special symptom complexes. At this level protrusions occur more frequently than at the C4–C5 level. Disc protrusion is much less commonly seen at the C2–C3 level, and, of course, at C1–C2 true disc protrusions cannot occur.

Cardinal Features of Root Involvement at Various Levels

The third cervical root, which makes its exit between C2 and C3, is rarely affected. The characteristic feature of its involvement is pain in the suboccipital and occipitoparietal regions in the realm of the sensory dermatome. The erector capitii muscles splint vigorously. Similarly, the fourth cervical root is infrequently implicated in true lateral disc protrusion. Splinting of the erector capitii muscles and myalgic type pain in the shoulder girdle muscles usually occur. Focal atrophies and sensory patterns of characteristic type are not necessarily present.

Encroachment on the *fifth cervical root* is not difficult to discern. The only confusion lies in shoulder cap pain due to cuff tears or inflammation of the bursae. The largest burden of motor supply of the deltoid muscle comes from the fifth cervical root. This muscle atrophies perceptibly and rapidly. Pain and sensory changes are noted over the muscle. The biceps jerk may be depressed. The presence of neck pain, and the absence of mechanical exacerbation on movement of the arm, help in the differential diagnosis from shoulder lesions.

Compression of the *sixth cervical root* may lead to atrophy in the realm of the pectoral, biceps, and triceps muscles, along with a sensory defect along the lateral side of the upper arm and in the thumb and possibly the first fingers. The biceps and possibly triceps reflexes may be depressed.

The *seventh cervical root* may manifest itself as the site of pathology by numbness in the thumb and in the first and possibly the second finger, along with wasting of the triceps and brachioradialis muscles, and the pectoral muscle. The triceps reflex may be depressed or absent. There may be obvious weakness in the extensors of the wrist.

The *eighth cervical root* has a characteristic pattern of involvement, with implication of the intrinsic muscles of the hand and sensory changes in the fifth and possibly the fourth finger. One looks carefully for the presence of Horner's syndrome, due to implication of the autonomic fibers coursing with the root. Narrowing of the palpebral fissure is the most obvious aspect of this syndrome. Its presence should also call to mind the possibility of a superior sulcus tumor of the lung as a major differential diagnostic possibility.

Diagnostic Aids

Roentgenographic examination, including anteroposterior, lateral, and oblique views, is all-important. Evidences of focal changes at a single level, such as disc narrowing, unique arthritic spurring, or foraminal encroachment, may be valuable in correlation with the clinical data. Loss of normal lordosis, indicating muscle splinting, may be a clue to the presence of a cervical rather than a shoulder girdle lesion. Spinal fluid studies per se are not very helpful. The protein may be elevated to a moderate degree.

Pantopaque myelography is the most valuable item in the final diagnosis (Fig. 20–4). Skillful myelography can determine the level of root impingement, its severity, along with the presence of cord widening or compression, and even resulting vascular distortion. All these factors enter into determination of the operative approach and the ultimate decision as to whether operation or conservative treatment would prove the wiser choice. Lateral roentgenograms are absolutely necessary to determine whether there is encroachment on the ventral aspect of the cord.

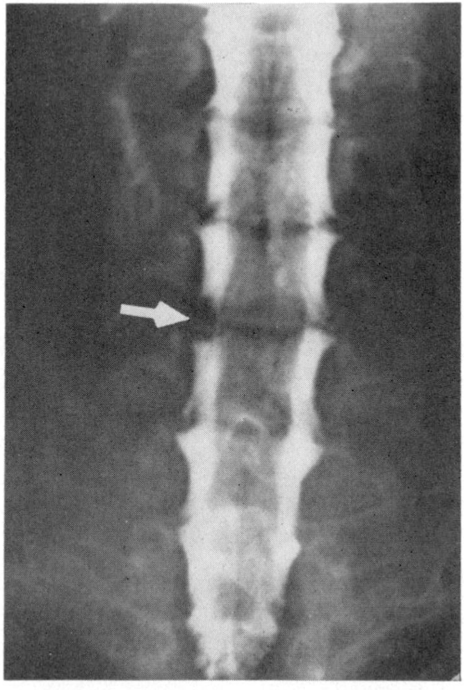

Figure 20–4. Herniated intervertebral disc at C5-C6 on the right side, placed laterally and producing a single root compression. Note the widening of the root shadow (arrow), in comparison with the appearance of the root shadows above and below and on the opposite side.

Treatment

There are only two types of treatment. One, specific treatment, involves decompression of the nerve or spinal cord by surgical intervention. This should be reserved for patients who obviously do not improve or, indeed, become worse on conservative treatment. Conservative treatment, unfortunately, is quite non-specific. Early careful attention is paid to attempts to reduce muscle splinting or spasm which creates the picture of stiff neck.

Any reasonable physiotherapeutic approach is valid here. Sometimes the dissipation of the splinting increases the symptoms of nerve root compression because the splinting is purposeful. However, if use of a collar or traction does relax the muscles and at the same time reduces the radicular pain, there is excellent hope for relief of symptoms by conservative means. The direction of traction must be related to the position of greatest comfort for the patient. Traction should never be abruptly exerted, and the force should not exceed 5 to 10 pounds. The goal of traction is to relax the muscles rather than to evoke a stretch.

Dry heat, for some reason, not only fails to help the patient with cervical radicular pain but often potentiates the pain. Wet heat, on the other hand, is usually gratifying. Massage and other forms of physiotherapy may or may not prove helpful, as may muscle relaxant drugs. At best, they are very inefficient forms of treatment.

Injection of so-called trigger points is commonly done, but falls in the aforementioned category of ineffectual or inefficient methods. Cortisone and its derivatives are widely used. One cannot attribute a specific value to these preparations. When there is an arthritic background to the complaints they may be of some value. Salicylates and other analgesics are a valuable part of treatment in tiding the patient over the acute phase in the hope of a conservative cure.

Operation. Operative intervention is reserved for patients who do not respond symptomatically to conservative treatment or who go on to show devastating signs of nerve root damage. One must qualify this point. Certain roots subserve important function and it is not conservative to allow their motor and sensory outflow to be destroyed. An example is the eighth root, which serves intrinsic hand function, and does not tolerate compression well. Long-standing compression of the *eighth nerve root* may lead to a picture simulating the post-traumatic dystrophic hand or the shoulder-arm-hand syndrome. When this happens the prospect of eventual recovery is very poor, even after successful operation.

The *fifth cervical nerve*, which largely supplies the deltoid muscle, likewise does not take kindly to compression. When the deltoid muscle atrophies rapidly an almost intractable frozen shoulder syndrome may appear. The *sixth and seventh cervical nerves* subserve rather gross muscle apparatus and one need not be too anxious about prolonging conservative treatment so long as its continuance is logical.

OPERATIVE TECHNIQUE. For the laterally placed disc lesion, operation consists in a unilateral approach involving stripping of the cervical musculature on the side of the lesion and exposing the laminae of the vertebrae above and below. Small portions of the abutting laminae are removed, exposing the nerve root as it courses to the foramen. When the root is adequately visualized the offending material is removed from beneath it and the roof of the foramen is removed in so far as it is necessary to afford adequate decompression. This may be an important part of the procedure if there is a marked arthritic reaction in the region of the joints of Luschka.

When a single joint is involved, fusion is almost never necessary, and the patients rarely complain later of neck pain. When the joints are involved bilaterally, fusion must be considered to avoid continuing neck complaints. Removal of a midline extruded disc or transverse ridge necessitates a complete laminectomy with a transdural approach to the lesion beneath the cord. It is a very different operation from the extradural removal of a laterally placed disc and carries much higher risks of complication. The dentate or denticulate ligaments may be cut to allow the cord to ride free over any residual ventral encroachment on the intraspinal space.

TRAUMA TO THE INTRASPINAL CONTENTS

Trauma to the spinal cord and nerve roots may be direct and due to actual penetration of the bony canal by foreign bodies or portions of the vertebral elements, particularly the laminae; or the cord and roots may bear the brunt of impact of massively extruded disc material at the time of fracture or fracture-dislocation of the body. The cord may be encroached upon by extradural bleeding secondary to vertebral trauma, or sustain a violent impact from abnormal vertebral excursion. The insult may be momentary, or a continuing one, as in bony impingement in fractures or fracture-dislocation. There may be an irreversible insult to the blood supply of the cord so that it continues to show increased evidence of destruction and edema in spite of removal of the original traumatizing forces. It is important here to emphasize certain desiderata of diagnosis and treatment.

For purposes of such presentation, let us consider a clinical problem as a means of developing a modus operandi in the management of acute cervical trauma. Let us attend a patient who has been found at the scene of an automobile accident. Naturally one's eye will take in the scene, the distance of the body from the car or site of impact, and other details of the actual accident. These are common-sense items and will enter into the final analysis of the mechanism and degree of violence of the injury. Assessment of the state of the patient and of the nature of his total injuries in terms of shock is paramount. If there is evidence of cord involvement, is it partial or complete? If it is complete, and the patient is conscious, it is important to find out from the patient or from any other competent observer whether there has been a change from partial to complete, or whether there has been some clearing of signs and symptoms. No information is more important in making a decision as to further treatment than knowledge of whether or not there was a complete transection at the moment of impact. Evidences of direct injury to the cervical region may allow one to make assumptions as to whether the injury to the cord was due to the

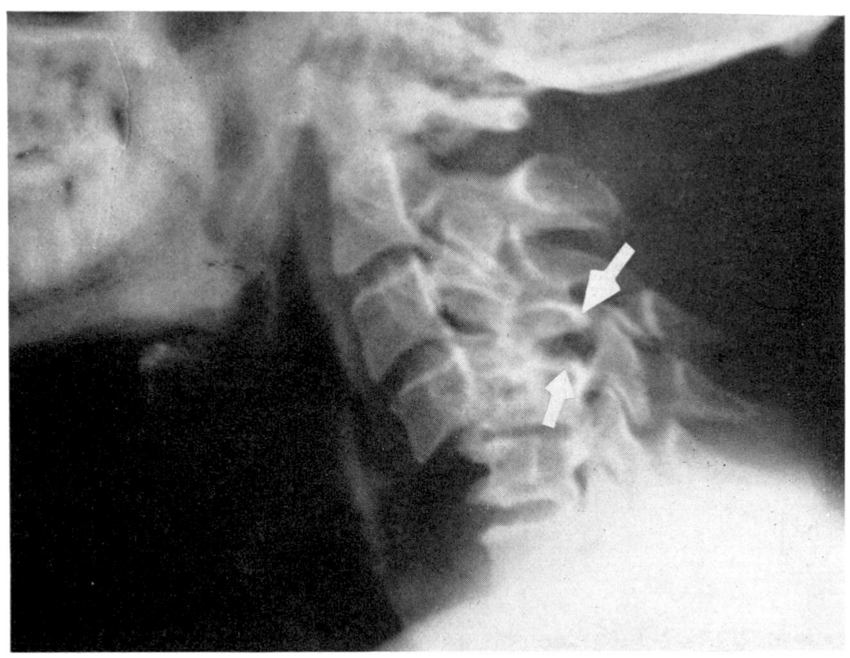

Figure 20–5. Fracture-dislocation of C4 on C5. Note that the posterior portion of the arch (upper arrow) comes to lie very close to the posterior margin of the vertebral body below (lower arrow). Although it is very easy to visualize fracture-dislocations roentgenographically at the higher levels, it is often difficult to visualize those situated below C6 because the shoulders obstruct the view. A great effort should be made to visualize down to T1 if nothing is seen above and a luxation is suspected clinically.

direct compression by fracture or was produced secondarily by abnormal excursion of the spine, as after frontal injury.

The next major problem is the transportation of the patient, assuming that all normal general principles of management of trauma have been carried out, including the reduction of shock. A great deal of educational data has been put forth on the proper transportation of patients with vertebral injury, with great detail as to the manner of movement and the position of the body. Unless an x-ray machine was available at the site of injury so that the exact damage and the nature of impingement on the cord could be determined, it would be difficult to predetermine the optimal position for carrying the patient. The only important principle is to avoid motion as much as possible and maintain the spine in the most fixed position possible during transportation of the patient, with a real attempt to avoid disturbing the status quo.

When the patient reaches his destination and further studies are feasible, roentgen examination must be carried out for intelligent and logical decisions to be made. There must be sufficient personnel so that the patient can be handled with the least possible disturbance of skeletal alignment. In the final decision as to treatment so much depends on x-ray findings that a diligent attempt must be made to get adequate roentgenograms with the least possible danger to the patient. Fractures and fracture-dislocations are usually easily seen (Fig. 20–5). However, laminar fractures are sometimes difficult to see, particularly when special techniques are made difficult (Fig. 20–6). When there is any suspicion of laminar fracture or impingement on the cord by bony elements, other things being equal, operation is a wise choice.

Let us assume that the x-ray films have been adequate and there is evidence of fracture or fracture-dislocation with a disturbance in vertebral alignment. In a patient with an incomplete lesion, the choice is cervical traction rather than operative intervention. Unless one has been intimately concerned with treatment of these injuries, one might casually assume that reduction of vertebral malalignment would be simple with the vertebral elements exposed. This is far from true, and traction is a much more efficient means of obtaining reduction in such cases.

Continuing with this same patient as an example, if reduction can be carried out by traction the long-term treatment is continued in the same fashion unless the patient shows signs of increasing cord involvement. In that event, operative decompression of the spinal cord is necessary to rule out residual compression by extradural bleeding or unrecognized fracture of the laminar elements with direct impingement on the cord. If x-ray films reveal no residual evidence of fracture-dislocation, especially in the presence of compression fractures of the vertebral body, one must seriously consider a disc extrusion or massive epidural hemorrhage. Significant disc

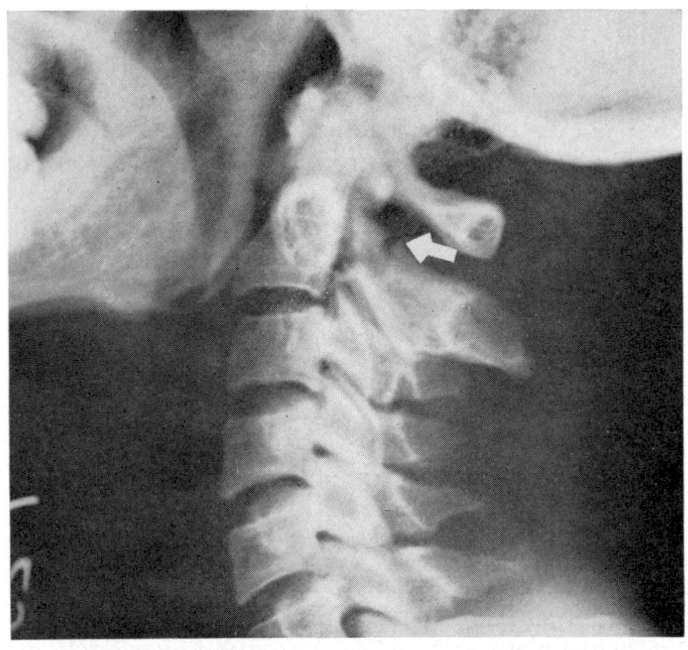

Figure 20–6. Fracture of the lamina of C2 (arrow) without significant displacement of the fragments. A fracture such as this, as well as fracture involving the pedicles, is easily overlooked on incomplete examinations of the cervical spine. A complete examination, including oblique and stereoscopic roentgenograms, is usually necessary when the pathology is not obvious.

narrowing will be an additional factor leading to the diagnosis of disc extrusion. In such cases a choice of operative intervention outweighs any considerations of conservative treatment.

In summary, when roentgenography does not allow one to make assumptions about the nature of the cord injury, it is wise to explore in the expectation of finding either unrecognized depressed fractures or disc extrusion and hemorrhage. Beyond that one gets more and more into the realm of philosophical decisions, based partly on personal experience and judgment, and partly on institutional points of view. When there is functional evidence of complete transection of the cord immediately after injury, without subsequent improvement, there is a good deal of debate as to the value of operation. In the past, it was easy to discount the value of surgical treatment because of the fear of the complications of shock. Today, with the able support of the anesthesia and shock teams, this factor cannot enter into a final decision.

There still remain secondary questions as to the effect of operative trauma and of the necessary intubation and positioning on the lesion. The ultimate question concerns the value of decompression if the cord has been severely damaged. Those who are against such operative procedures say that, if the dura is not opened to expose the cord, decompression is valueless. On the other hand, if the dura is opened and the cord is extremely edematous and protrudes through the dural incision, the damage may be irrevocable. Those who argue for operation answer by saying that, in this state of affairs, operation will have made no real difference in the outcome. However, they believe that opening the dura and giving a modicum of room to improve blood supply may lead to cord recovery, at least in part.

Various fine details of this argument may go on indefinitely. For example, there are constant family pressures to leave no stone unturned, and this may be a factor in eventual operative intervention. The presence of severe pain, particularly radicular pain suggesting foraminal encroachment by fracture-dislocation, would tend to sway the surgeon in the direction of decompression. It is only fair to say that many men, who have had a wide secondary experience during World War II and subsequently, are in favor of intervention under any circumstance. It should be borne in mind, however, that the completely transected cord, with a good history to document its existence, will not recover after any procedure, and the patient should not be subjected to unwarranted further trauma.

To sum up, exploration should be done in all patients with partial injuries of the spinal cord who subsequently become worse. Exploration should also be done in all patients with unexplained cord compression, signs, and symptoms; in all patients with compound injury; and whenever there is any question of laminar fractures. The course to follow in patients with immediate complete transection without any evidence of recovery falls in the realm of personal decision based on the individual attitude of the operator and his experience. When there is no question of progressive deficit or bony impingement by fracture particles, fracture-dislocation is best treated by external traction.

Special Features of Injuries at Level of Atlas-Axis Complex

The atlas-axis complex, as mentioned in the opening paragraphs of this chapter, makes up a highly specialized apparatus designed to allow a wide range of motion of the head upon the cervical spine. The atlas, upon which the head rests and upon whose co-joints the head may elevate or depress, revolves upon the odontoid portion of the axis. The odontoid at some time in its evolutionary past was actually the body of the first cervical vertebra. In order to maintain the proper relationship of atlas to axis, the odontoid must be held in check anterior to the spinal cord by strong ligamentous structures. These include the transverse and alar ligaments, which maintain the odontoid and the atlas on the horizontal plane, and the apical ligaments, which extend upward from the apex of the odontoid to the anterior margin of the foramen magnum.

These ligaments, particularly the former two, are very strong, and it is unusual for them to be torn. However, if they are avulsed, the odontoid during motion of the head and neck may come to lie against the ventral aspect of the spinal cord with devastating results. Actually, a trauma severe enough to tear these ligaments usually creates irreparable damage to the spinal cord.

Fracture of the odontoid may cause forward slipping of C1 on C2, with narrowing of the anteroposterior intraspinal space for the cervical cord, and subsequent marked signs of cord compression (Fig. 20–7). A great

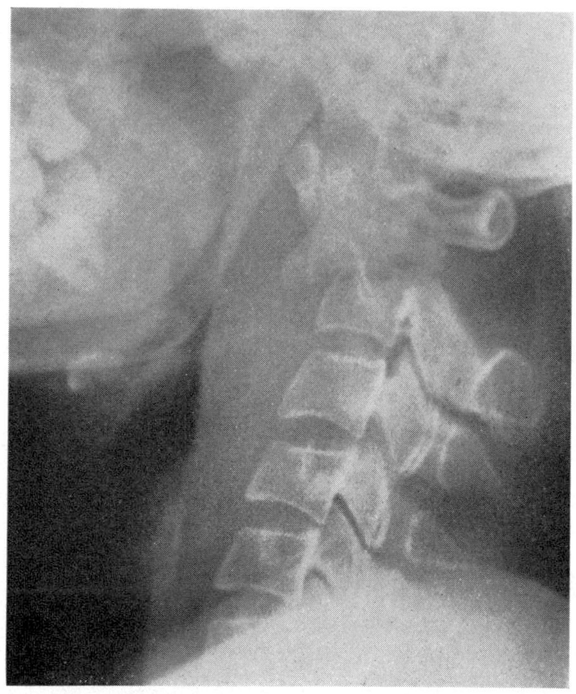

Figure 20–7. A fracture-dislocation of C2 at or just below the base of the odontoid process. Note the marked prevertebral soft tissue swelling.

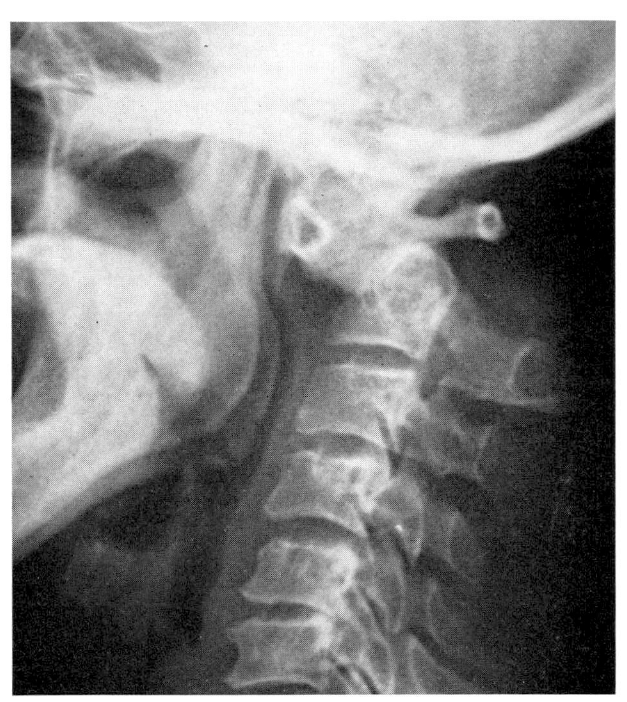

Figure 20–8. Congenital anomaly of C2—ununited odontoid process. There is a luxation of C1 on C2, which brings the posterior arch of C1 to a point fairly close to the upper portion of the body of C2. This is a potential cause of compression of the spinal cord. This type of anomaly is often confused with a fracture, particularly if the films are made after an accident.

many of the so-called fractures and fracture-dislocations of the odontoid complex are really congenital anomalies, without fusion of the odontoid to the body of the axis (C2), and a disturbance of relationship of the apex of the odontoid to the foramen magnum.

Various other anomalies occur, including very narrow diameters of the foramen magnum and the intraspinal space. These can lead to compression of the cord which is not clinically apparent except after injury. Soft tissue infections and nasopharyngeal infections anterior to the column may lead to ligamentous degenerative changes, caries of bone, and insidious dislocation of C1 on C2. Occasionally, a congenitally short odontoid process may slip under the check ligaments and come to press against the ventral aspect of the cord. This is the so-called somersault, or Marjolin, dislocation.

Adequate x-ray analysis is the major determinant in lesions of the atlas and axis. One must again emphasize the fact that an enormous range of congenital anomalies occur in this region. The presence of a fracture or fracture-dislocation must not be taken for granted merely because trauma to the neck has called attention to the region (Fig. 20–8). Careful measurements of intraspinal diameters, and preferably myelography, must be carried out when the condition is not too acute, to establish the need for decompression of the spine and foramen magnum as opposed to simple fusion or expectant care.

Supportive Care

There is probably no surgical problem which makes such high demands upon the combined medical team as injury to the spinal cord. The psychiatrist, neurologist, internist, urologist, orthopedist, and, most of all, the nurse, are crucially involved. Special problems are created by skin breakdown, loss of serum protein, and sphincteric disturbances. The patient with cord injury responds violently in emotional terms and generally withdraws from his environment. This makes care more difficult and militates against early rehabilitation into a more normal environment. Almost from the moment of injury the medical team must think in terms of preparing the patient for a well adjusted, socially normal, and vocationally efficient future.

Decubitus ulcers, contractures of joints, and bladder and renal infections extend the rehabilitation period by months and years. It is the responsibility of attending teams to think of possible complications early and to keep in mind the special psychological peculiarities of the ego-damaged paraplegic. Particularly in the male there is an immense feeling of shame and uselessness. Unless one has the patience and wisdom to make it clear to such a patient that these problems can be surmounted, one is likely to find him unconsciously sabotaging every effort at rehabilitation.

ROOT AVULSION

Root avulsion is an uncommon injury and usually implies force applied so that the shoulder moves in one direction and the head and neck in the opposite direction. Because of the nature of buffering of the brachial plexus, the impact or avulsive force often occurs at the level of the vertebral foramina. The roots may literally be pulled from the spinal cord. Careful examination may disclose evidences of long-tract involvement suggesting injury to the cord at the time of the avulsion. However, this may not occur, and there may be integrity of cord function with massive denervation at the root level. It is important to determine the level of injury since not only does the outlook differ, but exploration in the region of the brachial plexus and of the roots intraspinally necessitate totally different operative approach.

Electromyography may be helpful in delineating true root lesions as opposed to plexus lesions. There is a characteristic myelographic pattern based on meningeal herniations at the sites of dural tear (Fig. 20–9). Occasionally these avulsive lesions are followed by unpleasant and dysesthetic pain, almost of causalgic type, and it is important to recognize the level of injury in outlining efficacious treatment. It is obviously not possible to repair such roots under most circumstances.

The Brachial Plexus

The brachial plexus is a complex structure and the bane of most medical students. It consists chiefly in re-alignment of the elements of roots emerg-

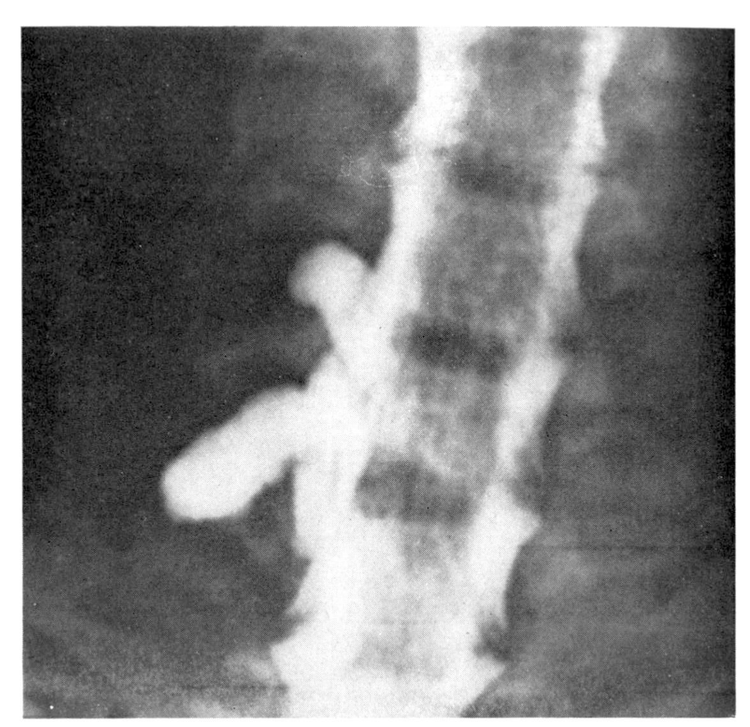

Figure 20–9. Avulsion of two of the roots forming the brachial plexus on the right side. Due to the tear of the dura, where the roots are pulled out, there is an outpouching of the arachnoid which is almost pathognomonic of avulsion of the root.

ing from C5 through T1, on their way to form the final peripheral nerves. There may be a cephalad shift for embryonic reasons, so that the fourth cervical root is also included in it.

Generally speaking, injury above the clavicular level affects nerve root, primary cord, or the direct muscular branches which take their origin from the nerve roots themselves or from their primary cords. Injury below the clavicle involves the secondary cords and their branches, so that the injuries would simulate an injury to one or more peripheral nerves. There are several important points to be brought out in order to better understand plexus lesions. The first is that the plexus is an unusually heavy structure in terms of its neural elements and its connective tissue sheathing. It is enwrapped in an ingenious fashion by fibrous tissue in such a manner that its terminations are snubbed, or, in other words, the fibrous covering tends to take up and diffuse any stretching or avulsive force. This mechanism plays a large part in protecting the plexus against injury.

In mammalia, generally, one finds a fascinating parallel between the nature and strength of the plexus sheath snubbing and the environment of the species. The gibbon, for example, has a most unusually strong and ropelike brachial plexus, since it is prone to be among the most acrobatic of the apes, using its long, thin arms to swing from tree to tree. The necessity of a heavily protected plexus is obvious, and nature has therefore responded with an adequate device. Nevertheless, severe blows which tend to separate the head and shoulder, depressing the latter and violently forcing the head to the opposite side, are likely to damage the plexus in spite of its excellent buffer. The upper fibers are more likely to be injured and occasionally even avulsed. Direct penetrating injuries to the plexus, as by knife wounds, are much more common.

In addition to the final elements, or peripheral nerves, which take their origin from the fused and reseparated portions of the plexus proper, there are a few branches from the nerve roots themselves and from the primary cords which should be noted. Their emphasis is important because they may suffer injury to which the carefully snubbed plexus is not vulnerable. They are the dorsal scapular, which innervates the rhomboids and levator anguli scapulae, and the long thoracic nerve of Bell, which supplies the serratus, along with the suprascapular nerve to the supraspinatus and infraspinatus muscles and the subclavian nerve to the subclavius and scalene muscle groups.

The latter three nerves arise high in the primary cords rather than from the plexus proper. Because they are small nerves, angling out from the plexus proper and unprotected by its sheathing, they are especially susceptible to injury both by direct violence and by unusual stresses. For example, the long thoracic nerve which is quite exposed as it travels posteriorly in the neck may be injured by direct pressure or by stretching in various vocational pursuits, such as hod carrying. During World War II, patients in large plaster spicas, lying prone, supported on their elbows, quite frequently showed injuries to the serratus from the abnormal lateral strain on the scapular muscles and concomitant traction on the nerve. Occasionally, secondarily after such an injury, the abnormal pull of the scapula away from the posterior chest wall is such as to throw stress on the suprascapular nerve and create sequential trauma and loss of function in the supraspinatus and infraspinatus muscles. Such injuries are often confused with congenital anomalies or muscular dystrophies.

In summary, the brachial plexus is carefully protected and only suffers avulsive injuries from blows of great violence tending to separate the shoulder and the head. Branches which take off from the roots early, or from the primary cords, are particularly vulnerable to special forms of injury and occupational hazards.

In terms of treatment, direct lacerative injuries of the plexus admit of early exploration and repair, with much more favorable results than avulsive injuries. Avulsive injuries infrequently involve the plexus, and the damage may be widespread, including vascular disruption. Exploration in a complicated field, without any definite evidence of exact site of injury, makes perfect repair almost impossible, and obtainable perhaps only at a price of damage to normally functioning neural tissue. Electromyography may be most helpful in clarifying the exact level of injury.

SCALENUS ANTICUS SYNDROME

For a long time the scalenus anticus syndrome was considered a major cause of so-called brachialgic pain, or symptom complexes now known to be much more compatible with cervical root compression. The actual syndrome consists in the clamping down of the scalenus muscle over the adjacent portions of the brachial plexus and major vascular trunks. Since the lower or inferior portions of the plexus are closest to the scalenus insertion, the neurological symptoms and signs are ordinarily confined to discomfort on the ulnar side of the hand and weakness of the intrinsic muscles.

Compression of the subclavian artery may lead to obliteration of the pulse in certain positions and pressure on the venous return to produce swelling and discoloration of the distal portion of the extremity. The scalenus syndrome is rarely a primary one; most frequently splinting of the scalenus muscle is sequential to a lesion elsewhere, very much as the low back muscles splint when there is root compression and radicular pain. It is most often a real entity in the presence of cervical rib. Generally speaking, it is not a major cause of root pain and most of the clinical patterns which were formerly thrown in with it have now been separated into better delineated syndromes.

CERVICAL RIB SYNDROME

The syndrome of the cervical rib is on firmer ground. Usually, the rib articulates with the seventh cervical vertebra (Fig. 20–*10*). It may have a

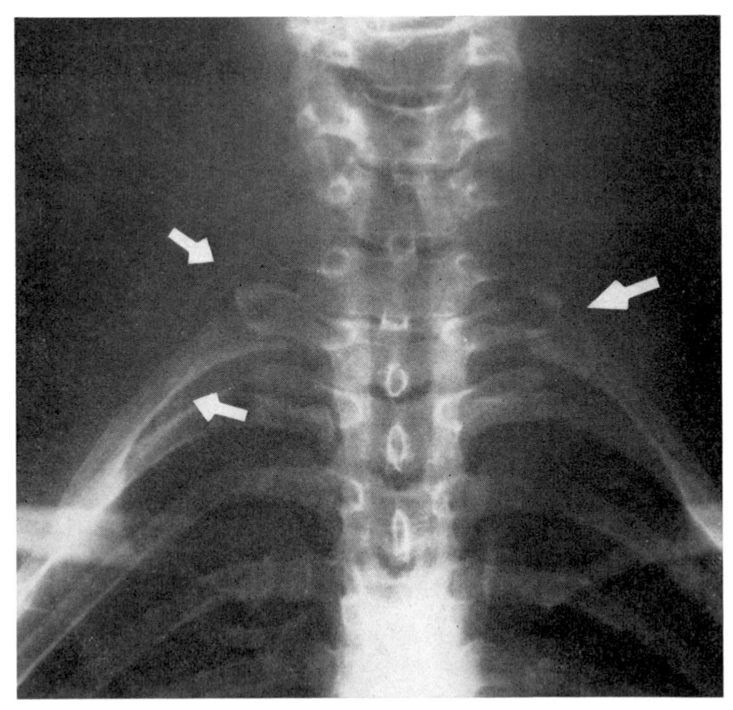

Figure 20–10. Anteroposterior roentgenogram of the cervicothoracic junction, demonstrating the presence of bilateral cervical ribs. On the patient's left side the anterior end of the rib cannot be visualized roentgenographically (arrow). On his right side one can see the posterior aspect of a rib (upper arrow), and then a segment where no rib can be seen, followed by another segment where again a fragment of a cervical rib can be visualized (lower arrow).

cartilaginous extension which is not obvious roentgenographically but manifests itself in the severity of symptoms. The anomalous rib causes pressure on the lower portion of the plexus with the most frequent symptoms in the realm of the eighth root, involving the intrinsic muscles of the hand and the ulnar side in terms of sensory defect. Compression of the subclavian artery may cause extensive vascular pathology, and acute trauma may aggravate the picture by causing thrombosis of the vessel at the site of impingement by the rib. The picture, when well established, is a clear cut one.

One must emphasize the importance of visualization of vascular structures at the same time as the brachial plexus is freed from compression. If a thrombosis is found it must be dealt with, or the entire picture will fail to improve. The gravest deficiency in treatment up to the present decade lay in the lack of recognition of the vascular factor in this syndrome. Operation must be radical so that there is no remaining question of relief of the compromise of neural elements by the rib and its fibrous attachments. Only under such circumstances can excellent results be achieved. The sudden appearance of the cervical rib syndrome after acute trauma, or its aggravation, should call to mind the possibility of thrombosis of the subclavian artery or severe stretching of the lower portion of the plexus over the anomalous rib.

CHAPTER 21

INJURIES TO THE LOW-BACK MECHANISM

By SAWNIE R. GASTON, M.D., and
EDWARD B. SCHLESINGER, M.D.

Low-Back Pain Due to Other Than Intervertebral Disc Injuries

By SAWNIE R. GASTON, M.D.

GRAVITY AND THE LOW-BACK MECHANISM

When man chose to stand erect and combat the laws of gravity with his quadrupedal motor-skeletal equipment, he fell heir to the ills inherent in the frequent inadequacies of that equipment. As the technical nature of the world we live in became increasingly more complex, and the mind of man turned to the production of labor-saving devices, the inadequacies of his structural equipment became intensified by the decline in his physical fitness. This has become apparent in our children, who suffer by comparison in muscle-testing examinations with children of other countries who live closer to the earth, with fewer conveniences of transportation and fewer sedentary diversions.

Man is a moving mechanism working against the effect of gravity upon his own weight and those additional weights he may carry, and he is obliged to fulfill tasks of varying muscular force in a patterned or in an unaccustomed way. To meet these demands he has an erect osseous framework with ligamentous attachments surrounded by a supporting muscular envelope and a covering of subcutaneous tissues and skin. The visceral, glandular, circulatory, and nervous systems nourish and motivate this musculoskeletal framework in a manner too complex for man ever to synthesize, or even fully comprehend. Above all, man is an individual with a mind, a personality, with work to be done and a life to live. This then is the subject of our study, and the focal point of our interest is a complaint of low back pain with or without radiation. This symptom cannot be dissociated from the foregoing considerations.

Whether it is abrupt or gradual, trauma plays a role in the genesis of low-back pain. Each individual possesses a physical endowment which permits a kinetic life within the boundaries of this endowment. Some by constitutional habitus and physical fitness enjoy a broad scope of physical activity without mishap. Others are strictly limited in performance, but within the confines of their limitation may also avoid mishap. Under such circumstances the motor-skeletal system is in a state of compensation. This balance can be disturbed by injudicious overloading of the ordinarily well-equipped performer or by less taxing provocation in the limited performer. Unfortunately, the precipitating event is most often completely unanticipated. The awareness of pain signalizes the failure of the motor-skeletal system to meet the demands placed upon it, and the cause of this failure is the cause of the pain. Our objective is to determine, if possible, where and why this failure occurred, and how to treat it.

TRAUMATIC ACUTE LOW-BACK PAIN

The usual history of traumatic acute low-back pain is one of an off-balance act of lifting by those accustomed to heavy labor, or an insignificant act of bending or turning by others not so accustomed. On occasion an unexpected cough or sneeze may initiate pain by indirect muscle violence. The patient is aware of sudden sharp pain in the low-back region, and may even be aware of a tearing sensation as though something gave way. Others state that pain was not remarkable, but they found it impossible to straighten up from a flexed position. The acute pain may subside and the patient may even complete the day's work. Usually, however, the trunk is immobilized immediately or some hours later, when pain on attempted movement intensifies to produce near or complete disability. What has happened to the low back structures to produce these symptoms? The multiplicity of anatomic potential makes identity of the specific tissue or tissues involved almost impossible; the immobilized patient is in such distress that examination is generally fruitless in localizing areas of tenderness and tests for localization of the pain cannot be performed. The sequence of events follows a primary and a secondary phase.

Pathogenesis

Primary phase. The original sudden pain is due to an injury to some anatomic structure in the low back. The tearing sensation may be a very accurate symptom of an actual tear of ligament, fascia, or muscle. The possible structures involved include the intimate ligamentous envelopment of the bony spine, articulations of the spine, or the muscle envelope. There may be a tear in the periosteum, at the site of origin or insertion of ligament, in muscle, or in fascia. Pain may be due to pressure on the posterior longitudinal ligament from a protruding disc, and, if there is nerve root compression as well, the pain may radiate into the buttocks, posterolateral thigh, and leg.

Secondary phase. Whichever tissue was injured, the pain provoked by this event acts as a trigger which sets off an immediate or delayed alteration in the physiology of the trunk musculature, known as muscle spasm, which, in turn, produces more pain which causes partial splinting of the back or total immobilization of the patient. This alteration of muscle physiology may be a purposeful protective reflex in some instances, but, with injuries to ligaments, muscle, and fascia in which the original pathologic process of injury readily gives way to the process of repair, the disability and distress caused the patient by this splinting mechanism appear out of all proportion to its usefulness. Elimination of muscle spasm is coincident with symptomatic relief of acute pain and restoration of trunk motion. The residual minimal soreness indicates the lesser degree of magnitude of the original injury which precipitated this explosive change in muscle physiology, and lends support to the concept that the secondary and not the primary phase of this reaction produces the major disability and deserves the earliest therapeutic attention.

Conversely, if the initial pain-producing stimulus is a continuing one, such as a fixed disc protrusion, which is not a readily reversible original injury, the muscle spasm and its concomitant pain and disability often persist despite the best or the most prolonged conservative treatment. These clinical observations give direction to diagnosis, treatment, and prognosis.

The Clinical Picture

Examination of the patient characteristically shows a list of the trunk to one side, with the erector spinae muscles on the convex, long side of the list palpable as a prominent, hard cord. These "frozen" muscle groups are in a position of maximum stretch and have lost their ability to contract and relax. The physiological explanation of this is obscure. If pain is unilateral, the list is generally away from the side of pain. If the offending lesion is a herniated disc, the list is most often away from the side of the disc protrusion. Occasionally, the patient is immobilized in a flexed position, and both erector spinae groups stand out as prominent cords. The muscle spasm in low back disorders creates a buttress of noncontractable muscle groups, which limits motion.

Tenderness may be localized, but more often the patient is in too much distress to localize tenderness, and tests performed to determine pain-producing sites by manipulation generally so intensify the patient's general discomfort that they confuse the issue, rather than clarify it. A complete examination after the muscle spasm is relieved affords much more accurate and useful information, and is much more humane. Early examination should, however, include a careful neurological examination of the lower extremities, particularly in the presence of sciatic pain. Alteration in reflexes, motor strength, or sensory perception, together with the pattern of distribution of pain, may indicate compression of a nerve root by a herniated disc. Such information alters both the treatment and the prognosis.

Diagnosis

Diagnosis begins with a searching history designed to reveal the mode of onset, whether abrupt or gradual; the absence or presence of previous back pain, and the nature of its occurrence and frequency of recurrence; and whether the pain has been incapacitating, partially disabling, or a nagging nuisance. In cases with abrupt onset, knowledge of the exact nature and force of the trauma, the patient's immediate response to trauma, and the interval between injury and the orderly succession of subsequent symptoms are diagnostically and prognostically significant. In cases of gradual onset and persistent pain, a daily calendar of the pattern of pain in relation to activity is most helpful. Information regarding the patient's ability to sleep and turn in bed, pain upon arising, pain after a short interval of activity, after prolonged activity, after long sitting, standing, or walking, upon bending or change of position, and the effect of rest upon pain often indicates what one may expect to find on physical and roentgen examination. The goal of diagnosis is specificity, and as much is to be gained from a careful history as from a thorough physical examination.

Physical examination is conducted first with the patient standing. The alignment of the spine, the level of the pelvis, the presence or absence of muscle spasm, and the mobility of trunk motion are investigated. Limitations of motion and pain-producing motions with localization of pain are recorded.

Dynamic structures often show tenderness which is absent with the patient lying prone. In the supine position the degree of straight-leg-raising is determined. The attachment of hamstring muscles to pelvis flexes the lumbosacral joint and stretches the paravertebral soft tissues. It also puts tension on the sciatic nerve. The exact location and degree of pain are recorded. The hips and trochanteric regions are examined, and the strength of the anterior antigravity trunk muscles is evaluated by tests to be described. Neurological examination of the lower extremities, including muscle atrophy and weakness, sensory disturbances, and deep tendon reflex changes, must not be omitted in the absence of sciatic pain. Information may be gained to explain back pain due to disc pressure on neural elements which supply local muscle groups.

In the lateral recumbent position hyperextension of the hip puts stress on the lumbosacral joint and gives more selective information concerning faulty mechanics at this site. The same maneuver with the opposite hip and knee held in flexion stabilizes the lumbosacral joint and places a shearing force on the sacroiliac joint. The sacroiliac joint, owing to its massive construction, is rarely the site of injury and pain. The structures of the lumbosacral mechanism are much more susceptible.

Examination is completed with the patient lying prone. Deep thumb pressure in the midline over the interval between the spinous processes of the lumbar vertebrae often indicates a level of tenderness with pathologic significance at L5–S1, L4–L5, or higher. Pressure is transmitted to produce intervertebral joint motion, and directly or indirectly affects their supporting ligaments. Superficial pinching locates "fibrositic" tenderness over the gluteal and lumbosacral areas and deep muscle tenderness of focal "trigger points." The posterior iliac spine is frequently the site of tenderness, and the interpretation of this finding is elusive. Its occurrence appears to be associated with faulty mechanics of the lumbosacral joint. Finally, the strength of the back-supporting musculature and the amount and location of pain produced by these tests are noted.

Roentgenographic examination should include the following films: anteroposterior and lateral views of the lumbosacral junction, right and left oblique views of the lumbosacral junction to show the pedicles and apophyseal joints, and a 35-degree anteroposterior tilt film to show the sacroiliac joints and sacrum.

Successful treatment depends upon accurate diagnosis. The examiner's vision should be broad to the etiological potential of back pain, and focal to the observed motor-skeletal signature of the cause of pain in the individual patient. Only then can a rational scheme of management be planned to meet the particular needs of each patient.

Treatment

Primary treatment of acute low-back pain is directed toward relief of pain and muscle spasm. As long as the initiating stimuli are readily reversible, relief of muscle spasm coincides with relief of pain, except for a mild residual soreness at the site of tissue injury. In the case of nerve root compression by a herniated or protruded disc, however, relief of muscle spasm may be much more difficult or impossible to achieve because the initiating stimulus persists. In fact, the pain may be intensified by relief of spasm due to further incarceration of the disc.

Relief of muscle spasm due to tissue injury, other than a disc, is relatively simple and usually produces a rapid response. One of several methods can be employed.

Rest. In patients with severe muscle spasm and marked disability, complete bed rest is indicated. To permit such a patient to remain ambulatory is to ignore the influence of the erect posture on the trunk musculature. The involved muscle groups are obliged to work against gravity, and, as relaxation of the muscles is the goal of treatment, the extra load thrown on the trunk musculature tends only to defeat the treatment. It so often happens that a patient on partial bed rest will feel comfortable lying down, only to have the list and pain recur after a few moments in the erect position. Complete bed rest can be augmented by constant moderate heat, as by a heating pad, to the low back area. This has a soothing and relaxing effect. Sedation is also helpful. The bed should be firm, with a board beneath the mattress to avoid sag and support the back. This treatment can be accomplished at home, with meals and bedpan provided. If the patient is hospitalized, bilateral leg traction, 5 pounds to each leg, or pelvic band traction provides a stabilizing effect on the back and aids in relaxation. Some patients find that the supine position and traction aggravate their symptoms. This is the exception, but, under such circumstances, use of the head and knee gatch often corrects their discomfort. The purpose of these measures is to afford relaxation and rest, and lessen the need of the splinting action of the frozen muscle groups, which respond with cessation of spasm.

Relaxants. An adjunct to bed rest in the hospital is the use of muscle relaxants to accelerate the relief of spasm, and to reinforce the effect of traction and recumbency. These agents include tubocurarine and mephenesin. Tubocurarine is administered intramuscularly in the buttock not more often than once every other day. The instructions as to preparation for injection, which come with the vial, must be closely followed. The physiological effect is a relaxing action upon the myoneural junction, partially blocking conduction of pain impulses. Unfavorable side-effects are few and uncommon, and consist chiefly of shortness of breath or excessive weakness. The antidote is 1 ml. of a 1:2,000 solution of neostigmine injected intramuscularly.

Mephenesin, known in this country as Tolserol or Lissephen, among various trade names, has an ephemeral action by vein, but produces a rapid, relaxing effect upon muscle spasm and, if such acceleration is considered important, it may shorten the period of recumbency. This drug should be used cautiously as directed, and proper judgment in selection of cases is considered essential. Its use is seldom indicated.

Surface anesthesia. Patients with less severe spasm and disability, or those who, on the merits of their signs and circumstances, are considered suitable for ambulatory treatment, can be managed in a different way. The principle of treatment is to interrupt the vicious cycle of pain, spasm, and more pain. Ethyl chloride as a surface anesthetic has proved its effectiveness over the years. The mechanism of its action, other than as a surface anesthetic, has been rationalized, but not documented. The technique is a combination of the use of the spray, together with gentle relaxing exercises. The patient assumes a lateral recumbent position with the extremity nearer the examining table extended, and the other flexed at hip and knee until pain is experienced (Fig. 21–*1*).

The area of subjective localization of pain by the patient is sprayed with ethyl chloride until skin blanching is obtained. The flexed extremity is then voluntarily extended and again flexed at the hip by the patient to determine if this exercise still produces pain. If so, the spray is repeated. If the pain has shifted, the new area is sprayed, and the exercise is repeated. No one area should be sprayed more than three times to avoid a skin burn, and not more than one treatment a day should be undertaken. The patient then lies on the other side, performing the exercise again with the uppermost leg, and the spraying is repeated. The patient is then instructed to rest as much as possible, and to repeat these gentle non-

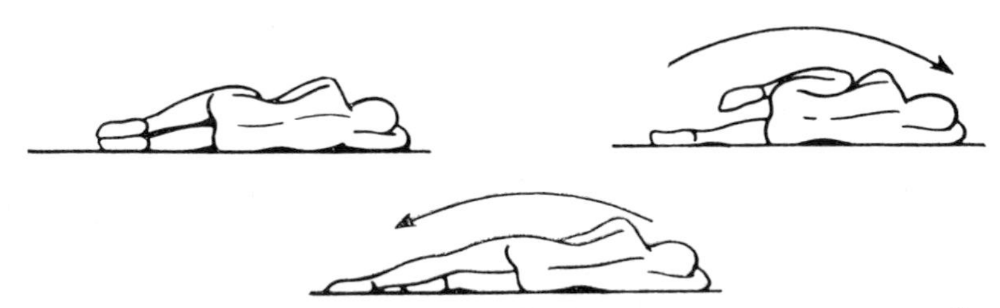

Figure 21–1. Treatment of muscle spasm. (From Kraus, Hans: Diagnosis and treatment of low back pain, GP 5:55, 1952.)

gravity lateral recumbent exercises every hour. These exercises provide gentle coordinated muscle action and allow re-education of purposeful movements within pain limits. As an office procedure, one must assess the benefit of the treatment against the stiffening and painful effects of travel between the patient's home and the doctor's office. This applies to any form of daily physical therapy. The journey may nullify any benefit of treatment, and the patient might be better off remaining in bed at home. In some cases, however, the effects of ethyl chloride spray verge on the spectacular.

Local anesthesia. Certain patients present, on early examination, a definitely localized "trigger point" area of tenderness at the site of their pain. This may represent a localized area of tissue injury, such as a tear or avulsion of fascia, ligament, or periosteum. In such cases injection of procaine hydrochloride until tenderness disappears may have an immediate beneficial effect upon relief of spasm and restoration of trunk mobility. The use of this drug deserves a mention of caution. Some patients have a sensitivity to procaine hydrochloride to a slight or to a serious degree. It may make them feel lightheaded and giddy, from which they recover within an hour, but which make it better to have them traveling with a companion than alone, or it may produce serious cardiovascular depression or a manic reaction. It is advisable to question the patient carefully about previous experiences with procaine hydrochloride and, if there is any question, to abandon the procedure or proceed with extreme caution. For this reason it is wise to prepare the patient with an oral or hypodermic barbiturate before the injection, and to use 1 per cent procaine hydrochloride rather than a stronger solution.

Aftercare

Once the patient has recovered from the acute phase of acute low-back pain there is generally complete symptomatic relief or an area of residual soreness which indicates the original site of tissue injury and repair. In either event, a careful examination should be made to determine, if possible, the cause of the failure of body mechanics which permitted the attack. Possibly there is no cause other than an overwhelming insult to otherwise normal motor-skeletal equipment. However, if this is the first indication of mechanical decompensation under stress, other attacks may follow, and prophylactic measures should be instituted when possible. Imbalance or inadequacy of the trunk musculature often can be corrected by exercises. Anomalies of the lumbosacral spine, such as a transitional presacral vertebra, spondylolysis, or spondylolisthesis, may be a predisposing cause. Herniation of a nucleus pulposus will require further conservative or subsequent operative treatment. A generalization can, however, be made. The optimal time to treat trauma is when the patient is first seen. The injured tissues are never again more receptive to repair. Adequate rest before the patient returns to work and proper protection at work should be provided, particularly with the first attack. Faulty body mechanics should be corrected by improving to normal strength and performance the first line of defense against subsequent recurrence of decompensation, the antigravity muscle envelope of the kinetic motor-skeletal frame. At times this implies the temporary use of a support as well as exercises. Acts of physical labor which exceed the ability of the patient's antigravity equipment should be prohibited until such time as the patient is able to perform them. For some patients this involves a change of occupation.

CHRONIC LOW-BACK PAIN

Chronic low-back pain indicates some inherent or acquired weakness in the osseous framework or its supporting structures. The grab bag of anatomic explanations is replete with combinations whose assembled mosaic satisfies some and dissatisfies other observers. The combinations are arranged and rearranged to serve experience and personal conviction. Many believe that low-back pain cannot be attributed with certainty to any specific anatomic feature. Accurate diagnosis, however, is the working tool of medicine and, despite the complexity of the problem, there still remains a responsibility to explain cause. Often the obsolete is a stepping stone to truth.

Categorically, chronic low-back pain will be discussed under the following headings:

(1) low-back pain of postural origin;
(2) myositis and fibrositis;
(3) osteoarthritis (with or without nerve root compression);
(4) unstable lumbosacral spine.

LOW-BACK PAIN OF POSTURAL ORIGIN

An intensive study of low-back pain was carried out in a large group of patients. Statistically, in the etiological analysis, the pain in one of the largest groups in this clinic was considered to be of postural origin. The history was one of non-disabling lumbosacral pain coming on in mid-morning, and increasing through the day in direct relation to activity and fatigue. Early in the course the pain would be relieved by rest but, as the symptoms persisted over a longer period of time, it would persist despite rest. The patients were women, and the onset of symptoms often followed some time after childbirth. This was thought to be related to relaxation or weakening of the abdominal musculature, and to the increased duties of attending the infant. There was generally a paucity of physical signs. Good trunk motion, absence of tenderness, and lack of roentgen findings gave no clue to the exact location or cause of pain. The possible relation of pain to muscle weakness and fatigue prompted the use of muscle tests to determine the strength of the antigravity trunk musculature.

Muscle Tests

These tests are performed as follows: With the patient supine (Fig. 21–2), the strength of the lower abdominal and hip flexor muscles is tested

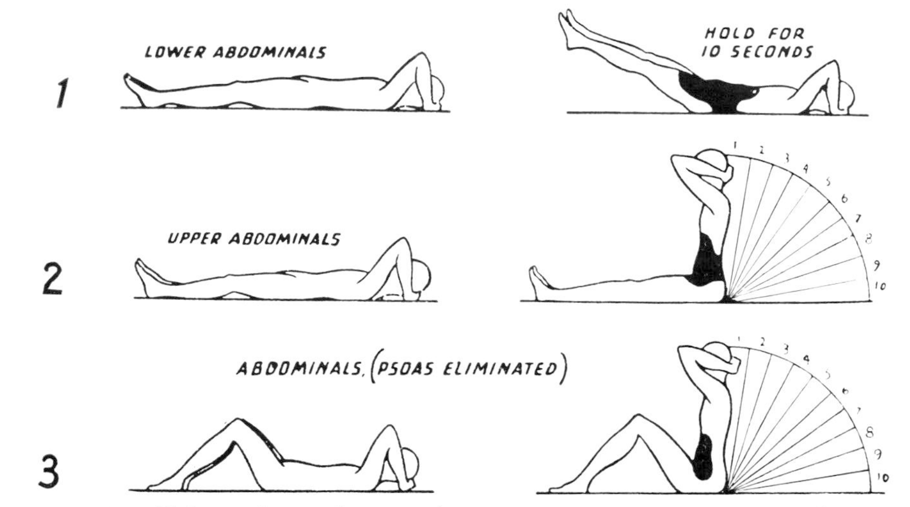

Figure 21–2. Abdominal muscle tests. (From Kraus, Hans: Diagnosis and treatment of low back pain, GP 5:55, 1952.)

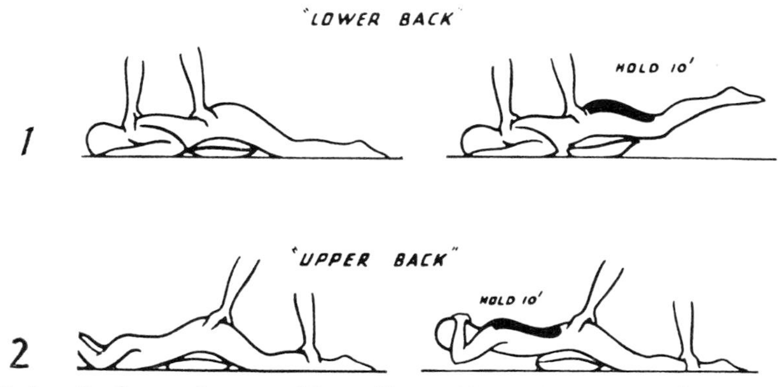

Figure 21–3. Back muscle tests. (From Kraus, Hans: Diagnosis and treatment of low back pain, GP 5:55, 1952.)

by bilateral straight-leg-raising maintained with the heels at a distance of 18 inches from the examining table for a period of 10 seconds. This can normally be performed without pain or effort. Next, the examiner steadies the patient's legs and the patient is instructed to sit up slowly to an erect sitting position with hands behind the head. Normally, this should be done without pain or effort. The abdominal musculature is further evaluated by performance of the same sitting-up test with the hips and knees flexed and the feet secured to the table by the examiner. The hip flexors are thus placed at a disadvantage.

The back musculature is tested with the patient prone and a pillow under the hips (Fig. 21–3). First, the legs are raised free from the table with the knees straight for a period of 10 seconds; then with the examiner holding the legs to the table for support, the patient, with hands behind the head, arches the upper trunk free from the table for 10 seconds.

The presence and location of pain produced by these tests is noted and, more often than not, the pain experienced by the patient will be identified with the pain of his chief complaint. These tests reproduce the patient's symptom complex, and the offending inadequate muscle groups can be identified. The tests are invalid in the presence of acute pain. A true evaluation of muscle strength cannot be determined until pain is minimal.

These tests provided such valuable information that this writer made them an integral part of the examination of all patients with low-back pain. It soon became apparent that weakness and imbalance of trunk musculature was a frequent finding in both sexes, and was not solely the aftermath of childbirth in certain women. Other findings added another facet to the pattern. The patient's ability to touch the floor with the fingertips without bending the knees demonstrated the tightness of the hamstrings and back muscles, and gave an indication of the reserve flexibility of the back in terms of sudden bending movements. Tight back and hamstring muscles not only contribute to the fatigue pattern, but delineate the point beyond which a patient may exceed the stretch of taut back structures and produce an acute insult to muscle, fascia, ligament, or other tissue.

For the present we are concerned with back pain directly related to effort, without acute disabling attacks and with only the muscle tests giving a clue to cause.

Treatment

It was postulated that weakness of the trunk musculature could cause an imbalance of the synergistic action of muscle groups with selective overloading which, in turn, could produce back fatigue and pain. If true, here was an entity identified with the supporting muscle envelope of the

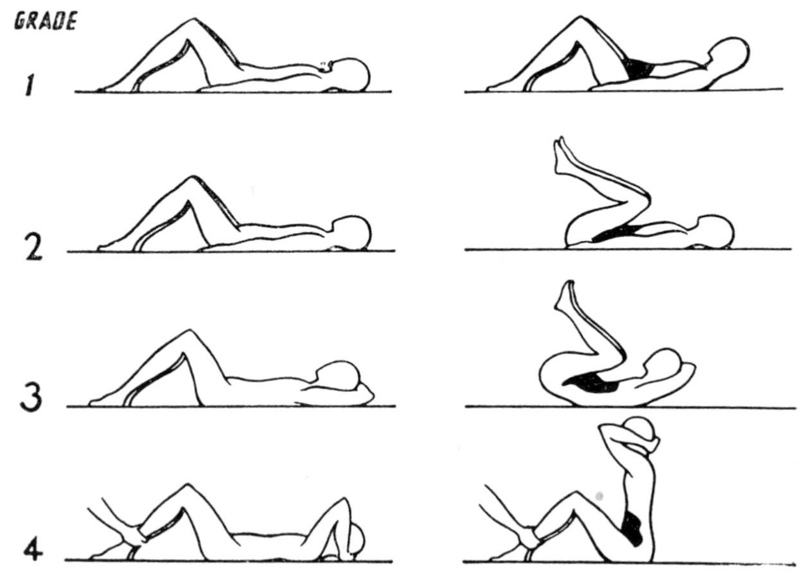

Figure 21–4. Exercises to build abdominal muscle power. (From Kraus, Hans: Diagnosis and treatment of low back pain, GP 5:55, 1952.)

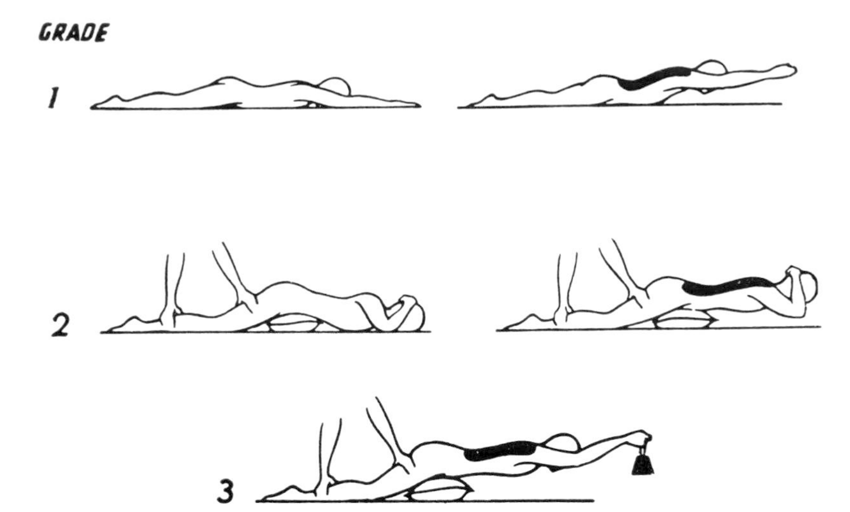

Figure 21–5. Exercises to build upper-back muscle power. (From Kraus, Hans: Diagnosis and treatment of low back pain, GP 5:55, 1952.)

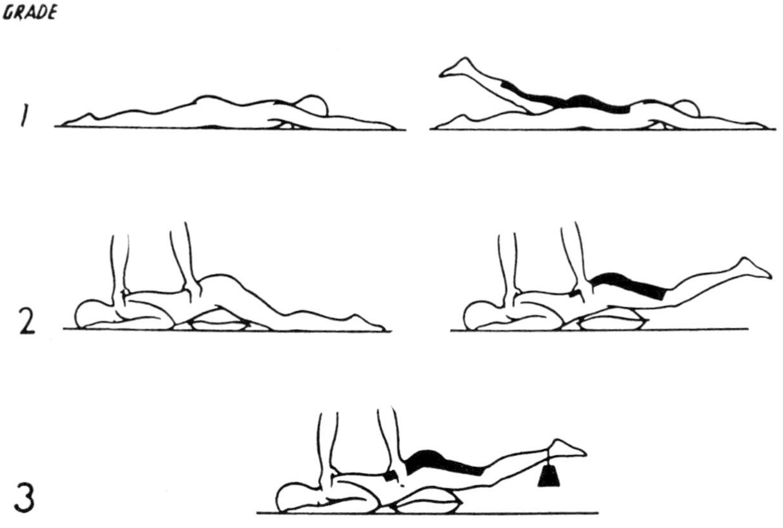

Figure 21–6. Exercises to build lower-back muscle power. (From Kraus, Hans: Diagnosis and treatment of low back pain, GP 5:55, 1952.)

trunk, and peculiar to its physiological state of fitness. To test the validity of this thesis, the empirical test of response to muscle-strengthening exercises was studied. When these patients regained normal muscle strength and balance, their pain disappeared. This program has been followed for almost ten years, and the results leave no doubt as to the cause of the back pain and its remedy in this group.

The program is as follows: The patient is advised of the cause of pain and assured of relief if the discipline of treatment is observed. A minimum of three months is required, and a patient who does not participate fully will not be benefited. Visits twice a week for supervised exercises are essential. Few people exercise adequately on their own. The exercises

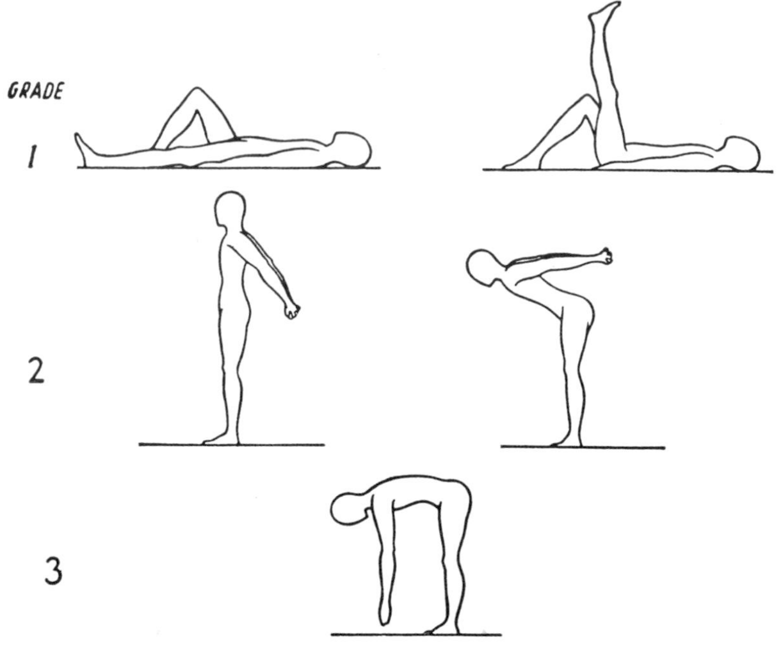

Figure 21–7. Exercises to increase elasticity of hamstrings and back muscles. (From Kraus, Hans: Diagnosis and treatment of low back pain, GP 5:55, 1952.)

are graded according to the exertion required, starting with gentle exercises, within the limits of pain. A daily program of home exercises is mapped out, starting with 10 minutes and increasing to 30 minutes twice daily. Very weak patients should exercise for a few minutes hourly throughout the day. These exercises are illustrated in Figure 21–4 (to build abdominal muscle power), Figure 21–5 (to build upper-back muscle power), Figure 21–6 (to build lower-back muscle power), and Figure 21–7 (to increase elasticity of hamstrings and back muscles).

Such a program, initially designed for postural low-back pain, has found application in the treatment of other categories of low-back pain to be described.

MYOSITIS AND FIBROSITIS

The multiplicity of structures in the low-back region which may be the site of pain has been mentioned. The skin and subcutaneous tissues are no exception. Examination by direct palpation may disclose a diffuse tenderness over the sacral and upper gluteal regions. Direct palpation, however, does not elicit the depth of such tenderness. Diffuse tenderness should prompt the examiner to lift and pinch the skin and subcutaneous tissues between thumb and fingers. The presence of exquisite tenderness when pinched indicates an inflammatory process in the skin and subcutaneous tissues referred to as fibrositis. Deep tenderness over the buttock and back muscles should also be investigated, and may represent an inflammatory lesion of muscle (myositis). This may be diffuse or localized. When it is localized, the areas of deep tenderness are referred to as trigger points. Fibrositis is treated by pinching massage, preceded by 15 minutes of gentle heat to make the procedure less painful. Diffuse deep-muscle tenderness is treated by deep kneading massage. Trigger points are injected with 1 per cent procaine hydrochloride and, if pain is persistent, the injections are repeated. These patients may require exercises for mobility and strength.

OSTEOARTHRITIS

Osteoarthritis is a disease of adult life, generally after the age of 40 years, which results from the wear and tear of everyday use and involves particularly the weight-bearing joints. Its natural history depends upon age, obesity, occupational strain and trauma, accidental injury, and faulty body mechanics. These factors also influence remissions and exacerbations of painful symptoms. Roentgenographic evidence of osteoarthritis of the spine is a common finding in patients over 40, but often exists in the absence of symptoms. Asymptomatic persons with osteoarthritis, however, are vulnerable to changes of occupation and trauma, which may precipitate painful symptoms, especially after rest, and which improve after moderate use during the day only to be worse again the next morning.

Treatment

The treatment of osteoarthritis is palliative. In essence, the pattern of treatment should include rest, heat, use of salicylates, and adaptation of the work load to tolerance. A bed board and lumbosacral support are often helpful. Compensatory mechanisms, such as the supporting musculature, should be tested and improved when necessary. Long periods of inactivity, such as prolonged sitting, should be interspersed with gentle activity to avoid stiffness. Heavy labor, once significant symptoms of osteoarthritis have supervened, may have to be discontinued.

OSTEOARTHRITIS WITH NERVE ROOT COMPRESSION

Fortunately, few patients with advanced osteoarthritis of the lumbar spine develop signs of nerve root compression with sciatic pain indistinguishable from the sciatic symptoms secondary to a protruded disc. Nerve root compression may be due solely to hypertrophic bony changes projecting into the spinal canal or encroaching upon the intervertebral foramina, or to a combination of bony encroachment and inflammatory edema of neighboring soft tissues.

Treatment

Conservative management of nerve root compression, secondary to osteoarthritis, warrants the use of a lumbosacral support if the symptoms are mild, or of complete bed rest with or without pelvic or bilateral leg traction, if severe. Radiotherapy may have a palliative effect. If the compression is due mainly to soft tissue inflammatory changes about the nerve root, x-ray therapy may be effective in shrinking the swollen tissues and relieving the compression. If compression is due to bony impingement and severe symptoms persist, nothing short of operative mobilization and freeing of the nerve root will be effective. This is rarely necessary, and should be considered only as a last resort.

UNSTABLE LUMBOSACRAL SPINE

The ambiguous term, "unstable lumbosacral spine," remains in common use, but is difficult to define except as a mechanical inadequacy of the low-back mechanism with a potential to produce painful symptoms. Often the exact site of weakness cannot be identified, but frequently the roentgenogram discloses a structural defect in the bone. The part played by many such congenital defects in the actual production of symptoms is open to some question, but it is generally conceded that gross congenital anomalies constitute a source of weakness in the vertebral column. Recurrent soft tissue injuries and abnormalities of the intervertebral disc often play an important part in the production of an unstable lumbosacral spine.

Recurrent Soft Tissue Injury

Significant tears of supporting ligaments, muscles, and fasciae render these structures, through a process of connective tissue repair, less well suited to their role of supporting the spine. Repair may elongate these structures, make them less elastic, or actually shorten them. Failure to provide adequate support through laxity or inelasticity, or a narrow reserve in flexibility if shortened, contributes to the ease of re-injury. Eventually, such a back may have such a narrow margin of performance without pain that nothing short of operative stabilization of the lumbosacral joint by spinal fusion will control the symptoms and overcome the disability.

Characteristically, the recurrent attacks of pain are sudden, severe, and disabling. The acute pain subsides with appropriate treatment directed toward control of muscle spasm and adequate rest and protection. During the interval between attacks, the patient is free of pain, examination is essentially negative, and roentgenograms of the lumbosacral spine are normal. Treatment between attacks is directed toward strengthening the trunk muscles, and stretching the tight back and hamstring muscles to increase flexibility and lessen the damaging effect of a sudden movement which may challenge these tight structures. Failure of this program warrants consideration of spinal fusion.

Congenital Anomalies

Anomalies of the lumbosacral spine are most commonly found in the lower lumbar segments. Four or six, instead of five, lumbar vertebrae may be present. It therefore becomes necessary, when identifying the level of the anomaly, to use a designation other than numerical for purposes of clarity. This is easily accomplished by referring to the last lumbar vertebra as the presacral vertebra, be it the fourth, fifth, or sixth lumbar vertebra by actual count. This designation is also helpful when identifying an interspace which is the site of nerve root compression.

Transitional presacral vertebra. The most common anomaly is the transitional presacral vertebra, which exhibits architectural characteristics of both a last lumbar vertebra and a first sacral segment. Such a vertebra is recognized by overdeveloped transverse processes, which abut on the sacrum to form a joint or actually fuse with the sacrum. This anomaly may be unilateral or bilateral. It is defined as incomplete sacralization if a joint is interposed between the transverse process of the presacral vertebra and the sacrum, or complete sacralization if this junction is a solid bony strut.

Clinical interpretation of the significance of this anomaly centers about its mechanical role as a pain-producing lesion. In short, is a transitional presacral vertebra an unstable vertebra predisposing to the penalties of an inherently weak back? The answer to this question is found in part in the correlation of symptoms with roentgen evidence of the presence of such a lesion, and also with the findings at operation for disc removal and/or spinal fusion in selected patients. The first offers this information. Many patients x-rayed for complaints other than back pain are found to have a painless transitional presacral vertebra. Secondly, at operation it is possible to demonstrate the degree of motion between the transitional vertebra and the sacrum. If the presacral vertebra is joined to the sacrum by one or both transverse processes, no motion can take place. In the absence of motion, no pain should occur. If it is connected to the sacrum by joints, motion is minimal or questionable. Consequently, the transitional presacral vertebra either is completely stable and innocent of pain, or permits minimal motion which may cause pain at its junction with the sacrum.

Major pain-producing stresses associated with a transitional presacral vertebra are believed to occur at the level above the anomaly. Disc protrusion associated with this anomaly most often occurs at this interspace, and rarely occurs between the transitional vertebra and the sacrum. This consistent finding suggests the transitional presacral vertebra to be more rather than less stable than the normal presacral vertebra.

Back pain associated with a transitional vertebra exclusive of disc protrusion rarely requires operative intervention. Treatment is directed toward the compensatory muscle envelope, with exercises directed toward restoring normal strength and elasticity, a bed board for night support of the trunk, and a supporting belt when required. Should such management fail and spinal fusion be contemplated, fusion should include the vertebra above the transitional segment.

Spondylolysis and Spondylolisthesis

Spondylolysis and spondylolisthesis most commonly occur in the presacral vertebra, but may occur in other lumbar vertebrae. Spondylolysis is defined as a unilateral or bilateral defect in the neural arch without forward slip of the vertebral body. Spondylolisthesis is a bilateral defect with forward displacement of the body of the vertebra. Whereas the lateral x-ray view is required to demonstrate the presence or absence of displacement, the defect is best seen in the right and left oblique views of the lumbosacral junction.

There is an inexact correlation between anomalies of the presacral vertebra and a painful back. There are many people enjoying a full, active life without back pain whose roentgenograms, taken for other reasons, disclose spondylolysis or spondylolisthesis. This observation is so common as to give the surgeon pause in interpreting the significance of this lesion. In the presence of chronic low-back pain which fits no pattern other than mechanical instability in a patient who has had an adequate course of conservative treatment without success, it is probable that the lesion revealed by x-ray is a cause of persistent pain. Such a patient should have a spinal fusion. The younger the patient, the less likely that a further program of exercises and support will relieve symptoms, and the more likely that the prospect of permanent partial invalidism will be unacceptable to the patient. The onset of symptoms after age 40, when the compensatory mechanisms are most likely to fail, justifies a more conservative approach. It is a characteristic of spondylolisthesis that, in addition to back pain, pain may radiate to both buttocks and thighs. Nerve root compression from a protruded disc can occur with spondylolisthesis, and it is the surgeon's responsibility to ascertain by careful examination and myelography if this is the case. However, nerve root traction on the cauda equina by the displaced vertebra can also account for the radicular distribution of pain. Under such circumstances relief can be obtained by spinal fusion alone. The fusion must include the posterior elements of the vertebral segments above and below the anomaly.

Herniation of the Nucleus Pulposus

Recognition must be given to the interrelationship between mechanical failures of motor-skeletal structures which produce disc disease, and the effects of disc disease upon the motor-skeletal structures. A normal disc functions as a hydraulic intervertebral bearing to facilitate mobility of the lumbar spine. A disturbance of its normal function affects the integrity of the contiguous vertebrae, together with their apophyseal joints and supporting ligaments, to produce an internal derangement of the intervertebral anatomy as a unit. Sciatic pain results from nerve root compression by a herniated or protruded disc, and back pain is frequently caused by the broad pressure of a bulging disc against the posterior longitudinal ligament. However, it is evident, by a process of elimination, that other elements in the intervertebral unit are also capable of producing pain. Back pain which exists prior to surgical removal of a disc often persists following disc removal. The exact site of the pain is uncertain. The intervertebral unit is unstable mechanically, and the signature of this instability is continued back pain. Stabilization of the involved segments by spinal fusion at the time of disc removal eliminates pain due to instability.

The practical application of these facts is of the utmost importance in advising a patient with disc disease when surgical intervention is compulsory. Should operation consist of removal of the disc alone, should the disc be ignored and only a spinal fusion performed, or should spinal fusion accompany every disc removal? The answers to these questions are a matter for mature judgment in each case, and are considered on page 645. Further elaboration is limited to a consideration of the second question. It is a grievous error to "pour the concrete" of a spinal fusion over symptomatic, uncorrected disc disease. On the other hand, one cannot help but anticipate the day when a "soft" degenerated disc can be accurately diagnosed and successfully treated by spinal fusion, without subjecting the posterior longitudinal ligament, disc, and nerve root to the needless trauma of exploration prompted by surgical curiosity.

Clinical practicability demands that there be a conservative method of managing patients with disc disease whose symptoms do not warrant operation, as well as patients with severe symptoms who decline operation. In the absence of evidence of progressing neural damage, the surgeon may temporize and employ conservative therapy. This is not always successful, but often convinces the patient that operation is necessary, and, as often, convinces the surgeon that the patient will recover without operation.

Conservative treatment is simple. Complete bed rest is indicated—in the most comfortable, relaxed position, whether with bilateral leg traction flat in bed or with a double back and knee gatch or whatever attitude the patient elects. The important purpose is to eliminate the load of gravity and put the involved disc at rest. Adequate sedation is essential. The imponderables include time, expense, and the uncertainty of the outcome. After painful symptoms subside, a brace should be provided when the patient is ambulatory. Operative intervention is indicated only if significant muscle weakness persists, or if the patient fails to achieve relief of pain commensurate with his threshold and obligations.

SPINAL FUSION

Indications

The indications for spinal fusion, from an orthopedist's point of view, include:

(1) x-ray evidence of degenerative or anomalous changes at the level of a disc removed for herniated nucleus pulposus, or clinical evidence of a pain-producing mechanism in addition to the protruded or herniated disc;

(2) pain-producing anomalies of the lumbosacral spine which fail to respond to conservative measures as outlined;

(3) recurrent attacks of severe lumbosacral pain due to soft tissue failures which interfere with the patient's obligations, and fail to respond to thorough conservative measures.

Technique

The basic type of spinal fusion herein described is known universally by the name of its originator, Dr. Russell A. Hibbs, who in 1911 first performed this type of fusion for tuberculosis of the spine at the New York Orthopaedic Hospital. Modifications have not altered the fundamental principles of the operation, although various additions have been evolved to ensure stability of the fusion in the immediate postoperative period. The Hibbs technique is designed to obtain a bony fusion not only between the laminae of contiguous vertebrae but through the apophyseal joints as well. Once the apophyseal joints and laminae are solidly united, no motion can occur between the vertebral bodies. It is the soundest in principle and practice of all posterior-type fusions.

The patient is positioned prone with hips and knees flexed in such a way that the lumbosacral region is flat, and the adjustable break in the table is at the level of the pelvis so that flexion and extension of the lumbosacral spine can be controlled during operation. Pressure on the chest and abdomen is eased by two large bolsters placed lengthwise on either side of the patient. Endotracheal intubation to assure an airway is advisable.

A midline vertical incision is made from the spinous process of the third lumbar vertebra to the midline crest of the sacrum (Fig. 21–8). The subcutaneous tissues are incised to deep fascia, and the fascia is incised over the tips of the spinous processes and the sacral crest. The spinous process and laminae at each level are then divested of erector spinae muscle by a subperiosteal dissection with a periosteal elevator, extending out to the apophyseal joint on each side. The ligamentum flavum is similarly exposed. The spinous processes, laminae, and apophyseal joints are completely divested of soft tissue by elevator and curet, leaving clean cortical bone (Fig. 21–9). As previously mentioned, a salient feature of the Hibbs fusion is inclusion of the apophyseal joints, which are prepared by excision

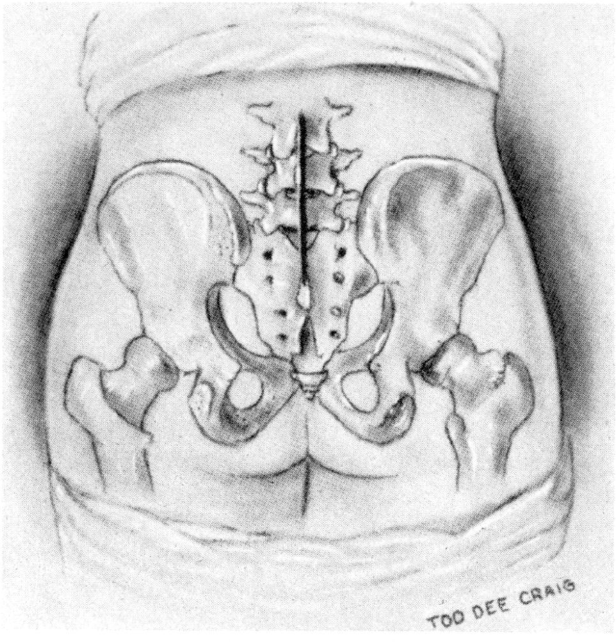

Figure 21–8. The skin incision.

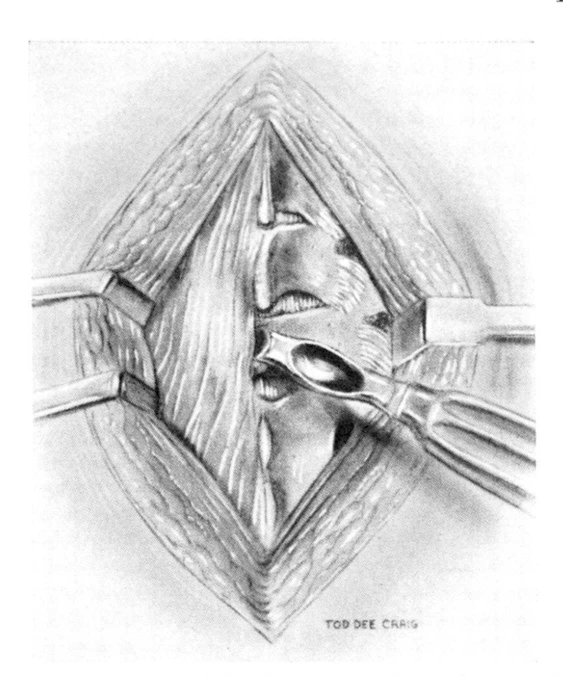

Figure 21–9. Exposure of the laminae and interlaminar ligaments.

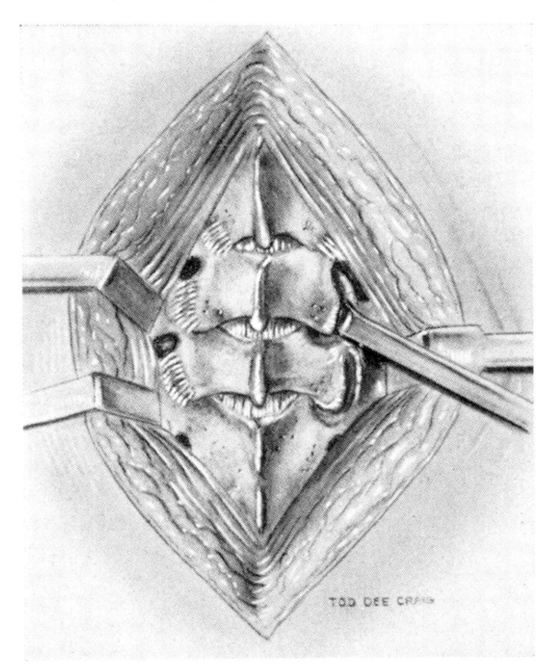

Figure 21–10. Excision of cartilage from lateral joints.

of their articular cartilage with osteotome and curet (Fig. 21–*10*). The final stage of the fusion is designed to fill the apophyseal joints with bone chips and bridge the laminae by turning bone chips up and down in an interlocking fashion from the laminae and sacrum by means of a gouge (Figs. 21–*11*, 21–*12*). Additional bone from the patient's posterior ilium, or from the bone bank, may be added in a vertical match-stick fashion. Modifications to ensure early stability of the fusion area consist of the use of screws across the apophyseal articulations, or of an H-type graft wedged between the spinous processes and overlying the laminae, in addition to the basic Hibbs fusion technique as described. The advantages of these

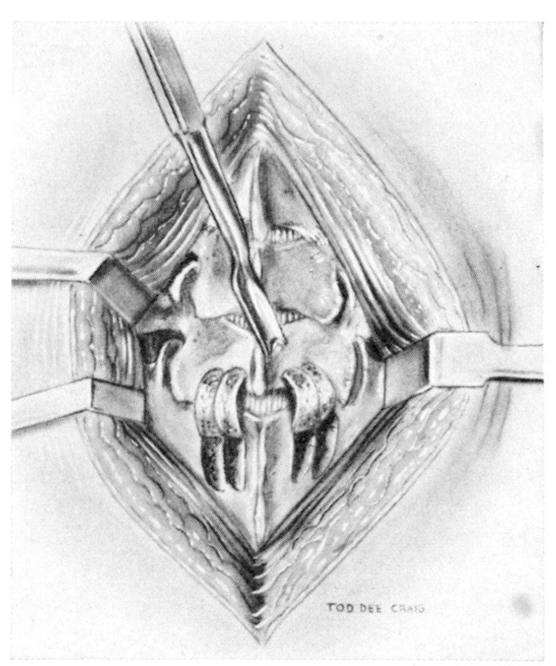

Figure 21–11. Bridging of the interlaminar spaces with bone chips.

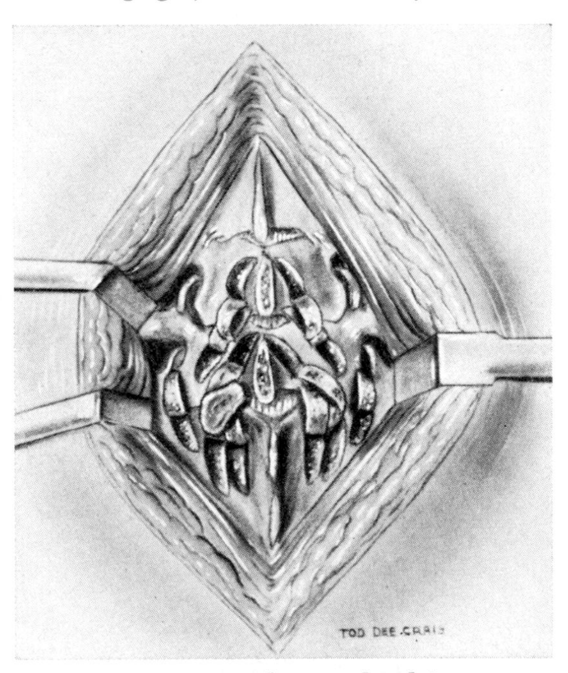

Figure 21–12. The completed fusion.

modifications are less postoperative pain, earlier mobilization of the patient, and possibly a higher rate of fusion.

Aftercare

Postoperative care permits free motion of the patient in bed within the limits of comfort, and out of bed with a Knight spinal brace or stout corset in one or two weeks. Approximately five months is required to obtain a "young" fusion, and during this period the patient's activities should be reasonably guarded. Return to light work in four to six weeks after operation is often possible, but lifting and bending are to be avoided. The relative maturity of the fusion in terms of heavy work can be assessed by x-ray after expiration of the five-month period.

Injuries of the Intervertebral Discs

By EDWARD B. SCHLESINGER, M.D.

THE BONY SPINE is much more than a static supporting structure. It flexes, extends, and rotates upon itself, and bears and distributes weight and force. One may anticipate that the actual mechanics by which all these functions are performed are ingenious and efficient. It is the modus operandi of nature that structure responds to the demands of function effectively or fails to survive. It is of more than parenthetical interest that the human spine has had to adapt to the change from quadrupedal to upright posture. Of equal clinical and pathological significance is the almost complete loss of muscular coat which has resulted from our urban pattern of life, along with such factors of minor disastrous significance as the automobile seat, high heels, and the debutante slouch.

ANATOMY OF THE INTERVERTEBRAL DISC

The actual structures which convey mobility upon the spine are the intervertebral discs, along with their limiting ligaments. These discs, which are fibrocartilaginous structures, lie between each two adjoining vertebrae in the cervical-thoracic-lumbar chain, except for the first two cervical vertebrae, which are subserved by a totally unrelated type of joint apparatus.

The disc consists of a gelatinous-elastic center eccentrically placed slightly dorsally within a tough, laminated casing of connective tissue known as the annulus fibrosus. The annulus abuts upon a cartilaginous plate at each vertebral body surface, and is firmly interwoven with the posterior and anterior longitudinal ligaments, which, posteriorly and anteriorly to the vertebral bodies, limit and bind the entire mobile spine. These ligaments are very strong and straplike throughout their course, but are most dense and broad over the intervertebral disc spaces. They tend, however, to attenuate laterally toward the region of the foramina of exit of the nerve roots.

The intervertebral space tends to rise, as a slight bulge, over the vertebral surface on either side, because of the attachments of the longitudinal ligaments and the annulus, along with the presence of the epiphyseal ring. Blood vessels penetrate the cartilaginous plate, but in the adult are not notably present in the disc itself. Nerve fibers of a type suggesting that they are chiefly designed to subserve pain can be found in the posterior longitudinal ligament and disc. Characteristically these fibers arise from the recurrent branches which re-enter the spinal canal through the intervertebral foramina after leaving the posterior primary branches two segments above their destination.

The nucleus pulposus consists of a gelatinous centrum of high water content, along with a network of connective tissue containing cartilage cells and large, clear, vacuolated cells reminiscent of notochordal origin. Actually, since the process of senescence begins at birth, the discs seen as pathological specimens are universally typified by degenerative changes, mechanical distortion, and loss of fluid content.

The cervical and lumbar discs are larger than are the thoracic, and wider anteriorly, which accounts for the normal lordosis in these regions. The thoracic spine, perhaps to protect the contents of the chest, has very little mobility. The overlapping of the posterior elements, the thin discs, and the heavy rib cage all contribute to this relative rigidity.

In terms of function, then, the cervical and lumbar discs bear the brunt of kinetic wear and tear, the thoracic discs sharing in the dissipation of force in even fashion. Since stress collects chiefly at the cervical and lumbar joints, it is here that pathological changes usually occur and clinical syndromes become obvious. Indeed, disc protrusion in the thoracic region depends upon a special and unusual set of circumstances, and is quite rare. Statistically, the sites of greatest motion and stress, as one might deduce, are in the midcervical and the lower lumbar region.

INJURY OF THE INTERVERTEBRAL DISC

Trauma is a relative term here since, unlike some self-regenerative organs, the disc (and its limiting ligaments) undergoes almost constant stress in its functions as the fulcrum of a lever, as a joint, or as a shock absorber. However, there are factors which unquestionably predispose to disc disease. One might list them as follows:

Poor structure—a fascinating array of inborn architectural defects come to mind, both bony and ligamentous. One young woman came to laminectomy for removal of herniated lumbar disc with a previous history of nine major operations in ten years of married life. These included surgery for abdominal and bilateral femoral hernia. She had four lumbar vertebrae, three completely extruded discs, and soft, oblong-shaped vertebrae of an unusual rarefied appearance. Yet, until she was injured in an elevator accident, she was free of back complaints!

Poor function—misuse of the low back as a lever in lifting heavy weights throws severe stress upon the lower lumbar ligaments and discs. If the muscular coat, in addition, is poor, the wear and tear upon the disc is abnormal.

Unphysiological abuse—actually a corollary of the above, but, as recordable incidents, injudicious stresses are prime examples of trauma. Any engineer can calculate the amount of stress which will collect at the lumbosacral joint when the back is used in weight lifting. Sudden strains are especially damaging when the muscular coat is unable or unprepared to dissipate the applied force.

Actual trauma—translation of acute force to the paravertebral muscles, ligaments, annulus fibrosus, disc, and bodies themselves; forceful shearing stresses, and acute flexion, extension, and rotation may cause tearing of the limiting ligaments, and severe damage to the disc itself. Sudden heavy weight bearing may cause similar pathologic changes.

HERNIATION OF THE INTERVERTEBRAL DISC

Mechanism

Having sustained repeated insults or a single drastic trauma, the annulus fibrosus and posterior longitudinal ligaments fray out, and the layers separating the disc from the spinal canal fray out almost to a membranous coat. Then, following even a trivial challenge to the joint by motion, the disc is squeezed into the canal. If the limiting ligaments are damaged but untorn, the intra-disc material bulges with them into the canal, and the condition is considered to be a protrusion of the disc. If, however, the outer layers and limiting ligaments are completely torn or membranous, the fragments of disc material may exude freely into the vertebral canal, and the condition is called a herniated or "extruded" disc. Ordinarily the more acute and intractable syndrome is associated with extruded discs. Chronic low back disease and repeated episodes of fragmentary radicular pain are more characteristic of protruding discs.

The posterior longitudinal ligament is least strong laterally and so is more vulnerable to disc protrusion there. The nerve root passes over this same weak zone on its way to its foramen of exit after it leaves the dural sac, and this is more likely to be involved than are the central contents of the dural sac. The canal is more shallow laterally and the exiting root may also be forced up and out against the unyielding wall of the canal. More medially placed lesions are unlikely to cause severe and constant pain, since they exert compression upon a dural sac consisting in roots surrounded by a fluid buffer. A median-placed disc lesion must be of fairly large size to be of clinical importance. The laterally placed lesion may produce symptoms when it is surprisingly small, if it is strategically placed under the root, especially at the foraminal level.

The Clinical Picture

Once the disc has herniated, multiple factors determine the individual characteristics of the syndrome. These include:

(1) the degree of tension on the root;

(2) the individual sensitivity of the root, and its ability to accommodate to stretch;

(3) the degree of embarrassment of the nerve's arterial supply and the amount of venous engorgement;

(4) the exact lie of the disc and nerve in so far as it determines the fibers (sensory or motor) sustaining the maximum compression;

(5) the degree of reactive muscle splinting;

(6) the nature of the lesion, its water content, rate of depolymerization, shrinkage, and its likelihood of remaining in a fixed position or increasing in bulk.

In the lumbar area the pattern of root compression by disc is ordinarily a single root syndrome. A large lesion may press on several roots, or create tension on one and direct pressure on another. A very large lesion may compress the entire dural sac and cauda equina. These latter events, however, remain the exception, and the uniradicular picture is the usual clinical entity. The greatest fulcral stress lies at the lower two lumbar joints, and they consequently bear the brunt of pathological change. Upward of 90 per cent of disc lesions occur at L5–S1 and L4–L5. The percentage drops rapidly, moving cephalad into the thoracic region, and involvement of thoracic discs is very rare and of special pathological significance. Accordingly, the two roots most frequently compressed are S1 (at L5–S1) and L5 (at L4–L5). The common muscle innervation by the lumbosacral roots is so widespread over the lower limb that the involved root is not easily identified by muscle examination. Sensory patterns are more discrete and reliable, and so have more value in determining exact root involvement. Nonetheless, certain motor clinical patterns prevail, which are useful to the clinician. The L5 root is far more frequently the cause of weakness of the calf muscle and great toe extensor, and generally the S1 root is less likely to cause any grave muscle changes.

The sensory pattern is quite helpful in localizing the exact root implicated in compression of the lower lumbar first sacral root. Symptomatically, the most common sensory complaint (other than pain) is tingling or "pins-and-needles." To most patients, this defines numbness. True numbness is infrequently noted. Physiologically, the sensory overlap is such that loss of sensation in a single dermatome is rarely perceived by the patient once actual loss of sensation prevails. During the earlier stages of nerve involvement and during recovery, however, positive sensations of single root origin are present, and the patient is aware of the exact realm of the involved root. This explains why, postoperatively, patients will often complain of sensations of numbness throughout the radicular area. One can easily reassure the anxious patient, given the preceding facts.

Grossly, the lateral aspect of the dorsum of the foot and the lateral three toes are in the sensory zone of the first sacral root. The great toe and, frequently, the second toe are in the realm of the dermatome of the fifth lumbar root. The radiation of pain and paresthesia is ordinarily clear-cut, and thus furnishes valuable clinical data. The radiation of pain of roots above L5 does not include the foot. Third and fourth lumbar root pain typically radiates across to the medial side of the thigh. Any pain which crosses the anterior thigh in a medial direction is highly suspected of being above the L4–L5 level in origin, and should be an adequate reason for myelography, no matter how classic the remainder of the syndrome.

The radiation of L5 or S1 root pain is ordinarily quite obvious, from the lower lumbar spine, buttock, hip, and posterolateral thigh, to calf and foot. Any or all of these areas may be skipped almost completely, and the patient may thus have seemingly focal pain in a single one of the above zones. The most diffuse and least clearly demarcated radiation is with the "bulging" disc and irritated root. Often, such pain is in the hip and upper thigh only, and is quite vague. Hard compression of the root usually has a more discrete and easily described radiation.

Depending on the "lie" of the root on the disc, however, the syndrome varies greatly. With great pressure against the posterior longitudinal ligament and irritation of the nerve fibers supplying it, the pain is usually in the erector muscles and deep in the buttock. The posterolateral ligament is supplied by the recurrent fibers of the posterior primary branch of the root two spaces above. This is the most atypical of the standard syndromes, and all the others generally have a radicular signature.

Tenderness along the course of the sciatic nerve is an unusual symptom and sign, and worthy of note. It denotes a true neuritic pathologic change, and signifies more than usual damage to the nerve and its nutrition above. Such neuritic tenderness also carries important evidence of possible irreversible changes in the root, and is of great prognostic importance.

In general, deep tendon reflex changes are useful in determining which root is involved, but have certain limitations in exactness of localization. For example, although the quadriceps is largely innervated by roots originating above L5, the patellar jerk (its stretch reflex) is frequently depressed and occasionally absent with compression of the fifth lumbar root. Compression of the first sacral root specifically seems to depress the Achilles reflex, but such depression may frequently be due to an L5 root lesion.

Because of the multiple innervation of lower limb muscles, atrophy and paresis are not always of firm localizing value. However, much more pronounced atrophy and weakness occur ordinarily with L5 than with S1 involvement. The quadriceps is largely supplied by roots originating above L5 and yet it will occasionally strikingly melt away with a lesion of the fifth lumbar root. In sum, motor changes are less useful as localizing data than are discrete sensory changes.

Differential Diagnosis

Disc compression as a cause of root lesions must be differentiated from:

(1) *extradural metastatic tumor;*
(2) *primary tumor*—especially neurofibroma—of the cauda equina;
(3) *neuritis*—especially diabetic;
(4) *lumbosacral plexus* invasion by extension of tumor of the bowel or pelvic contents;
(5) *obliterative disease* of aorta and iliac arteries;
(6) *myeloradiculopathies*—such as the Guillain-Barré syndrome.

Extradural metastatic tumor. Invasion of vertebral elements and the extradural space by metastatic tumor is probably the most important lesion to rule out as a cause of mechanically aggravated or constant back and limb pain. A complete clinical history and examination, along with careful consideration of the roentgenograms, blood count, and sedimentation rate, are mandatory and must precede the formulation of any decision about the nature of the pathologic process responsible for the syndrome.

Primary tumor. Except as an early neurofibroma, primary tumor is unlikely to create a uniradicular pattern. Pain is more consistent, and is less related to motion or position. Spinal fluid protein is usually significantly high.

Neuritis. True neuritis is infrequent, and is most commonly diabetic in origin. Paresthesias and dysesthesias, tenderness along the course of the nerve, and a peripheral nerve distribution, along with widespread involvement, are all atypical for the disc syndrome.

Lumbosacral plexus invasion by bowel or pelvic tumor. This is a common cause of intractable radiating pain. Once established, it is usually constant, unrelated (relatively) to mechanical signs, and of a distribution showing involvement of a plexus rather than of a single root. Early it may be a disheartening, baffling entity, affording no real opportunity for clinical diagnosis. At times, edema of the limb from interference with venous return is a diagnostic clue, as, of course, is the presence of a pelvic neoplasm. Any atypical, severe, intractable pain, particularly in the older patient, deserves very careful study before spinal operation is considered.

Obliterative disease of aorta and iliac arteries. Circulatory disorders of the lower limbs, both arterial and venous, deserve more consideration than they have commonly had. Aortography, in recent years, has made possible a clearer conception of the syndromes of occlusion of the lower aorta and iliac vessels. These syndromes are perfectly capable of simulating involvement of nerve roots.

Myeloradiculopathies. These diseases are not commonly uniradicular, but are capable of causing rapid atrophy, severe pain, and muscle tenderness and hyperesthesia with or without parallel general neurological signs and symptoms.

Clinical Examination

A brief summary of examination technique may serve a useful purpose. The patient's gait and stance are noted. Scoliotic tilt and its variation during bending gives information as to the acuteness of the attack, and the position of the lesion. Loss of lumbar lordosis denotes splinting of the erector spinae muscles. Difficulty in forward and lateral bending and hyperextension reveals the degree of root compression. Jugular compression by increasing the spinal fluid pressure may enhance the radicular pain and suggest a large and acute lesion. Straight-leg-raising, by making the root taut, may offer a gauge of the critical degree of nerve root compression. Observation of the comparative size of the buttock and limb muscles in the standing and in the lying position, along with a search for muscle flabbiness, fasciculation, and atrophy, affords a great deal of contributory data about chronicity, degree of damage, and level of involvement. Actual muscle power testing, except with the small muscles of foot and toes, is unrewarding because the muscles are too gross to show minor but important deficits. The sensory examination can be quite rapidly carried out, so long as the dermatomes are carefully compared, both in contiguity and in the two limbs. Examination moving across dermatomes is more likely to uncover changes than is comparison of like areas. The lumbosacral dermatomes over the buttocks should be checked for confirmatory evidence, especially when examination of lower dermatomes produces conflicting data. With it all, subjective sensory complaints reconcilable with anatomic structure are almost as valuable as, and are more common than, the finding of well-delineated areas of numbness on testing.

The reflexes are always tested in various positions with the patient relaxed, and the degree of their fatigability compared when possible. Muscles and nerves are palpated for soreness and discrete tenderness. Skin temperature is compared grossly, and all pulses are noted. The low back is palpated for tenderness, and the spinous processes are compressed for evidence of focal exacerbation of pain. Pressure lateral to a spinous process often elicits typical pain. The sciatic notch is also pressed upon, along with the sacroiliac joints and the gluteal and erector muscles. The hip joints and trochanters are palpated to rule out local disease.

Indications for Surgery

Indications for surgery are both absolute and relative. The former are easier to outline; the latter border on the philosophical, and depend upon an intimate understanding of motivation of the individual patient.

The specific indications include the following:

(1) intractable symptoms in the face of adequate treatment;

(2) progressive serious neurological deficit in spite of treatment;

(3) repeated attacks in spite of intelligent management—these may be not only physically incapacitating, but also economically disastrous.

Among the relative indications may be included the following:

(1) impending marriage or childbearing after at least several disabling attacks;

(2) occupations requiring absolute physical fitness;

(3) lack of response to a restricted existence and sound treatment over a long period of time.

All of the philosophical criteria can be summed up for the partially handicapped (with unquestionable personal integrity) in a single query: "Would you rather be dead than practice being dead indefinitely?"

Choice of Operation from a Neurosurgeon's Point of View

Simple disc removal is an unusually precise, atraumatic procedure, with no real price in terms of skeletal, neural, or general supportive structural damage. Convalescence is rapid and usually quite pain-free. Accordingly, one cannot be human and not think wistfully of it when contemplating the choice of a procedure of much longer duration, and far more traumatic and disorganizing to normal structure. After spinal fusion, the postoperative course is more painful and much more likely to be complicated by transient sphincteric disturbances, distention, and thrombophlebitis, and even personality disintegration. Convalescence is ordinarily longer and more confining.

Still, to allow such considerations to weight the decision (given proper indications) between simple disc removal and disc removal with spinal fusion is just as illogical as offering a patient with carcinoma of the stomach a gastrostomy instead of a gastric resection, because it is simpler to perform and allows a more rapid convalescence. There are *absolute* and *relative* indications for adding fusion to simple disc removal.

The absolute indications include:

(1) a well-documented history of back symptoms preceding nerve root pain;

(2) real structural weakness, shown on roentgen and clinical examination;

(3) marked *local* arthritic changes at the level of the disc herniation;

(4) multiple lesions.

The relative indications include:

(1) vocations requiring great muscular effort;

(2) involvement of the proximal joint (L4–L5 or L5–S1) in the local degenerative pathologic process.

The neurosurgeon generally feels that the well muscled spine of normal architecture which sustains disc herniation secondary to acute unphysiological stress will be restored to normal functioning by simple disc removal.

Lesions above L4–L5 are deliberately eliminated from this discussion because the technical aspects of the problem actually outweigh the clinical indications, and constitute a special problem.

Technique of Surgery of the Intervertebral Disc

The protruded disc is approached through the interlaminar space, with additional exposure gained, where needed, by biting away the edges of the adjacent laminae. The ligamentum flavum which stretches across the space is removed to the laminar margins, exposing the epidural space and the underlying dura covered more or less by a fatty areolar layer interlaced with veins. The ease of access and visualization of the root depend upon:

(1) The position of the patient on the operating table. An attempt is made to flex the lumbar spine to increase the interlaminar spaces. If there is pressure upon the abdomen from below, the epidural veins will be large and the areolar tissue full; however, if such a technical error is avoided, the veins are almost "potential" structures.

(2) The size of the lesion and the crowding of the space.

(3) The anatomical features of the spine. There is a striking variability in interpedicular distances or the roughly cross-sectional area of the epidural space. With narrow measurements the dural sac is crowded in the lateral diameter, and the lesion further narrows the space. The root may then come to lie pressed hard against the shelving lateral wall of the interspace. Parallel variations include steeple-like laminae so that the interspace is almost vertical, and close application of the laminae to one another, making lateral access to the root very difficult. Also, the intervertebral space, because of unusual obliquity of the laminae, may lie beneath the rostral laminae, making access difficult and crowding the root further.

The root is identified from its exit from the dura proper to the foramen below. It is separated gently from the lateral wall of the interspace, exposing the intervertebral space and the site of the protruding disc. With the root gently retracted medially, the bulging intervertebral space is visualized and the lesion dealt with, using delicate rongeurs and dental chisels to remove all the accessible disc material. The course of the root is then followed right into the foramen, until the operator is assured there are no fragments remaining free which might compromise the root. All that remains to be done is a careful toilet of the wound to prevent, as far as possible, oozing of blood and subsequent scar formation.

Myelography

The myelogram, in sophisticated hands (where it belongs), is an important preliminary to disc surgery. It is never to be considered a diagnostic or screening test, but its value lies in revealing the exact nature of the problem preoperatively. Knowledge that no other pathology exists above or below is almost mandatory before fusion is contemplated. Multiple lesions are quite common, and the second lesion may be masked initially but become anything but silent later. All in all, the risks and inconvenience of myelography are far outweighed by its value, presuming expertness on the part of the technician.

It might be said, parenthetically, that the results of desultory study are becoming tragically obvious after two decades of disc surgery. Undoubtedly greater conservation will follow the appearance of careful statistics on the over-all picture. One almost daily sees more and more cases for reappraisal or re-operation. The odds against successful rehabilitation rise steeply after an initial operation. It is the considered opinion of this writer that careful myelography can reduce enormously the percentage of poor results by offering precise preoperative information to the surgeon.

Other Laboratory Studies

There is no real general usefulness to lumbar puncture without myelography. The spinal fluid protein may or may not be elevated, the level depending chiefly on the degree of mechanical block to the movement of the spinal fluid. Generally, it is well below the value found when tumors are present in the same region. Complete block is unusual, as is cellular reaction. In a difficult diagnostic problem, lumbar puncture may have an indication, but should not be done separately if a myelogram is contemplated, since the puncture will greatly increase the possibility of a technically poor myelogram by subdural injection of dye. In essence, if one does not need a myelogram for diagnosis and localization, spinal puncture similarly has little to contribute.

Part V

THE HEAD AND SPECIAL SENSES

CHAPTER 22

INJURIES OF THE SKULL AND BRAIN

By LESTER A. MOUNT, M.D.

ANATOMY

The scalp is composed of skin, subcutaneous fat, superficial fascia, galea aponeurotica, and pericranium (Fig. 22–*1*). The skin is thick and is held firmly to the galea aponeurotica by the superficial fascia, but is separated from the galea by the subcutaneous fat. The main blood vessels, nerves, and lymph vessels are found in the subcutaneous fat. The galea aponeurotica is loosely attached by areolar tissue to the pericranium, which is really the periosteum of the bone. The periosteum is not firmly attached to the bone except at the sutures, where it blends with the fibrous tissue between the adjacent bones.

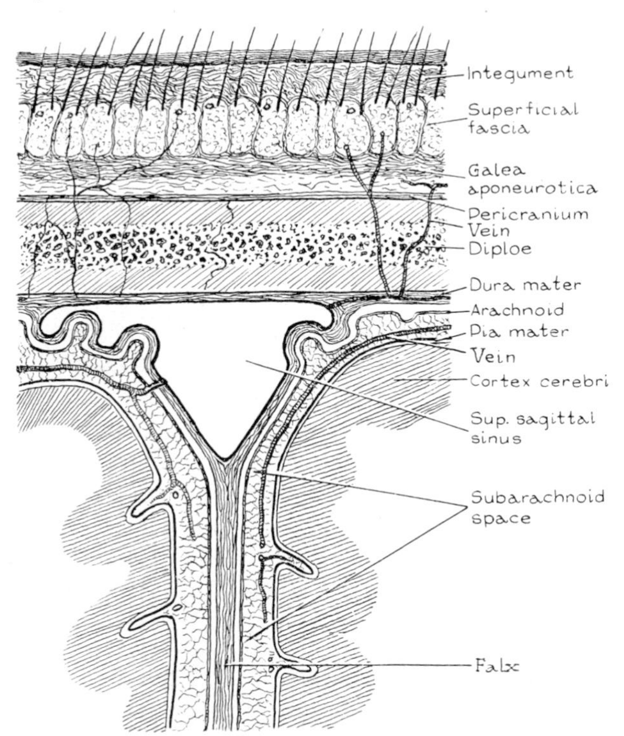

Figure 22–1. Layers of the scalp, skull, meninges, and cortex of the brain.

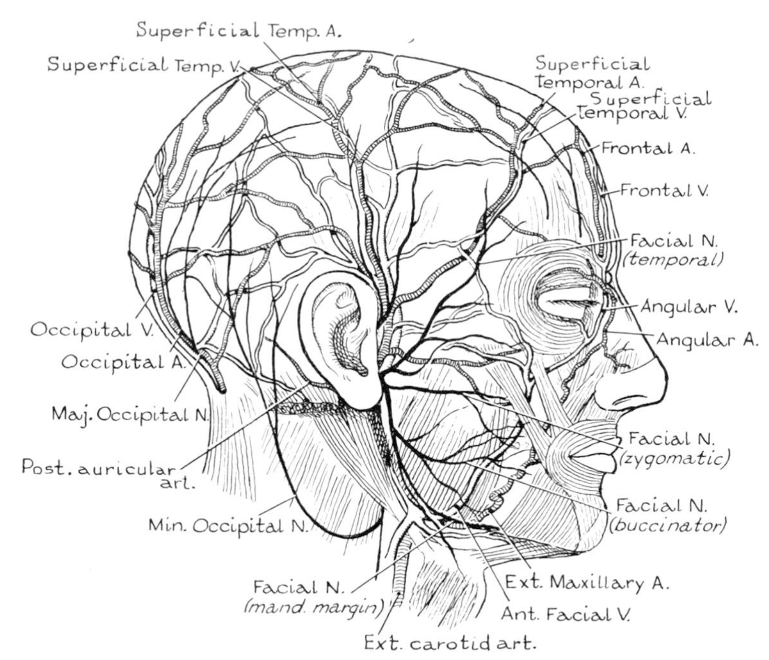

Figure 22–2. The main arteries, veins, and nerves of the head. Every scalp flap should have a main artery supplying it.

The galea aponeurotica is a thick, fibrous layer which extends over the top and sides of the head. It acts as a broad, flat tendon for the occipitalis and frontalis muscles. It is attached posteriorly to the superior nuchal line, and ends laterally over the temporal fascia, having no definite margin; anteriorly, it envelops the frontalis muscles and ends by blending with the fascia covering the corrugator supercilii and orbicularis oculi muscles.

The scalp is richly supplied with blood by branches from both the internal and external carotid arteries (Fig. 22–2). The frontal region is supplied by the frontal and supraorbital branches of the ophthalmic artery (from the internal carotid artery). The temporal and parietal regions are supplied by the deep and superficial temporal arteries (branches of the external carotid artery). The occipital region is supplied by the occipital and posterior auricular arteries, both of which are branches of the external carotid artery. The various arteries supplying the scalp anastomose freely. The venous drainage follows closely the arterial supply. The vessels empty into the external jugular vein, except for the occipital vein, which drains into the vertebral or deep cervical veins. The veins of the scalp anastomose with the internal jugular vein by way of the common facial vein, with the cavernous sinus by way of the superior ophthalmic veins, with the superior sagittal sinus by way of the parietal emissary veins, with the lateral sinuses by way of the mastoid emissary veins, and with the veins of the dura and all of the dural sinuses by way of small veins which perforate the bone to join the diploic veins and extend inward through the inner tables, or by way of other veins which penetrate the bone at the sutures (see Fig. 22–*1*).

The lymph vessels of the front part of the scalp empty into the preauricular lymph nodes; those of the middle part of the scalp empty into the postauricular nodes, and those of the back of the scalp into the occipital nodes.

The nerve supply of the scalp is from the three branches of the trigeminal nerve and the second and third cervical nerves (Fig. 22–3).

The cranium is composed of eight bones: one frontal, two parietal, two temporal, one occipital, one ethmoid, and one sphenoid. The bones are united by sutures which commonly close by the middle of the second decade but sometimes remain open throughout life. They are composed of two compact layers separated by more spongy bone, called the diploe. The diploe is absorbed in the frontal, ethmoid, and sphenoid bones to form the paranasal sinuses. The bones are relatively thick over the top, front, and back of the cranium, but are thin on the sides, under the temporal muscles.

The brain is covered by three layers of membrane, the dura mater, the arachnoid, and the pia mater. The dura, a tough fibrous layer covering the inner table of the bone, possesses a thickened extension, the falx cerebri, which separates the two lateral hemispheres of the brain, and another thickened extension, the tentorium, which stretches like a tent across the posterior and inferior one-third of the cranial cavity to support the occipital and temporal lobes and to separate them from the cerebellum. The falx holds up the midsagittal portion of the tentorium. The falx is divided into two parts just before it joins the dura on the inner surface of the skull, thus forming the superior sagittal venous sinus, and

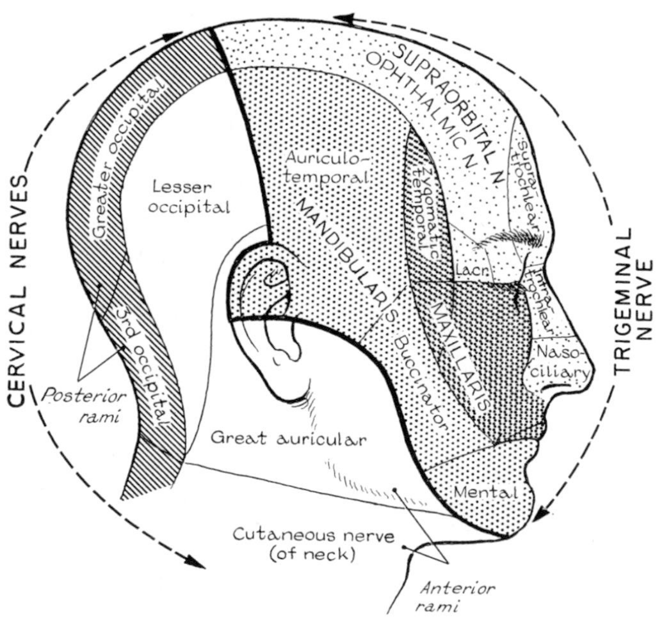

Figure 22–3. The sensory nerve supply of the scalp and face.

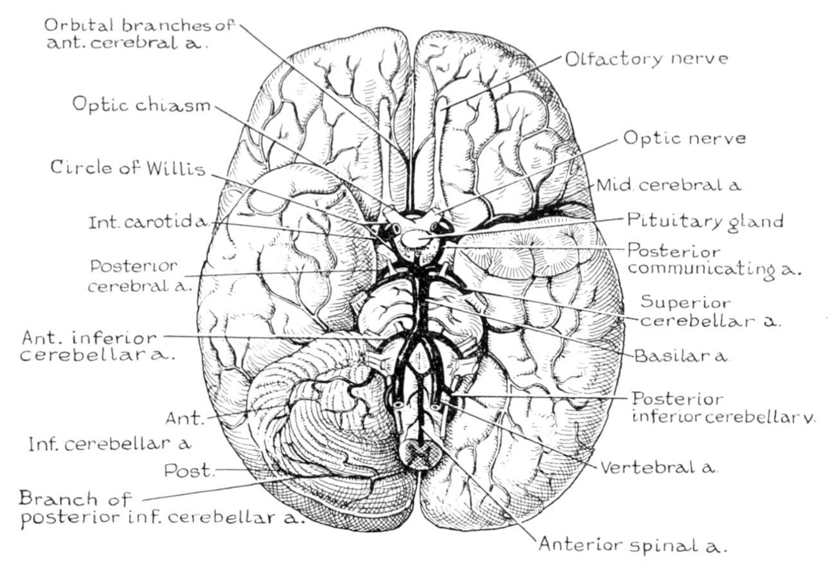

Figure 22–4. The main arteries at the base of the brain.

similarly, where the tentorium joins the dura, the lateral sinuses are formed.

The brain is a soft mushy structure composed of nerve cells, the gray matter, and their axons, the white matter, both of which are supported by the glia, all of these being derived from the ectoderm. It consists of two cerebral hemispheres, the basal ganglia, the cerebellum, and the brain stem. The cerebral hemispheres are divided into the frontal, temporal, parietal, and occipital lobes. Inside the brain are cavities, called ventricles, containing cerebrospinal fluid. The ventricles are in continuity with each other, either directly or indirectly, and the fourth ventricle empties into the cisterns at the base of the brain. The basal cisterns are in continuity with the subarachnoid spaces within the spinal canal and over the surface of the brain. The cerebrospinal fluid is largely secreted within the ventricles and is largely absorbed over the surface of the cerebral hemispheres, although there is a constant osmotic exchange going on in the ventricles and basal cisterns, as well as in the subarachnoid space. Obstruction to the flow of cerebrospinal fluid results in increased intracranial pressure, as does also a decrease in the rate of absorption.

The brain receives blood by way of the internal carotid and the vertebral arteries. The vertebral arteries join together anterior to the medulla to form the basilar artery. The carotid and basilar arteries at the base are joined together by communicating arteries to form the circle of Willis (Fig. 22–4). The vertebral arteries and basilar arteries supply the brain stem, cerebellum, the occipital lobes, part of the basal ganglia, and the posterior inferior surface of the temporal lobes. The internal carotid arteries supply the frontal lobes, the parietal lobes, the remainder of the basal ganglia, and the rest of the temporal lobes.

Venous blood (Fig. 22–5) is drained by way of the large dural sinuses and the cavernous sinus, which empty into the internal jugular veins. The superior cerebral veins draining the upper third of the cerebral hemi-

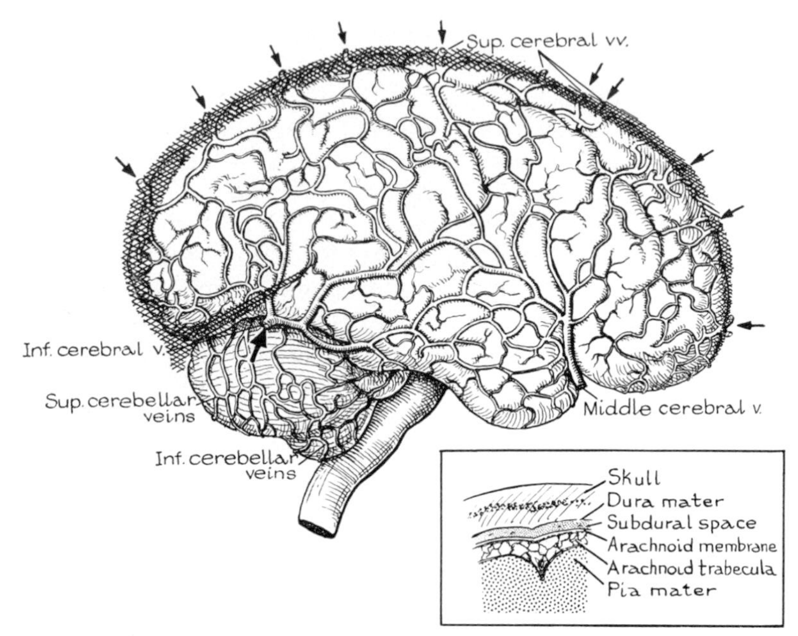

Figure 22–5. Veins of the lateral surface of the brain. It is the superior or the inferior cerebral vein (indicated by arrows) which is torn as it crosses the subdural space. The resultant bleeding forms a subdural hematoma. (See also Figure 22–1.)

spheres empty into the superior sagittal sinus. The middle cerebral veins, which empty into the cavernous sinus, drain the middle third of the hemispheres. Other veins emptying directly into the lateral sinuses drain the inferior third of the hemispheres. The great vein of Galen drains the interior and inferior parts of the cerebral hemispheres and basal ganglia and empties into the straight sinus, which in turn drains into the lateral sinuses. The cerebellum is drained by veins which empty into the straight, the petrosal, or the lateral sinuses.

The dura mater is supplied mainly by the middle meningeal artery, but it also receives blood from the ophthalmic, internal carotid, occipital, ascending pharyngeal, and vertebral arteries. The veins draining the dura parallel the arteries supplying it.

EXAMINATION OF PATIENT AND INTERPRETATION IN TERMS OF PATHOLOGICAL PHYSIOLOGY AND PATHOLOGICAL ANATOMY

The patient, when first seen, is often in *shock* and consequently has low blood pressure, rapid pulse, and a low temperature. The low temperature may be due partially to exposure. At this time the patient should be treated for shock and nothing beyond a cursory examination should be made. However, gross fractures, pneumothorax, ruptured viscera, or continuing hemorrhage should be found at this time.

The patient may be in *coma*, which is a state of unconsciousness from which he cannot be aroused even by powerful stimuli. This, of course, is due to injury to the center of consciousness, which many neurophysiologists believe is located in the diencephalon, but the exact site is not known. After the initial period of coma the patient becomes *semiconscious*. In this state he reacts to painful stimuli but does not speak. The next step in recovery is the *state of confusion*, in which the patient responds by carrying out simple commands, or speaks, but is not clear mentally. There are different degrees of confusion, and the patient may fluctuate between confusion and full consciousness. From the state of confusion he ultimately becomes *fully conscious*. The duration of each of these states varies with the severity of brain injury, and the stages of semiconsciousness and confusion may be so brief as to be unrecognized. The patient is in a dangerous condition as long as he is comatose and the longer this state lasts the poorer is the prognosis, although patients have made good recovery after long periods of unconsciousness. If a patient recovers consciousness and then lapses again into unconsciousness, some new condition has arisen, such as hemorrhage into the epidural space, subdural space, or the brain itself. Occasionally cerebral edema will be responsible for the second loss of consciousness.

Increased intracranial pressure, which develops in most patients following head injuries, produces abnormal responses in the pulse, respiration, and blood pressure. At first the increased intracranial pressure is compensated for by displacement of cerebrospinal fluid without production of any clinically demonstrable effects. As the pressure increases, the venous pressure is increased and the patient complains of increasingly severe headache and may become increasingly restless and vomit. As a result of the pressure on the vessels, some anemia of the brain is produced and the autonomic medullary centers respond by slowing the pulse, slowing and deepening the respiration, and raising the blood pressure. With still further increase in intracranial pressure, the blood pressure is raised still more, the pulse becomes full, bounding, and rapid, and the respiratory rate is increased. The temperature meanwhile is rising. When compensation fails the blood pressure falls, the pulse becomes even more rapid and thready, the respirations become stertorous, shallow, and irregular, and death soon follows if the pressure is not relieved.

As mentioned earlier, the temperature is frequently low on admission, and later it rises, its height being an index of the amount of brain injury and hemorrhage. A *progressively rising temperature* is a very grave prognostic sign.

Subconjunctival hemorrhage may occur as a result of direct trauma to the eye, but uniform, *widely distributed hemorrhage far back on the eye* is strongly suggestive of a basal fracture of the skull in the frontal region.

The pupils may be normal in size, constricted, or dilated. *Constricted pupils* are suggestive of pressure upon or hemorrhage into the pons or midbrain, especially when associated with bilateral pyramidal tract signs. The pupils react to light by constriction, either directly or indirectly from the other eye. *Bilateral pupillary dilatation* points to brain stem injury. A *unilaterally dilated and fixed pupil* is indicative of herniation of the uncus, the medial part of the temporal lobe, over the edge of the tentorium through the incisura with pressure on the third nerve and on the brain stem. This is usually due to an ipsilateral extradural or subdural hematoma, but it may be due to an intracerebral hemorrhage or to cerebral edema. Dilation, constriction, and inequality of the pupils, and poor reaction to light, are grave prognostic signs, especially dilatation accompanied by fixation.

Papilledema, an important sign of increased intracranial pressure, is seldom seen early. *Conjugate deviation of the eyes* to one side and inability to move the eyes to the opposite side is due to injury to the second frontal convolution on the side toward which the eyes are looking. *Convulsive jerking of the eyes* to one side is due to injury to the brain stem. The appearance of *bleeding from the ear, of blood behind the ear drum,* or of *cerebrospinal fluid otorrhea* is indicative of a basal fracture of the skull. One must be careful to determine that the blood has not run into the ear canal from the outside or that there has been no local trauma to the external auditory meatus itself. *Ecchymosis over the mastoid process* is also evidence of a basal fracture (Battle's sign).

Cerebrospinal fluid rhinorrhea is usually indicative of a basal fracture through the nose or the paranasal sinuses, but occasionally the fracture may be through the petrous pyramid with drainage of the fluid through the eustachian tube into the nose (see discussion in Chapter 23).

Drooping of one side of the mouth, blowing out of one cheek on respiration, and *incomplete closure of the lids of one eye* are signs of facial paresis. If the motor pathways are intact, even an unconscious patient will not allow his own hand to be dropped on his face, unless the coma is very deep. A paralyzed lower extremity will tend to lie in an everted position. A lesion high in the brain stem produces *decerebrate rigidity,* a condition from which few adults recover. In this state the extremities are all extended and spastic, the back is arched, the forearms are pronated so that the back of each hand rests against the thigh, and the feet are maintained in plantar extension. When this occurs almost immediately after trauma it is the result of direct injury to the brain stem. When it occurs later it is the result of pressure on the brain stem by herniations of the uncus secondary to hemorrhage or edema or to delayed midbrain hemorrhage. When the basal ganglia are involved, there is rigidity, often of cogwheel type, and there may be a tremor. Regardless of the location of brain injury, there is likely to be complete flaccidity of the extremities at first, but this may change very rapidly to spasticity.

Twitchings of the muscles or *convulsive seizures* on one side indicate injury to the contralateral motor area of the cerebral cortex. The *reflexes* may be hyperactive to absent, and the Babinski sign may be present or absent when the motor pathways are injured. Abnormal reflexes are of pathological significance. When the patient is able to move his extremities in a coordinated, purposeful manner there is no serious injury to the motor system.

Lack of response to painful stimuli may signify either motor paralysis, absence of pain sensation, or coma.

When there has been subarachnoid hemorrhage, the neck is usually stiff and there is usually a *positive Kernig sign.*

INJURIES OF THE SCALP

Abrasions and contusions of the scalp are treated in the same way as those elsewhere in the body. The open areas should be cleansed carefully with soap and sterile saline solution. All dirt must be removed, and the area painted with Zephiran solution.

Lacerations of the scalp bleed profusely because of the rich blood supply. The arteries often retract into the subcutaneous fat, so that ends of the vessels are difficult to find. The rich blood supply is instrumental in preventing infection. Large areas of the scalp may be stripped from the skull, remaining attached only by a narrow pedicle, and they may still be sutured back and remain viable. The lacerated wounds should be sutured as soon as the patient is out of shock and his condition otherwise permits. In the nonsensitive patient procaine penicillin, 400,000 units, and streptomycin, 0.5 gm., are given intramuscularly before the operation is

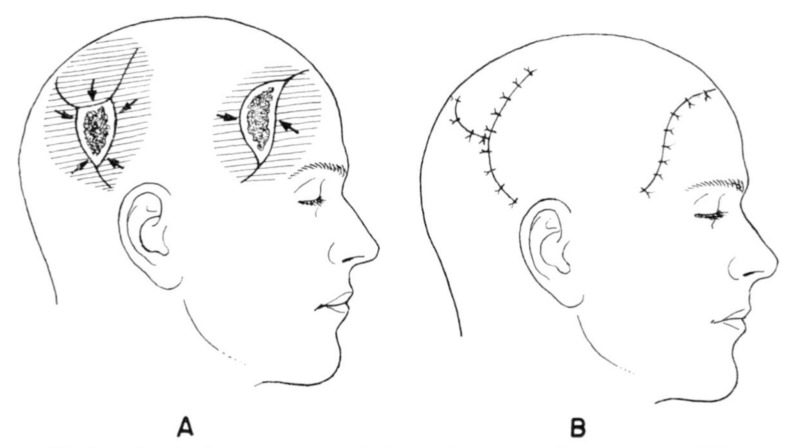

Figure 22–6. Scalp lacerations with loss of tissue. The areas of debridement and undermining of the scalp beneath the galea are shown, as well as the relaxing incisions which are made in order to allow closure. The arrows indicate how the scalp is shifted to effect closure.

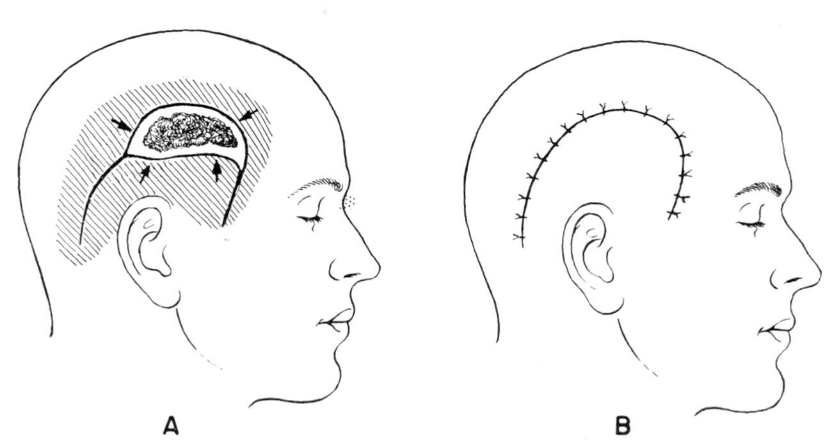

Figure 22–7. A large scalp wound with loss of tissue. Another method of making relaxing incisions is shown. The shaded area represents the undermined scalp.

started. The hair must be shaved widely around the laceration; the scalp should be perfectly cleaned with soap and plenty of sterile saline, and then painted with Zephiran solution. Procaine, 1 per cent, is then injected into the scalp around the laceration before the wound itself is similarly cleansed and debrided. Only when preparations for operative treatment have been completed should the lacerations be deeply explored for fractures or foreign bodies. When extensive debridement is necessary, the galea aponeurotica may be undermined, relaxing incisions made, and scalp flaps shifted, in order to bring the edges of the wound together (Figs. 22–6, 22–7). When a great amount of tissue has been lost it may not be possible to approximate all the edges. In such event the important areas are covered by making relaxing incisions (Figs. 22–8, 22–9) and the denuded areas are covered with Thiersch grafts. The scalp is closed with fine plain catgut or silk, using interrupted sutures with buried knots in the

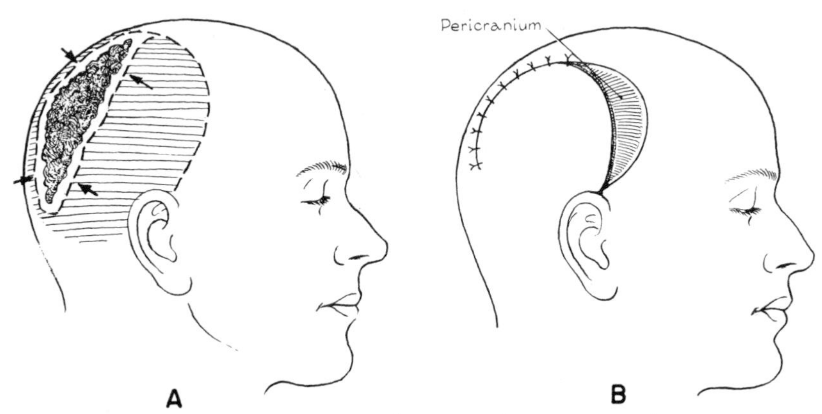

Figure 22–8. The loss of tissue in this wound is so great that, in spite of undermining and shifting of the scalp flap, it is not possible to close the scalp completely. A Thiersch graft is used to cover the denuded area.

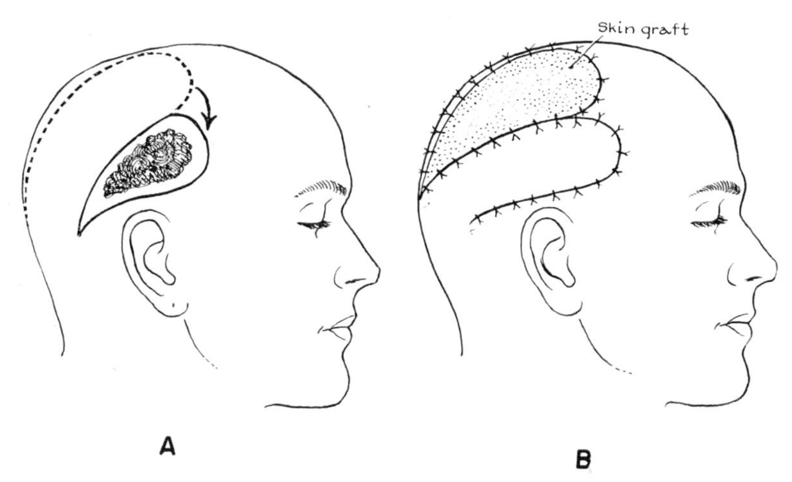

Figure 22–9. Another wound in which loss of tissue is great and another type of shifting of scalp is done. The occipital artery would supply this flap of scalp. A Thiersch graft is used to cover the denuded area.

galea and interrupted sutures of fine silk in the skin (see Fig. 22–*13, E*). When exposed areas, i.e., those not covered by hair, are sutured, the skin edges should be carefully approximated, as in plastic surgery, with frequent sutures placed in the skin. These should be removed in 24 hours to prevent scars of suture holes or transverse scars across the incision. In areas covered by hair, the skin and galea are frequently closed with one suture of silk through both layers. The sutures are then left in place for one week. If the patient has been previously immunized, a booster dose of tetanus toxoid should be given. If the patient has not been immunized, he should be tested for sensitivity to horse serum and, if not sensitive, be given tetanus antitoxin.

Great care should be taken in treating lacerations of the scalp, since infection may spread to the skull or intracranially, through the veins penetrating the bones (see Fig. 22–*1*), and produce osteomyelitis, cavernous sinus thrombosis, superior sinus thrombosis, lateral sinus thrombosis, subdural abscess, meningitis, and/or brain abscess. Hence, in addition to careful technique in operative treatment, as a further precaution against infection the patient should be given procaine penicillin, 400,000 units, and streptomycin, 0.5 gm., twice daily for five days.

A hematoma of the scalp may be very extensive and spread beneath the galea over most of the skull. Its firm edge often feels like the edge of a depressed fracture of the skull, and only roentgenography will reveal whether or not a depressed fracture is present. These hematomas are not serious. They usually absorb spontaneously, but can be made to disappear more quickly by use of a pressure bandage. Pressure disseminates the blood and hence promotes more rapid absorption. It is rarely necessary to aspirate such hematomas, and this should be done only if the overlying scalp is becoming thin. When aspiration is necessary, it should be done with a freshly boiled or autoclaved needle inserted into the hematoma through adjacent normal scalp which has been cleansed with soap and water and painted with Zephiran solution.

A cephalhematoma is a hemorrhage beneath the pericranium. It is found most frequently in the newborn. Its extent is limited by attachment of the pericranium to the fibrous tissue between the sutures. It is almost always absorbed without assistance.

FRACTURES OF THE SKULL

Fractures of the skull are important, primarily, in that they are an index of the severity of the trauma, and hence of the probable brain injury, and, secondarily, because they may lead to infection of the skull, meninges, or brain. Thirdly, a fracture in the temporal region or across a venous sinus may result in an extradural hemorrhage, and, lastly, fragments of bone may be depressed into the brain.

Fractures of the skull may be classified as follows: (*a*) Simple: linear, comminuted, depressed; (*b*) compound: linear, comminuted, depressed (gun shot), extending into nose or accessory nasal sinuses, extending into ear.

Simple linear (Fig. 22–*10*) ***and comminuted fractures*** require no special treatment; it is, however, best to keep the patient from lying on the fracture site.

A depressed fracture (Figs. 22–*11*, 22–*12*) can be fully evaluated only by x-ray examination. When there is a depressed fracture, elevation should be performed as soon as the patient's condition permits. This is done by turning a scalp flap (Fig. 22–*13, A*) around the depressed area under local anesthesia, if the patient is sufficiently cooperative, or under local and Pentothal anesthesia with the precautionary use of an endotracheal tube. The incision is made through the skin and galea aponeurotica. Bleeding is controlled by Michel clips or clamps, and the flap of scalp is elevated. As much of the pericranium as possible is spared. If the fragments cannot be lifted out, a trephine or burr hole is made next to the depression. When a laceration of the dura, and hence of the underlying brain, seems unlikely, the depressed fragments of bone may be elevated by inserting a blunt instrument, such as a periosteal elevator, under the fragments and elevating them. Such fragments are often so impacted that upon elevation they remain nicely in place. This maneuver is especially useful in "ping-pong" depressed fractures in young babies. It should be remembered that depressions of the inner table are often greater than those of the outer table. Before the depressed fracture over a dural venous sinus is elevated a large piece of muscle or Gelfoam should

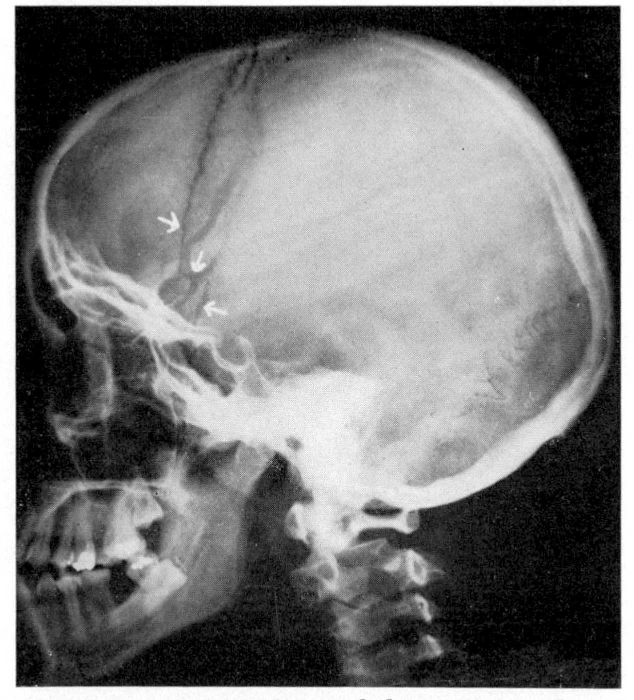

Figure 22–10. Roentgenogram of a simple linear fracture along the coronal suture, then crossing the middle meningeal channel and extending down into the base. A fracture extending across the middle meningeal channel in this region is likely to tear this artery, producing an extradural hemorrhage.

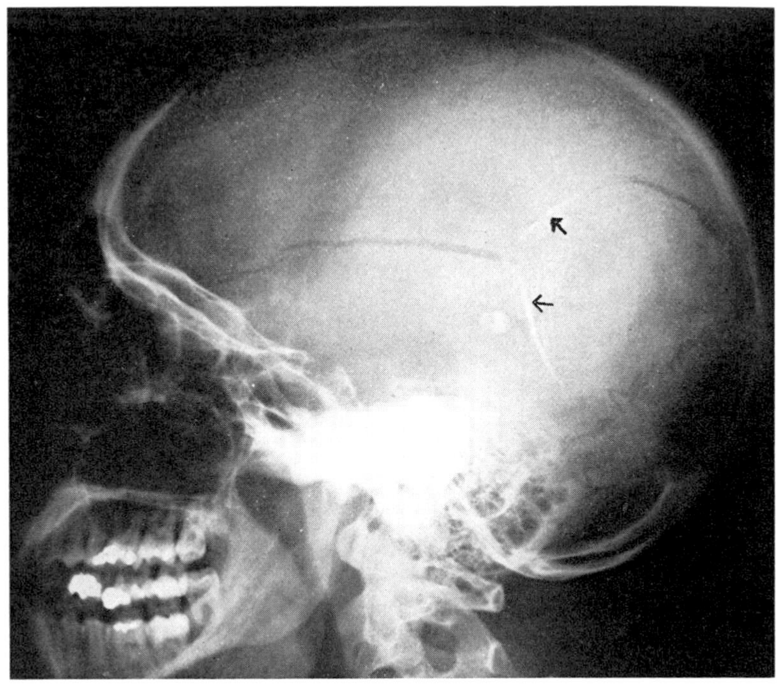

Figure 22–11. Roentgenogram of the skull with multiple fractures, including a depressed fracture (white line indicated by arrows). The overlapping of the bone produces the increased density. The linear fractures extending forward and backward from the depressed area are readily seen.

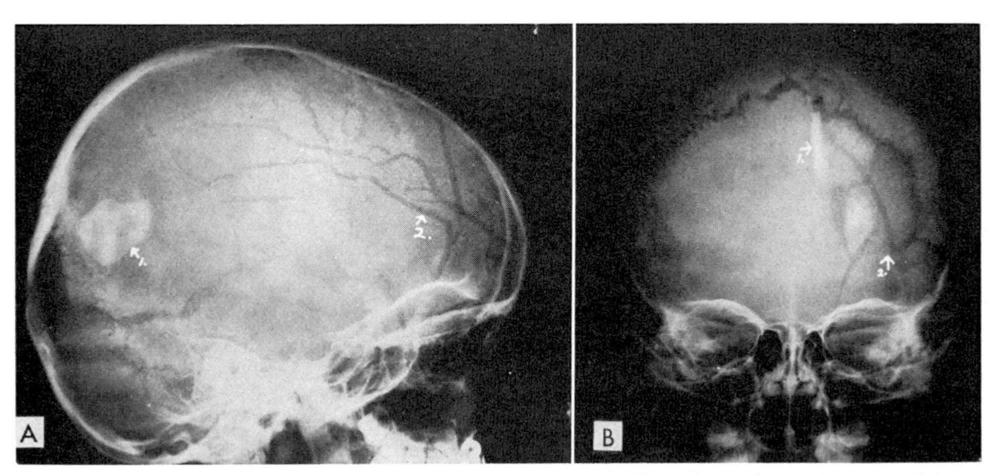

Figure 22–12. Multiple linear fractures of the skull and one large depressed fragment.

A. Lateral view showing depressed fragment (arrow 1). Arrow 2 points to one of the many linear fractures. The dark area in the posterior occipital region is the site from which the bone fragment has been dislocated.

B. Anteroposterior view showing the depressed fragment of bone (arrow 1) and the site (arrow 2) from which it was dislocated. About this site linear fractures radiate like the spokes of a wheel from the hub.

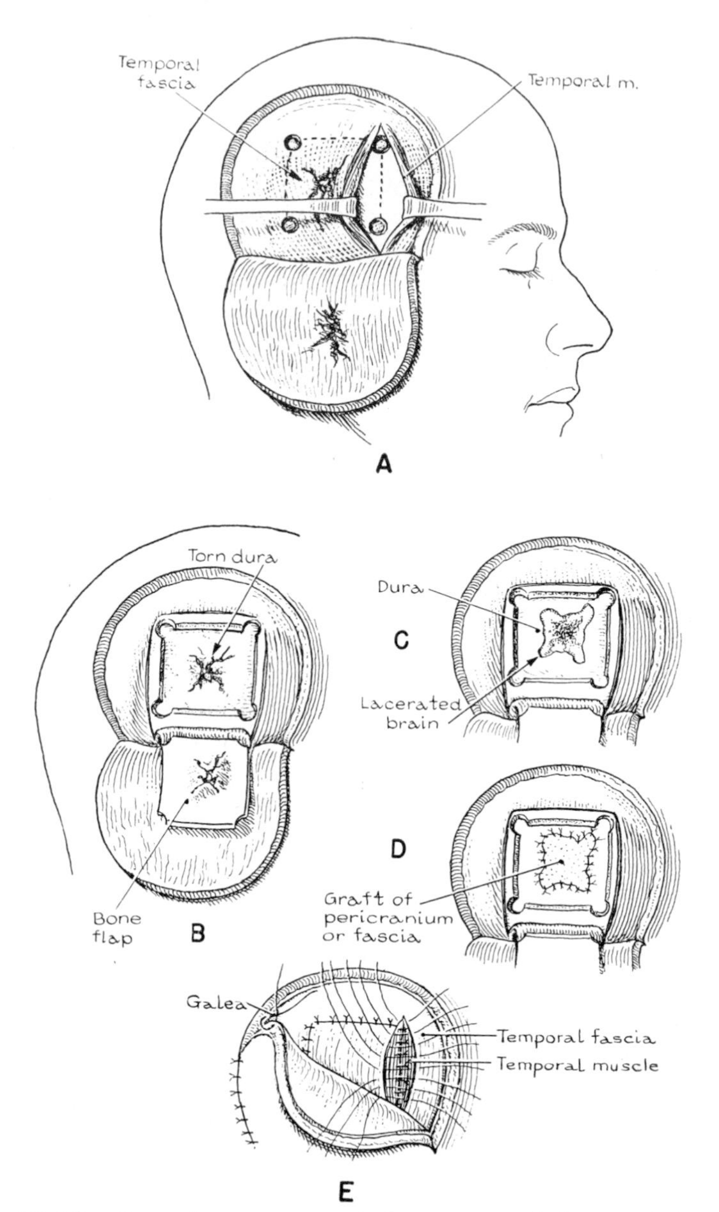

Figure 22–13. Steps in treatment of the compound depressed fracture of the skull shown in Figure 22–12.

A. The scalp flap has been turned around the site of fracture. The temporal fascia and temporal muscle have been incised and retracted in anterior part, and two trephine openings have been made. The proposed posterior trephine openings and lines where the skull is to be sawed have been indicated. Debridement of the wound in the scalp, temporal fascia, and temporal muscle is done before the scalp flap is turned, but was omitted in the drawing to better indicate the position of the scalp and the bone flaps in relation to the wound.

B. The bone flap has been turned, revealing a spicule of bone projecting into the brain.

C. The bone spicule has been removed, and the dura has been debrided.

D. Debridement of the brain has been done, and the dura has been closed by means of a graft.

E. The temporal muscle, the temporal fascia, the galea, and the skin are closed. The knots in the galea are tied and buried beneath the galea.

be available to control hemorrhage from the sinus, as the bleeding may be very profuse and the patient may quickly become exsanguinated. When bone fragments are projecting into the brain, less trauma to the brain will be done if the fragments are removed under direct vision. The brain is gently retracted to prevent additional damage to it during removal of the bone. The dura is repaired with interrupted black silk sutures, and pericranial fascial grafts are used if necessary. If a subdural hematoma is suspected, the dura should be opened to permit inspection of the brain and then closed.

At times better visualization will be obtained and less trauma done by use of a bone flap around the depressed fragments. A bone flap is made by placing four or more trephine openings through the skull. These are then connected by use of a wire saw which is threaded between bone and dura by means of a dural guide. This guide then protects the dura from laceration while the bone is being sawed. The edge of the bone is bevelled so that the flap may be replaced without danger of its being depressed into the cranial cavity. After the four sides have been sawed, the flap may be carefully lifted. The temporal muscle, if attached to the flap, is protected when the sawing is done and is left attached when the bone flap is turned (Fig. 22–*13, B*).

Use of the bone flap will also allow remolding of the impacted fragments by forcing them back into their original position. If necessary, these fragments of bone may be wired to each other and to the edges of the bone around the depression. If this is not possible, the defect may be plated. If the defect is not more than 2 cm. in diameter, tantalum or steel wire mesh may be used to cover it, and the pericranium sutured over the mesh. If the diameter is more than 2 cm., a stainless steel or tantalum plate is used. The plate is wired in place, and the wound is closed by interrupted fine black silk or fine plain catgut in the pericranium and loose areolar tissue over it, in the temporal muscle, in the temporal fascia, and in the galea aponeurotica, and silk is used in the skin. The sutures are so placed in the galea that the knot is buried beneath the galea (Fig. 22–*13, E*).

Compound linear and comminuted fractures are treated in the same way as lacerations without fractures, with the same preliminary care to make the wound as clean as possible. If the bone is abraded, the abrasions should be curetted until clean; if the bone is grossly contaminated, debridement is necessary. Loose fragments of bone should be removed. Bacitracin-neomycin solution, 1,000 units per milliliter, should be instilled in the wound before each layer is closed. However, the cortex of the brain should be protected from the antibiotics for fear of producing convulsive seizures. Procaine penicillin, 400,000 units, and streptomycin, 0.5 gm., should be given intramuscularly before operation and then twice daily for five days or longer if indicated.

Compound depressed fractures (Fig. 22–*12*) are treated as early as possible in the same manner as simple depressed fractures. In addition debridement of all layers, including the bone, dura, and brain, should be carefully done. Care must be taken to remove all foreign bodies, such as

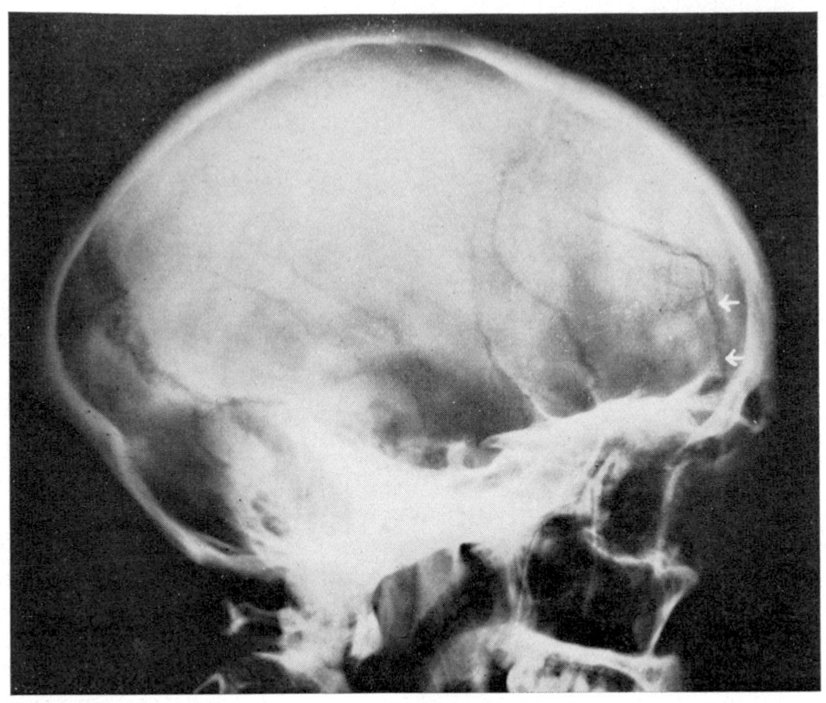

Figure 22–14. Lateral roentgenogram showing a linear fracture which extends into the frontal sinus. Such a fracture is really a compound, or open, fracture.

dirt, sand, hair, and bone. The wound is then carefully irrigated with quarts of saline or Ringer's solution. Defects in the dura are closed by grafts of pericranium, temporal fascia, or fascia lata, using interrupted fine silk sutures, so that a water-tight closure is effected (Fig. 22–*13, E*). The galea is closed with fine plain catgut or silk, and the skin with silk. Each layer is carefully irrigated with bacitracin solution, 1,000 units per milliliter, before the sutures are tied. Procaine penicillin, 400,000 units, and streptomycin, 0.5 gm., are given intramuscularly as in compound linear fractures.

Fractures extending into the nose or paranasal sinuses (Fig. 22–*14*) are compound fractures because of connection with the exterior of the body. As a result, there is danger of infection, and this danger is increased if the patient has sinusitis. Roentgenography may not reveal the fracture but may show gas in the brain substance or ventricles, that is, pneumocephalus, which of course indicates an open fracture. These patients should be given large doses of chemotherapeutic and antibiotic drugs for ten days or longer, if indicated by the clinical course. Sulfadiazine gets into the cerebrospinal fluid better than any of the other drugs, and hence sulfadiazine, 2 gm., with 2 gm. of sodium bicarbonate, should be given at once and then 1 gram of each every four hours. The dosage should be regulated to maintain a blood level of 12 to 15 mg. per 100 ml. Penicillin, 800,000 units, and streptomycin 0.5 gm., are also given twice daily. If upper respiratory tract infection is present or if the rhinorrhea is persistent, operative treatment becomes necessary. This consists in turning a scalp and bone flap, finding the dural tear, and repairing it with a flap of dura, a piece of fascia lata, or a muscle stump. (See also discussion of fractures of the nose and paranasal sinuses in Chapter 23.)

Fractures extending into the ear, that is, across the petrous pyramid, are usually associated with severe brain injury and are potential sources of meningitis or brain abscess. Hemorrhage into the middle ear occurs and blood may be seen behind the drum. If the tympanic membrane is torn, blood will drain from the ear. If the dura and arachnoid are torn, cerebrospinal fluid also will leak from the ear when the drum is ruptured. When the drum is not ruptured, cerebrospinal fluid will escape through the eustachian tube and drain from the nose or may run down the esophagus unnoticed. Large doses of antibiotics should be given, as recommended later for patients with cerebrospinal fluid rhinorrhea. Surgical repair is almost impossible in these patients, because, first, patients having fracture of the base of the skull usually have serious injury to the brain and their condition does not permit a major intracranial operation, and, second, the tear in the dura and arachnoid could be in either or both the middle and posterior fossae and hence exploration in both areas is necessary. (See also Chapter 23.)

Complications of Fractures of the Skull

Most of the complications of fractures of the skull are related directly or indirectly to the presence, or possibility, of intracranial infection. Bacteria from infected lacerations of the scalp may spread to the skull by direct extension or by way of the veins which extend into or through the bone and produce osteomyelitis. Further extension of the infection may result in an epidural abscess. Rarely subdural abscesses, meningitis, sinus thrombosis, and/or brain abscess may be caused by spread of the infection in the scalp or skull through the veins without producing osteomyelitis. A compound fracture of either the cranial vault or base immediately introduces the danger of intracranial infection.

Cerebrospinal fluid rhinorrhea is the result of a fracture of the base of the skull which extends into the nose, nasal sinuses, or ear. In the latter instance the cerebrospinal fluid reaches the nose by way of the eustachian tube. In addition to the fracture, there must be a tear of the dura and arachnoid, thereby leaving a passageway for bacteria to enter and produce a meningitis or a brain abscess, or for air to enter and produce pneumocephalus (see Case I, infra).

TREATMENT of cerebrospinal fluid rhinorrhea consists in the administration of antibiotics and chemotherapeutic agents as described under Fractures Extending into the Nose, supra (see also Chapter 23). When the rhinorrhea is the result of a fracture extending into the nose or nasal sinuses, serious consideration of operative repair should be given if the amount of fluid is copious or if it persists longer than one week. Operative therapy consists in a frontal craniotomy, opening of the dura, identification of the fracture and the tear in the dura, covering the tear with a piece of muscle, holding the muscle in place by silver clips or sutures, and closure of the wound.

Cerebrospinal fluid otorrhea is the result of a fracture of the petrous pyramid in association with tearing of the dura and arachnoid and rupture of the tympanic membrane. It has been discussed in the preceding paragraph.

Cranial aerocoele consists of gas within the scalp, usually beneath the pericranium, or within the skull in the extradural space, in the subdural space, in the subarachnoid space, in the brain substance, or in the ventricles, any combination of the above areas being theoretically possible. Cranial aerocoele is caused by penetrating wounds or by fractures through the paranasal sinuses, the mastoid cells, the tegmen tympani, or the calvarium itself. Treatment consists in the repair of the opening through which the gas enters, as described above.

Pneumocephalus. Following injury air is found more frequently within the brain substance and/or ventricles than it is in any of the other spaces (Fig. 22–*15*). This condition is commonly called pneumocephalus, which literally means air within the brain. It is the result of a compound fracture of the skull, usually extending into the paranasal sinuses or the nose. In addition there must be a laceration of the meninges and the brain. The brain becomes adherent at the site of fracture, and air is forced into the lacerated brain by hard respiratory expiration or by blowing the nose. (A patient with cerebrospinal fluid rhinorrhea should be cautioned not to blow his nose.) The symptoms of pneumocephalus are increasing intracranial pressure, headaches, nausea, vomiting, visual disturbances, drowsiness, and occasionally convulsions. Cerebrospinal fluid rhinorrhea is not necessarily present. Pneumocephalus is usually found within the first few weeks after injury, but is occasionally discovered months later. Roent-

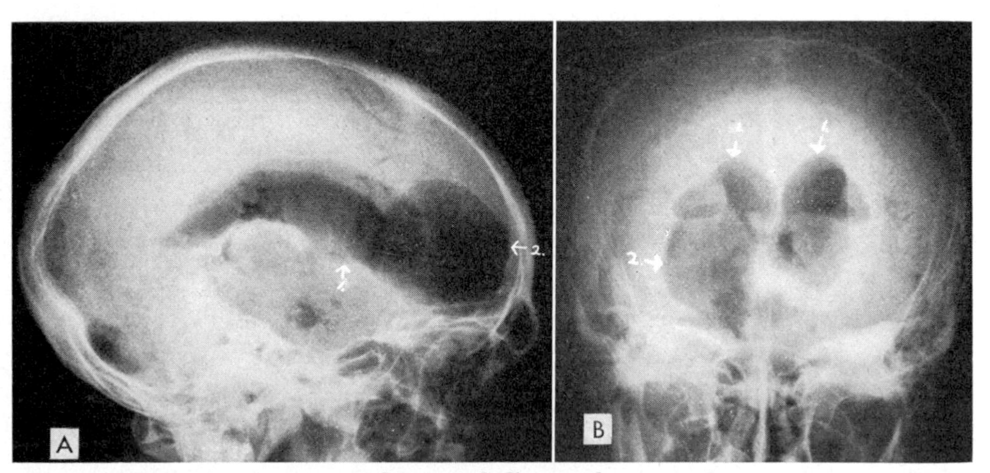

Figure 22–15. Fracture of base of skull extending into the nose.

A. Lateral roentgenogram showing air in the brain (arrow 2) and the lateral ventricle (arrow 1).

B. Anteroposterior roentgenogram showing the lateral ventricles (arrow 1) and the air within the substance of the brain (arrow 2).

genography of the skull will establish the diagnosis (Fig. 22–*15*). The treatment is repair of the dural tear and evacuation of the air within the brain. Infection of the brain may be associated with this condition, but early treatment will tend to prevent its occurrence.

Case I (Pneumocephalus)

History. This 33-year-old man was first seen 25 days after the automobile in which he was sitting was struck from the rear. His head struck the windshield as he was thrown from the car. He was dazed but not unconscious, but headache had developed, which continued up to the time of admission. For the first two days after injury, brownish watery fluid had drained from the nose. Two days before admission he became depressed and had difficulty in speaking. His gait became unsteady, his memory poor, and his headache increased.

Examination. Pulse 96, respiration 22, blood pressure 130/74, temperature 99.2. The positive signs were fullness in midportion of forehead, alternating tremor of the right upper extremity, and ataxia on heel-to-knee test bilaterally. The deep tendon reflexes were hyperactive bilaterally, with a transient triceps clonus and left ankle clonus. Hoffman and Oppenheim signs on the left were positive. The nasal margins of the optic discs were blurred, and there was a left central facial paresis.

Course in hospital. Roentgenograms of the skull (Fig. 23–*15*) showed a slightly depressed fracture involving the left frontal bone and the left frontal sinus. The ventricles were filled with air, and there was an aerocoele in the left frontal lobe, measuring 5 by 5 by 4 cm.

The patient was placed on penicillin 100,000 units every three hours, with sulfadiazine 1 gm. and sodium bicarbonate 2.4 gm. every four hours. Surgery was performed the day after admission, a bone flap being turned in the left frontal region. Yellowish fluid and gas were recovered from the ventricle, as well as from the aerocoele. The fracture was found to extend into the ethmoid sinuses as well as into the frontal sinus, with an opening into these sinuses which measured 1.5 by 0.5 cm. The brain had herniated into this opening and was densely adherent to the dura around it. When the brain was separated from the opening a sinus was found which extended into the frontal lobe, and yellowish fluid escaped from this sinus. There was no purulent material. Penicillin solution, 1,000 units per milliliter, was instilled into the opening in the frontal and ethmoid sinuses, and the opening was covered by muscle held in place by silver clips. Gelfoam saturated with penicillin solution was placed over the muscle, and the wound was closed in layers. The patient was allowed out of bed on the fifth postoperative day. Temperature returned to normal two days later. The penicillin and sulfadiazine were discontinued, and the patient was discharged from the hospital 11 days after surgery, free of symptoms, except for a slight left central facial paresis.

Cerebral fungus, or herniation of the brain, is the result of a compound fracture in which the dural and scalp tears were not repaired, and is usually associated with intracranial infection. Such a fungus is treated by elimination of the cause. Ventriculography may be advisable to rule out a brain abscess, and repeated lumbar punctures to relieve pressure and reduce bulging of the ventricle and brain in the region of the fungus in order to prepare the way for repair of the scalp and dural defects or perhaps for placing a graft on the fungus.

Meningitis secondary to head trauma is the result of inadequate early treatment of scalp wounds or compound fractures. It is treated by elimination of the focus of infection, culture of the cerebrospinal fluid for identification of the causative organism, and administration of the proper antibiotic in large doses by mouth or parenterally, but not intraspinally.

Brain abscess following fractures of the skull is almost always due to fragments of bone or other foreign material being driven into the brain, but it may be the result of fractures extending into the frontal sinuses or nose. The brain abscess may be associated with or follow a subdural abscess. The symptoms and signs are those of increased intracranial pressure: headache, nausea, vomiting, disturbances in vision, and papilledema. Other symptoms and signs depend on the area of brain involved and may consist of convulsions, weakness, paralysis, sensory disturbances, reflex changes, unsteadiness in walking, and ataxia. Abscess can be prevented by early definitive treatment, including complete debridement, removal of foreign bodies, closure of the dura and scalp, and antibiotic therapy.

TREATMENT after abscess has developed consists in accurate localization of the abscess by arteriography or ventriculography and complete removal when possible, tight closure, and vigorous antibiotic therapy and chemotherapy with those agents effective against the organisms cultured from the abscess. Catheter drainage is used when the abscess cannot be removed because of its location and when free exchange by way of the catheter is possible. At times open drainage must be performed.

Osteomyelitis of the skull following head injury is the result of direct contamination of the bone. Infrequently it may be due to spread from an infected hematoma without a scalp laceration. In such cases the hematoma has become infected by way of the blood stream or by extension from a superficial infection in the scalp, such as a furuncle. It can be prevented by early definitive treatment, with adequate debridement and antibiotic therapy. On examination there is swelling and tenderness of the scalp over the infected bone. The diagnosis is made by visualization of moth-eaten areas in the x-ray films.

TREATMENT is by complete removal of the involved bone plus local and general antibiotic therapy. The type of organism should be determined by culture before operative therapy is undertaken, so that the most effective antibiotic and chemotherapeutic agents can be used before and during surgery.

Arteriovenous fistula between internal carotid artery and cavernous sinus (see Fig. 22–*16*) is an infrequent complication and occurs in some patients with fractures in the middle fossa extending into the region of the cavernous sinus. The internal carotid artery is torn and the escaping arterial blood passes into the cavernous sinus. Occasionally this occurs without a skull fracture, as a result of rupture of an aneurysm of the internal carotid artery within the cavernous sinus. Symptoms of a carotid-cavernous fistula are a noise in the head synchronous with the pulse, unilateral chemosis, unilateral proptosis, and at times a unilateral pulsating exophthalmos. Extraocular muscle weakness and impairment of vision develop later. The diagnosis is verified by carotid arteriography; the treatment is ligation of the internal carotid artery in the neck and intracranially.

Case II (Carotid artery–cavernous sinus fistula)

History. A 54-year-old right-handed white woman was admitted to the Neurosurgical Service of the Neurological Institute on October 21, 1951. Her chief complaint was a pounding noise inside her head, related mostly to the left ear, of almost 18 months' duration. On May 30, 1950, approximately at midnight, and for an unknown reason, she had fallen while going up the front stairs of her house. She was unconscious for

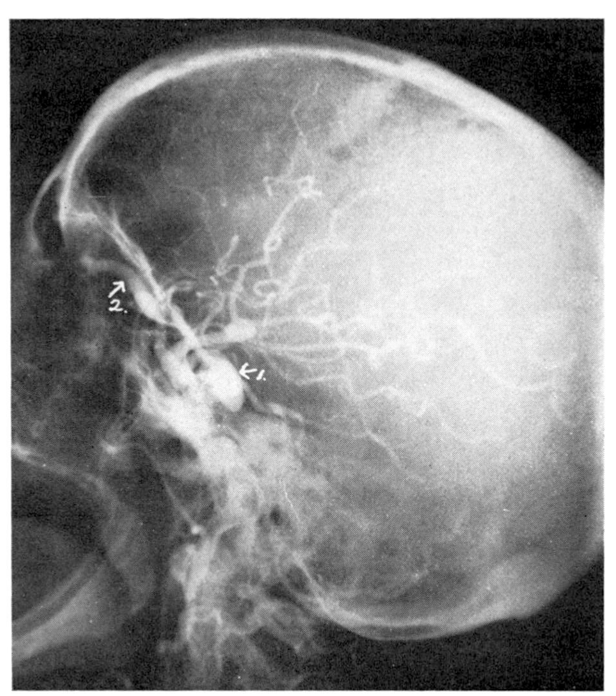

Figure 22–16. Lateral arteriogram showing a traumatic arteriovenous fistula between internal carotid artery and cavernous sinus. The carotid syphon may be seen above and in front of the cavernous sinus (arrow 1). The dilated ophthalmic vein (arrow 2) is carrying arterial blood from the cavernous sinus. The dilated ophthalmic veins are responsible for the exophthalmos, and, because they are carrying mostly arterial blood under pressure, the eye pulsates.

two to five minutes, but no apparent injury resulted from the fall. The patient went to sleep and went to work as usual the next day. During the whole day she complained of headache and pain over her eyes, and the left eye began to feel "swollen." She returned home and about 10:00 P.M. that evening she noticed the sudden onset of a pounding noise "like hammering" inside her head, mostly localized to her left ear. This was a continuous noise, with exacerbations synchronous with her pulse. Immediately afterward her left eye became "harder" and was completely closed, remaining that way for about five days. At the same time there was marked ecchymosis around the eye, which progressively subsided in a few days. The left-sided ptosis gradually improved during the next four months. When her left eye began to open she noticed double vision. This disappeared within a period of two months.

Examination. Visual acuity: O.D. 20/20; O.S. 20/70 (not corrected). Visual fields were normal. Ophthalmoscopic examination showed engorgement of the veins of the left fundus. There was no papilledema. The third, fourth, and fifth cranial nerves showed no abnormality. There was no diplopia, but there was weakness of the left external rectus muscle. The rest of the cranial nerves were also normal.

Laboratory studies. Findings of complete blood count, urinalysis, sedimentation rate, and Mazzini test were normal, as were the cerebrospinal fluid pressure, cytology, and chemistry. Caloric and audiometric tests were essentially normal. Roentgenography of the skull, including special projections, revealed no pathologic findings.

Impression. Considering the history and physical findings, the diagnosis of arteriovenous fistula of the left internal carotid artery and left cavernous sinus was made by all observers.

Arteriography. On October 23, 1951, under local anesthesia, left common carotid percutaneous arteriography was performed. This failed to show any abnormality. The right common carotid artery was then injected, and films revealed a large arteriovenous fistula in the right cavernous sinus. This drained through the posterior portion of the circular sinus into the left cavernous sinus and the left superior ophthalmic vein (Fig. 22–*16*). Since the bruit was not obliterated by bilateral common carotid compression, percutaneous right vertebral arteriography was done. This showed a tremendous right posterior communicating artery supplying part of the carotid circulation, and explained why the bruit could not be eliminated by bilateral carotid compression.

First operation. Two days later, on October 25, 1951, the right internal carotid artery was exposed in the cervical region and a Selverstone clamp was applied. The right internal carotid artery was completely closed with the Selverstone clamp 17 hours after the artery had been exposed.

The postoperative course was uneventful. One examiner was still able to hear a bruit, which was very soft, compared with the preoperative one. The patient, however, still complained of the "annoying noise" inside her head. The tools attached to the Selverstone clamps were removed 72 hours after the right internal carotid artery had been completely obliterated.

Second operation. On October 31, 1951, through a right temporal craniectomy, the right internal carotid artery was ligated intracranially. During the operation the corresponding posterior communicating artery was well visualized.

Course. The patient showed remarkable improvement, which has persisted. The bruit objectively disappeared, although the patient described a very faint "sizzling" noise in her left ear. The conjunctival chemosis subsided, as well as engorgement of the veins of the left fundus, and the fullness previously noted in the veins of the left upper eyelid disappeared. The left proptosis clinically improved, although exophthalmometer readings remained the same. Visual acuity and visual fields were unchanged.

INJURY TO THE BRAIN

Cerebral concussion is an injury to the brain sufficient to produce a disturbance in the physiological function of the brain, but not sufficient to produce anatomical disruption in the brain tissue. It is characterized by an injury to the head, followed by unconsciousness, which is momentary or which may last for an hour. Neurological signs are absent, or are minimal and transient. On regaining consciousness, the patient may have a headache, dizziness, nausea, and vomiting; however, after a brief period, lasting under ten days, the patient usually makes a complete recovery. Only in the apprehensive, anxious, nervous patient or the compensation case are there likely to be residual symptoms.

Treatment is symptomatic, and the doctor should convey his optimism to the patient. (See details of treatment under Management of the Patient with Head Injury, page 683.)

Case III (Cerebral concussion)

History. A 38-year-old obese man had been beaten up by several men about 1 hour before admission. He was unconscious for 4 or 5 minutes. On regaining consciousness he noted dull occipital headache, blurring of vision, and bleeding from the nose.

Examination. Pulse 80, respiration 18, temperature 98.6, blood pressure 140/85. The patient was mentally clear, with superficial laceration of the left forehead, and the left eye was closed by periorbital swelling and ecchymosis. The nose was swollen and there was dried blood on the right side. There was no bleeding from the ears or blood behind the tympanic membranes. There was some unsteadiness in walking and a tremor of the outstretched fingers. Examination was otherwise normal.

Roentgenograms of the skull were normal.

The patient was free of symptoms in three days, and the neurological signs disappeared.

Cerebral contusion is caused by an injury to the brain sufficient to produce bruising of the brain with small hemorrhages. These petechiae are usually scattered, but may become confluent, and a small amount of blood may escape into the subarachnoid space. Swelling is always present around the site of the contusion, but in some cases it becomes more generalized. As a result of the bruising, swelling, and hemorrhage, the injured parts may become pulpefied, i.e., necrotic and liquefied. This occurs most frequently in the anterior part of the temporal lobes, and the anterior and inferior parts of the frontal lobes. Intracranial pressure is always increased. Cerebral laceration and hemorrhage are always accompanied by varying amounts of cerebral contusion; hence the clinical differentiation is one of degree. Therefore, clinical findings in both will be discussed together.

Case IV (Cerebral contusion)

History. Seventeen hours before admission, this 30-year-old woman pulled the chain of a water closet, and the tank, weighing about 30 pounds, came loose and fell three or four feet, striking her on the right side of her head and right shoulder. She was unconscious 10 minutes, and then had headache, with pain in the area where she was struck, and dizziness. Two hours after injury she vomited. Weakness of the right upper extremity was apparent at that time, and she became drowsy. She was unsteady when she walked.

Examination. Pulse 68, respiration 20, temperature 98.8, blood pressure 150/96. Neurological signs were right hemiparesis, right hyperreflexia, and right central facial paresis.

Course in hospital. Roentgenograms of the skulls were normal. Lumbar puncture showed an initial pressure of 180 mm. of water. The fluid was slightly blood tinged, containing 950 red blood cells, 85 per cent of which were crenated. She progressively improved in the hospital. The drowsiness disappeared. The strength improved gradually, but there was some residual weakness and hyperreflexia in the right extremities when she was discharged from the hospital 19 days after injury.

Cerebral laceration and hemorrhage, as the terms indicate, consist in disruption of the substance of the brain with extravasation of blood from the torn arteries and veins. Lacerations are most frequent at the base of the brain. The amount of hemorrhage depends on the size and position of the vessel torn. Traumatic rupture of an aneurysm which had been silent, or of a large blood vessel, may result in severe bleeding into the subarachnoid space, the subdural space, the substance of the brain, or a combination of all three.

The healing of contusions, laceration, and hemorrhage of the brain is similar to that in other parts of the body. First liquefaction and phagocytosis of the devitalized tissue and blood occur. The microglia become the phagocytes of the brain, and the astrocytes form a glial scar. Their presence has been found within a few days after injury. Fibrous or mesothelial scar extends outward from the blood vessels. It is the mesothelial scar which is more likely to cause the convulsions following trauma. When there is anatomical disruption of nerve cells in the brain, atrophy occurs, since the nerve cells and their processes within the central nervous system do not regenerate. In the early stages it is not possible clinically to distinguish between anatomical disruption and a temporary interruption of physiological function by pressure or swelling, as the neurological signs are the same.

In patients having cerebral contusion or cerebral laceration and hemorrhage the history is one of severe trauma to the head, and most often there is a fracture of the skull. The period of unconsciousness varies, but it usually lasts a minimum of 30 minutes and may continue for days. The longer it lasts the more serious is the brain injury likely to be, and the greater the possibility of sequelae. One must be alert in observing the depth of unconsciousness, as partial or incomplete recovery of consciousness followed by retrogression is indicative of a new pathological process, such as hemorrhage or edema, added to the initial brain injury.

The clinical signs which the patient exhibits depend on the location of the injury. A large hemorrhage into a silent area of the brain, such as the right frontal or right temporal lobe, produces increased intracranial pressure, but there may be no focal neurological signs. Injury to the motor cortex or motor pathways results in weakness or paralysis, and increased deep tendon reflexes and pathological toe signs such as a positive Babinski or Chaddock reflex. Injury to the sensory cortex or pathways results in numbness and impairment in sensation. Injury to the speech areas produces aphasia, and injury to the visual cortex or pathways is followed by impairment in the visual fields and visual acuity. Ataxia, decreased muscle tone, and nystagmus are caused by injury to the cerebellum. Diabetes insipidus and high temperature characterize injury to the hypothalamus. Cranial nerve signs suggest injury to the brain stem. Any combination of these symptoms and signs may be present; the greater the number, the more serious the injury.

In addition to the direct trauma to the brain, another hazard is produced when there is greatly increased intracranial pressure on one side as a result of either hemorrhage or edema. This hazard is a herniation of the uncus through the incisura. When this happens the uncus is pushed against the midbrain, displacing and squeezing it against the opposite edge of the tentorium. The herniated uncus presses upon the ipsilateral third nerve and posterior cerebral artery, and indirectly upon the contralateral posterior cerebral artery. It interferes with the venous drainage from the midbrain and causes hemorrhage into the midbrain. The pressure on the midbrain may produce decerebrate rigidity. Pressure on the third nerve produces dilatation of the pupil. Pressure on the posterior cerebral artery produces homonymous visual field defects. Hemorrhage into the midbrain may produce dilatation of one or both pupils, decerebrate rigidity, coma, and death. Evidence of midbrain involvement is, therefore, very serious, and death may be imminent. (See details of treatment under Management of the Patient with Head Injury, page 683.)

Extradural hemorrhage of clinical significance is commonly arterial in nature, resulting from a tear of a branch of the middle meningeal artery, usually in the anterior temporal region where the artery is embedded in bone. Occasionally extradural bleeding is venous in character, originating in a tear of one of the venous sinuses. In each instance there is a fracture of the skull. In the former event the fracture extends across the squamous part of the temporal bone or the greater wing of the sphenoid bone (Fig. 22–*10*); in the latter the fracture extends across the superior sagittal sinus or lateral sinus. Extradural hemorrhage rarely occurs without a fracture of the skull. Extradural hemorrhage of venous origin is infrequent, and the clinical course closely resembles that of an acute subdural hematoma.

The typical history of an extradural hemorrhage of arterial origin is one of an injury resulting in unconsciousness, followed by a lucid interval or at least partial recovery of consciousness, which is then succeeded by increasing stupor progressing to coma, increasing weakness beginning in the face or arm on the side opposite to the hemorrhage and spreading to the leg, dilatation of the pupil usually on the side of the hematoma, and, if the hematoma is unrelieved, bilateral dilatation and fixation of the pupils, decerebrate rigidity, and death due to uncal herniation. If the injury to the brain is sufficiently great, the unconsciousness due to the injury itself and that due to pressure of the epidural hemorrhage may overlap, and hence there will be no lucid interval. Early convulsive movements may appear in the contralateral extremities. The pulse and respiration are slow, and the blood pressure becomes elevated. The stage of the slow pulse and respiration may be of very short duration and never recognized. The pulse and respiration then become rapid, and the blood pressure continues to rise, as does the temperature. In the terminal stages the blood pressure falls, the pulse becomes thready, respirations become shallow and rapid, and the temperature continues to rise.

TREATMENT consists of emergency operative therapy, usually under a local anesthetic. The whole head should be prepared and draped. A straight incision is made in the temporal region, beginning at the zygomatic process and extending upward 10–12 cm. The incision is carried right down to the temporal bone through the temporal fascia and the temporal muscle. The muscle is then separated subperiosteally from the bone, and a self-retaining retractor is inserted to hold back all of the layers (see Fig. 22–*17*). A trephine opening is then made in the temporal bone and enlarged to 5 or 6 cm. by means of rongeurs. The extradural clot is seen immediately beneath the bone and it is removed, the bleeding point is located, and bleeding is stopped either by electrocautery or by silver clips. At times it may be necessary to ligate the middle meningeal artery as it enters the skull through the foramen spinosum. This is done by silver clips, silk ligatures, or electrocautery. If a subdural hematoma is suggested by a bluish discoloration of the dura, the latter should be opened to permit inspection of the brain and evacuation of the hematoma. The patient should show signs of improvement. If he does not, and if there are indications of herniation of the uncus, the temporal lobe of the brain should be gently lifted upward and the uncus lifted out of the incisura. When the uncus is released, there is usually a gush of fluid from the incisural region. The wound is then closed in layers with interrupted sutures of black silk in the dura, temporal muscle, temporal fascia, galea aponeurotica, and skin.

The unconscious patient operated on under a local anesthetic will often recover consciousness as soon as the extradural clot is evacuated. Also the signs of midbrain compression (uncal herniation) will rapidly improve. This is well demonstrated by the following case.

Case V (Extradural hemorrhage)

History. This 15-year-old boy, while playing football, five hours before admission, was hit on the left side of his head by an opponent's knee. He was not dazed by the blow and continued to play for several minutes. After resting 10 to 15 minutes, he began to complain of pain in the left side of his head and of some dizziness. On the way home he felt dizzy and drowsy and "acted as if he were drunk." One hour after injury he began to vomit, and vomited three times at 30-minute intervals. His family physician advised hospitalization.

Examination. Pulse 60, respiration 20, blood pressure 118/60. The patient was drowsy. There was tenderness and slight redness in the left frontoparietal region. There were no focal neurological signs.

Laboratory studies. Roentgenograms of the skull were normal. Hemoglobin was 10.2 gm.; erythrocytes were 4,250,000; leukocyte count was 21,150, with 91 per cent polymorphonuclears and 9 per cent lymphocytes.

Course. The patient, admitted at 9.00 P.M., remained drowsy but responded readily during the night and continued to complain of headache. The next morning a spinal puncture was done. The fluid was clear; the pressure 190 mm. of water. There were one white blood cell and three red blood cells. The total protein was 31 mg. per 100 ml. The colloidal gold and Wassermann tests were negative. Following the spinal puncture the headache became more severe. One hour later the pulse fell to 50, blood pressure rose to 170, and the patient vomited and became restless. Two hours after the puncture, he had become unresponsive verbally, very agitated, and moved his right arm less than the left. The left pupil was slightly smaller than the right, but both reacted briskly to light. The deep tendon reflexes were hypoactive throughout. There was a positive Babinski sign on the right. The patient was taken to the operating room where the right pupil became dilated. A trephine opening was first placed on the right side because of the dilated pupil, but there was no evidence of extradural or subdural bleeding. A trephine opening was then made in the left temporal region and a large extradural clot was found. The opening was enlarged by performing a subtemporal craniectomy. Both liquid blood and solid clot were found and removed. The clot was 4 cm. thick. Bleeding, from the middle meningeal artery 4 cm. from the foramen spinosum, was stopped with silver clips. The brain did not expand to its normal position immediately, and a drain was placed in the extradural space.

The patient was operated on under local anesthesia and as soon as the clot was removed he began to respond and the pupils became equal. He continued drowsy for two days, and a nominal type of aphasia, right hemiparesis, and a positive Babinski sign on the right were observed. Seven days after surgery the neurological signs had disappeared, and the patient was asymptomatic on discharge from the hospital on the fifteenth postoperative day. When last seen one year later, he had no complaints, and there were no positive neurological signs.

Comment. It was fortunate that this patient was in a hospital where emergency neurosurgical procedures could be performed. The spinal puncture, a dangerous procedure in head injury cases, resulted in herniation of the uncus and midbrain compression. Had this patient not been operated upon so promptly, he would not have survived.

This case illustrates that a patient may remain conscious after the initial injury and have no fracture of the skull yet still have a ruptured artery or vein with resultant severe intracranial hemorrhage.

Subdural hematoma may be acute or chronic. *Acute subdural hemorrhage* may result from tearing of one or more superior cerebral veins or of the Labbé vein, but it is usually due to laceration of the brain, including

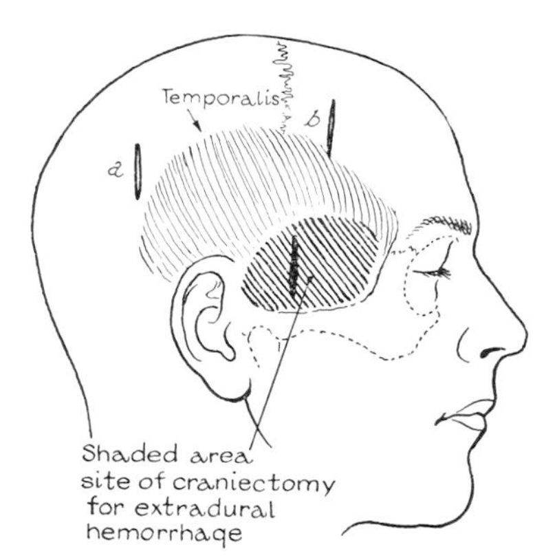

Figure 22–17. Sites of skin incisions for making the trephine openings for a subdural hematoma (a, b, and the vertical black line in the shaded area).

the pia and arachnoid, with tearing of arteries and veins at the site of laceration. It is associated with very severe and most often fatal injury to the brain, the clinical picture being that of cerebral laceration and hemorrhage. Occasionally when injury to the brain is not serious, the superior cerebral veins may be torn and a large hemorrhage into the subdural space occur.

Such a hemorrhage has been found in fighters who have not regained consciousness after being "knocked out" or who have regained consciousness for a short period only. In these cases the signs and symptoms resemble closely those of an extradural hemorrhage, but usually the neurological signs are more diffuse.

TREATMENT is immediate operation preceded by bilateral carotid arteriography if the patient's condition permits. This will determine the side on which the hemorrhage occurred, and if it is bilateral. Two or three liters of cross-matched blood should be available, as a great amount of blood may be lost before the bleeding point is located and bleeding stopped. The operation is performed under a local anesthetic or none at all. The entire head is prepared and draped. Trephine openings are made in the posterior parietal region on the dorsolateral surface of the skull and a comparable one on the lateral surface in the posterior frontal region (Fig. 22–*17*). If the hemorrhage is not found on one side, similar openings are made on the other side. In fact, both sides should always be opened since the hemorrhage may be bilateral. If the hemorrhage is not found in the frontal or parietal region, trephine openings are made in the low temporal regions. Although in acute subdural hematoma there will be some liquid blood which can be evacuated through trephine openings, it will be necessary to turn a bone flap in order to evacuate a solid clot and to locate and control the bleeding point. In placing the bone flap, the sites at which bleeding is likely to occur must be kept in mind. The bleeding points may be difficult to locate and to control. Bleeding may be stopped by means of silver clips, electrocautery, Gelfoam, or oxidized cotton. The wound is then closed in layers.

If the acute subdural hematoma is due to laceration of the brain the prognosis is very poor, since the brain injury will be marked.

Case VI (Acute subdural hemorrhage)

History. This patient was a man 68 years old who had difficulty in hearing. At 11:00 P.M. the day before admission, he did not see his wife approaching him and was startled by her touch, lost his balance and fell, striking the back of his head in the midline against the wall. As he fell to the floor he was not unconscious, and he had no bleeding from the cranial orifices. He got up and lay across the foot of the bed before continuing to undress and to go to bed. He said that he was all right. At 2:00 A.M. he wakened, complaining of headache. He vomited and became very restless. These symptoms continued, and a physician was called at 4:00 A.M. Morphine sulfate, 0.01 gm., was given without effect on the headache. At 9:00 A.M. the patient became comatose and remained so.

The past history revealed only a blood pressure at times as high as 180, albumin in the urine, and evidence of cerebral arteriosclerosis.

Examination. The patient was comatose and cyanotic. Respirations were labored at 28, the pulse was 124, and the blood pressure was 180/96. There was an abrasion 1 cm. in diameter, and edema of the scalp in the left posterior parietal region. There was no blood in any of the cranial orifices or behind the ear drums. Contusions and ecchymoses were present over the ulnar sides of both forearms at the junction of the middle and lower thirds. The pupils were dilated and fixed. The veins of the retina were dilated, and the arteries were pale. Two small hemorrhages were present near the right optic disc. The deep tendon reflexes were hyperactive in the left upper extremity and in both lower extremities. There was an equivocal Babinski sign bilaterally, and the abdominal reflexes were absent. No eversion was present in either lower extremity. There was slight stiffness of the neck. The Kernig sign was negative. The muscle tone was normal.

Roentgenogram of the skull showed no fracture.

Course. Because of the patient's poor condition, relief of the intracranial pressure offered the only chance of survival. A trephine opening was first made on the left side, but no hematoma was found, and the pressure was found to be greatly increased. A solid clot was found on the right side in the subdural space, and it was necessary to turn a small flap in order to evacuate the clot. The clot, 3 cm. thick, covered the right hemisphere from the frontal to the occipital pole. There was evidence of cerebral arteriosclerosis, and the brain did not re-expand after the clot was removed. His condition did not improve after evacuation of the clot, and death occurred 3½ hours after completion of the operation.

Chronic subdural hematoma is the result of tearing of one or more veins which extend from the brain across the subdural space to the various dural sinuses. The veins there are fixed at both ends, but are free where they extend across the subdural space. When the brain moves within the intracranial cavity, as it does with every movement of the head, these veins are stretched. When a head injury occurs, movement of the brain within the skull may be great, and if the veins cannot stretch sufficiently they tear and blood escapes into the subdural space. The hematoma is usually within the subdural space supratentorially but may be within the posterior fossa.

The cause of the late development of increased intracranial pressure is liquefaction of the inner part of the clot, with a subsequent increase in the size of the liquid mass, due to osmosis. The clot is gradually organized by the ingrowth of capillaries and fibroblasts from the dura. This layer, next to the dura, is called the outer membrane. The inner membrane of the hematoma is a thin, transparent layer of mesothelium.

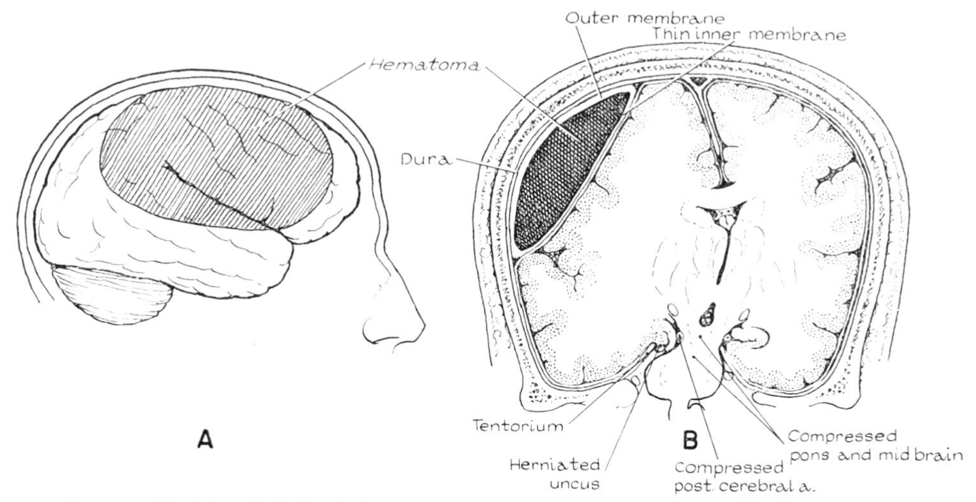

Figure 22–18. Subdural hematoma.

A. The usual location of a subdural hematoma on the dorsolateral surface of the cerebral hemisphere.

B. Coronal section, showing the hematoma, with resultant displacement of the brain to the opposite side, herniation of the uncus, and compression of the posterior cerebral artery, as well as of midbrain and pons.

The history is that of a head injury which may be insufficient to cause loss of consciousness or clinical signs. In alcoholics the injury may even be forgotten. The patient continues to complain of headache from the time of injury, although it may vary in severity, and there may be periods of freedom from it. Days, weeks, or even months later evidence of increased intracranial pressure develops, with severe headaches aggravated by change of position, nausea, vomiting, mental changes, and disturbances in vision.

There may be no neurological signs, but one pupil is often dilated and this is usually but not always on the side of the hematoma. Low-grade papilledema is frequently present. Ataxia is usually present when the hematoma or hygroma is in the posterior fossa (see Case VIII). The patient becomes drowsy, and the state of consciousness may show remarkable variation within a few minutes. At this stage the pulse and respiration are usually slow. With further advance in pressure the patient becomes comatose, the tone in the muscles increases, the deep tendon reflexes become hyperactive, the Babinski reflexes become positive, and one or both pupils become dilated and fixed. Decerebrate rigidity appears. At this stage the pulse and respiration become accelerated, the blood pressure falls, and the temperature rises. If the hematoma is not evacuated, the patient will die as a result of herniation of the uncus into the incisura.

Such herniation of the uncus takes place in the presence of a large hematoma and produces many of the signs exhibited. It causes pressure upon the midbrain, third nerve, posterior cerebral arteries (Fig. 22–*18*), and the veins draining the midbrain, resulting in hemorrhage into the midbrain and infarction of occipital lobe. Inequality of the pupils is an early sign of herniation of the uncus. The larger pupil is most often found on the side of the hematoma, but it may be on the opposite side. With greater herniation the pupil becomes dilated and fixed, and both pupils may be involved. The mental responses become less active, and the patient becomes comatose. Hemiparesis progresses to hemiplegia and quadriplegia. The tone of the extremities increases, decerebrate rigidity occurs, and, unless the pressure is relieved, death soon follows.

It is axiomatic that patients with a history of head injury who later develop headaches and mental disturbances, and whose roentgenograms show a shift of the pineal gland, have a subdural hematoma until it is proved otherwise. It must be emphasized that the hematoma may be found on the side opposite to that suggested by the clinical findings and also that subdural hematomas are often bilateral. X-ray films are normal unless the pineal gland is calcified and is found to be displaced. The electroencephalogram is usually not helpful.

The presence or absence of a subdural hematoma may be determined by carotid arteriography (see Fig. 22–*19*), but it can also be found by multiple trephinations. If the condition of the patient permits, it is preferable to do bilateral carotid arteriography before resorting to operative therapy. It will show the site or sites of the hematoma, and it may also demonstrate the presence of an intracerebral hematoma, a possible vascular abnormality, or an area of pulpefied and swollen brain.

Treatment. Surgery is performed under local anesthesia if the patient is manageable, or with local and intravenous Pentothal anesthesia, with an endotracheal tube, if he is not. The entire head is prepared and draped. If there is ataxia or nystagmus, the patient should be placed face down so that trephine openings can be made in the suboccipital region. If these signs are not present, the supine position is preferable. If arteriography has been done, the site of the hematoma will already be known. Should the patient's condition be too critical for preliminary arteriography, the first trephine opening should be placed in the posterior frontal region just above the upper attachment of the temporal muscle (Fig. 22–*17*). The dura is usually bluish when a subdural hematoma is present, but a blue color may also be produced by a cortical vein. When the dura is opened, the outer layer of the hematoma is encountered and, when this is opened, the liquefied hematoma is found and is gradually evacuated. A rubber catheter is gently inserted into the subdural space and the cavity is irrigated with Ringer's solution until the return is clear. A second trephine opening is placed in the posterior parietal region and the dura opened to explore further for subdural hematoma and to facilitate its removal. A third opening may be made in the inferior temporal region, for the same purpose. Frontal, parietal, and temporal openings should be made on both sides, because of the frequency of bilateral subdural hematomas.

The outer layer of the subdural hematoma is disturbed as little as possible, as it is vascularized and may continue to ooze blood. The thin, transparent inner membrane rarely requires any consideration in adults, but in children, especially infants, it may hold the brain down, inhibit its growth, and allow space for re-formation of the hematoma. In such cases

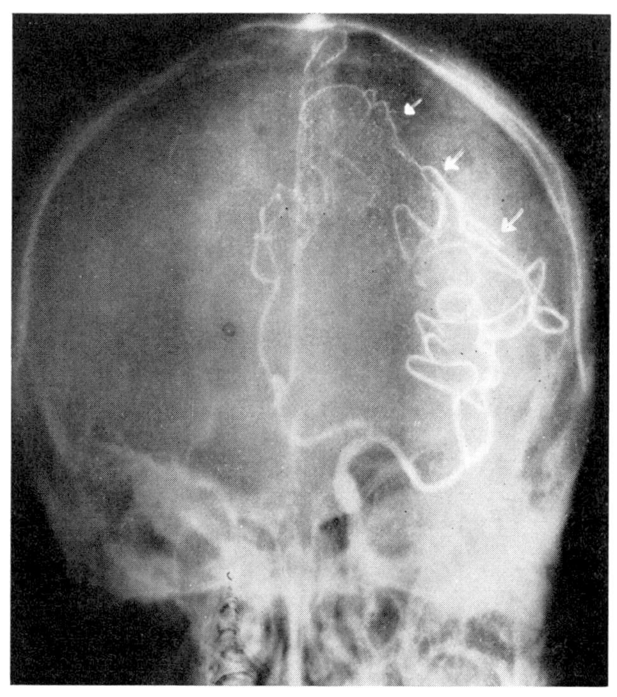

Figure 22–19. Anteroposterior arteriogram showing large subdural hematoma. The arrows indicate depression of the cortical vessels from the inner table of the skull. The anterior cerebral artery seen in center of the film is displaced to the opposite side.

it is necessary to turn a flap and to incise the inner membrane widely. This is rarely necessary in adults. In adults, when the brain does not promptly re-expand to eliminate the subdural space, a Penrose drain is left in place for 24 hours and the patient is kept as much as possible with the side of the hematoma down, to allow gravity drainage and to promote re-expansion of the brain. The closure is routine, with interrupted black silk sutures in the galea and skin. The dura is rarely closed.

The patient most often improves immediately after the hematoma is evacuated. Even unconscious patients will frequently regain consciousness. The course is usually one of progressive improvement, but in patients with arteriosclerosis the brain may not re-expand and the hematoma may re-form.

Case VII (Subdural hematoma)

History. Three months before admission this man fell 9 feet when the ladder on which he was standing broke. He was unconscious for about 30 minutes. He sustained a laceration in the right frontal region, fracture of the right wrist, and multiple contusions and abrasions. He had rather vague complaints in addition to headache, but two months later he developed weakness in the right extremities, numbness in the right upper extremity, forgetfulness, and inability to walk.

Examination. Pulse 64, respiration 18, blood pressure 168/96, temperature 99.6. The significant neurological findings were spastic right hemiparesis, right central facial paresis, indistinctness of the margins of the optic discs, impairment of hearing on the left, mildly hyperactive deep tendon reflexes, more noticeable on the right, and loss of sensation to pin prick on the right.

Course in hospital. Roentgenograms of the skull were normal. The pineal gland was not visualized in the anteroposterior view. The electroencephalogram showed a focus in the left temporal region. Bilateral carotid arteriography (Fig. 22–*19*) showed depression of the vessels from the inner table of the skull on the left side, indicating subdural hematoma. There was no evidence of a mass on the right.

Bilateral parietal, frontal, and temporal trephine openings were made. When the dura was opened on the left side, a large liquefied subdural hematoma was found and was evacuated. The cavity was carefully washed until the return was clear. The brain fortunately re-expanded, eliminating the hematoma cavity in the subdural space. There was no hematoma on the right side. The patient improved immediately after operation and was discharged nine days later.

Subdural hygroma is the result of tear of the arachnoid in such a manner that there is a ball-valve–like action which permits escape of cerebrospinal fluid into the subdural space but prevents its return. In addition, there is frequently some hemorrhage into the subdural space. The increased protein in the fluid, which is the result of associated subdural hemorrhage, draws more fluid into the subdural space by osmosis. As in the case of subdural hematoma, a subdural hygroma may be either acute or chronic, and the clinical picture and therapy are exactly the same as those of a subdural hematoma. Like subdural hematoma, subdural hygroma may be found in the posterior fossa as well as above the tentorium.

Case VIII (Subdural hygroma)

History. This 13-year-old boy was jolted out of the rumble seat of an old car during a bumpy ride 18 days before admission. He was unconscious for 12 hours and semiconscious 4 days, and then gradually regained a normal level of consciousness. Headaches gradually increased. Diplopia developed, and his doctor observed increasing papilledema. He was then transferred to this hospital.

Examination. Pulse 98, respiration 24, blood pressure 115/68, temperature 100.4. The patient was alert, cooperative, and unsteady in walking. The left ankle jerk was hyperactive. There were two diopters of papilledema, and nystagmus on lateral gaze to either side. Weakness of the external rectus muscles was present on both sides, but was more pronounced on the right.

Course in hospital. Roentgenograms of the skull were normal. A ventriculogram, performed after biparietal trephination showed no subdural fluid, was normal. Because of the nystagmus and increased intracranial pressure, trephine openings were made on both cerebellar hemispheres, and, when the dura was opened, 15 ml. of clear fluid was recovered from the left subdural space. The patient's symptoms disappeared, and he was discharged from the hospital on the tenth postoperative day. The only finding at that time was resolving papilledema, which subsequently disappeared.

Massive intracerebral hemorrhage occurs in the first 24 hours after injury and is the result of laceration of the brain or of rupture of an intracranial aneurysm or an arteriosclerotic artery. Hemorrhages due to the latter two, associated with head injury, are rare. Acute massive traumatic intracerebral hemorrhage is associated with extensive and widespread injury to the brain. In such event the patient is deeply unconscious from the time of injury. The pulse is rapid and weak early, and becomes progressively more so. The respiration, which early may be regular, although increased in rate, becomes irregular and gasping. The blood pressure is usually low from the beginning. Complete flaccidity associated with absence of deep tendon and corneal reflexes is the rule. The pupils are dilated and fixed, or soon become so. In these cases operative therapy offers little help to the patient. In the first place, it usually is contraindicated by the presence of shock, and in the second place, the extensive brain injury makes it fruitless. Operation on these patients is usually done in the hope of finding a subdural or epidural hematoma.

Bilateral carotid arteriography should be performed before any operative therapy if the patient's condition permits. This will allow accurate localization of the hemorrhage (see Fig. 22–*20*) and will demonstrate the presence of an associated subdural hemorrhage or extradural hemorrhage.

If arteriography cannot be done, the procedure is that described for a subdural hematoma. When the hemorrhage is located, it is necessary to turn a bone flap or perform craniectomy in order to open the dura and remove the clot. After the dura is opened, a transcortical incision is made, the clot is removed, the bleeding points are controlled by silver clips, electrocautery, oxidized cotton and/or Gelfoam, and the wound is closed in layers.

Less extensive intracerebral hemorrhage may occur, and may be associated with subdural hemorrhage, as is well demonstrated by the following case.

Case IX (Subdural and intracerebral hemorrhage)

History. This 60-year-old man fell 20 feet, striking his head. He was immediately unconsciousness for perhaps 20 minutes. He then regained consciousness, but three or four hours later he became drowsy and developed increasing weakness on the left side, which progressed to a left hemiplegia, and the right pupil became dilated. The patient was taken to the operating room where bitemporal and right frontal trephination was performed, and 20 ml. of liquid and clotted blood was removed from the right subdural space and 4 or 5 ml. from the left subdural space. A small incision in the right temporal lobe revealed a small amount of fresh blood which was also removed. The intracranial tension seemed relieved. The pupils became equal, but the hemiplegia did not improve, and the patient remained semicomatose. He was given oxygen and gastric feedings. He remained the same for one week, and then became comatose and had difficulty in breathing. A tracheostomy was performed and he was transferred to the Neurological Institute.

Course. As soon as he was admitted, a right common carotid arteriogram was made (Fig. 22–*20*), using 35 per cent Diodrast. This showed a large upward displacement of the middle cerebral artery and its branches, and the anterior cerebral arteries were displaced to the left. This suggested an intracortical hemorrhage in the right temporal region.

A craniotomy was immediately performed. The dura was under great pressure. A transcortical incision was made in the middle temporal gyrus and 60 ml. of solid currant jelly–like clots was removed. The patient improved immediately. The day after operation he began to respond to the spoken voice. He was continuing to improve six months after operation when he died suddenly of a coronary occlusion. At that time he was able to walk, but had no voluntary movements in his right hand.

Gunshot wounds of the head (Fig. 22–*21*) are treated the same as any other compound fracture. It is imperative that all foreign bodies, such as fragments of hair, skin, dirt, and the bullet itself, as well as blood clots and pulpefied brain, be removed. After debridement of the scalp, bone, and dura, suction is used to remove the foreign material scattered in and along the walls of the pathway of the bullet. A head light is the most effective means of assuring visualization of the pathway of the bullet.

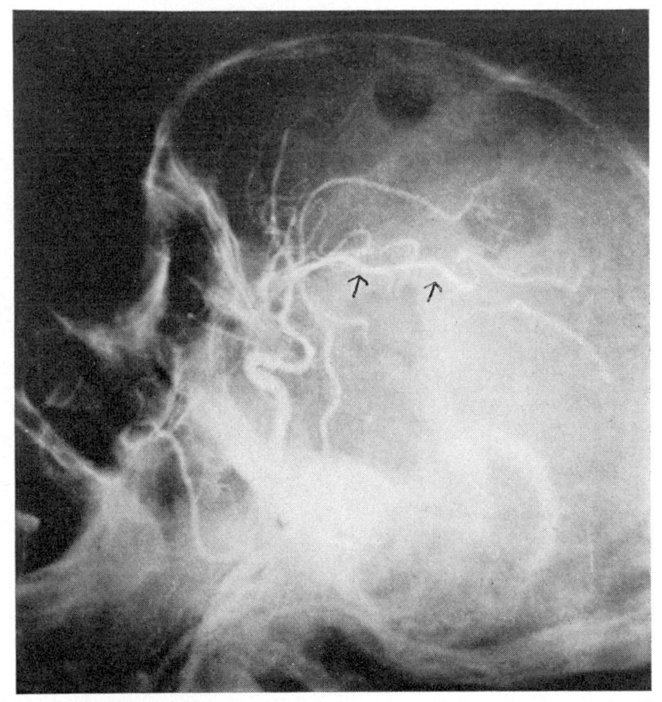

Figure 22–20. Lateral carotid arteriogram showing upward displacement of middle cerebral artery and its branches as indicated by the arrows in a patient having a large intracerebral hemorrhage in the temporal lobe. The anteroposterior view (not shown) revealed marked displacement of the anterior cerebral arteries to the opposite side.

At the operating table the Berman-Moorhead locator is the best means of localization of metal objects within the brain. (The approach of this instrument to a metal object causes an increase in sound.) It must be remembered that all other metal objects, such as towel clips, Michel clips, or hemostats, must be out of the field.

After debridement of the brain and irrigation of the bullet tract with quarts of saline or Ringer's solution, the dura and remainder of the wound are closed in the same manner as described for Depressed Fractures (p. 661).

MANAGEMENT OF THE PATIENT WITH HEAD INJURY

A detailed account of the accident itself as well as of what happened thereafter is necessary to evaluation of the type as well as of the degree of injury. The patient must be treated for shock before anything more than a superficial examination is performed. This examination should rule out the presence of pneumothorax, ruptured abdominal viscus, and major fractures. After the patient is out of shock, the spine, chest, abdomen, and extremities should be checked for evidence of injury, and then as nearly complete a neurological examination as possible should be performed. If

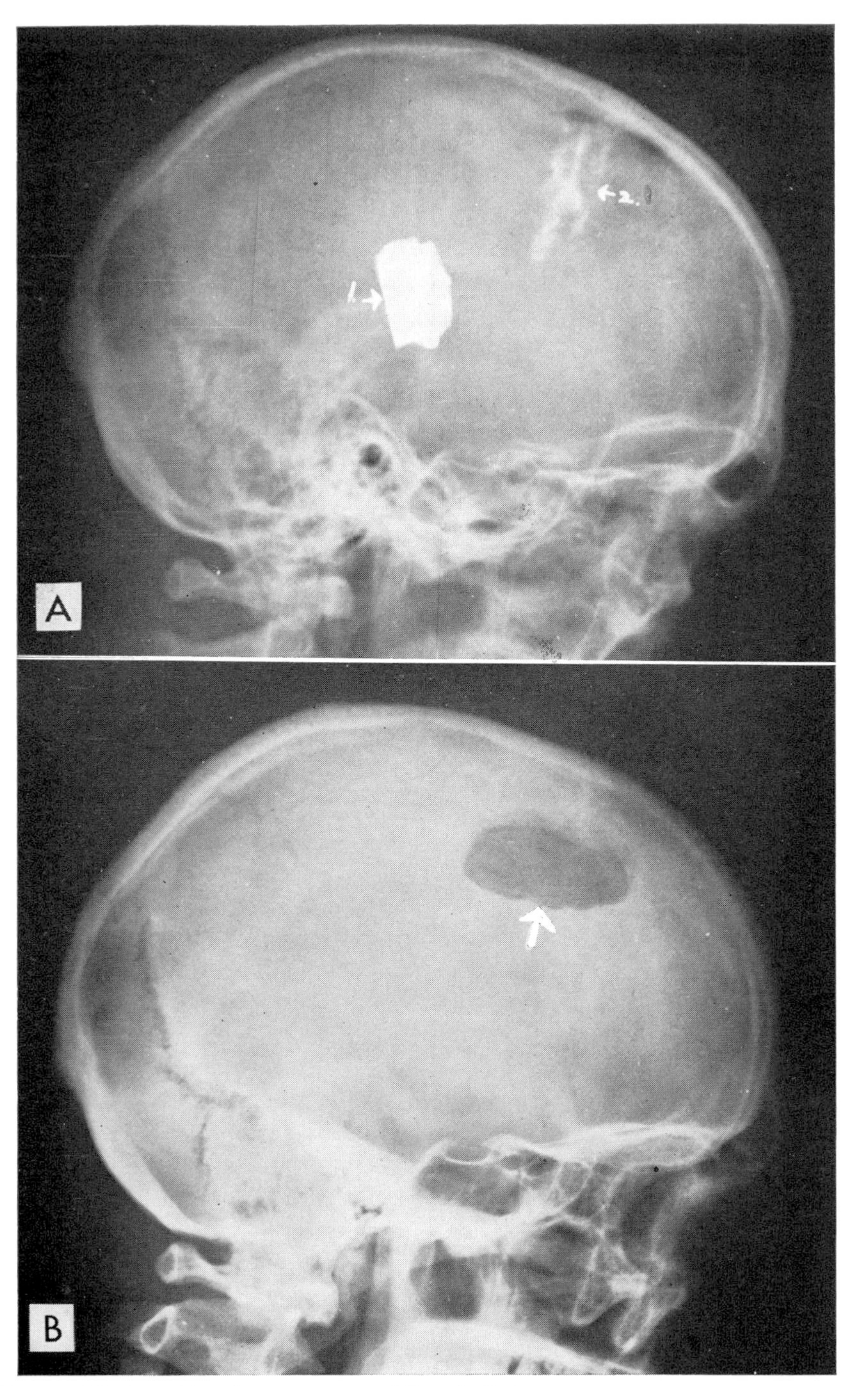

Figure 22–21. Head injury caused by shell fragment.

A. Roentgenogram showing shell fragment (arrow 1), the bone and metal debris along the tract of the fragment (arrow 2), and the opening in the skull made by the fragment.

B. Roentgenogram after operative therapy. Note absence of shell fragment and of bone and metal debris, as well as the craniectomy opening. Plating was done later.

the patient is unconscious the examination will be limited, but it does reveal important neurological data. Examination of the scalp will reveal contusions, lacerations, hematomas, or depressed fractures, but it must be remembered that the edge of a hematoma of the scalp often feels like a depressed fracture, and also that the inner table of the skull is frequently depressed more than the outer table. The eyes can be checked for evidence of hemorrhage, for position, for pupillary equality, size, shape, and reaction to light, and for condition of the eyegrounds. Blood in the nose is suggestive of fracture of the base of the skull in the anterior fossa if there is no evidence of direct trauma to the nose. Cerebrospinal fluid draining from the nose is definite evidence of a basal fracture of the skull. It represents a fracture in the cribriform plate, in the sphenoid or frontal sinuses, or in the petrous pyramid, with fluid draining into the middle ear and then into the eustachian tube, pharynx, and nose. Blood in the external auditory meatus without local trauma in or immediately outside the ear, or blood behind the tympanic membrane, is indicative of a basal fracture of the skull. Cerebrospinal fluid draining from the ear is, of course, diagnostic of a basal fracture, with tearing of the overlying dura and arachnoid. Drooping of one corner of the mouth, flattening of the nasolabial fold, blowing out of one cheek with expiration, and widening of one palpebral fissure are all signs of facial paresis. Stiffness of the neck suggests bleeding into the subarachnoid space.

The deep tendon, abdominal, and cremasteric reflexes, as well as the various pathological toe signs, should be checked. Decreased reaction to painful stimuli in the incompletely unconscious patient is helpful in localization.

In the conscious patient one can check the strength, muscle tone, coordination, reflexes, sensation, and speech, as well as the cranial nerves.

It is extremely important to have a baseline neurological examination that is as complete as possible in order to evaluate the findings of later examinations.

Lacerations should not be explored until preparations are ready for definitive treatment, and the skin around the laceration is cleansed and painted with Zephiran solution to prevent introduction of bacteria into the wound. Roentgenograms of the skull are important to determine the presence of a depressed fracture, a fracture passing across the middle meningeal artery or one of the major venous sinuses (the latter could be associated with an extradural hemorrhage), or a fracture extending into the petrous pyramid or into one of the paranasal sinuses. Fractures extending into the paranasal sinuses, the inner ear, or the mastoid sinuses are actually open fractures. If the pineal gland is shifted from its normal position, an intracranial mass must perforce be present, and this is most likely to be a hemorrhage, either extradural, subdural, or intracerebral. Therefore, roentgenography should be done as soon as the patient's condition warrants it, and certainly before any surgical treatment is undertaken.

When the patient is sent to his room, the following order should be written:

1. Bed rest.
2. Elevate head of bed 30 degrees (for better venous drainage).
3. Pulse and respiration and blood pressure should be recorded every 15 minutes for 4 hours, then every half hour (to demonstrate early any evidence of increasing intracranial pressure.)
4. Temperature should be taken every 2 hours.
5. Notify doctor (*a*) if pulse goes below 60 or above 120; (*b*) if blood pressure goes below 100 or above 160; (*c*) if there is any progressive deterioration in the state of consciousness.
6. Ice caps to head.
7. Aspirin, 0.6 gm., and caffeine citrate, 0.12 gm., for headache, if the patient is not nauseated.
8. Sodium phenobarbital 0.12 gm. every 2 hours for restlessness, if necessary, or paraldehyde 4–8 ml. intramuscularly.
9. No opiates (these cause slowing of the pulse and respiration and constriction of the pupils).

If maintenance of an adequate airway is difficult and is not readily achieved by turning the patient on his side with face turned downward toward the bed so that the tongue will drop forward, a tracheostomy should be performed.

A good airway is extremely important. An accumulation of carbon dioxide raises the intracranial pressure and promotes intracranial bleeding as well as swelling of the brain. Prolonged unconsciousness (12 hours) is an indication for tracheostomy.

Fluid intake should be maintained at 1500 ml. per day, and more than this if the patient has fever. This is best done by hypodermoclysis, using 500 ml. of 5 per cent dextrose in physiological saline solution and 1,000 ml. of 5 per cent dextrose in water. As soon as the patient ceases to vomit, a nasogastric tube can be inserted and the food and fluid intake can be readily maintained.

If the patient is not doing well and there is concern about the possibility of hemorrhage into any of the spaces or into the brain, bilateral carotid arteriography by an experienced surgeon and x-ray team offers an excellent means of determining what is taking place intracranially with a minimum of risk to the patient and without altering intracranial pressure relationships.

In the first 24 hours one must be most concerned about intracranial hemorrhage. The changes in vital signs associated with increasing intracranial pressure, as previously discussed, consist in early slowing of the pulse and respiration, and later rise in the pulse, respiration, blood pressure, and temperature. A patient who has regained consciousness shortly after injury and then in the next 24 hours has a decrease in consciousness which progresses to coma has intracranial bleeding, most probably of arterial origin, and most likely has an extradural hemorrhage, but possibly a massive subdural hematoma or an intracerebral hemorrhage. Such a patient is in urgent need of exploration in the temporal regions, for the purpose of evacuation of the clot and control of the bleeding points. Quick action in such cases is life saving. The whole head should be prepared and draped so that further surgical measures can be undertaken if necessary (see Extradural Hemorrhage—treatment, p. 673).

A deepening of the state of unconsciousness indicates an additional pathological process, such as hemorrhage or edema. In such a patient, if an extradural hematoma is found, there must also be severe injury to the brain to account for the prolonged unconsciousness before it could have been produced by extradural hemorrhage.

Inequality of the pupils developing in the first 3 to 24 hours is also suggestive of extradural hemorrhage. At first the pupil on the side of the hemorrhage may be smaller, but later it becomes dilated and sluggish in its reaction to light. At this stage decerebrate rigidity may appear, and the patient is in critical condition.

Twitching or real clonic movements or focal convulsive seizures may herald the onset of extradural hemorrhage. Such movements occur on the side opposite the hemorrhage and are followed by increasing weakness in these extremities. The deep tendon reflex changes are less informative, as they are as apt to be decreased as increased following injury, but it is helpful when they can be compared with findings of the baseline examination. Actually, shortly after injury the deep tendon reflexes are more apt to be depressed on the side opposite the site of the injury. Sensory changes or homonymous hemianopia are rare in patients with subdural or extradural hemorrhage.

The appearance within the first 24 hours of signs of focal involvement of the brain which were not present immediately after injury is also suggestive of intracerebral hemorrhage. This is the result of injury to an artery, the rupture of an abnormal vascular structure such as an aneurysm, or the coalescence of multiple petechial hemorrhages. In the last instance, neurological signs are present on admission and these become more marked.

It is usually unnecessary to evacuate these hemorrhages within the first 24 hours, but at times prompt operation is imperative.

Acute subdural hematomas within the first 24 hours are associated with severe brain injury, i.e., laceration of the brain. Early operative removal usually does not save the patient, but is the only hope for his survival.

After the first day following injury, one must watch for evidence of subdural hematoma or hygroma, intracerebral hemorrhage, extradural hemorrhage of venous origin (infrequent), cerebral edema, and of course the possible development of meningitis in the event of compound fractures.

In a patient developing a subdural hematoma there are signs of gradually increasing intracranial pressure, such as slowing of the pulse and respiration, diminishing consciousness, deepening coma, and evidence of midbrain pressure, inequality in the size of the pupils, decreased pupillary reaction to light, and eventually dilatation and fixation of the pupils. When this stage is reached decerebrate rigidity may develop and the patient is in imminent danger of death. Operation should be performed before decerebrate rigidity appears.

Cerebral edema may cause the same neurological signs as a subdural hematoma, and a positive diagnosis is possible only after multiple trephine openings have been made or bilateral carotid arteriography has been performed. Edematous pulpefied brain can sometimes be removed, with relief of increased intracranial pressure and benefit to the patient.

The signs of an extradural hemorrhage of venous origin are similar to those of a subacute subdural hematoma with increasing signs beginning 2 to 5 days after injury. Roentgenography usually demonstrates a fracture of the skull which passes across one of the dural venous sinuses, and carotid arteriography will show the presence of the mass.

There are focal neurological signs when an intracerebral hemorrhage or laceration of the brain is present, unless it has occurred in a silent area of the brain, such as the anterior parts of the right frontal or temporal lobes in right-handed patients. The signs present depend upon the region of the brain involved by the hemorrhage.

From the first week up to months after the injury, one must watch for a chronic subdural hematoma. The signs are first headache, then nausea, vomiting, and papilledema, and later fluctuation in the state of consciousness. The neurological examination may show no focal signs, but there may be inequality of the pupils. Roentgenography may show a lateral shift of the pineal gland when the hematoma is on one side only or is greater on one side.

The key to ultimate success in the management of the patient with head injury is the earliest possible medical as well as occupational rehabilitation. Every patient who has had a brain injury, including those with minor concussions, is worried about the possibility of physical or mental sequelae even when he is making a very satisfactory recovery. It is easy for these patients to become psychoneurotic. They need frequent reassurance and encouragement. They should become ambulatory and return to work as early as possible. A patient who has been unconscious for only a few minutes and who has no positive neurological signs may be up as soon as he feels like getting up and may return to work within a few days or a week; actually, as soon as he is symptom free he may be discharged from the hospital and return to light work, and within two weeks he may return to heavy work.

A patient who has residual symptoms and signs should have every helpful form of physiotherapy and occupational therapy to hasten his recovery and to make it as nearly complete as possible. Being with other disabled patients helps to prevent the patient from feeling sorry for himself. It affords an opportunity for one patient to learn from another, which they do eagerly, and it fosters a spirit of competition on the road to recovery. A patient whose disability is such that he cannot resume his previous occupation can be tested for his aptitude and then taught a new and suitable occupation in accordance with his physical and mental capacities. He should also be placed in a proper job.

It cannot be too strongly emphasized that any litigation should be concluded as early as possible by a lump sum settlement. Symptoms are known to remain as long as the patient may benefit from any litigation because of their presence. Rehabilitation is also more quickly accomplished when the patient has nothing to gain by remaining sick.

Electroencephalography is of little practical value in the first week after injury, except as a basis for comparison when future studies are made. Clinical and electroencephalographic improvement usually run parallel courses, but at times the patient may be well by clinical examination and still have some electroencephalographic abnormalities. This is believed to indicate cerebral dysfunction. A normal electroencephalogram is indicative of no abnormal cerebral tissue in 87 per cent of the cases. This is of value in separating patients with hysteria or malingering from those with organic cerebral dysfunction resulting from trauma. Further, it is believed that the electroencephalogram indicates the degree of cerebral dysfunction. Focal electroencephalographic signs are associated with persistent clinical signs. Serial electroencephalograms are of value in predicting those patients who will develop signs.

SEQUELAE OF HEAD INJURY

The most common unfavorable sequel of head injury is the so-called "postconcussion syndrome." This is a symptom complex consisting of headache, dizziness, nervousness, forgetfulness, personality changes, difficulty in concentration, and frequently insomnia. It is poorly named because it is not the result of a concussion but is due to diffuse injury to the brain. Neurological examination and electroencephalography show a few scattered signs. Pneumoencephalography will demonstrate atrophy of cortex and subcortical tissues by an increase in the size of the ventricles and of the sulci on the surface of the brain. The duration of these symptoms is dependent upon the severity of the injury, personality factors, work situation, and litigation status.

Localized injury to the brain may result in varying grades of loss of strength, sensation, coordination, vision, mental powers (post-traumatic neurosis or psychosis as in Case X), or in epilepsy (post-traumatic epilepsy).

Injury of the cranial nerves usually occurs in thin channels of exit from the cranial cavity as a result of fractures or hemorrhage. The nuclei or the end-organs such as the labyrinth may also be injured. The first eight cranial nerves, nuclei, or end-organs are the ones usually injured, the last four rarely being involved. The hearing apparatus is the organ most frequently injured. (See discussion in Chapter 23, under Injuries to the Auditory Apparatus.)

Case X (Post-traumatic psychosis)

History. A white man, 46 years old, fell down fourteen marble steps, striking his head on the steps on the way down. He was immediately unconscious and was still comatose one hour later when he was admitted to the hospital.

Examination. The patient was deeply comatose; temperature was 99, pulse 84, respiration 24, blood pressure 85/50. Pupils were equal and reacted sluggishly to light. The deep tendon reflexes were absent. There was no stiffness of the neck. There was a hematoma of the scalp in the left temporal region, and blood behind the left ear drum. Roentgenograms showed multiple linear fractures of the skull without depression.

Course in hospital. Fifteen minutes after admission, the patient reacted slightly to pain but did not move the right upper extremity. Preparations were being made to operate for an epidural hematoma about 4 hours after injury when he became semiconscious and moved his right arm. He was then placed in an oxygen tent, although his color was good. He was incontinent of urine. Movement in the right arm continued to improve, and the patient became more responsive. Nineteen hours after injury he became very noisy and restless, and paraldehyde, 4 ml., was given intramuscularly. The vital signs were well maintained. By the second day after injury, the patient responded to simple commands and took fluids by mouth. He moved all extremities well, except for some residual weakness in the right upper extremity. For the first 16 days he remained alternately somnolent and extremely restless, in a confused mental state. He was cooperative within the limits of his restricted comprehension and short attention span. He had regained bladder and bowel control and was up in a wheel chair. Shortly thereafter he was able to talk. However, he remained confused and disoriented and had no insight. He was euphoric and wandered about the floors. It was impossible to keep him in one place. As he made no improvement in a two-week period and would not stay in one place, he was transferred to a mental institution 34 days after the injury.

The patient improved very slowly and was discharged from the psychiatric hospital four months after injury. He was able to return to his former trade as a printer and has continued to remain well.

CHAPTER 23

INJURIES TO AUDITORY APPARATUS, NOSE AND PARANASAL SINUSES, LARYNX AND TRACHEA

By FRANZ ALTMANN, M.D.

AUDITORY APPARATUS

Auricle and External Auditory Meatus

THE GENERAL PRINCIPLES of treatment of wounds of the auricle are the same as of that of wounds elsewhere in the body. In tears, cuts, or lacerations, primary closure of the wound should be attempted after the wound has been properly cleaned. In more extensive injuries, severely traumatized tissue, including cartilage, should be excised, but great care should be taken not to remove more tissue than is absolutely necessary, since the blood supply of the auricle offers favorable chances for recovery. If larger parts, even the entire auricle, are completely severed, they should be sutured into place, if possible, after exact apposition of the skin margins. Prevention of infection is the most important point in treatment of injuries to the auricle. Chemotherapy and the common antibiotics usually will prevent development of wound infections of the ordinary type, but they will not always prevent occurrence of the most unpleasant complication, that of perichondritis of the auricular cartilage. This infection is characterized by redness, diffuse swelling, and marked tenderness of the auricle, followed by circumscribed fluctuation when an abscess has formed. Perichondritis is often caused by *Pseudomonas aeruginosa* (*Bacillus pyocyaneus*), which is resistant to sulfonamides and such antibiotics as penicillin, Terramycin, or Achromycin. Local application to the wound of solutions of bacitracin or of polymixin B will, in many instances, prevent further complications. If, however, a wound infection develops despite these precautions, cultures should be taken and sensitivity of the causative organism determined to permit proper treatment (see Chapter 3).

If perichondritis progresses to abscess formation, larger areas of the cartilage may become necrotic, and sequestration eventually take place. Since this may lead to marked deformities of the auricle, it is advisable to treat such abscesses adequately in the early stages by making one or

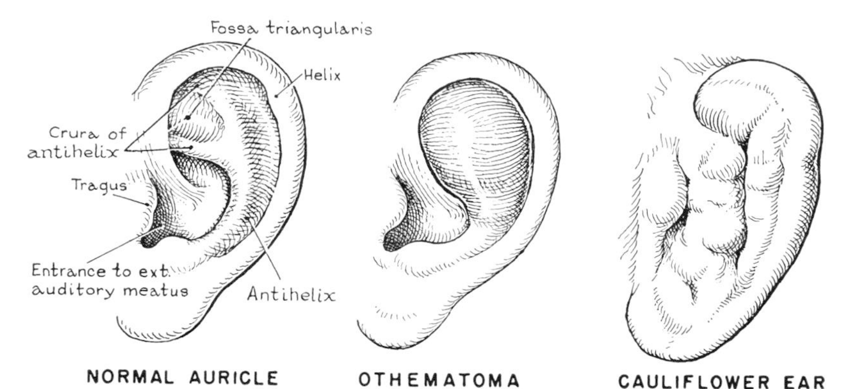

Figure 23–1. The external ear, showing one normal auricle and two which have been injured.

several incisions through the entire thickness of the auricle from one side to the other. The incisions should run, if possible, parallel to one of the grooves of the normal ear. Drains should be introduced and the wound irrigated with a solution of the appropriate antibiotic, provided the causative organism is found sensitive to local application. If the injury causes marked deformity of the auricle, plastic surgery becomes necessary, particularly in men in whom the deformed auricle cannot be hidden by the hair.

When trauma is caused by a blunt object hitting the auricle in a tangential direction, blood may accumulate between the cartilage and perichondrium on the lateral surface of the auricle, frequently in the fossa triangularis. This condition, called othematoma (Fig. 23–*1*), is often combined with a diffuse hemorrhagic infiltration of the overlying soft tissues. Othematoma is frequently seen in boxers, wrestlers, acrobats, and inmates of mental institutions, or in people who carry on the shoulder heavy loads which rub against the ear. In patients who are debilitated or who show abnormal fragility of the blood vessels, othematoma can occur from a relatively insignificant trauma, such as a slight slap with the hand, or from lying on a hard pillow. An early othematoma has the appearance of a hard, elastic, non-tender swelling. If it is not disturbed, the hemorrhagic exudate organizes, with the growth of connective tissue, followed by shrinkage. This leads to thickening, or even to marked deformity of the auricle—the so-called cauliflower ear (see Fig. 23–*1*). The deformity is particularly marked when the exudate has become infected and perichondritis developed.

In early stages, when the blood is still fluid, treatment consists in aspirating the exudate with a short needle of large lumen under strict aseptic precautions, followed by application of a pressure bandage. Often, especially in the later stages, aspiration alone is insufficient, and one or several incisions will be necessary, preferably parallel with the border of the helix. The coagula are aspirated with a cannula, or removed with a curette. Then a simple pressure bandage is applied and left on for at least one week, until the detached perichondrium again adheres to the cartilage. In some instances the use of a mold or dental stent, plaster of paris or plastic, is helpful. If the blood is aspirated and secondary infection prevented, the auricle will regain its original shape, except possibly for some thickening at the site of the hematoma.

Injuries to the external auditory meatus are caused more often by foreign bodies than by direct blows or by chemical burns from fluids which have penetrated into the meatus. Foreign bodies should be removed very gently with small hooks or blunt ring curettes and, if necessary, under general anesthesia. Removal by canal irrigation with warm saline solution is contraindicated because of possibility of the simultaneous presence of a tear in the drum and a secondary infection of the middle ear. If the skin of the canal is lacerated, the edges should be trimmed down, avoiding unnecessary removal of skin.

Infections should be prevented or controlled by use of appropriate antibiotics. The most unpleasant complication of an extensive wound in the canal is the development of stenosis or even of complete atresia of the lumen, which can occur in injuries involving larger parts or the entire circumference of the lumen. Attempts to prevent such stenosis by tight packing of the canal, by introduction of a plastic mold, or by skin grafts held in place with a hollow plastic obturator are often unsuccessful. If stenosis has already developed, the only way to achieve a permanently patent ear canal is by a modified radical mastoidectomy, with formation of a tympanomeatal flap and skin grafts applied to the canal.

Tympanic Membrane

Injury to the tympanic membrane is the result of either a direct blow or a sudden change of air pressure in the external auditory meatus or middle ear. Direct trauma is rare because of tortuosity of the lumen of the external auditory meatus. It is most frequently observed in persons who have scratched the skin of the canal with a wooden stick or a metal needle

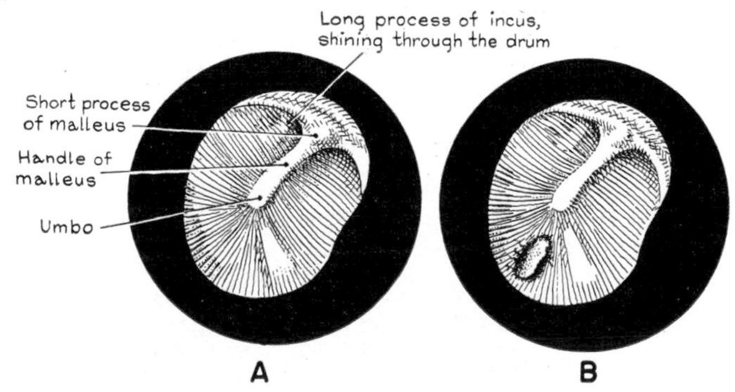

Figure 23–2. Otoscopic view of drum membrane.
A. Normal tympanic membrane.
B. Tympanic membrane with traumatic perforation.

and suddenly moved the head to the side on which the object was introduced. In such cases the object which penetrated into the middle ear may also injure the facial nerve or the promontory. Much more common is rupture of the drum membrane as a result of sudden increase in the air pressure in the external auditory meatus caused by blows to the ear, by high diving, and, particularly in war time, by blasts from explosives. Even a marked increase of the intratympanic pressure, as from violent blowing of the nose or therapeutic air inflations, will not produce rupture of a normal drum membrane, but it can cause rupture of atrophic scars in the drum. Injuries to the drum frequently seen in longitudinal fractures of the temporal bone will be discussed later.

The most common site of ruptures of indirect origin is the inferior half of the drum, particularly in the anterior quadrant. The perforation may range from a small linear tear to a very large defect, especially when caused by blast injury. The perforation usually lies within the pars tensa of the drum membrane and does not extend to the bony margins. The edges of the perforation are either clean cut or somewhat ragged, and are often slightly hemorrhagic. Occasionally small suffusions are seen in other parts of the drum.

The signs and symptoms are pain at the time of injury, often followed by a slight hemorrhage of short duration and a feeling of fullness in the ear. The perforation of the drum per se will hardly cause any significant hearing loss, but if the perforation is the result of exposure to a blast a more marked "traumatic" deafness, tinnitus, and, in some instances, vertigo with nausea are noted.

Traumatic perforations of the drum membrane, in the great majority of cases, close spontaneously, provided they do not extend to the bony tympanic sulcus and no infection of the middle ear supervenes. The latter complication will probably occur unless preventive measures are taken. The infectious material is, in most instances, brought into the middle ear from outside, either directly by the object which injured the tympanic membrane and penetrated the middle ear, or secondarily through irrigations, attempted instrumental removal of blood coagula, or instillation of ear drops. If rupture of the drum resulted from high diving or from a blow to the ear sustained while swimming, water may enter immediately. Another possible source of infection is suppuration in the nose, the paranasal sinuses, or the nasopharynx.

In the early stages treatment of traumatic perforation consists mainly in prevention of secondary infection. Proper management includes prophylactic use of antibiotics for several days following injury, abstinence from any manipulations in the external auditory meatus, and treatment of any existing nasal or nasopharyngeal infection.

If, despite absence of infection, perforations show no tendency to close, cauterization of the margins with trichloracetic acid or a 5–10 per cent silver nitrate solution, followed by application of a prosthesis (cigarette paper, cellophane, gold foil, etc.), will, in some instances, succeed in bringing about a closure. Sometimes closure of the perforation with a free skin graft (myringoplasty) becomes necessary.

Temporal Bone

Injuries to the temporal bone may occur alone or in association with injuries to other parts of the skull. Injury may affect each of its three main components—the petrous, squamous, and mastoid portion—alone or in combination, but most frequently the petrous portion is involved.

In direct injuries to the mastoid portion, foreign bodies, splinters of bone, and debris should be removed as soon as possible to prevent infection or, if infection has already developed, to provide adequate drainage. Prophylactic or therapeutic use of antibiotics is indicated. In the event of profuse bleeding the sigmoid sinus should be exposed and, if found injured, packed. Complete mastoidectomy for mastoiditis developing from wound infection will rarely become necessary today.

Fractures of the petrous portion are usually part of more extensive fractures of the base of the skull, and are present in about one third of the patients with such injury. There are three main types of fractures of

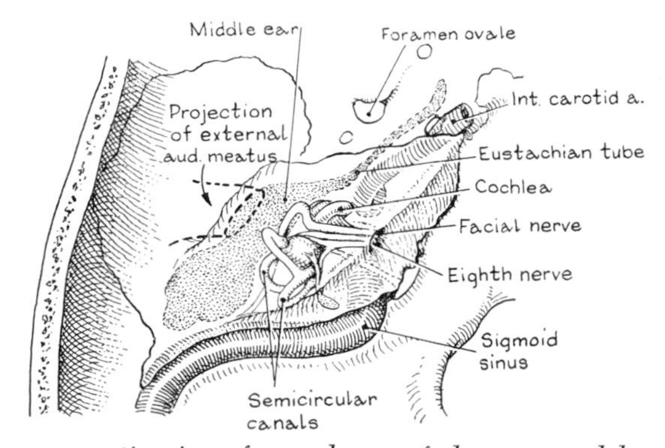

Figure 23–3. Diagrammatic view, from above, of the temporal bone and its contents.

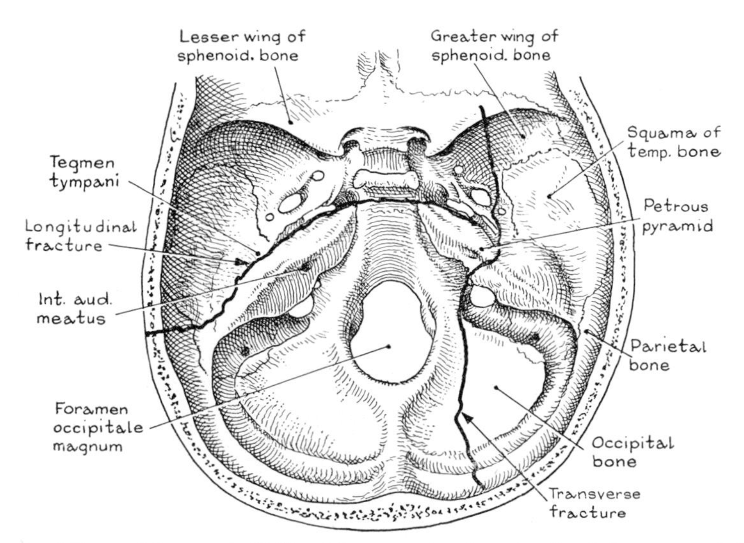

Figure 23–4. View of base of skull with extensive longitudinal fracture of the petrous portion on the left side and a transverse fracture on the right side.

the petrous portion—longitudinal, transverse, and combined fractures (Fig. 23–4). Of these three, the longitudinal type occurs most frequently, the fracture line extending into the middle fossa from the squama temporalis, or from the parietal or occipital bone through the mastoid into the tegmen tympani and from there along the superior petrosal ridge forward to the level of the geniculate or even the gasserian ganglion. The fracture line sometimes extends through the osseous portion of the external auditory meatus and the tympanic sulcus, which causes tears in the tympanic membrane and in the skin of the external meatus. The ligaments of the auditory ossicles are often torn, and the ossicles themselves luxated, or even fractured. In about 15 to 20 per cent of the cases the facial canal is injured, usually in the region of the geniculate ganglion, with subsequent hemorrhage into the nerve. The bony labyrinthine capsule is not affected in typical longitudinal fractures, although through the impact of the blow hemorrhages may occur in the perilabyrinthine spaces, particularly in the scala tympani at the basal coil of the cochlea. In the internal auditory meatus the nerves may be damaged by overstretching, which causes hemorrhages or even outright tears. The vestibular nerve is most frequently affected, occasionally being torn completely, particularly at the point of its ramification. At this location the cochlear nerve is affected less frequently, and the facial nerve rarely.

In early stages of longitudinal fractures the main clinical symptom, aside from the general symptoms of skull fracture, is bleeding from the external auditory meatus, with the hearing at least partially preserved. The bleeding indicates either a tear in the skin of the external auditory meatus or a hemorrhage extending into the middle ear, which penetrated through a tear in the drum membrane into the lumen of the external auditory meatus. In the much rarer cases, in which the drum remains intact, the blood accumulates in the middle ear (so-called hematotympanum). On otoscopic examination a bluish discoloration of the drum membrane is noted. Another possibility, which should always be considered when blood is found in the external auditory meatus, is a depressed fracture of the anterior wall of the bony canal caused by the capitulum of the mandible, with laceration of the overlying skin, when the capitulum has been pushed backward through the wound by the trauma. The fracture line occasionally radiates from the mastoid toward the bony canal in the form of several small fissures, causing a bloody suffusion at the posterosuperior wall without a tear. If the fracture line goes through the cortex of the mastoid, within a few days ecchymoses develop in the overlying skin, together with marked tenderness. More extensive hematomas are found if the sigmoid sinus, which lies on the inner surface of the mastoid, has been injured. Facial paralysis, as previously mentioned, is found in about 15 to 20 per cent of the cases. It need not follow the accident immediately, but may develop many hours or even several days later, since it is generally caused by hemorrhages into the nerve fibers and not by tears of the fibers.

Roentgenological demonstration of the fracture line is difficult, especially when the line extends into the temporal squama. It is successful in approximately one third of the cases. Bleeding from the ear canal is of short duration. If it is followed by a serous secretion of longer duration, the possibility of escape of cerebrospinal fluid through a tear in the dura should be considered, although such an occurrence is rare in a purely longitudinal fracture. In some of these cases air may enter the cranial cavity from the middle ear (pneumocephalus).

After disappearance of the blood crusts from the lumen of the external auditory meatus, which sometimes takes considerable time, characteristic changes may become visible in the contour of the tympanic ring and in the drum. The regular contour may be interrupted by a step-formation, most frequently in the posterosuperior part of the circumference, indicating that the fracture line has gone through this area. The tear or tears in the drum, if present, extend from this area inward. Traumatic perforations of the drum show a good tendency toward healing and are, after a short while, transformed into scars radiating from the site of the fracture of the bony margin into the drum. Perforations rarely persist unless secondary infection prevents healing of the tears.

The facial paralysis in longitudinal fractures shows, in the majority of cases, a tendency toward complete recovery.

The hearing loss is marked, especially soon after injury. In rare instances only is it a purely conductive loss; more often it is a combined conductive and perceptive, a so-called mixed, loss. This is explained by the fact that one usually finds in these cases not only middle ear changes, but also hemorrhages into the inner ear, in addition to the changes in the cochlear nerve within the internal auditory meatus. The perceptive component is of two types—either a sharp tonal dip at or around c^5 (4,000 dv), or occasionally a more or less uniform hearing loss throughout the entire tonal range. The uniform loss is explained by multiple bleeding extending into the cochlea or into the cochlear nerve, the sharp tonal dip at c^5 resembling very much the dips seen in blunt injuries without fracture to the head or the dips from exposure to over-loud sound. Its mechanism of development will be discussed later.

The middle ear component of the hearing loss generally disappears in several weeks, following resorption of the blood from the middle ear. Persistence of conductive deafness for more than eight weeks is probably the result of either the persistence of perforations in the drum, fractures of the ossicles, or perhaps the formation of adhesions in the oval window niche from organized coagula in the middle ear.

The perceptive component also shows a marked tendency toward recovery. The tonal dip at c^5 improves, usually in the first weeks, although in many instances part of it persists permanently. The more uniform losses throughout the entire tonal range show a slower rate of improvement.

It has been found that almost half the patients with longitudinal fractures eventually regain normal hearing, while the others show a hearing loss of only slight or moderate degree. Severe loss or complete deafness is rare. If it occurs, it is probably the result of a complete tear of the cochlear nerve in the internal auditory meatus.

Two points of great importance for correct evaluation of these cases must be considered. Initial improvement of hearing may be followed by a gradual secondary decrease which, in rare instances, may lead to complete deafness. The audiometric examination of the uninjured ear sometimes also shows a dip at c^5, with a good tendency for remission.

Peripheral vestibular symptoms, such as vertigo, nystagmus, past-pointing, and the tendency to fall, are quite common in the first days after a longitudinal fracture. The frequency of the vestibular symptoms is explained by hemorrhages in the vestibule, or by damage to the vestibular nerve or some of its branches within the internal auditory meatus. Complete loss of vestibular function because of a tear of the nerve in the internal auditory meatus is very rare.

In some cases it is very difficult or even impossible to differentiate between peripheral and central vestibular changes. If the vestibular symptoms are of peripheral origin, they usually disappear within a few weeks. If they persist for a longer period, the possibility of post-traumatic central vestibular changes should be considered, particularly changes in the brain stem in the region of the vestibular nuclei and the posterior longitudinal fascicles, resulting from petechial hemorrhages.

The second type of fracture of the petrous portion, the transverse fracture, occurs less frequently. Two forms can be distinguished. In one, the fracture line extends from the posterior or, less frequently, from the middle cranial fossa through the bony labyrinthine capsule. In the other type, single or multiple fractures are confined to the bony capsule of the labyrinth without involvement of the other parts of the petrous pyramid or parts of the base of the skull.

Unlike the findings in longitudinal fractures, the membranous labyrinth is torn in transverse fractures and blood is found in the perilymphatic and endolymphatic spaces. The changes in the middle ear are less significant. Small hemorrhages are frequently seen at the medial wall of the tympanic cavity, and often there is accumulation of blood in the middle ear and the adjacent pneumatic spaces. In other cases, one may find in the middle ear and the pneumatic spaces a mixture of blood and cerebrospinal fluid or cerebrospinal fluid alone. Sometimes the cerebrospinal fluid drains from the middle ear through the eustachian tube into the nasopharynx, and from there it may get into the nasal cavity and appear at the nostrils. The ossicles and the drum membrane, as a rule, remain intact.

Transverse fractures of the labyrinth cause, with rare exceptions, complete deafness and complete loss of vestibular function. After injury the patients evidence the typical signs and symptoms of acute labyrinthine destruction, complete loss of hearing, horizontal rotatory nystagmus of third degree to the opposite side, as well as vertigo, nausea, and often vomiting. The vestibular symptoms usually disappear within a few weeks, the consequence of central compensation, but the deafness remains complete. Facial paralysis is seen in about half of these cases and is, as a rule, noted immediately after the injury. It is usually caused by severe injuries or tears of the nerve in its course across the labyrinth, and shows a very poor tendency toward improvement.

X-ray examinations, particularly in Stenvers' position, will show the fracture line in about half of the cases. Absence of visualization, however, is no proof a fracture is not present. This is particularly true when multiple fissures are confined to the labyrinthine capsule itself.

The main danger from transverse fractures, aside from the complete and lasting loss of cochlear and vestibular function, and the often permanent facial paralysis, is the development of meningitis. The danger of an early meningitis is particularly acute when the fracture involves a temporal bone and there is acute or chronic otitis media. Unlike the longitudinal fractures which pass through periosteal bone, and which heal in the usual way with bony callus formation, the transverse fracture involves periosteal, enchondral, and sometimes also endosteal bone. Within the enchondral capsule the fracture does not heal with the usual bony callus, but, instead, the fracture line becomes filled only with connective tissue. This explains why transverse fractures, unlike longitudinal fractures, remain visible in x-ray pictures for years. The connective tissue in the fracture line represents a potential pathway of infection from the middle to the inner ear, and from there to the meninges, which may lead to development of meningitis even after many years.

In rare instances the fracture line traverses the cochlear or, in exceptional cases, the vestibular portion only, causing an isolated or major loss of cochlear or vestibular function. In a few such cases diagnosis was confirmed by roentgenological and histological examination.

Combinations of longitudinal or oblique and transverse fractures are less common; in some of them a complete avulsion of the petrous pyramid has been observed.

Occasionally one sees a partial or complete avulsion of the mastoid process or combinations of oblique fractures of the posterior fossa with longitudinal or transverse fractures of the petrous pyramid.

The symptoms in every event are determined by the extent of the injury and the parts involved in the particular case.

The management of fractures of the temporal bones consists in measures for treatment of craniocerebral injuries in general, as discussed in Chapter 22, and treatment of the fractures themselves.

The immediate mortality from basal skull fractures, caused by severe brain injuries, hemorrhages, or shock, is still high. With elimination of these factors, the prognosis for fractures of the temporal bones is improved considerably since chemotherapy and antibiotics have greatly reduced the mortality caused by meningitis, the most dreaded complication. If signs of increased intracranial pressure are noted in fractures of the temporal bones, the possibility of an extradural hematoma from a torn middle meningeal artery, or of a hemorrhage from a torn sigmoid sinus, should be considered. The fracture line should be exposed and the blood clots removed as soon as the initial shock has been overcome and the general condition of the patient has sufficiently improved.

In non-infected cases mechanical cleansing or irrigation of an ear discharging blood or cerebrospinal fluid should be avoided. Prophylactic use of chemotherapy and antibiotics is advisable, particularly in transverse fractures where, as already mentioned, the danger of meningitis is very great. If infection has already developed, chemotherapy should be started at once. If the infection does not respond to treatment immediately, operative treatment is advisable. Surgery is still indicated, despite the progress of chemotherapy, if a transverse fracture occurs through an ear with a chronic middle ear infection. At least a radical mastoidectomy, with exposure of the fracture line and removal of all the infected tissue, should be performed as soon as the patient's general condition permits. When intracranial complications have already developed, even more radical surgery may become necessary, depending on the type and extent of the injury, and the type of endocranial complication. Another indication for operative intervention is the escape of cerebrospinal fluid from the wound for more than two or three weeks without signs of infection. This situation should suggest a tear in the dura, which must be exposed and sutured, if necessary with the help of a piece of muscle tissue or fascia lata. Pneumocephalus, if present, will usually clear up.

Persistent facial paralysis in transverse fractures where the nerve is torn, either in the internal auditory meatus or in its course across the labyrinth to the geniculate ganglion, can rarely be treated surgically. In most cases the facial paralysis in longitudinal fractures shows a good tendency toward recovery. In certain cases, however, when injury to the nerve within the middle ear or mastoid can be suspected from the clinical symptoms and the roentgenological evidence, operative exposure of the nerve and appropriate treatment of the injury may be indicated.

A still unsolved problem is presented by the cases in which a transverse fracture heals without immediate complications, with the fracture line remaining visible on x-ray examination for many months or years. Because of the danger of late development of meningitis, prophylactic labyrinthectomy should still be seriously considered during the course of otherwise insignificant middle ear infections, despite the great improvement in the prognosis for meningitis.

In a given case it is sometimes difficult to determine clinically or roentgenologically if a head injury has caused a fracture of the petrous portion of the temporal bone. If injury has been followed by a complete or marked loss of hearing of the perceptive type on one side, without loss of the vestibular function, two possibilities should be considered—an occult longitudinal fracture with stretching or partial tearing of the cochlear nerve, or the presence of fissures in the cochlear capsule or in the spiral lamina, the result of a sudden increase of the intralabyrinthine pressure from the trauma. Unilateral loss of the vestibular function, together with some perceptive hearing loss, could, on the other hand, be caused by fissures in the wall of the vestibule.

Effect on hearing of blunt head injuries without fracture of temporal bone. In order to evaluate properly the effect of a given injury, repeated hearing tests are indispensable. They should be started as soon as the condition of the patient permits. In a considerable number of cases, especially following blunt injuries to the occipital region, a hearing loss is noticed immediately after injury. The hearing loss is characterized by a bilateral and more or less equal circumscribed dip around c^5 (4,000 dv), or by a steep drop in hearing above c^4 (2,000 dv), the dip remaining

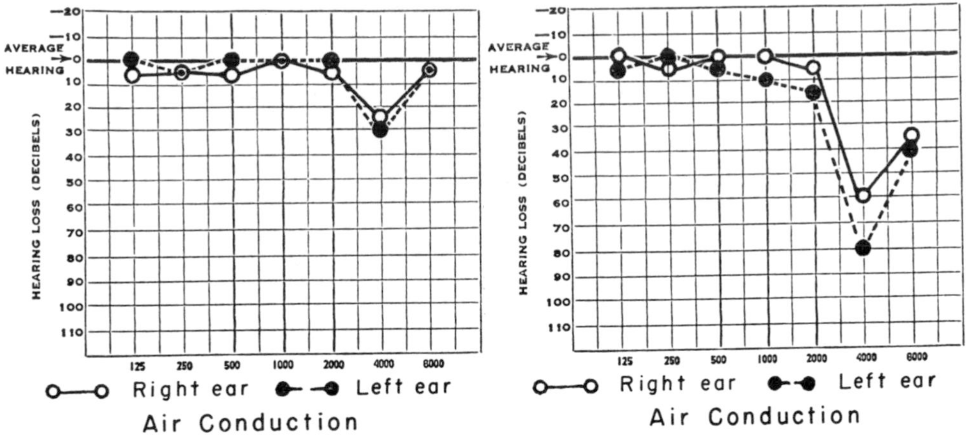

Figure 23–5. Typical audiograms after blunt head injury.

around c⁵. The hearing loss shows a tendency toward partial recovery within a few weeks; it is sometimes accompanied by a slight tinnitus.

The changes are explained by the assumption that a blow to the head creates in the skull bones a pressure wave which is transmitted through the bone to the cochlea in the same manner as a pressure wave in air is carried by the conductive mechanism. Within the cochlea the pressure wave produces a violent displacement of the basilar membrane, particularly in the upper half of the basal coil, with subsequent injury to the organ of Corti at the point where stimuli producing sounds of the approximate pitch of c^5 are perceived.

The hearing losses from blunt blows are similar to those observed in trauma resulting from exposure to loud sounds and gun fire, without any direct injury to the head. Immediately after exposure, hemorrhages may be seen in the drum, or even small perforations which, however, heal within a short time. The effect on hearing is usually very slight.

Explosions, as a rule, cause more extensive perforations in the drum membrane, which may be permanent, particularly when the middle ear has become infected. Under the impact of the explosion the stapes may be fractured and dislocated, and hemorrhages may extend into the perilymphatic spaces of the vestibule. Reissner's membrane, or even the basilar membrane in the cochlear duct, may show ruptures. Hearing loss is determined by extent of permanent damage to the middle as well as the inner ear. The inner ear recovers completely, if the trauma is slight; otherwise a marked loss in the upper tonal range remains permanently, or may even increase slightly within the first few months following the accident.

Post-traumatic cochlear and vestibular disorders of central origin. Post-traumatic deafness is not necessarily the result of damage to the organ of Corti, the spiral ganglion, or the fibers of the cochlear nerve. In certain cases of brain injury, such as concussion, either alone or combined with a fracture of the base of the skull, the neurological symptoms, together with the results of the vestibular tests, point to a more central seat of auditory damage—brain stem, midbrain, or subcortical or cortical centers. Escher, in his 1948 review of the known facts on central deafness, states that lesions of the cochlear nerve during its course from the fundus of the internal auditory meatus into the brain stem and to the tuberculum acusticum usually produce a hearing loss involving the whole tonal range, in contradistinction to labyrinthine lesions which, in most instances, produce a more circumscribed hearing loss. If the hearing loss is quite pronounced, examination with tuning forks shows the upper tone limit to be lowered considerably and the lower limit to be raised; the auditory field evidences a so-called "concentric narrowing." Damage to the trapezoid body in the brain stem may result in bilateral hearing loss. Since the main part of the cochlear nerve eventually crosses over the midline to the opposite side, lesions higher up in the brain stem or in the midbrain are characterized by a predominantly contralateral deafness. This is particularly true of lesions in the lateral lemniscus. In damage to the medial geniculate body there is unilateral deafness for speech with preservation of hearing for pure sounds and unilateral loss of caloric vestibular responses. The functional losses resulting from damage to the subcortical and cortical centers are still the subject of much controversy.

The audiometric curves in lesions of the central auditory pathways are not sufficiently characteristic to permit the diagnosis of a central lesion with any degree of certainty. A further complication lies in the fact that peripheral and central auditory lesions may very well be present simultaneously in a given case.

Vestibular symptoms commonly follow brain concussion. Shortly after the accident the symptoms observed are either a feeling of unsteadiness or true vertigo, particularly in movements of the head or change of body position, so-called positional or postural vertigo. On examination spontaneous as well as positional nystagmus may be noted. Peripheral vestibular disturbances subside, usually within a few weeks, whereas central disturbances may persist for a long time. Late symptoms may include unsteadiness in walking, bending, and lying down, as well as occasional attacks of rotatory vertigo, particularly of a postural character. If spontaneous nystagmus is present, which is the case more often in the weeks following the accident than later, it differs somewhat from the nystagmus occurring in peripheral vestibular disorders. One finds, for example, marked nystagmus with past-pointing and falling but with normal hearing, or marked nystagmus without past-pointing and falling, or nystagmus in an abnormal direction.

Vestibular tests may also show perverted nystagmus, direction being different from that normally induced, or they may reveal any one of the following: conjugate deviation of the eyes, the eyes moving in the direction of the slow component of the nystagmus normally induced by the particular test and then remaining fixed in the end-position for the duration of the stimulation; loss of vestibular responses on both sides without loss of cochlear function; loss of postrotatory nystagmus with normal caloric nystagmus, or loss of both postrotatory and caloric nystagmus; dissociated eye movements, the direction and amplitude of nystagmus being different in the two eyes; nystagmus preponderance to one side (that is, nystagmus being elicited more easily to one side than to the other).

Especially important is the presence of positional vertigo and nystagmus, which may remain as the only symptoms of damage to the vestibular system. Of particular diagnostic significance is positional nystagmus which either changes its direction in different positions, beats in a vertical direction, or shows no regularity at all.

The presence of normal hearing will, in many instances, facilitate the diagnosis of central vestibular disorders, particularly if the neurological examination reveals certain localizing signs.

Abnormal vestibular signs and symptoms are, in many instances, best explained as the result of damage from petechial hemorrhages to the brain stem in the region of the vestibular nuclei and their connections with the nuclei of the nerves to the eye muscles.

The diagnostic difficulties are often still further increased by combinations of peripheral and central vestibular disorders, such as fracture of the base of the skull with severe brain concussion. Intensity of the vestibular symptoms seems to depend to a certain extent on severity of the trauma, and is especially marked following trauma to the occipital region.

Furthermore, one must bear in mind that disturbances of the vestibular function may be combined with peripheral or central auditory disturbances, or a combination of both, factors which will make proper evaluation of these cases still more difficult. Thorough and repeated tests of hearing and of the vestibular function are essential in all cases of trauma to the head. The vestibular tests are particularly important because pathological vestibular symptoms, especially the anomalies of nystagmus and responses to stimulation, cannot be influenced voluntarily by the patient. The possibility of simulation, therefore, can be eliminated.

NOSE AND PARANASAL SINUSES

Nose

In direct blows to the face the nose is the part most frequently involved. The type and extent of the resulting injury varies with site of the injury and direction of the striking force. The bony as well as the cartilaginous portions may be affected.

In direct frontal blows, the most common injury is a transverse fracture of the nasal bones at the border between the thicker upper segment and the thinner lower segment (Fig. 23–6). Very heavy blows may result in comminuted fractures. A lateral blow to the nose may produce a fracture of only one nasal bone, or there may also be a fracture of the frontal process of the maxilla. In other instances the entire bony arch may be dislocated from its attachment at the base and be pushed to the other side. Fracture or dislocation of the nasal septum is common in nasal injuries. The septal cartilage may be fractured in a vertical or horizontal direction, and the fragments may protrude into or obstruct the lumen of one or both nasal cavities. In some instances the anterior end of the

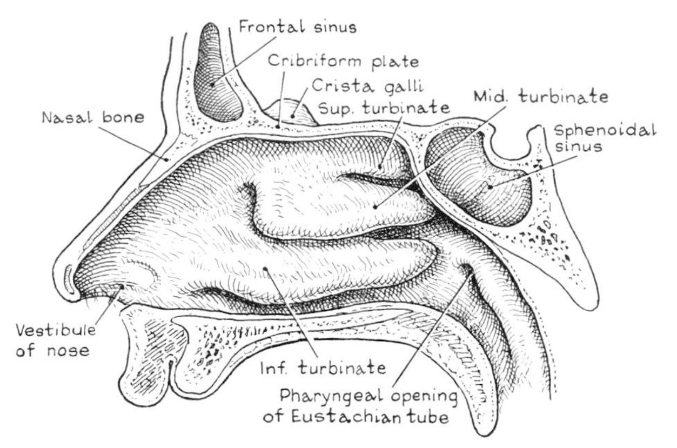

Figure 23–6. Paramedian sagittal section through nasal cavity.

cartilaginous septum is forced out from its groove in the underlying bone and dislocated laterally (Fig. 23–7). It then becomes visible in one of the nostrils beside the columella. In blows against the lip and the columella, the mucosa is often lacerated below the edges of the nasal bones, with backward dislocation of the lateral cartilages over the nasal bones. When the nasal bones are not yet intimately fixed in the midline, as in children, depressed fractures in only one nasal bone or infraction at its junction with the frontal process of the maxilla is frequent. Severe frontal blows may cause dislocation of one or both nasal bones outward over the frontal processes of the maxilla or backward between the processes. Each type of injury results in a considerable flattening of the nasal bridge. Dislocation and fracture of the anterior (lower) end of the septum is especially frequent in children, produced by either a blow or a fall, or at birth by passage of the infantile head through the genital canal.

In nasal fractures a marked swelling of the soft tissues is usually noted within the first 24 hours, accompanied sometimes by ecchymoses of the eyelids and of the conjunctivae. Fractures of the nasal bones generally cause bleeding from the interior of the nose, due to tears in the nasal mucosa, and often produce nasal obstruction. Such obstruction can be caused by accu-

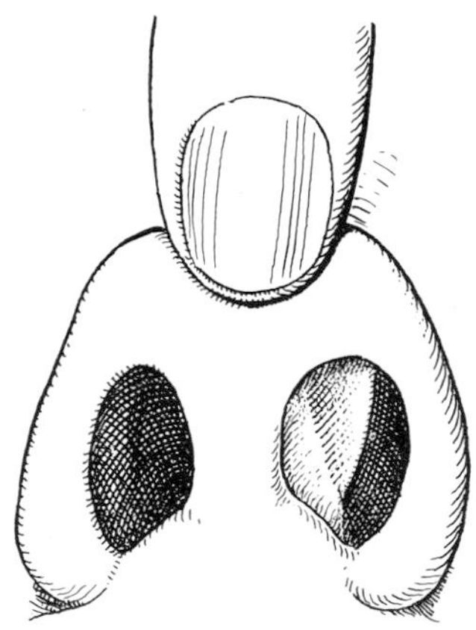

Figure 23–7. Dislocation of anterior (lower) end of nasal septum.

mulation of blood in the passages, by hematomas in the septum, or by septal fractures with displacement of the fragments and protrusion into the lumen of the nasal cavities. The configuration of the nose may be changed as the result of fracture, but it is sometimes difficult to recognize slight changes, particularly after swelling has developed. Palpation may reveal marked tenderness even on light pressure, bony crepitation, or subcutaneous emphysema. X-ray examination of the nasal skeleton is invaluable in the diagnosis of fractures with dislocation, which require immediate treatment.

The proper recognition of fractures in children is of special importance. They are often overlooked and, if the nasal bones are left in a wrong position, the deformity may progress with the growth of the facial skeleton. X-ray examination is less dependable in small children. For this reason bleeding from the nose after even slight trauma should always be regarded as a possible sign of nasal fracture, and a careful examination and search for fractures should be made.

Fractures should be treated, if possible, within the first 24 hours, before swelling and bleeding change the normal contour of the nose and before infection occurs. If the patient is seen after swelling has already developed, it may be advisable to wait until the swelling has subsided somewhat before reducing the fracture. Local anesthesia is usually used in adults; general anesthesia of short duration is used for children.

In uncomplicated fractures, such as depressed fractures of the tips of the nasal bones, the fragments are readjusted with an appropriate instrument, preferably a Walsham forceps. If this instrument is not available, a periosteal elevator, a Freer elevator, or even a Kelly clamp covered with cotton soaked in mineral oil or covered with rubber tubing can be introduced into the nasal cavity under the depressed bone. The latter is then elevated and brought into proper position. At the same time, the fracture of the septum, if present, is reduced. If the septum has slipped out of the septal groove, it is put back into place. After the displaced bones and the dislocated lateral cartilages, if any, have been repositioned, an external splint is applied for a few days to maintain the nasal bones in the correct position. The nasal cavities are packed with gauze to keep the septum and the torn mucosal flaps in place.

Hematomas of the septum, with accumulation of blood between the cartilage and the perichondrium, are seen not only after fractures but also after forced bending of the septum. The hematomas may appear on both sides of the septum and may cause considerable nasal obstruction. The treatment consists in incision and drainage, followed by packing of the nose in order to press the mucosa against the cartilage and prevent re-formation of the hematoma.

More complicated, particularly comminuted, fractures of the nasal bones present a more difficult problem. It is generally easy to bring the fragments into proper position as long as they are still loose, but it is difficult to maintain them there. This can sometimes be achieved by packing the nose with gauze, but in most cases an intranasal splint suspended to an external bar will prove more effective.

Some authors recommend open reduction in these fractures. The nasal pyramid is exposed, using the same approach as in a rhinoplasty. The displaced parts of the osseous and cartilaginous skeleton are then loosened and reset. After reduction, the incision in the mucosa is closed with sutures. This method permits reduction of the fracture at any time, regardless of the state of the overlying soft parts.

In severe open, comminuted fractures, which are often accompanied by extensive lacerations of the skin or of the mucosa, a careful primary repair of the soft parts is necessary, in addition to the repositioning and immobilization of the dislocated bony parts. The most dangerous complication in these cases is fracture of the cribriform plate of the ethmoid bone and tearing of the covering dura. It can be diagnosed by escape from the nose of blood with cerebrospinal fluid or of cerebrospinal fluid alone. If, under prophylactic antibiotic therapy and the avoidance of cleansing and blowing of the nose, the leakage does not stop in 10 to 14 days, it may be necessary to try to elevate the frontal lobe of the brain by external approach, expose the tear in the dura, and then close it either with sutures or by application of a piece of fascia lata or muscle to the upper surface of the tear.

Paranasal Sinuses

The paranasal sinuses (Figs. 23–8, 23–9) are frequently involved in direct craniofacial trauma. Most commonly the maxillary sinus, less often the frontal, and rarely only the ethmoid sinuses are affected.

The main danger in a sinus injury is the possibility of an ascending infection from the nose, which is particularly serious if the fracture penetrates the posterior wall of the frontal sinus or the roof of the ethmoid.

The maxillary sinus is often involved in fractures of the maxilla and malar bone, particularly in those which pass through the floor of the orbit. In addition to an accumulation of blood in the sinus, sometimes together with bony fragments or foreign bodies, one may find a step-formation in the infraorbital margin with deformity, particularly flatness in the zygomatic region, ptosis of the eyeball, diplopia, or anesthesia in the infraorbital region, if the infraorbital nerve is injured. X-ray findings will confirm the diagnosis and give information which will be of great help if reduction of the fractured parts becomes necessary. If the floor of the orbit is fractured and needs repositioning, or if the sinus contains bony fragments or foreign bodies, repositioning and removal of the fragments can best be achieved by a Caldwell-Luc approach, in which the sinus is entered from the oral cavity through the canine fossa. A wide opening into the inferior nasal meatus should be made, and the sinus tightly packed with gauze to keep the fragments in place. The end of the packing should be brought into the nose before the incision in the oral mucosa is closed. After a few days, the packing is removed from the nose.

The frontal and ethmoid sinuses may be involved in severe injuries, particularly in direct blows to the forehead and the middle part of the face, which also cause fractures of the maxilla and of the nasal bones. The overlying tissues may be lacerated or remain intact. Non-depressed fractures of the anterior wall of the frontal sinus, even if comminuted, do not present any serious problems. Open depressed fractures are much more serious and require operative treatment because of the possibility of a dural tear. Such a tear may permit escape of cerebrospinal fluid or inflow of air to the cranial cavity (pneumocephalus). The danger of infection (meningitis or even brain abscess) is acute.

In fractures of the posterior wall of the frontal sinus, the fracture line may extend inward to the region of the cribriform plate, to the roof of the orbit, or even to the optic canal. Locally one finds abrasions or lacerations of the forehead and ecchymoses around the eye. There may be temporary or permanent loss of the sense of smell and damage to the optic nerve, accompanied sometimes by complete loss of vision.

If the force is applied mainly to the interorbital space, as is often the case in airplane accidents, the nasal bones and the frontal processes of the maxilla are pushed back into the ethmoidal labyrinth, with possible fracture of the cribriform plate. The dura in this region is very easily torn, since it is much thinner than that in the frontal area. Tearing is made more likely by the fact that the dura is firmly anchored by its ex-

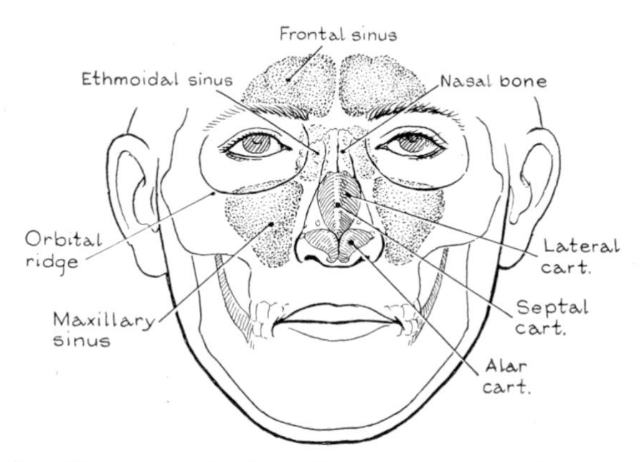

Figure 23–8. Diagrammatic frontal view of nose and paranasal sinuses.

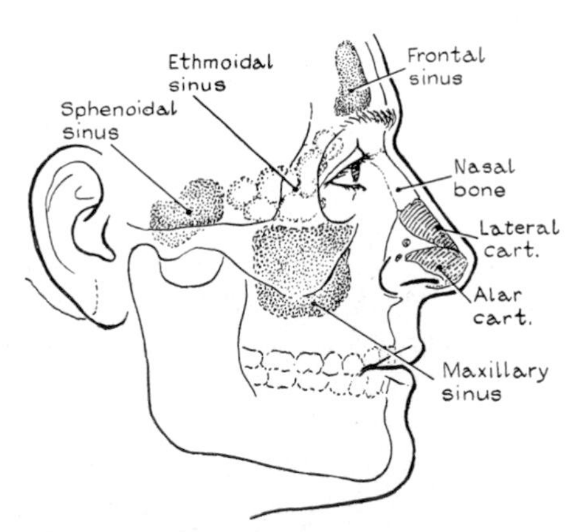

Figure 23–9. Diagrammatic lateral view of nose and paranasal sinuses.

tensions through the bone along the olfactory nerves, which pass through the cribriform orifices, whereas it strips off easily in the frontal region.

In fractures of the maxilla, in which the entire middle portion of the face is detached from the skull and pushed upward and backward, a cerebrospinal fluid rhinorrhea is produced by fracture of the cribriform plate, the result of the impaction and comminution of the interorbital space.

Clinically these patients show bruising and swelling of the cheeks, abnormal motility of the upper jaw in the skull, alterations of the bite, and more or less complete loss of the sense of smell.

In the first stages of cerebrospinal fluid rhinorrhea the fluid is often mixed with blood and, when the brain is simultaneously injured, with particles of cerebral substance. Later the fluid becomes clear, and its flow is increased by bilateral jugular compression. Chemical analysis, particularly if sugar is present, will confirm the diagnosis. Clinically the presence of cerebrospinal fluid can often be suspected when a handkerchief moistened with the fluid does not stiffen after drying. It will, however, stiffen when moistened with fluid produced by the nasal mucosa. In some instances cerebrospinal fluid rhinorrhea is not observed as long as the patient lies in bed, but develops as soon as he sits up. If the tear in the dura is below the frontal pole, the rhinorrhea may not develop because the subarachnoid space is narrower at this site than it is on the inferior surface of the lobe over the cribriform plate. Also, the dural opening may be plugged by brain tissue.

X-ray pictures, particularly stereoscopic views, will often, but not always, reveal the fracture line. They may also show the presence of air in the cranial cavity or even in the ventricles. The demonstration of a fracture line in the ethmoid is particularly difficult.

A dural tear can sometimes be suspected even without the escape of cerebrospinal fluid, when the films show any one of the following: a wide gap in the posterior wall of the frontal bone, or a marked displacement in that area; a fracture across the base from one anterior fossa to the other; sharp fragments of the posterior wall of the frontal sinus projecting posteriorly; a fracture line that widens as it descends along the posterior wall into the ethmoid sinus; displacement of the frontozygomatic synostosis associated with tilting of the crista galli.

Treatment should be started as soon as hemorrhage and shock are controlled and the extent of bone injury is determined. The treatment, assisted considerably by chemotherapy and antibiotics, consists in adequate exposure, removal of devitalized tissue and foreign bodies, reduction of the fractures and, if the dura is torn, exposure and suture of the tear. The need for immediate treatment is less urgent in injury resulting from blunt violence without laceration of the soft tissues than it is in a penetrating wound.

In blunt injuries with cerebrospinal fluid rhinorrhea it is sometimes difficult to decide whether to expose and close the dural tear or await spontaneous closure by treating the patient with strict bed rest and chemotherapy, and forbidding any cleansing or blowing of the nose. The latter course can be followed only if the x-ray pictures do not show large gaps, dislocations of bone, or spicules protruding into the brain. In most cases the rhinorrhea will stop spontaneously in one or two weeks, but even then great caution is necessary. An insufficiently consolidated tear represents, however, an extremely great danger, since meningitis or even a brain abscess may develop after a simple cold or sinus infection, sometimes years after the trauma. Recurrence of the cerebrospinal fluid rhinorrhea after several weeks of bed rest is suggestive of the presence of a latent communication between nasal or paranasal cavities and endocranium; surgical treatment is necessary before infection has occurred.

Air may enter the cranial cavity through a dural tear at the time of the injury or, more frequently, a few days later. In rare instances pneumocephalus may appear many weeks, or even months, after injury. Pneumocephalus as a rule, but not necessarily, is combined with cerebrospinal fluid rhinorrhea. The entrance of air into the cranial cavity is usually caused by a sudden increase in intracranial pressure from either sneezing, blowing the nose, or coughing. The air generally accumulates in the subdural space, but may penetrate into the cerebral substance, or even into the ventricles. Pneumocephalus can cause headaches or localized pressure symptoms. It is easily demonstrated in x-ray pictures. Since pneumocephalus is indicative of an at least temporarily open communication between the nose or the paranasal sinuses and the cranial cavity, conservative treatment should be tried only in acute cases in which the air penetrated at the time of injury or within the first few days. In late or recurrent pneumocephalus, operative closure of the dural opening is imperative for prevention of endocranial infection.

The dural tears can be exposed through the sinuses or by an intradural route. The location of the tear and the extent of sinus involvement in the injury will determine choice of the route. Consultation with a neurosurgeon is advisable in doubtful cases.

When approach is made through the frontal sinus, at the close of the operation either the sinus should be obliterated or an adequate communication into the nose should be secured with the help of a plastic tube introduced from the sinus into the nose. The tube can be left in place for many weeks or months. If the pathologic process extends into the ethmoid sinus, the latter can be exenterated through the frontal sinus. The primary objective in every case is to prevent the persistence of any pocket or air-containing cavity without provision of a channel for free drainage into the nose.

If bullets, shell fragments, or other radiopaque foreign bodies have penetrated into one of the sinuses, an attempt should be made to determine their exact location by means of x-ray pictures, particularly stereoscopic views. When found in the maxillary sinus, as is frequently the case, they are removed through a Caldwell-Luc approach; in the frontal, ethmoid, or sphenoid sinus, through an external operation. If they have penetrated into the pterygomaxillary fossa, they can be reached through a transantral approach with removal of the posterior wall of the maxillary sinus. If the foreign bodies are not radiopaque, their presence may be revealed through suppuration or fistula formation, which may indicate the need for an exploratory operation.

LARYNX AND TRACHEA

Injuries to the larynx and trachea are relatively rare because of the protected position, the resilient suspension, and the elasticity of the component parts of the two organs. Such injuries occur in peacetime mainly in accidents (automobile, airplane, railroad, industrial, sport, etc.), brawls, attempted murder, particularly with mugging, and attempted suicide.

In contusions one finds bloody suffusions of the skin and hematomas in the mucosa, especially in the aryepiglottic folds, the ventricular bands, and the arytenoid cartilages. The trauma itself may cause, at the time of accident, a severe shock quite out of proportion to the relatively mild degree of injury. The prognosis of simple contusions is good when the effects of shock are under control. The hematomas generally are absorbed quickly when bed rest, cold compresses, liquid or soft diet, voice rest, and, if necessary, antibiotic therapy are used. Tracheostomy will rarely be necessary unless the hematomas are very large.

Fractures of the laryngeal cartilages occur in sagittal blows to the larynx when the cartilages are pressed against the vertebral column, in lateral compression of the larynx, or through direct impact of foreign bodies. Fractures are rare in children, since the entire larynx is cartilaginous; they occur with more frequency in the third decade of life, as ossification sets in. They decrease in frequency with advanced age, because ossification is generally completed.

The thyroid cartilage is most frequently fractured because it is most prominent (Fig. 23–*10*). Longitudinal fractures are found in the midline or, more laterally, at the border between the ossified and cartilaginous parts of the wings. Fractures of the superior cornua are also quite common, and are a typical finding in hanging or strangulation. The arytenoid cartilages may be dislocated anteriorly in thyroid fractures. Next in frequency of occurrence are fractures of several cartilages. Isolated fractures of the

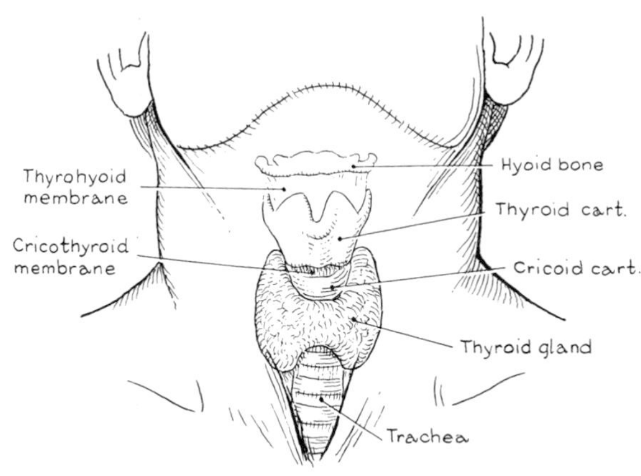

Figure 23–10. Diagrammatic frontal view of larynx and trachea.

cricoid or arytenoid cartilages, of the inferior cornua of the thyroid cartilage, or of the hyoid bone are rare.

The main symptoms are tenderness and swelling over the larynx caused by either hemorrhage into the tissues or edema, with hoarseness, or even aphonia and pain, which is more pronounced in talking and swallowing. If the mucosa is torn, blood may be coughed up. Emphysema may develop in the deep tissue spaces and in the subcutaneous tissues of the neck. The emphysema may become quite extensive. It may extend into the mediastinum and the interstitial tissue of the lungs and cause considerable dyspnea. Dyspnea may also be caused by extensive mucosal edema, hematomas, or narrowing of the airway by displaced fragments of the laryngeal cartilages.

The characteristic crepitation and abnormal motility of the fragments are difficult to elicit soon after injury because of the swelling and tenderness of the overlying tissues. X-ray examination, especially laminography, may help in revealing the fractures, the extent of displacement, the degree of narrowing of the airway, and the presence of emphysema in the deeper structures. Roentgenography will also facilitate recognition of small fractures without displacement, which otherwise might be mistaken for simple contusions. External examination several days after the accident, when the swelling has subsided and the tenderness has decreased, is generally more revealing.

The larynx should be examined as soon as the condition of the patient permits it. The extent of injury to the interior of the larynx, the site of hematomas, the amount of edema, the motility of the vocal cords, displacement of fragments, and, above all, the width of the airway, can be ascertained by indirect laryngoscopy (Fig. 23–*11, A*).

The most important early complications of laryngeal fractures are dyspnea and bleeding. Late complications, such as perichondritis and

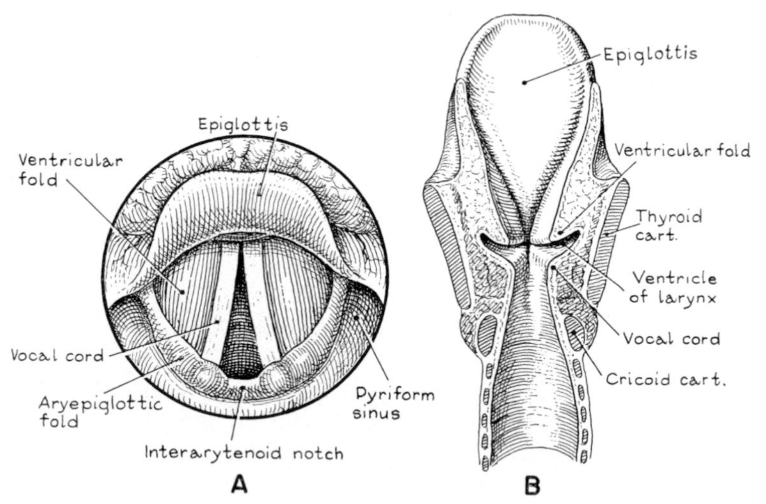

Figure 23–11. Anatomical relations of larynx.
A. Larynx seen by indirect laryngoscopy.
B. Frontal section through the larynx and the trachea.

abscess formation with subsequent cicatricial stenosis of the lumen, have become less common with the advent of chemotherapy and proper management of the fractures themselves.

Patients with laryngeal fractures must be carefully watched for signs of laryngeal obstruction, manifested by retraction at the suprasternal notch, the supraclavicular fossae, and the intercostal spaces. If even a slight sign of obstruction becomes evident, tracheostomy must be performed immediately, especially if emphysema is present, because dyspnea often increases rapidly and necessitates a hasty emergency tracheostomy. The stoma should always be created some distance below the site of injury.

Hemorrhages may originate from an external wound or from the interior of the larynx. External bleeding can easily be stopped when the wound is taken care of. Internal bleeding, if slight, usually stops spontaneously after a while. If it is more severe, tracheostomy should be performed and the larynx packed through a direct laryngoscope. Laryngofissure, or even ligation of the main stem of the superior thyroid artery, may become necessary in rare instances. If blood was aspirated into the lungs, aspiration through the tracheal stoma should be performed.

If the cartilages are severely dislocated, a core mold should be introduced as soon as possible after tracheostomy. It serves as an internal splint which tends to preserve the natural shape of the laryngeal lumen and prevents cicatricial stenosis. Sometimes, however, laryngofissure must be performed to remove detached pieces and to reset the dislocated cartilages. This again should be followed by insertion of a core mold.

Fractures of the hyoid bone cause pain and sometimes crepitation at the site of injury, expectoration of blood if the pharyngeal mucosa was torn, and pain on swallowing and lateral movements of the tongue. The fractures heal either spontaneously or after the fragments are wired.

Late complications are treated as they arise in the same manner as infectious diseases of the larynx.

Stab and incised wounds are the result of attempted suicide, self-mutilation, or accidents.

Self-inflicted wounds usually run across the neck. Because of retraction of the platysma and the muscles of the neck in deeper wounds, the tissues usually gape widely. In most cases the deeper wounds penetrate the hyothyroid membrane between the thyroid cartilage and the hyoid bone. They may stop in the fatty tissue in front of the epiglottis, or pierce the epiglottis and open the hypopharynx, or possibly penetrate the posterior pharyngeal wall to the vertebral column. Incisions above the hyoid bone, through the cricothyroid membrane or the upper rings of the trachea, are much less common.

The main danger in these injuries again is dyspnea and hemorrhage from veins and branches of the superior thyroid artery. The large vessels in the carotid sheath usually are not injured, even if the cut penetrates to the spine, because at the time of injury the head is deflected backward and the large vessels are shifted posteriorly. Injuries to the inferior (recurrent) and superior laryngeal nerves can occur in rare instances.

In stab wounds the small visible surface wound may be out of proportion to and not indicative of the tissue damage at the depth of the wound.

Accidental wounds show a great variety as to location, extent, depth of penetration, and involvement of laryngeal structures.

The main symptom of incision wounds is bleeding; emphysema is less common. In stab wounds bleeding is less conspicuous externally because it extends more into the tissue spaces or into the larynx. Emphysema is usually present if the larynx was opened.

The primary aim in treatment again is control of bleeding, relief of dyspnea, and aspiration of blood from the lungs, if necessary. The external wound is cleansed and devitalized tissue removed; injuries to the cartilages are taken care of. If the laryngeal, pharyngeal, or esophageal wall has been opened, the opening is closed with sutures. The patient is fed through a gastric tube or by intravenous drip. If the neck wound is not infected, it is closed in layers and Penrose drains are introduced. Infected wounds are left open and packed until the infection is controlled and all the devitalized tissues are removed.

The main task of treatment during the later stages is prevention of a cicatricial stenosis and preservation or restoration of the voice. To achieve the latter, speech therapy is often required.

Stab wounds of the trachea usually heal without any special treatment. If, however, emphysema develops, immediate tracheostomy may become necessary. If the trachea was opened by the injury, the edges are sutured together after a low tracheostomy is performed.

Wounds from metallic foreign bodies occur mostly in war time. They may be caused by bullets, shrapnel, or splinters from grenades, bombs, etc. Bullets usually leave a much cleaner wound because of their smooth surface. They cause less extensive damage to the tissues than shrapnel and other foreign bodies with a rough or ragged surface. The laryngeal injuries are very often accompanied by profound shock.

The direction taken by the projectile is important in determining extent of the injury, whether it is transverse, sagittal, or oblique. Bullets may traverse the tissues of the neck without injuring the laryngeal skeleton and still cause mucosal hemorrhages; in other instances they travel in a tangential direction just through the outer layers of a cartilage, or traverse the lumen completely, entering the wall on one side and leaving on the opposite side. Occasionally a spent bullet lodges in the wall and may, still covered with mucosa, protrude into the lumen. Bullet wounds are usually relatively harmless, unless the large vessels of the neck are injured or the esophagus is opened. On the whole, they do not cause such excessive damage to the soft tissues or shattering of the cartilages as is caused by shrapnel or projectiles with ragged surfaces.

Treatment follows the same principles prescribed for other injuries. It consists in management of shock, control of bleeding, and maintenance of an adequate and dry airway, with a low tracheostomy, if necessary. Further treatment depends on the type and extent of the injury. Antibiotics and chemotherapy have greatly improved the prognosis. Such extensive injuries as shattering of the cartilages still present formidable problems to the laryngologist, and often necessitate repeated operative intervention. Aside from infections, the greatest danger is the development of stenosis of the lumen, particularly when parts of the cricoid cartilage are lost. Without further detail, it should be noted in passing that either excision of webs, dilation of the lumen with core molds, excision of scar tissue after laryngofissure, and application of skin grafts, or even the use of more complicated plastic procedures may become necessary. Loss of larger parts of the cricoid or thyroid cartilage necessitate use of cartilage implants to prevent collapse of the lumen. Restoration of the airway alone, however, is not sufficient for complete rehabilitation of the patient. The surgical treatment must, whenever necessary, be supplemented by appropriate speech therapy to improve and correct phonation as much as possible.

CHAPTER 24

MAXILLOFACIAL INJURIES

By MAURICE J. HICKEY, D.M.D., M.D., and
STANLEY L. LANE, M.D.

Fractures of the Mandible

By MAURICE J. HICKEY, D.M.D., M.D.

THE MANAGEMENT OF MANDIBLE FRACTURE is greatly simplified by adherence to two fundamental principles. *Reduction of the fracture* is synonymous with normal occlusion of the teeth. *Fixation in normal occlusion* must be maintained until the fracture has united. Selection of the best method of treatment is predicated upon determination of the simplest technique that will accomplish these two objectives.

DIAGNOSIS OF FRACTURE OF MANDIBLE

Examination of the patient may reveal swelling, ecchymosis, or an external wound. Drooling of saliva is common. Malocclusion of the teeth signifies displacement of a fractured segment of jaw. The mucous membrane may be lacerated. Swelling and ecchymosis in the floor of the mouth are quite common, and when accompanied by an adequate history of trauma are pathognomonic of mandible fracture.

Abnormal mobility between two segments of the mandible clinches the diagnosis. When the fragments are not displaced and the occlusional relationship of the teeth is normal, attempts to educe false motion should be made, but never with enough force to produce crepitus. The mandible is grasped firmly, but gently, on each side of the suspected fracture. A gentle bending motion then will usually disclose the presence of false motion at the fracture site without creating additional tissue damage.

Active movement of the jaw is defective, and a semiopen mouth position often is perpetuated by involuntary muscle spasm. Surprisingly little pain may be present, except when the mandible is moved.

Some combination of these signs usually will establish the diagnosis.

It should be confirmed by roentgenograms, which must include the entire mandible and both condyles. Fracture of a mandibular condyle should always be suspected and ruled out when the body of the bone has been broken.

DISPLACEMENT IN FRACTURE OF MANDIBLE

The problems, and a choice of method for reduction, of a mandibular fracture depend upon the amount and direction of displacement of the bone fragments. Displacement depends upon the force and direction of the offending trauma, the amount of soft tissue damage, and the pull of the muscles attached to the fracture fragments. A relatively consistent pattern of deformity can be anticipated according to the location and number of fractures present.

Fracture at Angle of Mandible

The posterior fragment, which is the ascending ramus of the mandible, is pulled upward, forward, and inward by the action of the pterygoid and temporal muscles (Fig. 24–*1*, *A*).

Fracture of Body of Mandible

The posterior fragment tends to become displaced upward and inward, as in fractures of the angle of the mandible. However, upward displacement may be limited when teeth in this fragment are opposed by upper teeth. The anterior fragment often is depressed and rotated (Fig. 24–*1*, *B*).

Fracture of Midline of Mandible

In this fracture the two fragments are counterbalanced by paired muscles. Consequently both fragments tend to displace toward the mid-

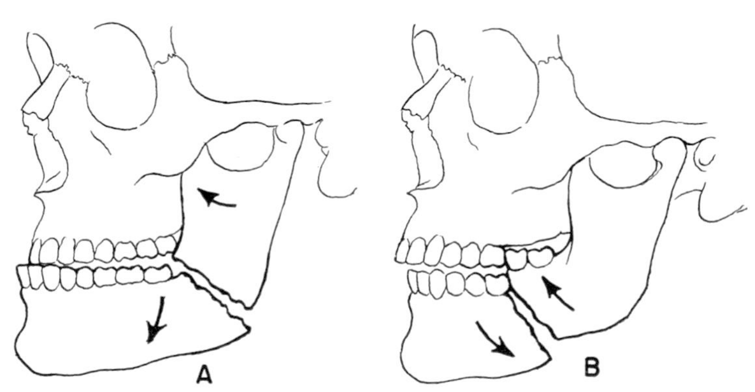

Figure 24–1. Fractures of the mandible.

A. Fracture at angle of mandible. Body of mandible may be depressed; the ramus is elevated upward and inward by the pterygoid and temporal muscles.

B. Fracture through body of mandible. Anterior fragment is depressed; posterior fragment is elevated. Opposing teeth in the maxilla may prevent elevation of the posterior fragment.

line. If the fracture is sufficiently oblique to permit overriding, severe overlapping may occur (Fig. 24–2). When the fracture line is at right angles to the mandible displacement is uncommon. Comminution of the fracture allows both fragments to collapse toward the midline.

Fracture of Neck of Mandibular Condyle

In unilateral injuries, displacement of the body of the mandible does not occur if there are opposing molar teeth (Fig. 24–3). When there are no opposing molar teeth the body of the mandible in the molar area is elevated, with a consequent opening of the bite in the region of the anterior teeth. When there are bilateral condylar fractures the body of the mandible is pulled backward and elevated to lower the symphysis and produce an increased "open bite."

Fracture of Body of Mandible and Opposite Condyle

The bone fragment between the two fractures will be displaced downward and backward at the symphysis by the hyoid muscles, and elevated at the ramus (Fig. 24–4). The bone fragment posterior to the fracture through the body of the mandible is displaced inward by the pterygoid

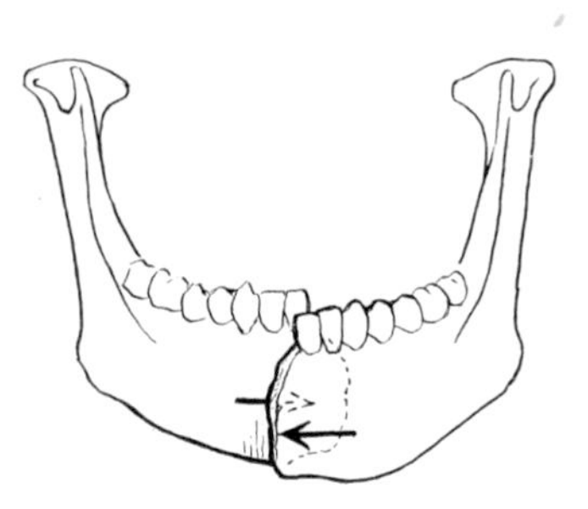

Figure 24–2. Fractures in the midline of the mandible. Displacement is toward the midline.

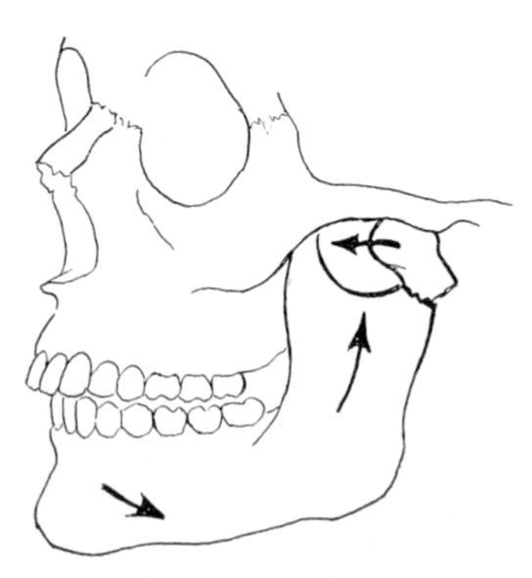

Figure 24–3. Fracture through neck of condyle. Displacement of the body of mandible may be prevented by opposing molar teeth.

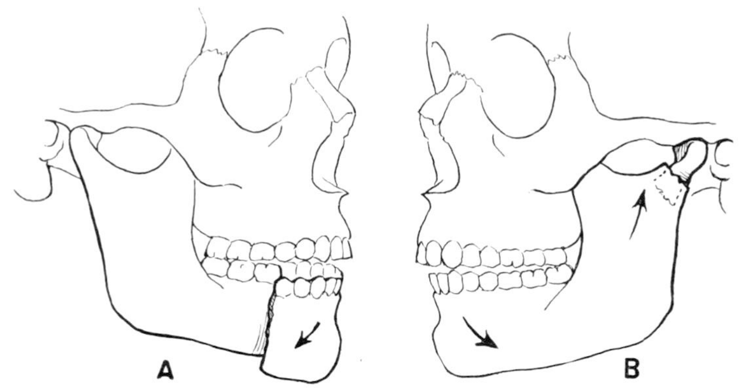

Figure 24–4. Fracture of body of mandible and contralateral condyle. A. The mandible anterior to the body fracture is displaced downward. B. The ramus on the side of the condyle fracture is elevated.

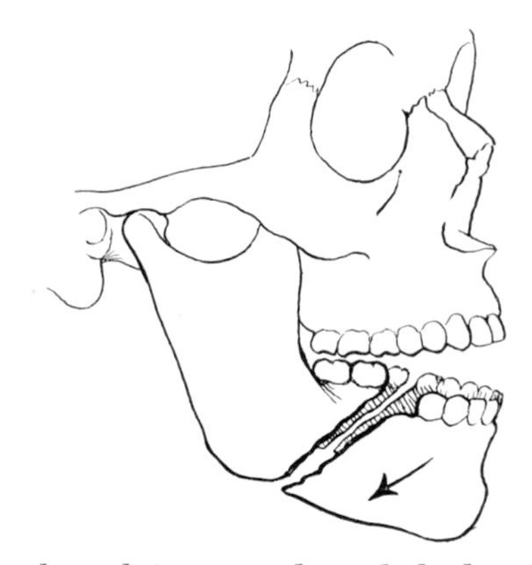

Figure 24–5. Bilateral fracture through body of the mandible.

muscles. Elevation of this fragment will occur if there are no opposing teeth.

Bilateral Fractures of Body of Mandible

The anterior fragment will be displaced downward and backward by the hyoid muscles (Fig. 24–5). The posterior fragments are displaced inward and upward, unless this deformity is prevented by opposing teeth.

Fractures of Edentulous Mandible

Fractures of the edentulous mandible are subject to the same displacing forces as when teeth are present, but the absence of teeth permits a much greater displacement than would occur otherwise (Fig. 24–6). Without teeth, displacement is limited only by the continuity of intact periosteum and the thick mucoperiosteum investing the visible intraoral portion of the mandible.

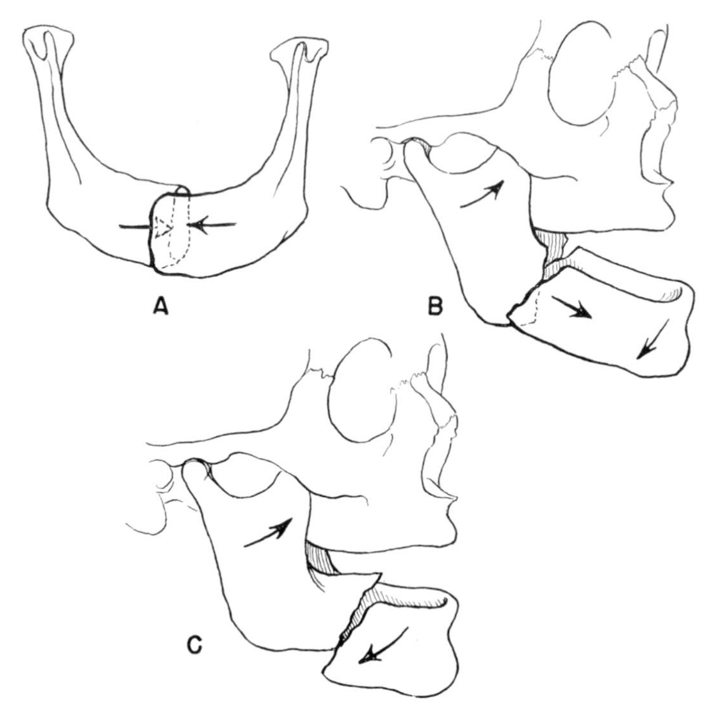

Figure 24–6. Fractures of the edentulous mandible.
A. Fracture at midline with overriding of fragments.
B. Bilateral fracture through body of mandible.
C. Unilateral fracture through the body of mandible.

TREATMENT OF FRACTURE OF MANDIBLE

Reduction and fixation with the teeth in normal occlusion usually can be accomplished by some method of treatment which immobilizes the fractured mandible against the intact and immovable maxilla. A single technique may be suitable for both reduction and fixation, but these two requisites to a happy result should not be confused.

Reduction and Immobilization

All fractures of the mandible should be reduced and immobilized as soon as possible. Delay may be justified by concomitant severe injuries to the brain, but whenever the operative risk permits surgical treatment of any kind an attempt to reduce the mandible fracture should be carried out. Early reduction usually can be accomplished by some simple method. Delayed reduction and fibrosis may necessitate extensive surgery in order to prevent facial deformity.

Manual replacement of the fracture fragments in normal position with good occlusion of the teeth is often possible when reduction is performed soon after injury, and the displacement is small in amount. Manipulation is greatly facilitated by mandibular nerve block, which obliterates pain and reduces muscle spasm.

In the presence of gross displacement perpetuated by muscle spasm, elastic traction is required for gradual reduction. Elastic bands, stretched between the wired teeth of the upper and lower jaws, will usually pull the displaced fragments into normal alignment, and the teeth into proper occlusion, without pain or additional trauma.

Of all the mechanical methods introduced for reduction and immobilization of a mandibular fracture, only intermaxillary wiring has withstood the test of time. Its application is simple, and excellent immobilization is provided. When reduction by elastic traction is necessary, intermaxillary wiring serves as the instrument both for reduction and for immobilization.

Simple intermaxillary wiring. This technique is useful for simple fractures with little or no displacement, and when there are teeth on both sides of the fracture. The wires should be applied to the teeth on each side of the fracture, and to the opposing teeth of the upper jaw. When wires are applied to molars and bicuspids they can be placed around single teeth, but, if immobilization requires that the incisor teeth be utilized for fixation, this method should not be used.

Multiple 8-inch pieces of 016 or 020 stainless steel wire will be needed. The end of a wire is passed through the interdental space in a buccolingual direction. The wire is bent and brought back through the next interdental space. The projecting ends are then twisted in a clockwise direction until a snug grasp on the tooth is accomplished (Fig. 24–7, *A*). When anterior teeth are implicated paired wires should be twisted together (Fig. 24–7, *B*). The opposed teeth of the upper jaw are wired in the same way. When sufficient wires have been placed on upper and lower teeth

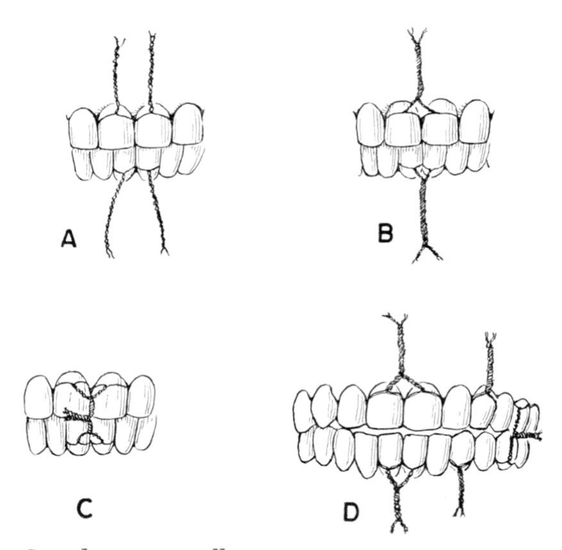

Figure 24–7. Simple intermaxillary wiring.
A. Placing of the individual wires.
B. Twisting upper and lower wires to form single wires.
C. Upper and lower wires twisted to provide fixation.
D. Additional wires may be placed to ensure adequate stabilization.

to maintain secure fixation, their ends are twisted together with the teeth in normal occlusion (Fig. 24–7, *C*, *D*).

Eyelet wiring (Ivy). This technique provides attachments for elastic traction designed to produce gradual reduction. Following reduction the eyelets provide attachments for fixed wires designed to provide immobilization.

Stainless steel wire of 016 or 020 gauge should be cut in pieces about 8 inches long. These are then bent in the middle and twisted to form a loop at the doubled end. The two ends of the eyelet wire are then passed together through the space between the teeth selected for wiring (Fig. 24–8, *A*), from the outer surface of the teeth. The free ends are then separated, one being passed back through the interdental space at the other side of the anterior tooth, and the other through the interdental space at the other side of the posterior tooth. One end of the wire is then passed through the loop and the ends are twisted tight. At this time care should be taken not to draw the eyelet loop into the interdental space. As many loops as necessary are prepared in the manner described. Rubber bands can then be placed between opposing eyelets to reduce the fracture or, if gradual reduction is not required, short pieces of wire can be passed through upper and lower opposing eyelets and twisted tight (Fig. 24–8, *B*).

This method of wiring provides a series of loops along the buccal surface of the teeth formed from a continuous piece of wire. The method has the advantage of providing many points for attaching elastic traction and distributes the pull of the elastics over a number of teeth. This reduces the possibility of loosening teeth by the pull of the elastic bands.

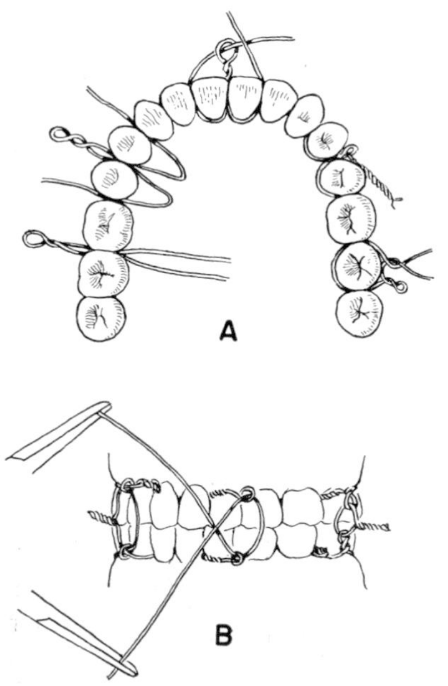

Figure 24–8. Eyelet wiring (Ivy).
A. *Inserting wires and twisting to form eyelets.*
B. *Twisting ligature wires to provide intermaxillary fixation.*

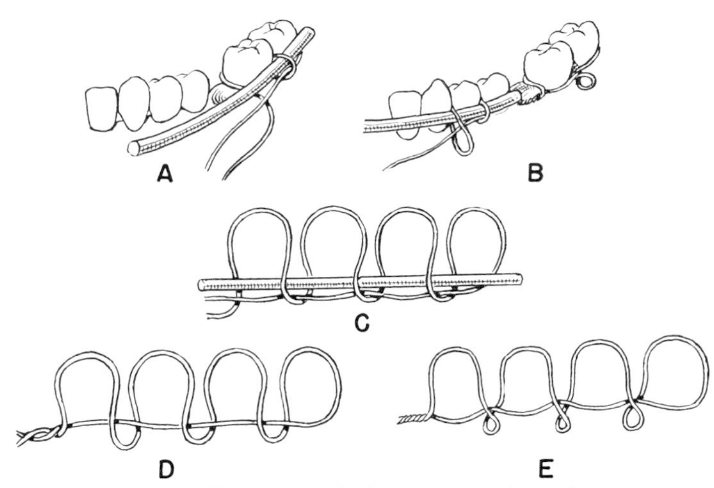

Figure 24–9. Intermaxillary multiple-loop wiring (Stout).
A. Utilizing lead bar in formation of loop.
B. Continuation of loops and twisting of wire to fill space of missing tooth.
C. Details of loop formation.
D. Twisting ends of wire to end a series of loops.
E. Final two turns to complete the loops.

Intermaxillary multiple-loop wiring (Stout). This technique requires the presence of three or more adjacent teeth. A stainless steel wire is passed through the interdental space separating the last two teeth in the arch. The buccal arm of this wire is placed against the necks of the teeth and a lead bar about 3 mm. in diameter is placed next to this wire (Fig. 24–9, *A*). The stick of a cotton applicator can be substituted for the lead bar. The lingual arm of the wire is then passed through the next interdental space, over the bar, and back through the same space. This forms a loop next to the gingival margin of the tooth (Fig. 24–9, *B*). This procedure is continued until the anterior teeth are reached, and the two ends of the wire are then twisted tight (Fig. 24–9, *D*). The bar is then removed, and each loop is given two turns (Fig. 24–9, *E*). On the lower jaw the loops are bent downward to form hooks, and on the upper jaw they are bent upward. If the space of a missing tooth is encountered, the two arms of the wire are twisted to fill the space and the looping procedure is continued (see Fig. 24–9, *B*).

Arch bars. The use of preformed arch bars affords some advantages. These bars are made to mold to the contour of the upper and lower jaws. They are ready-made with preformed hooks. In mandibular fractures it is often advantageous to utilize these on the maxillary teeth. They should not be used as a continuous bar crossing a mandibular fracture, if any reduction by traction is required. They may be used on the mandibular teeth if they can be applied after the fracture is reduced, or if sufficient teeth are available on either side of the fracture line to make it possible to cut the bar at the line of fracture. The arch bars are molded to the contour of the teeth and held in position by single wires passed over the bar, through the interdental space, around the lingual surface of the tooth,

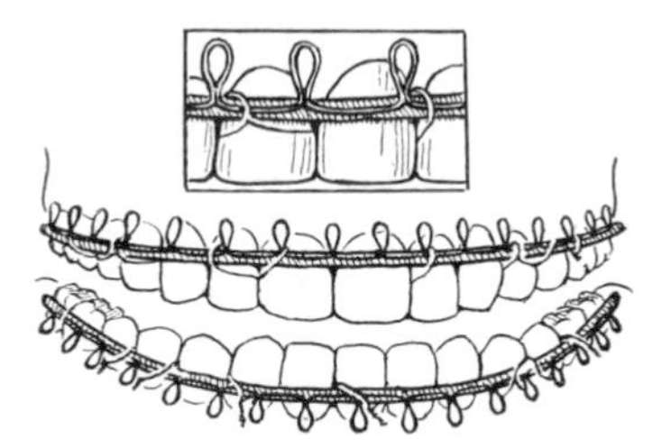

Figure 24–10. Arch bars. Preformed arch bar is wired to the teeth as shown in rectangular inset.

back through the interdental space, and under the bar, and the ends twisted tight (Fig. 24–*10*). Enough single wires must be used to anchor the bar firmly. The principal anchorage should be to molar and bicuspid teeth. If the bar is fastened to the anterior teeth with insufficient attachment, the anterior teeth may be loosened or even avulsed.

Open Reduction

On occasion, usually because of overriding fragments and insufficient teeth to provide anchorage for intermaxillary wiring, open reduction and interosseous wiring may be required. This technique is often advantageous in fractures through the angle or body of the mandible, especially when there are no teeth in the posterior fragment, in which event there may be extensive upward and inward displacement of the posterior fragment. Before surgical intervention is decided upon, the displacement must be carefully evaluated. If displacement is so slight that future function will not be impaired, surgical intervention is contraindicated. In such cases the anterior fragment should be immobilized in normal occlusion. If the displacement is severe enough to produce facial deformity or interfere with function, the posterior fragment must be reduced and immobilized.

Open reduction and interosseous wiring is best accomplished by an external incision deepened to expose the fracture line. Drill holes are placed on either side of the fracture (Fig. 24–*11*), and stainless steel wire

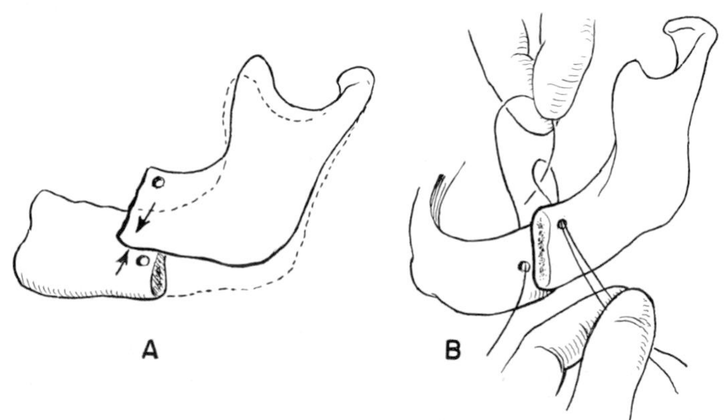

Figure 24–11. Open reduction of fracture of body of mandible.
A. Location of drill holes.
B. Passage of stainless steel wire through drill holes.

is passed through these holes and tightened. It must be remembered that the posterior fragment tends to ride upward, so that the drill hole in this fragment should be placed at a higher level than the drill hole in the anterior fragment. Whenever interosseous wiring is used, intermaxillary fixation should also be provided, if possible.

Other techniques for the reduction of fractures of the mandible include the use of cap splints, circumferential wiring, external pin fixation, and the use of Kirschner wires. These techniques all have a place in fracture therapy, but should be considered as auxiliary aids to be used in special situations.

FRACTURES OF MANDIBULAR CONDYLE

Fracture of the mandibular condyle occurs at the neck of the condyle and may vary from a simple fracture without displacement to complete dislocation of the condylar head from the glenoid fossa (see Figs. 24–3, 24–4). These fractures are usually the result of a blow on the chin and may be unilateral or bilateral. A single condyle fracture often is accompanied by a fracture through the body of the mandible on the opposite side. Any fracture through the body of the mandible requires examination for the possible presence of a condyle fracture. Any disturbance of the normal occlusion without fracture of the body of the mandible indicates a condyle fracture.

Disturbance of occlusion as the result of a unilateral condyle fracture will usually be reflected in an open bite. Contact of the teeth on the injured side may be restricted to the molar region. The jaw may be deviated to the injured side. In bilateral condyle fractures the entire mandible may be displaced backward. In these cases open bite may be quite pronounced.

Treatment

Treatment consists in restoring normal occlusion and immobilizing the mandible in the position of occlusion. Simple intermaxillary wiring is often all that is required. If immediate restoration of occlusion cannot be obtained, wiring with elastic traction should be used.

Often attempts are made to reposition the condyle by manual manipulation. These efforts are rarely, if ever, successful and are unnecessary. If occlusion is restored and immobilization maintained for about four weeks, good function will be obtained. Occasionally there will be moderate limitation of lateral movement, but this is unimportant.

Open surgical procedures have been advocated for repositioning of the condylar head. The operation is difficult and not without risk. The results obtained by open reduction are similar to those obtained by intermaxillary wiring.

AFTERCARE IN FRACTURE OF MANDIBLE

Once the fractured mandible has been reduced and immobilized, the problems of the patient's care become largely those of nutrition and mouth cleanliness.

As long as the jaws are immobilized, food must be provided that can be swallowed without chewing. If teeth are missing in the arches, soft foods such as puréed vegetables and finely chopped meats can be taken through the spaces. If a liquid diet is required, adequate food intake can be provided by the use of a mechanical food blender. Food prepared in the normal way can be liquefied in the blender. In this manner the normal dietary requirements can be satisfied.

Mouth cleanliness is most important. A warm saline mouth wash after meals is helpful. However, once full immobilization has been obtained, the outer surfaces of the teeth can be brushed regularly. It is often more convenient for the patient to use a toothbrush of the size designed for small children.

Immobilization of mandibular fractures is usually maintained for five or six weeks. After this period the tie wires or elastic bands are removed without disturbing the wires attached to the teeth, and the fracture lines are tested for absence of mobility. If the fracture is solid when bending force is applied, it is considered healed. If there is motion at the line of fracture, the mandible should be re-immobilized to the maxilla. The fracture lines can be tested at weekly intervals until healing is complete.

COMPLICATIONS IN FRACTURE OF MANDIBLE

Nonunion

This is a rather uncommon complication, but may occur in fractures at the angle of the mandible, or in the region of the symphysis. If healing is not complete by the eighth week of immobilization, nonunion must be presumed to exist. Operation designed to freshen the bone ends must then be considered.

Infection

This complication can be prevented or controlled by the use of antibiotics. All fractures of the mandible must be considered open fractures, and antibiotic therapy should be used until immobilization is complete.

Teeth in Line of Fracture

There is a wide range of opinion about what to do with teeth in the line of fracture. In general, if the tooth in a line of fracture is useful for immobilization it should be retained as long as possible. With antibiotic therapy the likelihood of infection is reduced. In some cases a single tooth in the posterior fragment may be all that is preventing severe upward displacement. Even though it is in the line of fracture, the retention of this tooth may avoid open reduction. If teeth in the line of fracture are retained, they should be watched carefully, and extracted if abscess formation appears imminent.

Asphyxiation

This is a prereduction complication and may occur when the fractures are in the region of the symphysis. Backward displacement of the symphysis permits the hyoid group of muscles to pull the tongue backward. Forward traction on the symphysis will relieve obstruction to the airway. In severe injuries manual traction on the symphysis may be required to preserve life until tracheostomy can be done.

Fractures of the Facial Bones

By STANLEY L. LANE, M.D.

INJURIES TO THE FACE are considered according to their anatomical location. For convenience the face can be divided into three parts.

The upper third of the face, above the level of the eyes, involves the base of the skull and the cranial cavity, and is within the province of the neurosurgeon. The lower third of the face consists essentially of the mandible, and has been dealt with in the first half of this Chapter. The middle third of the face (Fig. 24–12), which can be considered surgically the "upper jaw," includes the two maxillas, two nasal bones, two zygomatic bones and arches, two lacrimal bones, and portions of the ethmoid and sphenoid bones. It is bounded posteriorly by the pterygoid processes of the sphenoid bones (Fig. 24–13).

The nasal bones are the most frequently fractured bones of the face. In many injuries there is little displacement, and frequently the patient never seeks treatment. The mandible is the second most frequently fractured bone of the face. The zygomatic arch is third in frequency, and, unless there is marked deformity or interference with mastication, such fractures may be unrecognized and untreated. The maxilla is the fourth, and as a general rule this bone is fractured only in event of severe extra-

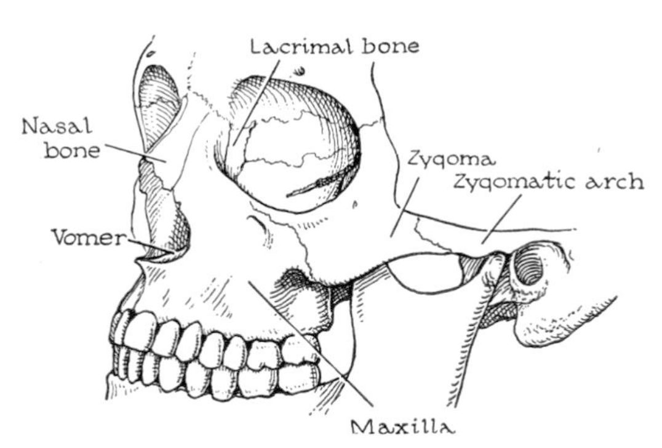

Figure 24–12. The bones of the middle third of the face.

oral trauma. The zygoma is fifth. Complicated fractures often involve several of the facial bones.

In every fracture of the mandible or maxilla the possibility of an associated fracture of the skull should be investigated. The presence of periorbital or perimastoid ecchymosis and of cerebrospinal fluid rhinorrhea or otorrhea should arouse a strong suspicion of skull fracture. Roentgenograms of the skull should be taken when fracture is suspected. Assessment of neurological damage is important in deciding upon a plan and schedule of treatment.

The causes of fracture are related to trauma which varies from blows of the fist to falls, and which may occur both in the home and in industry. In this day of high speeds, trauma related to transportation is becoming more common, and automobile accidents constitute the most frequent cause of complicated fractures of the middle third of the face. The front seat passenger, projected against the instrument panel by a sudden stop, is the most frequent victim. The fracture occurs most often on the right side, as the patient's face is turned toward the operator of the car.

ANATOMICAL CONSIDERATIONS

Normally there should be no mobility of the bones of the face, except for the mandible. This is the basis for diagnosis of fractures of the middle third of the face. Any mobility of the bones or of a portion of bone is pathognomonic of fracture. Malocclusion of the teeth is very suggestive. After a fracture or dislocation of the mandible has been ruled out, any acute change from a pre-existing occlusion implies a fracture of the middle third of the face. Another aid in diagnosing facial fracture is a change in contour or outline. There are many surface landmarks in the face that are readily palpable and bilaterally symmetrical. Palpation of the zygomatic arch, of the outline of the rim of the orbit, of the nasal bridge, and of the zygoma itself, all will aid in the diagnosis of fracture, when the palpation is performed simultaneously on both sides of the face. Other signs aiding in fracture diagnosis, such as ecchymosis, edema, nasal bleeding, and numbness will all be discussed under the sections dealing with the different types of fracture.

The bones of the face form a complex network and interpretation of x-ray films is difficult because of overlapping shadows, but multiple films, including stereoscopic views, usually disclose evidence of most fractures.

Structure

Fifteen bones make up the framework of the face. The lines of their junction, known as suture lines, are immobile.

There are two palate bones, each with a horizontal and a vertical plate. The horizontal plate has a superior surface, which forms the posterior part of the floor of the nose, and an inferior surface, which forms the posterior part of the roof of the mouth (Fig. 24–*13*). The vertical plate forms a partition between the nasal cavity and the sphenomaxillary fossa.

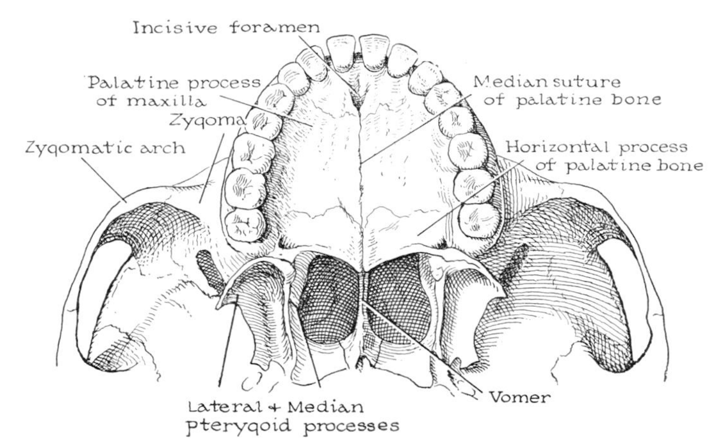

Figure 24–13. The inferior aspect of the bones of the middle third of the face.

The posterior border articulates with the pterygoid process of the sphenoid and presents the tuberosity of the palate. The posterior surface is the location of attachment of part of the origin of the internal pterygoid muscle.

The vomer is a quadrilateral plate forming the posterior part of the septum of the nose.

The maxillas comprise two symmetrical bones, each with a body and four processes—malar, nasal, palatal, and alveolar. The body is a hollow pyramid, and the large air cavity is the maxillary sinus, or antrum of Highmore. There is an opening from the sinus into the middle meatus of the nose located at the upper anterior portion of the nasal wall. The base of the pyramid forms the outer wall of the nose, and the apex articulates with the zygomatic bone. It is attached to the base of the skull by suture connections with many of the other bones.

The base of the maxillary pyramid articulates with the ethmoid and lacrimal bones and with the vertical plate of the palate bone. The superior surface aids in the formation of the floor of the orbit. Thus, each maxilla assists in forming three cavities—the orbit, and the nasal and oral cavities. It forms a large part of the palate, one-third of the floor of the orbit, and the floor and outer wall of the nasal cavity and pyriform aperture.

The malar process articulates with the zygomatic bone. The nasal process forms the inner margin of the orbit and articulates with the nasal, lacrimal, and frontal bones.

The alveolar process acts as the supporting structure for the upper teeth. It is made up of two plates, an external and an internal, consisting of thin layers of dense compact cortical bone and underlying cancellous bone. The outer plate merges with the outer surface of the true maxilla. The inner plate extends upward and is continuous with the palatal process of the palate bone and maxilla. The alveolar process, which holds the teeth, tends to disappear after the teeth are lost. The palatal process on either side forms the anterior part of the hard palate, and constitutes the roof of the mouth and the floor of the nose.

The two nasal bones are quadrilateral plates articulating with each other and forming the bridge of the nose. Each also articulates with the maxilla and the ethmoid.

There are two zygomatic bones. Each has a body, which is rarely fractured, and four supporting processes. These form the prominence of the cheek, part of the outer wall and floor of the orbit, and the floors of the temporal and zygomatic fossae. They are strong, quadrilateral bones on fragile supports. The posterior part provides attachment (origin) for some of the fibers of the temporal and of the masseter muscles.

Each frontal process articulates with the frontal bone at the supero-external orbital margin. Each orbital process articulates with the maxilla and frontal bone, and the greater wing of the sphenoid. It forms part of the zygomatic and temporal fossae, and part of the orbit. Each maxillary process articulates with the maxilla, and forms part of the anterior wall of the antrum. The zygomatic process articulates with the ipsilateral zygomatic process of the temporal bone, and completes the zygomatic arch. It is the site of origin of the masseter muscle.

The masseter muscle has superficial and deep fibers. The outer or superficial portion is the stronger, and its origin is a tendinous aponeurosis from the zygomatic process of the maxillary bone, and also from the anterior two-thirds of the inferior border of the zygomatic arch. The deep fibers form the smaller portion of the muscle, and arise from the entire deep surface of the zygomatic arch.

Because of the pneumatization of the bones, the middle portion of the face retains a great deal of elasticity. This allows it to absorb many traumatic insults which otherwise would be transmitted directly to the cranial contents. The maxillas are situated beneath the walls of the anterior fossa of the skull, and are rather loosely attached by "buttresses and flying buttresses." These aid in dissipating and diffusing the shocks of trauma. They will withstand a blow of great force received through the lower jaw, from in front or from the side; in a forward or downward direction, however, relatively little force is necessary to detach the maxillas from the cranium.

THE NOSE

The nose is made up of an osteocartilaginous framework with an outer covering of skin and muscular tissues, and an inner lining of skin and mucosa. The base of the osseous bridge of the nose is formed by the frontal processes of the maxillas. A narrow thick upper portion of the nasal bones rests on the medial portion of the nasal margin of the frontal bone and the frontal spine. The pyramidal framework of the nose is supported by a central septum which is both osseous and cartilaginous.

Fractures of the Nasal Bones Not Involving Base of Skull

The nasal bones may be fractured and pushed backward with or without comminution. The septum may be crushed or buckled. The bones may be displaced to one side or the other. It is desirable to replace the fragments before swelling masks the deformity. When possible this should be done within the first few hours after fracture.

In children, the nasal bones are separate and, therefore, may be fractured independently. Usually a direct blow fractures the frail inferior edge of the nasal bone. More than three-quarters of nasal fractures occur at the junction of the thick upper and thin lower portion of the nasal bones. A side blow may fracture only one side. Nasal fractures may cause soft tissue swelling and edema, ecchymosis, and conjunctival hemorrhage, tenderness, and crepitus. There may be a change in nasal contour, often masked by edema. Roentgenography aids in the diagnosis of nasal fractures. Reduction is usually simple, if done quickly. General anesthesia may be necessary. Local anesthesia is used in adults. Use of 10 per cent cocaine topically and of 2 per cent procaine hydrochloride by injection is appropriate; 2 per cent Xylocaine is effective and can be used both topically and by injection. Unless contraindications exist, 1:1,000 epinephrine may be added, 0.5 ml. to the ounce. Intraoral endotracheal anesthesia may be necessary in more complicated fractures.

Reduction. When there is little or no displacement, no treatment is necessary. If injury was recent, the bone fragments can be elevated with a closed pair of curved forceps placed in the nostril, coincident with external molding of the contour of the nose with the fingers. Cotton and petrolatum gauze placed over a blunt long elevator or forceps may be used for the same purpose, particularly when the septum has been fractured. The nasal arch is raised and the displaced bone is reduced by digital pressure. Overriding of the fragments is corrected when necessary, and the septum is restored to its groove in the vomer.

Fixation. An external splint may be necessary to prevent the nasal arch from reverting to a displaced position. A flat soft metal splint, covered with moleskin adhesive tape, or a dental compound splint which is molded while warm and then cooled, may be held in place with adhesive tape. Plaster of paris bandage strips may also be made into a splint. A Kazanjian splint, consisting of a frame and a bar by which continuous elastic pressure is maintained, exerts a continuous lateral force. Intranasal splints are not satisfactory as a rule, but petrolatum gauze packing for 24 to 28 hours to maintain elevation and control hemorrhage is often useful. If the nasal bones tend to sag, a mattress suture of fine wire passed through the skin from side to side and placed over buttons will often aid in preserving the prominence of the bridge of the nose.

A suspension method with a wire appliance used as an internal support to elevate and immobilize the comminuted fragments may be used. A firm wire is used, the intranasal portion of which is covered by dental compound, and an elastic band is used to attach it to a head support. This support may be a plaster of paris head cap, or a manufactured framework head cap with skeletal fixation.

THE MAXILLA

There are no powerful muscle attachments to the maxilla, only those for the muscles of facial expression. Therefore, except for the force of gravity, when fractured fragments are replaced they tend to remain in position. The internal pterygoid muscle is attached to the pterygoid process, and may tilt the maxilla backward, if the fracture includes the pterygoid wall. Fractures of the upper jaw may involve one of the walls of the antrum, causing hemorrhage or infection in its cavity. A diagnostic aid of importance is percussion of the teeth. In the absence of a dead or loose tooth, a dull note implies an antrum filled with blood or pus.

The maxilla has a very extensive vascular supply from the external carotid artery through the internal maxillary artery. Repair of injury is rapid and complete.

The sensory nerve supply is the maxillary, or second, division of the fifth cranial nerve (the trigeminal or trifacial). It supplies all structures about the maxilla, after leaving the cranium through the foramen rotundum in the greater wing of the sphenoid. It terminates by emerging through the infraorbital foramen as the infraorbital nerve.

Fracture of Alveolar Process

The most frequent fracture of the maxilla is a fracture of the alveolar process. This may be caused by trauma to the teeth due to a blow or fall, or it may occur during the extraction of teeth. The roots of teeth may be fractured, or the crowns broken. It may occur in relation to one tooth or to a segment containing several teeth. The external cortical plate of the alveolus usually is the portion detached.

Treatment. Complete detached fragments and fractured teeth and roots should be removed. The mucoperiosteum may be sutured after removal of the free fragment of bone.

If the entire alveolus is loose as a segment with several teeth included, the diagnosis is usually implied by malocclusion, and should be confirmed by intraoral x-ray pictures, both occlusal and periapical views. If the fragment is still attached to the mucosa and periosteum, union may be obtained by immobilization. A splint or arch wire, fixing the fractured segment to the sound portion of the maxilla, is the treatment of choice (see Fig. 24–17). A continuous figure-of-8 loop wire, extending between the stable and movable teeth, may be all that is necessary. Antibiotics should be used as indicated. It must be remembered that all fractures in the line of teeth are compound, or open, fractures, and must be treated as such. With infection or abscess formation, it may be necessary to remove the segment, but this complication is the exception rather than the rule.

Fracture of Tuberosity of Maxilla

This common fracture occurs during the extraction of molar teeth, most frequently in elderly patients who have some rarefaction of the bone. Such a fracture is usually associated with a single isolated molar tooth. There is firm attachment, and the force of mobilization for attempted removal, which need not be great, may cause fracture through the entire tuberosity area, including the floor of the maxillary sinus. It is not unusual for a dentist to find the entire tuberosity and floor of the sinus in the forceps clamped to the tooth.

Treatment. If the fragment is completely free, it should be removed, and the mucosa and periosteum sutured together, to close the opening of the floor of the sinus. The patient should be instructed not to blow his nose for at least a week or ten days. Antibiotics are usually indicated.

Fracture of Horizontal Portion of Maxilla

With trauma involving a complete segment of anterior teeth and applied leverage, the horizontal portion of the maxilla, forming the anterior part of the palate, may be fractured as a unit. This usually occurs as a fracture through one of the suture lines of the palate.

Treatment. The palate can be reduced and held in place by an acrylic tray, plate, or splint. It may be held in place by replacing the teeth in the alveolar arch and maintaining reduction of the fracture with the use of an arch wire fixed to the labial surfaces of the teeth.

Unilateral Fracture of the Maxilla

This may be caused by direct force from in front or from one side. The fracture extends along the median suture line of the palate, and also extends through the walls of the maxillary sinus. The fracture line, therefore, involves the lateral wall of the nasal cavity, and the anterior, lateral, and posterior walls of the maxilla. This may be associated with a fracture of the zygomatic bone and, if so, the fracture line would then involve the ipsilateral orbit and zygomatic process of the temporal bone.

The fractured maxilla may be depressed. In these cases there is likely to be thickening of the palate due to overlapping at the palatine suture line. Occasionally the fragment may be forced outward with a resultant spreading of the dental arch.

Diagnosis. The diagnosis of unilateral fracture of the maxilla may be based on the following clinical and laboratory findings:

(1) malocclusion and irregularity of the dental arch, or incorrect articulation with a history of trauma;

(2) mobility of the fragment and crepitus, if the segment is not impacted;

(3) dull note to percussion of the teeth;

(4) numbness of the infraorbital area, if the fracture involves the infraorbital foramen and injures the infraorbital nerve;

(5) impaired function and inability to chew;

(6) x-ray evidence of fracture;

(7) clouding of the maxillary sinus, which fills with blood, apparent by roentgen ray or by transillumination;

(8) nasal bleeding;

(9) facial deformity—change of contour of the face with flattening or fullness of the cheek;

(10) periorbital ecchymosis;
(11) tenderness and pain on movement, as in eating or chewing;
(12) diplopia, if the floor of the orbit is depressed.

Treatment. The mandible and noninvolved part of the maxilla are used as splints. The fractured fragment is replaced by manipulation. The mandibular arch is fixed to the firm part of the maxilla, and the displaced portion of the maxilla is then fixed to the remainder of the mandible. An arch wire is fixed to the mandible, or continuous or segmental loop wiring may be used. The uninvolved part of the maxilla may have a segment of arch wire or continuous wire loop fixed to the contained teeth, and intermaxillary fixation is then accomplished by wire. The movable fractured segment then can be wired, and reduction is obtained by elastic intermaxillary traction, later replaced by intermaxillary wire. After reduction the two maxillary segments may be united by a wire or arch. A cap splint made up of either coin silver or acrylic may be used. The occlusal surfaces of the teeth are exposed so as to allow good occlusion.

Overlapping of the segment, or spreading of the maxillary arch, may be corrected by elastic traction (Figs. 24–*14*, 24–*15*), or by use of a jack screw. The teeth in the collapsed segment may be fixed to hooks by buccal arch wires or by orthodontic bands. A palatal jack screw may be used to separate the segments. Elastic bands spread across the palate may be used, if the arch is separated. By overlapping wire hooks, elastic bands can also be used to spread an overlapped collapsed arch.

All fractures are contaminated, as there is a pathway to the fracture

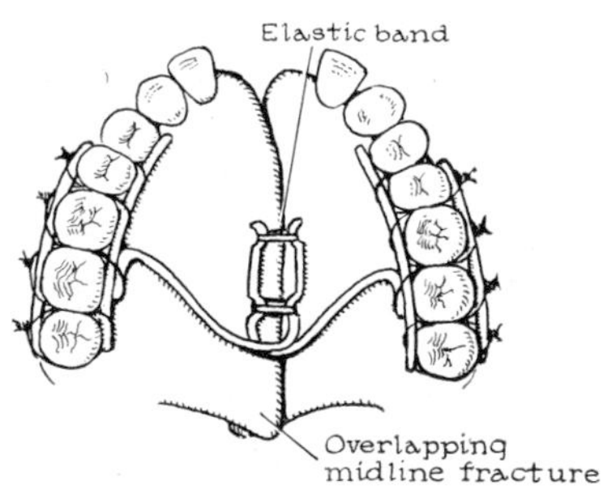

Figure 24–14. Overlapping fracture in midline of palate treated by elastic intermaxillary traction.

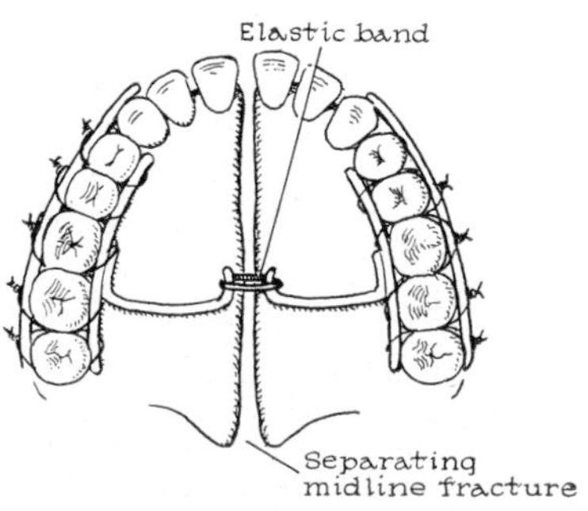

Figure 24–15. Separated fracture in midline of palate treated by elastic intermaxillary traction.

site either along teeth or through the maxillary sinus or the wall of the nasal cavity. Antibiotics should be used, at least during the acute episode.

In edentulous patients acrylic base plates can be used, or splints can be fashioned from plaster impressions. If the patient has an upper denture, it can be used for fixation of the fragments. Fixation is by direct wiring of the denture to the alveolar process.

Complete Horizontal Fracture of Maxilla

In this type of fracture the entire maxillary arch is displaced as a unit. It may be impacted upward or floating downward. This type of fracture is commonly referred to as a "floating maxilla." There is no muscle pull, and displacement is due to the force of gravity. There may be an associated longitudinal median fracture through the palate with either spreading or narrowing of the dental arch.

Treatment. A complete arch wire is fixed to the maxilla and to the mandible, or loop wires may be placed about the teeth (Fig. 24–*16*). Intermaxillary reduction is first accomplished by elastic traction. After reduction of the fracture the elastic bands are replaced by wires. After the normal intermaxillary relationship is established, in order to prevent the movable mandible with its depressor muscles from causing further separation and dropping of the maxilla, fixation should be augmented by a modified Barton head bandage or head-chin support. This forces the mandible and maxilla toward the base of the skull. Stainless steel wires may be attached to the dental arch in the bicuspid area, and brought out through the zygomatic portion of the cheek. They then are attached to a head cap, which may be made of plaster of paris. These wires may be fixed through small operative incisions to drill holes along the lateral walls of the orbit, or to the zygoma, if that bone is still attached to the skull.

If the maxilla is in good position, it may be maintained by a Kingsley splint attached to a head cap. This is a cap splint which is cemented to the teeth with heavy wires coming out of the mouth anteriorly and bent backward horizontally so as to allow them to be hooked to the head cap. This allows for direct upward traction. A similar type of fixation can be accomplished by preparing a labial arch wire, to be fixed to the teeth, with sol-

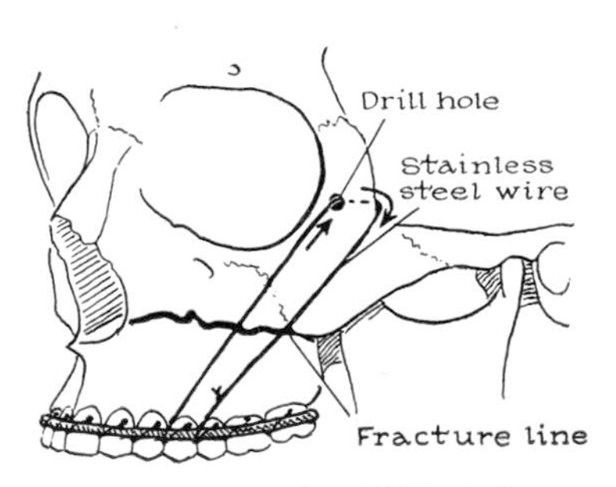

Figure 24–16. Stabilization of "floating maxilla" by wire suture after reduction by elastic traction.

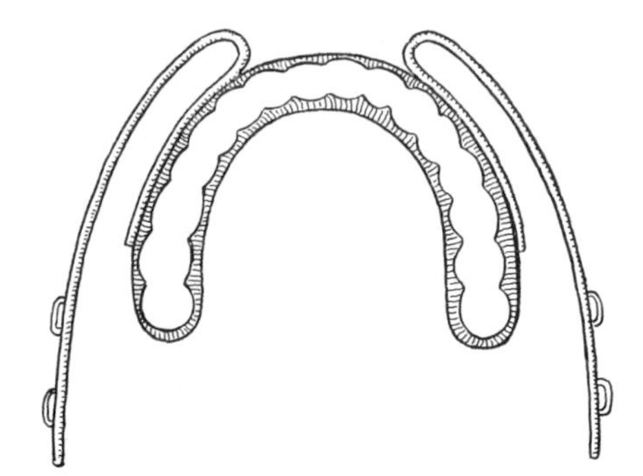

Figure 24–17. Labial arch wire with projecting anterior branches for use in stabilizing the maxilla. The projections are connected to a head cap.

dered anterior components to allow the upward traction (Fig. 24–17). The same type of splint is used in edentulous or partially edentulous patients.

In the edentulous patient, a denture can be used for fixation. The denture can be fixed to the maxilla by placing screws or pins through the flange in the denture directly into the maxilla. Circular intra-osseous stainless steel wires may be used to fix the denture to the maxilla. Then the denture and maxilla unit can be placed in proper position and maintained by mandibular fixation or by attachment to a head cap.

Comminuted Fracture of Anterior Maxilla

The fragments are reduced and a maxillary tray or Kingsley splint is used. A cap silver or acrylic splint may be used to hold the dental arch in position. To form these splints an impression of the maxillary arch is taken and plaster models are made which show the abnormal displaced alignment. The models are then sectioned through the fracture site, and replaced in normal position, with proper alignment. Splints can then be made from the aligned models to maintain the fragments in normal position, and these can be fitted in the mouth. Labial arch wires may also be used to maintain fixation in the simpler cases.

ZYGOMA AND ZYGOMATIC ARCH

Fractures of Zygoma and Zygomatic Arch

These injuries may be unrecognized, as the swollen soft tissues often conceal the existing deformity. There is usually little deformity other than a slight flattening of the upper part of the cheek. The patient may have diplopia if the orbit is involved, or restricted mandibular function if there is pressure on the coronoid process of the mandible.

Blows by direct violence, falls, and automobile accidents, in which the face hits the instrument panel of the car, are the most common causes. The injury is usually unilateral. The zygomatic arch is the weakest portion and the most frequent site of fracture. The infraorbital area, the frontal process, and the maxillary area follow in order of frequency of involvement.

Zygomatic fractures are almost always multiple, and are seldom open fractures. When the zygoma itself is involved, the body is depressed downward and inward, and there are breaks in all four areas.

Diagnosis. The signs and symptoms of fracture of the zygoma and zygomatic arch include the following:

(1) periorbital swelling and ecchymosis;

(2) local tenderness on palpation;

(3) depression beneath the eye, and flatness of the side of the face (this may not be noticed, because of swelling of the overlying soft tissues);

(4) pain may be present, but usually there is little discomfort;

(5) marked reduction of space between coronoid process of ramus of the mandible and the zygoma (this can be felt digitally by placing a finger in the mucobuccal fold; it should be checked by bilateral examination);

(6) epistaxis—bleeding into antrum and nose;

(7) anesthesia below the eye, tingling, and burning sensation due to pressure or injury to the infraorbital nerve;

(8) conjunctival hemorrhage;

(9) visual disturbances—blurred vision or diplopia may be present (this may be transitory and due to soft tissue and extraocular muscle edema and injury);

(10) drooping of face and lip;

(11) difficulty in opening mouth;

(12) mobility or crepitus.

Clinical examination may reveal one-sided flatness of the face. There may be flattening of the upper part of the cheek and fullness below. The distortion may be concealed by soft tissue swelling and pass unnoticed until the swelling subsides. However, if the eyeball is misplaced downward, the skin fold in the upper lid may be deepened. The outer canthus of the eye may be lower than that on the opposite side. On palpation one can usually define the fracture. The examiner should palpate both sides simultaneously. The entire outline of the orbit should be followed, and the levels of each infraorbital margin compared. There may be restriction of motion of the mandible caused by pressure against the coronoid process or temporal muscle. There may be trismus (inability to open the mouth fully), or restricted side-to-side motion, or even difficulty in closing the mouth. Function may be impaired by pain accompanying attempted use of the masseter muscle. Palpation intraorally in the superior buccal sulcus may show a lack of space between zygoma and maxilla, and between the coronoid process and the zygomatic arch.

Examination by palpation from in front may show an abnormal irregularity of the infraorbital margin above the outer canthus, and sometimes in front of the ear. Roentgenography is an important aid in determining the type and extent of the fracture; the maxillary sinus may be cloudy and filled with blood, due to injury of the mucosa. Transillumination may show a cloudy antrum, due to the presence of blood in the sinus.

Depressed Fracture (Limited to Zygomatic Arch)

There are usually three fractures, one at each end of the arch and one in the center. Actually, the arch is buckled, and should be reduced in order to correct the cosmetic deformity and the inevitable impairment of mandibular function.

Treatment. A heavy curved needle is passed from above downward through the skin beneath the depressed fragment to emerge below the arch. A wire is then passed and twisted together. Traction is used to elevate the fragment. If there is a tendency for the displacement to recur, the wire can be twisted over a glass slide or tongue depressor, which is placed so as to act as a horizontally placed bridge between the normal ends of the arch. A towel clip may be used, directly grasping the depressed bone and elevating it. Infiltration of a small amount of local anesthetic may be the only anesthesia necessary.

OPERATIVE REDUCTION (TEMPORAL APPROACH). The hair over the temporal region is shaved. A 2-cm. incision is made obliquely forward and upward, beginning 3 cm. above and in front of the upper attachment of the ear. The dense temporal fascia is exposed and then split vertically, exposing the temporalis muscle. A flat elevator is passed beneath the fascia on the surface of the temporalis muscle. It is directed behind the zygoma and under the arch. The bone or arch can then be elevated to any desired position (Fig. 24–*18*). Gauze or a towel is placed against the temporal area to prevent bruising of the scalp, and also to protect the thin portion of the skull against too much pressure which may cause a fracture.

OPERATIVE REDUCTION (INTRA-ORAL APPROACH) (Batson). An incision 2 cm. long is made in the buccal fold in the molar region and distal to the zygomatic process of the maxilla. An elevator is then inserted to the lateral side of the ascending ramus of the mandible and deep to the fractured arch. The arch is elevated upward and outward with the lateral wall of the maxilla being used as a fulcrum (Fig. 24–*18*). A Penrose drain is inserted and the mucosal incision is partially closed with fine chromic catgut.

Most simple zygomatic arch fractures remain in position following re-

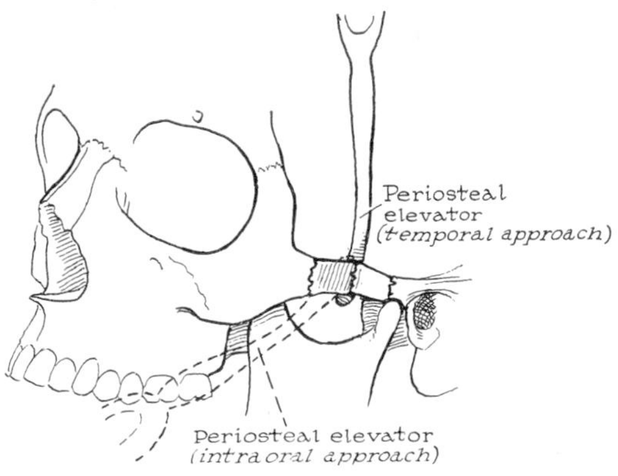

Figure 24–18. Elevation of a depressed zygomatic arch by a temporal incision and insertion of a lever. Broken line shows intraoral approach.

duction. However, it may occasionally be necessary to immobilize the mandible for at least two weeks by intermaxillary fixation to prevent masseter pull on the arch.

Displaced Fracture of Zygoma

The zygoma is usually fractured at its attachments to the frontal and sphenoid bones, the zygomatic arch, and the maxilla, and is displaced downward, inward, and backward. Occasionally there may be lateral displacement. The body of the zygoma itself is rarely fractured, but is usually separated and displaced as a unit. The walls of the maxillary sinus may be comminuted into many small fragments.

Treatment. Depressed fractures of the body of the zygomatic bone should be elevated to normal position as soon after injury as possible. After ten days the bones become fixed and reduction becomes difficult. There are several methods of treatment.

1. Manual manipulation from within the mouth may reduce the fracture. If so, no other treatment may be necessary.
2. A wire may be passed around bone, with a needle or a carrier, and the bone elevated by traction.
3. A tenaculum, hook, or screw may be passed through the skin into the bone, and it may be elevated by direct traction. This requires local anesthesia. Traction may be applied by means of an overhead pulley or head cap to maintain reduction and fixation.
4. Oral approach—under adequate anesthesia the mucobuccal fold lateral to the maxillary tuberosity is exposed. An incision is made through the mucosa. A short stout elevator is passed behind the fractured zygoma and it is elevated upward, outward, and forward. The buccal incision may be left open for drainage.
5. Temporal approach—as described above under the treatment of fractures of the zygomatic arch.
6. Trans-sinus approach—an incision is made in the mucobuccal fold in the cuspid-bicuspid area. An opening may be made through the anterior wall of the sinus (Caldwell-Luc), or entrance can be made through the comminuted fracture segments. A heavy elevator is passed into the maxillary sinus in the canine fossa area. The zygoma is then elevated by pressure from within the sinus. An intranasal window approach may also be used to elevate the bone.

Comminuted Fracture of the Zygoma

Fractures of this type may need additional support after reduction. With the floor of the orbit severely comminuted, the maxillary sinus must be evacuated of bone fragments and the displacement of the zygoma corrected and supported. These fractures are usually combined with fractures of the maxilla.

Treatment. Several methods of treatment of comminuted fracture of the zygoma are available.

1. Maxillary sinus approach—the anterior wall of the maxilla is exposed, and the spicules of bone are removed. The hematoma is evacuated from the sinus, and the bone fragments are manipulated into position. A naso-antral opening is made under the inferior turbinate, and petrolatum gauze strip packing is used to support the fragments and maintain an elevated floor of the orbit. The end of the packing may be brought out the nasal opening. The mucobuccal fold incision is then closed. Occasionally it may not be necessary to make the intranasal window, and the gauze packing is brought out the mucobuccal fold incision. The packing is removed gradually from one to two weeks postoperatively. Antibiotics are indicated.

2. Suspension method (Kazanjian)—the infraorbital ridge is exposed through the mucosa of the canine fossa, and a hole is drilled in the bone. A steel wire is brought out through the skin and placed with hooks to a head gear for a two-week period.

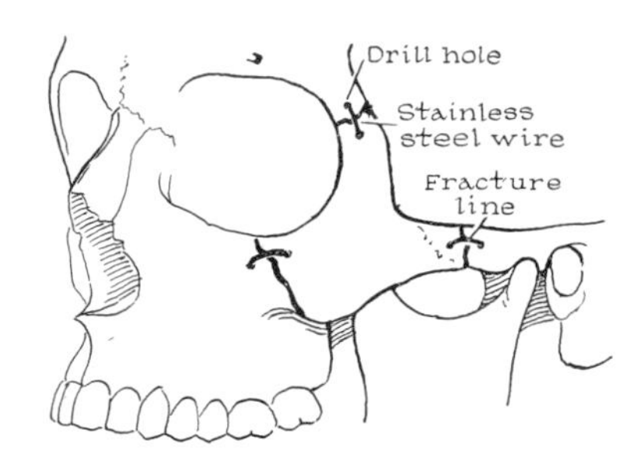

FRACTURE OF ZYGOMA

Figure 24–19. Fractures of the zygoma which may require internal fixation.

3. Direct interosseous wiring—a small external incision is made to expose the fracture site, and fine stainless steel wires are placed through drill holes in the bone. Internal fixation is usually required for fractures in certain areas: one at the outer rim of the orbit where there is separation at the frontal line suture, and the other along the infraorbital ridge at the maxillary suture line (Fig. 24–*19*). Occasionally a third point of fixation is at the zygomatic arch. This may be supplemented by antral packing, if necessary to maintain elevation of the floor of the orbit.

CHAPTER 25

INJURIES TO THE EYE

By J. VINCENT FLACK, M.D.

THE EYE is exposed by necessity of its function, but it is also well protected against external injury. Nestled in soft and yielding fat within the cavity of the bony orbit it is shielded above by the overhanging ridge of the frontal bone, below by the bony rim of the orbit and the prominence of the maxilla, and medially by the nose (Fig. 25–*1*). The lateral rim of the orbit is recessed and, depending upon its position in the orbit and the depth of the orbital cavity, the eye is more exposed. Additional protection is derived from the recoil of the head and neck reflexes and the extremely sensitive and rapid blink reflex. Finally, the protective mechanism is completed by a spontaneous lavage of the exposed surface of the eye with a profuse flow of tears in response to any irritation.

Occurrence of ocular injury depends largely upon environment, and is six to eight times greater in the male than in the female. In one city where metal work predominates, 53 per cent of all eye problems encoun-

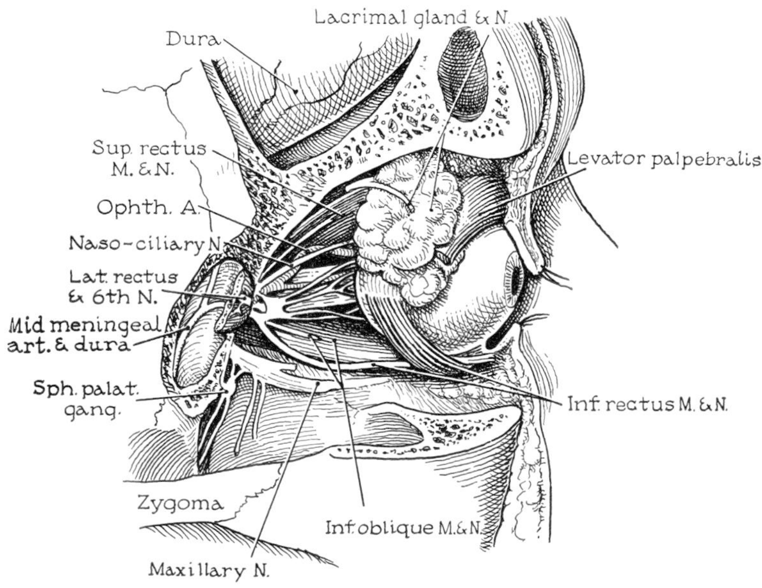

Figure 25–1. Normal anatomy of the eye and orbit.

tered in a large hospital were the result of trauma. There are indications that about 50 per cent of all unilateral and 20 per cent of all bilateral blindness is produced by accidental trauma.

BIRTH INJURIES

Retinal hemorrhage. Retinal hemorrhage occurs at birth as a result of increased intraocular pressure. This condition occurs in almost 50 per cent of primiparous births; it occurs more frequently than this when labor is long and difficult, and may be encountered less commonly after easy and rapid labor, and after the uncomplicated delivery of small premature infants. Both eyes are involved in about 50 per cent of the cases. Rapid spontaneous cessation of bleeding is the rule, and the retina is clear and devoid of any perceptible hemorrhage within seven to ten days. Permanent damage is to be feared only when severe hemorrhage involves the macula lutea.

Corneal opacities. Diffuse milky corneal opacities, almost always associated with swelling and ecchymosis of the ocular adnexa, are the result of edema. The cornea clears spontaneously and becomes transparent within a few days. Occasionally this is followed by the appearance of fine lines reflecting ruptures of Descemet's membrane. As these tiny defects are repaired, hyaline strands may arch over the posterior cornea and form bizarre patterns in the anterior chamber of the eye to produce subsequent strabismus, high myopia, or corneal irregularities.

Orbital hemorrhage. Hemorrhage into the orbit may occur during labor, and usually produces some proptosis of the globe of the eye. Among the causes of this phenomenon is fracture of the orbital wall by forceps, and this injury may produce concomitant damage to the ocular neurologic mechanism. Hemorrhage ceases spontaneously. Extravasated blood is absorbed quickly, but ocular aberrations consequent to the neurological injury may persist.

Treatment of Birth Injuries

Birth injuries to the eye are common, but self-limiting. The newborn infant has an enormous capacity for repair and recovery. Active treatment is unnecessary, and permanent damage is rare.

INJURIES TO THE EYELIDS

Contusions. The skin of the lids is very thin, abundant, sparsely supported by subcutaneous tissues and loosely connected to the deeper tissues. Very slight trauma produces rapid swelling which usually involves the entire lid. Hemorrhage spreads rapidly and extensively through the loose subcutaneous tissues so that a "black eye" is often accompanied by ecchymosis in the lid of the other eye. This should not be construed as reflecting bilateral injury. The extravasation is continuous, but ecchymosis is masked over the bridge of the nose by thicker skin.

Lacerations. Lacerations and puncture wounds often penetrate into the deeper structures of the eyelid. Division of the levator palpebrae muscle produces partial or complete ptosis. Damage to the lacrimal canaliculi produces epiphora. Lacerations across the fibers of the orbicularis oculi muscle tend to gape, but wounds parallel to the fibers are effectively closed by contraction of the muscle.

FOREIGN BODIES may be implanted to complicate the recovery from a laceration or puncture wound. Inert small foreign bodies, in the absence of infection, may become encapsulated by scar and cause little or no difficulty, but organic materials, such as wood splinters, often incite a granulomatous reaction eventuating in a cyst. As in other parts of the body, infection is the most common factor complicating an embedded foreign body. Suppuration, abscess formation, and the development of a fistula which remains patent pending spontaneous discharge or operative removal of the foreign body are not uncommon.

TREATMENT of a lacerated eyelid should be preceded by thorough cleansing of the surrounding skin. Early accurate primary suture of the wound should be done. A precise repair is of the utmost importance when the laceration involves the lid margin. Repair of a divided levator palpebrae muscle should be attempted, but usually is difficult due to retraction of the proximal cut end. Continuity of a severed lacrimal canaliculus may be reestablished by passing a small probe through the punctum and canal of the distal into the open cut end of the proximal segment. The probe is then passed through the proximal segment of the canaliculus into the lacrimal sac, where it is allowed to remain. Repair sufficient to permit removal of the probe usually occurs within ten days. Difficulty in locating the cut ends of the canaliculus may be overcome by injecting dye or sterile milk into the punctum of the intact canaliculus or the lacrimal sac, or both. The rich blood supply of the eyelid promotes rapid healing, and provides a strong defense against aerobic infection, but tetanus antitoxin or toxoid should be administered (see Chapter 3). Except when readily localized and easily accessible, embedded foreign bodies should usually be left undisturbed so long as infection does not supervene.

INJURIES TO THE CORNEA

The cornea (Fig. 25–2) constitutes the structural coat of the anterior (exposed) surface of the eyeball. Physiologically it transmits light rays and also has the major responsibility for their proper focus. Owing to an absolute uniformity of cellular pattern it is clear and transparent. It has a richly endowed nerve supply, but is devoid of circulation and depends upon diffusion from limbal vessels and upon the aqueous for cellular nourishment. The external corneal layer is a specialized epithelium, six or seven cells deep. These cells are of ectodermal origin, and the cells of the four deeper layers are of mesodermal origin. Only the surface (ectodermal) layer is capable of cellular replacement and rearrangement without scar formation. The repair of injuries to the deeper layers (Bowman's membrane) is characterized by scar formation.

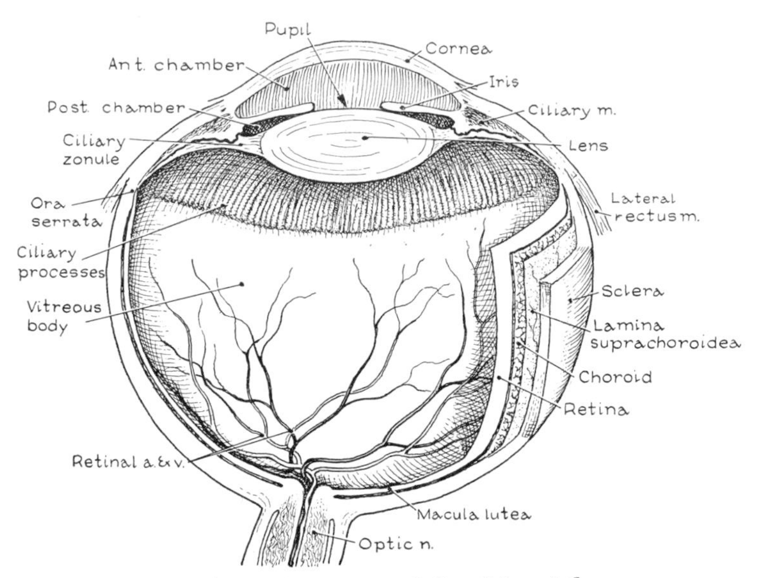

Figure 25–2. Structures of the globe of the eye.

Superficial abrasions and embedded foreign bodies constitute the bulk of corneal injuries. In the absence of infection and local anesthetics healing is complete within several days after injury. Healing is delayed when the abrasion is deep enough to implicate the underlying Bowman membrane. All corneal abrasions are attended by pain and excessive lacrimation, which may persist until repair is complete. When, in addition to the abrasion, a small foreign body has become embedded in the cornea, symptoms may be severe until it has been removed, and healing often is delayed by the presence of a residual foreign body stain.

Concussion of the cornea may disturb its endothelium and permit the entrance of small quantities of aqueous through resultant apertures. Linear or lattice-like opacities in the stroma may result, but usually disappear within a few days.

Laceration of the cornea heals rapidly when the wound edges have been perfectly approximated. Prolapsed iris or lens material should be ablated before the laceration is repaired, lest cyclitis, leukoma adhaerens, ingrowth of epithelium, or fistulization of the wound delay and complicate the healing process. Uninfected puncture wounds heal rapidly. Depending upon the depth and size of the wound, some resultant opacity follows most lacerations of the cornea.

Rupture of the cornea requires a force of sufficient magnitude to disrupt other components of the globe, and is usually a cause for concern. Small peripherally placed ruptures often implicate the iris, and larger lesions may result in extrusion of the lens, vitreous, or ciliary body.

Treatment of Corneal Injuries

Local anesthetic agents delay epithelialization, and should not be used unless necessary. Tetracaine hydrochloride (0.5 per cent) is least harmful to repair, and is the agent of choice when pain cannot be controlled by opiates. Atropine is not necessary. Ophthalmic ointments containing appropriate chemotherapeutic agents are the most effective defense against infection, but must not be used until the wound has been repaired sufficiently to seal off the anterior chamber of the eye. Until local treatment becomes permissible, oral or parenteral chemotherapy should be administered. The indications for tetanus antitoxin or toxoid obtain as in wounds of all other tissues. Embedded foreign bodies should be gently removed with a cotton applicator moistened in tetracaine hydrochloride solution (0.5 per cent) when necessary. The removal of foreign bodies with a corneal spud or curet should be done only by a competent ophthalmologist.

INJURIES TO THE SCLERA

The sclera (see Fig. 25–2) is an opaque continuation of the transparent corneal stroma. Structurally it is a tough inelastic external envelope which encloses and supports the contents of the globe. Lacerations and penetrating wounds of the sclera heal readily, provided the potential ravages of infection are anticipated and prevented by appropriate surgical and chemotherapeutic measures.

Embedded foreign bodies are encountered only about 0.5 per cent as often in the sclera as in the exposed cornea. Small particles, unless composed of iron or copper, usually become encapsulated, are well tolerated, and should be left undisturbed. Iron or copper particles of any size produce a chemical inflammation and must be removed. Larger foreign bodies of any material should be removed with forceps, curet, or magnet. When a foreign body has penetrated deep into the sclera, removal should not be attempted except by a competent ophthalmologist in a surgical environment adequate to prevent or cope with displacement of the embedded body into the vitreous chamber.

Rupture of the sclera occurs only as a result of a concussion injury violent enough to affect all components of the globe. The human fist has replaced the cow's horn as the instrument most commonly producing this lesion, which is always a cause for grave concern. The sclera usually bursts in its superior and medial quadrant at some distance from the point of direct impact, and in a line concentric with and 2 to 4 mm. from the limbus.

The eyelids are ecchymotic and swollen. Chemosis is marked, especially if the conjunctiva is intact over the rupture. Uveal tissue and vitreous may be seen in or prolapsing from the scleral wound. The lens often is displaced. Orbital hemorrhage with proptosis is common. In small lesions only the iris may be prolapsed or dialyzed, but some subluxation of the lens is almost always present. Hypotony and collapse of the globe are invariably present.

TREATMENT. A completely disorganized globe should be enucleated as soon as possible.

If no uveal tissue can be seen in the wound, and the edges of the rupture are not gaping, complete rest of the eye should be maintained, even in the presence of lens displacement. A gaping wound usually contains uveal tissue and vitreous matter which must be excised before repair is carried out. Occasionally a small prolapse of the iris or ciliary tissue may be replaced rather than excised. The rent in the sclera must be securely and accurately closed with fine sutures inserted by a technique which inflicts minimal additional trauma. Imperfections of repair produce delayed healing and usually result in staphyloma and eventual loss of the eye. The external surface of the operative site should be sealed with a flap fashioned from adjacent conjunctiva. Appropriate antibiotic and antitetanus therapy should be used in all cases.

THE PROGNOSIS is poor. Recovery of some vision is obtained in 30 per cent or less of all cases. Subsequent uveitis and secondary glaucoma are frequent. Sympathetic ophthalmia of the other eye is a constant potential complication which may occur in any case without relation to the severity of the original injury.

INJURIES TO THE IRIS AND CILIARY BODY

The mobility of the iris (see Fig. 25–2) allows for adjustments in the size of the pupil. This in turn governs the amount of light entering the eye, and facilitates synchronization of the focus mechanism which is dependent upon changes in the shape of the lens produced by the ciliary muscle. The iris may also assist in the absorption of aqueous humor which is secreted by the ciliary body. Both iris and ciliary body are richly endowed with nerves and blood vessels.

Concussion of the iris evokes an initial response characterized by a transient spastic miosis and an associated accommodative spasm. These are produced by parasympathetic irritation, and are to be differentiated from the identical result of sympathetic paralysis consequent to brain damage, and certain perforating injuries of the globe. Following the initial irritative miosis a paralytic mydriasis, associated with a paralysis of accommodation, is common. Occasionally iridoplegia may occur independently of the accommodative failure. In either event, the prognosis is uncertain and maximum recovery may not occur for several months. Some permanent defect, usually due to the iridoplegia, is not uncommon.

Hyphema, a condition which is characterized by hemorrhage into the iris and by a water-level accumulation of blood in the anterior chamber of the eye, often follows a mild concussion and almost always is produced by more severe injuries. Usually this condition is transient, and clears spontaneously within several days. Persistent hyphema is indicative of continued or recurring hemorrhage rather than faulty absorption of the extravasated blood and, when prolonged for more than three weeks, justifies a guarded prognosis and a suspicion of irreversible damage. Secondary glaucoma is common, and the combination of increased pressure and hemorrhage in the anterior chamber not infrequently may produce a blood pigment stain of the cornea.

TREATMENT OF HYPHEMA. Complete rest of the eye usually results in rapid recovery from traumatic hyphema. Cold compresses may be used for comfort and reduction of bleeding in the early stages following injury, after which warm compresses have a soothing effect. Atropine is unnecessary, and may have an adverse effect upon an already overburdened drainage system. Prevention of increased tension by miotics is usually more effective than an attempt to accelerate decompression by mydriatics. Eserine may be used at the onset of secondary glaucoma, but a persistent increase in tension should be decompressed—by repeated paracentesis if necessary. Attempts to lavage the blood from the anterior chamber of the eye at the time of paracentesis are unnecessary and unwise. Persistent glaucoma after repeated decompression and the use of miotics usually is indicative of some additional but unrecognized lesion.

Laceration of the iris due to accidental or operative causes does not heal. Obviously, this does not reflect any intrinsic defect in the reparative powers of this structure because, in response to inflammation or abnormal contact with the posterior surface of the cornea following a perforating injury, granulation tissue develops in a normal manner. Presumably repair of a lacerated iris is prevented by some influence of the surrounding aqueous humor which bathes the edges of the wound.

Laceration of the pupillary margin is common and, when the sphincter is involved by the wound, some resultant distortion of the pupil is to be expected. Multiple tears are usually present when the full thickness of the iris is lacerated, but severe injuries by a flying rock or ball often separate the iris root from the ciliary body by a single avulsed laceration. This is reflected by a black, crescentic defect through which the ciliary zonule and lens edge may be seen, and into which the vitreous may herniate. Occasionally the entire iris may be avulsed from the ciliary body, producing traumatic aniridia, the anterior and posterior layers of the iris may be separated, or the entire thickness of iris may be retroflexed and folded back on the ciliary body. Both iris and ciliary body may be displaced into the globe. Rupture or avulsion of the ciliary body from its scleral attachments, usually but not always associated with a rupture of the sclera, may occur.

An accurate assessment of the nature and extent of the iris injury is rarely possible until dispersion of hemorrhage from the anterior chamber has taken place. Late surgical repair is not indicated, except for relief of severe diplopia or dazzling resulting from a localized avulsion of the iris root from the ciliary body (iridodialysis).

INJURIES TO THE LENS

The lens (see Fig. 25–2) is a circular, transparent, double-convex structure composed of an elastic capsule, a semisolid cortex, and, in the adult, a fairly firm nucleus. Devoid of intrinsic circulation, it extracts nourishment from the surrounding intraocular fluid. It is held in position by the suspensory ligament which, in response to motivation by the ciliary muscle, alters the tension of the elastic capsule to influence the lens shape and control the focusing of transmitted light.

Traumatic cataract may result from concussion or laceration of the lens. Concussion may alter the permeability, or create a small bursting wound of the lens capsule. In either case the entrance of fluid into the lens substance produces a cataract. The nature and size of such an opacity depends not only upon the extent of the capsular damage, but also upon its location and the age of the patient. If the injured capsule recovers its normal semipermeable state rapidly, or a small rent is quickly sealed by fibrin or iris tissue before the entrance of fluid has caused irreversible damage to the lens substance, recovery and clearing of the opacity may occur. The prospects for such a spontaneous recovery are fairly good in the young, but the prognosis must be guarded in the adult, and especially in the aged patient. A minor injury to an elderly patient often results in a progressively increasing opacity or precipitates a senile cataract, whereas in the young a traumatic opacity clears or remains stationary. In the latter event, its position deepens with the growth of the lens while its size remains constant, but its presence constitutes infallible evidence of previous injury.

A rosette-shaped cataract results from diffuse changes in the anterior or posterior lens cortex; it may appear within hours or not until weeks after injury. Mild translucent opacities of this type occasionally clear spontaneously, but as a rule such lesions are permanent and stationary. A diffuse cataract is the inevitable result of a gross wound of the lens capsule, whether or not the wound becomes closed. The resulting opacities are bizarre in shape and variable in size; in the young, the lens matter may be completely absorbed to produce an aphakic eye.

The treatment of traumatic cataract is conservative, whether or not this injury may be somewhat obscured by edema of the cornea and extravasation of blood into the anterior chamber during the early stages following injury. Rest is essential. Atropine is contraindicated, and may reopen a capsular rent previously sealed by the iris. Miotics may relax the lens capsule sufficiently to allow closure of a small aperture. When the resultant opacity remains stationary and does not reduce vision, no further treatment should be carried out. When vision is permanently deranged, the patient's age is an important factor in determination of treatment. Discission is usually the method of choice in a child; linear extraction of the cataract may be successful in a young adult; and intra- or extracapsular extraction is indicated in elderly patients when the visual or cosmetic defects caused by the cataract are sufficient to justify operative treatment.

Displacement of the lens may result from rupture of the suspensory ligament at its lenticular attachments. As a consequence of this injury the lens may disappear into the vitreous or, less frequently, present in the anterior chamber of the eye. Depending upon the degree of injury to the ligament, it may remain in the position of original displacement, or move about from place to place. Symptoms and signs are quite variable and depend upon the degree and direction of displacement. When the displaced lens remains in its primary axis the resulting defect may be nothing more than lenticular myopia, but if it is displaced laterally or tilted from its primary axis, astigmatism requiring correction by lenses is the usual result. Monocular diplopia follows gross lateral displacement. Deficient lens support of the iris causes it to tremble on movement of the eye (iridodonesis).

The treatment of minor lens subluxations should be expectant. When correction of visual defects is necessary due to an inadequate other eye, a cataract lens is sometimes beneficial. Mydriatics may be required for iridocyclitis. Secondary glaucoma may supervene to produce a serious and sometimes insoluble complication.

Dislocation of the lens into the anterior chamber where it appears like a drop of oil or, if opaque, as a white disclike object, is rapidly followed by a severe cyclitis, corneal dystrophy, and severe secondary glaucoma. The dislocated lens should be removed as soon as possible. Posterior dislocation of the lens into the vitreous, on the other hand, is often well tolerated and, barring complications, the lens should be allowed to remain in its displaced position. Occasionally such a posteriorly displaced lens will pass through a dilated pupil into the anterior chamber by gravity, if the patient is placed in a prone position. Surgical removal of the loose lens then may be successfully accomplished. Unless this maneuver is successful, lens removal should be attempted only as a last resort.

INJURIES TO THE CHOROID

The choroid may be lacerated or implicated by a penetrating wound, but is most commonly damaged by hemorrhage consequent to a blow against the globe. The choroid may be detached by extravasating hemorrhage, or may rupture even in the presence of intact sclera. Concentrically placed indirect ruptures are common, prone to occur on the temporal aspect of the choroid, and may damage the macula lutea. The overlying intact retina becomes afunctional, and a scotoma develops. Treatment is expectant.

INJURIES TO THE RETINA

The retina which is derived from neural ectoderm is essentially an anterior projection of the brain, and fulfills the function of acceptance and transmission of light impulses. In common with all nerve tissue, this structure responds to trauma with hemorrhage, edema, and atrophy.

Retinal edema (Berlin's opacity, or commotio retinae) is a common result of concussion of the globe. The edematous expanse of the posterior retinal area surrounds the macula, which stands out like a bright red spot against a milky white background. Central vision is poor, but usually clears progressively as the edema subsides. Occasionally degenerative or pigmentary changes may supervene to produce a permanent defect in central vision.

Retinal hemorrhage may be intraretinal, preretinal, or subhyloid. Extravasation of blood, or even reparative fibrous tissue, may invade the vitreous. Hemorrhage is absorbed over a period of several weeks, but areas of retinal atrophy with scotomas may occur to produce permanent and, when the macula is involved, quite disabling defects.

Retinal detachment and its relation to trauma has been a subject for many arguments. It is notable that the violent athletic activities of youth, when the eye is young and healthy, are virtually unattended by this injury, and that countless parachute jumps by young healthy individuals are made without any recorded retinal separations. Only a violent and direct injury, such as a blow on the eye by a fist, baseball, or tennis ball, is adequate to detach a young and healthy retina. Under normal circumstances choroidal ruptures spare the retina, even when the sclera is also ruptured. It is reasonably certain that a healthy retina cannot be detached except by direct and adequate trauma. However, it is equally clear that a minor and indirect injury is capable of producing retinal detachment in the presence of cystic degeneration and vitreous changes consequent to age or atrophy accompanying high myopia. Regardless of the cause, retinal detachment requires operative repair.

INJURIES TO THE OPTIC NERVE

Optic nerve damage most commonly results from a penetrating injury. Massive intraocular hemorrhage effectively prevents early diagnosis. After the extravasated blood has been absorbed, and it is once again possible to examine the fundus, the evidences of optic nerve damage are apparent. Marginal rupture of the nerve produces an arcuate hemorrhage extending into the retina around the periphery of a fairly normal disc. An incomplete nerve rupture usually produces a depression of the lower half of the optic disc which resembles a coloboma. Complete rupture produces a disc that appears like a bottomless pit, and the vascular channels of the fundus are sparse or absent.

Occasionally optic nerve damage results from a severe contusion to the eyeball. Less severe contusions often produce considerable optic edema without gross damage to the nerve and, whenever the choroid or retina has been damaged, some optic atrophy is to be expected. Optic atrophy may indirectly follow an injury to the forehead, usually a fracture, which produces optic nerve compression by hemorrhage, or damage to the nutrient vessels supplying the optic nerve. Immediate loss of vision and of pupillary reaction to light may precede optic atrophy by several weeks. A fracture through the optic canal may or may not be visible on roentgenograms.

Optic nerve damage warrants a guarded prognosis, and expectant treatment.

INJURIES TO THE VITREOUS

Some changes in the vitreous are to be expected following any forceful concussion of the globe of the eye. A plasmodial diffusion of proteins from the uveal and retinal vessels is a common finding, which is recognizable by an increased vitreous flare. This is often associated with a liquefaction of the vitreous framework and the deposition of bright red pigment granules on the vitreous skeins. Hemorrhage into the vitreous chamber is common, and, when it is large in amount, the chamber of the eye appears black to ophthalmoscopic examination. Small hemorrhages usually are located in the anterior vitreous and tend to migrate toward the posterior lens capsule. Severe concussions may detach the vitreous, except from the ora and the optic nerve head, and occasionally complete detachment may allow the entire vitreous gel to move forward as the posterior chamber fills with intraocular fluid. Herniation of a portion of vitreous into the anterior chamber of the eye is an occasional concomitant of severe injuries in the region of the zonule.

TRAUMA AND OCULAR TENSION

Transient alterations of intraocular tension are among the constant and normal physiological reactions of the eye to trauma, and reflect spontaneous readjustment of a functionally intact neurovascular mechanism. Excessive or prolonged changes reflect some irreversible neurovascular damage.

Ocular hypertension (concussion glaucoma). Concussion alters and produces a temporary instability of ocular tension. A concomitant, but less marked, similar disturbance of the uninjured eye is common. Usually these products of some ill-defined autonomic vasomotor response are transient. Prolonged or excessive increase of ocular tension occurring early, or not for some time after injury, and often in the absence of any demonstrable intraocular lesion, is known as concussion glaucoma. The resultant severe ocular pain, accompanied by nausea and vomiting, usually can be relieved rapidly with miotics, but occasionally operative measures may be required for the reduction of intractable ocular hypertension.

Ocular hypotension. Transient hypotony may follow ocular concussion and, in some instances, reduced ocular tension associated with myopia and mydriasis may persist indefinitely. Papillary and retinal edema may become evident as a secondary product of prolonged hypotony. Some time may elapse before visual impairment occurs, but eventually degenerative changes, quiet iritis, and cataract are to be expected. No treatment is effective.

INTRAOCULAR FOREIGN BODIES

A foreign body within the eye is inevitably a serious injury. When it has passed through the ocular tissues without causing more than a small penetrating wound, the threat of early acute infection or chronic inflammation is imminent. More extensive laceration of the ocular tissues consequent to passage of the foreign body may be immediately disastrous to the eye. Even after recovery from the initial injury and avoidance of infection, ocular function may subsequently be destroyed by some adverse chemical property of the foreign body. Occasionally the late development of sympathetic ophthalmia or of intraocular cysts may destroy vision. Nevertheless, it is sometimes possible for ocular function to continue normal despite a retained foreign body.

About 15 per cent of penetrating foreign bodies come to rest in the anterior chamber, and 70 per cent enter the vitreous chamber. About 8 per cent are stopped and held by the lens, and the remainder pass com-

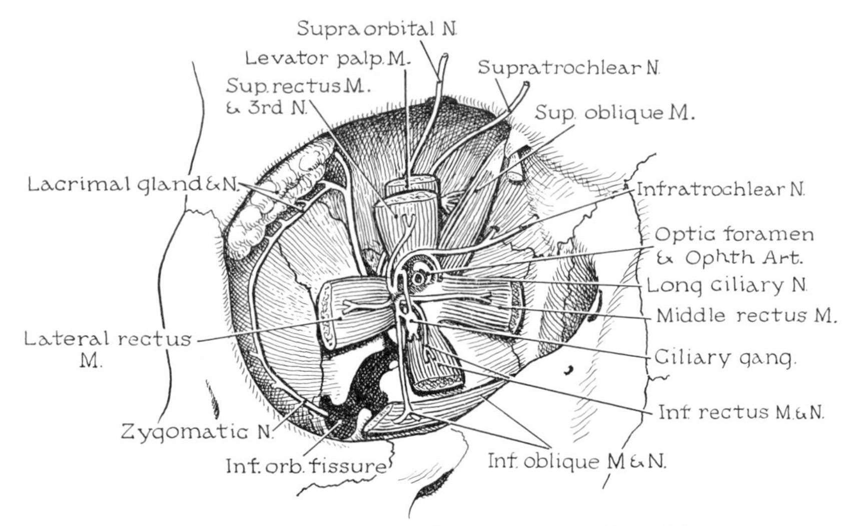

Figure 25–3. Extraocular contents of the orbit.

pletely through the eye and come to rest in the orbit (Fig. 25–3). The majority of foreign bodies are metallic and penetrate the eye with great velocity. Heat generated by the force of the blow may make the particle virtually sterile, and reduce danger of infection. On the other hand, penetration of the eye by organic matter, such as wood splinters, is commonly the precursor of frank suppuration. Penetrating missiles greater than 2.5 mm. in diameter usually destroy the eye; those less than 2 mm. in diameter usually do not have sufficient velocity to penetrate the ocular coats. Consequently, the majority of retained foreign bodies vary from 2 to 2.5 mm. in diameter. Elongated bodies, such as particles of wire, metal slivers, or a segment of needle, penetrate readily without gross laceration of the ocular walls.

The various tissues of the eye react in different degrees to the irritation of any foreign body. The lens has a low metabolic rate and is the most tolerant to foreign material of all ocular tissues, except when a gross laceration of its capsule permits free entry of aqueous. The anterior chamber may show little or no reaction to a particle of sterile foreign matter. Even the reaction of the vitreous may be slight in amount. However, the uveal tissues are more intolerant of foreign material and usually respond rapidly with a proliferative inflammatory reaction. The iris, on the other hand, may harbor a foreign body for a prolonged period without evidencing more than an occasional attack of iritis.

THE NATURE OF THE FOREIGN MATERIAL

The nature of the foreign body is of great importance. Sterile and chemically inert material excites a minimum tissue response. Gold, silver, platinum, sand, coal, stone, glass, plastics, porcelain, and rubber are inert materials. Gunpowder and cordite, when sterile, are also inert when contained within the eye. All such inert particles usually become insulated from the adjacent ocular tissues by encapsulation in a fibrous envelope after they have remained in the eye for any prolonged period. Of the various metallic substances which may penetrate the eye, zinc, lead, and aluminum usually are relatively inert; iron and alloys of copper are toxic; mercury and nickel rapidly excite violent inflammatory reactions.

Foreign Bodies of Iron, Steel, or Copper

Flying particles of iron or steel constitute the offending missiles in the great majority of intraocular foreign bodies. The deposition of iron pigment in the ocular tissues (siderosis bulbi) is a common and serious late complication of the prolonged ocular retention of ferrous materials. Ferrous metals can be magnetized. These three facts attest to the tremendous clinical importance of ferrous intraocular foreign bodies. When the ferrous content of an iron alloy is low, the risk of siderosis is correspondingly reduced, but so also are the effects upon such an alloy of the surgeon's magnet. Attempts to remove an intraocular foreign body which cannot be magnetized, except from the anterior chamber or lens, are formidable and hazardous procedures often entailing a risk of complications more serious than those of a retained foreign body.

Siderosis bulbi. An intraocular foreign body containing iron produces a gradual chemical change in the ocular tissues which probably results from ionization of the base metal, followed by its dispersion and deposition in the surrounding tissues. The resulting rusty appearance of the iris, cornea, and lens is a visible manifestation of the deposition of iron pigment in these tissues, and constitutes the clinical entity known as siderosis bulbi. A similar deposition of pigment in the retina is accompanied by a gradual loss of vision consequent to retinal degeneration. This phenomenon is almost always irreversible, and not infrequently is followed by retinal detachment and secondary glaucoma.

Chalcosis. Pure copper, or an alloy containing more than 85 per cent of copper, quickly excites a violent suppurative inflammation which usually destroys the eye. Alloys containing a relatively small amount of pure copper react by ionization, dispersion, and deposition of copper in the ocular tissues, to produce the condition known as chalcosis. A greenish blue ring is seen in the depths of the periphery of the cornea, and a colored sunflower cataract forms in the anterior cortex of the lens. The development of these phenomena may be prolonged over a period of years, but occasionally occurs within a period of months. Chalcosis is usually not as destructive to vision as is siderosis, and may sometimes be reversible following complete absorption or removal of the offending material.

DIAGNOSIS AND LOCALIZATION OF A FOREIGN BODY IN THE EYE

A detailed history is essential. All available information about the source, size, and nature of the penetrating agent should be educed and recorded. The direction and position of the wound of entry should be noted and reconciled with the history. Occasionally the intraocular foreign body can be visualized through the ophthalmoscope, but as a rule this is precluded by intraocular hemorrhage. A Berman-Moorhead locator is useful for the detection, but of relatively little value for the exact localization, of metallic foreign bodies in the eye. Detection of a magnetic body is possible within a range about ten times its diameter, but this range is reduced markedly when the foreign body is of nonmagnetic material.

Biplane Roentgenography

Biplane roentgenography is the most accurate and least complicated method for plotting the exact position of an intraocular foreign body. Posteroanterior and lateral films are taken (Fig. 25–4), and the position of the foreign body (Fig. 25–5) is charted in relation to a previously inserted contact lens containing four lead markers to designate the limbus (Fig. 25–6).

Bone-Free Roentgenograms

Whenever there is a possibility of an intraocular foreign body of questionable opacity, a bone-free film should be made (Fig. 25–7). These films may disclose foreign bodies of almost any density greater than that of the soft tissues. Minute particles of glass or metal, whose shadows would be lost in the grain of ordinary films, often are revealed clearly.

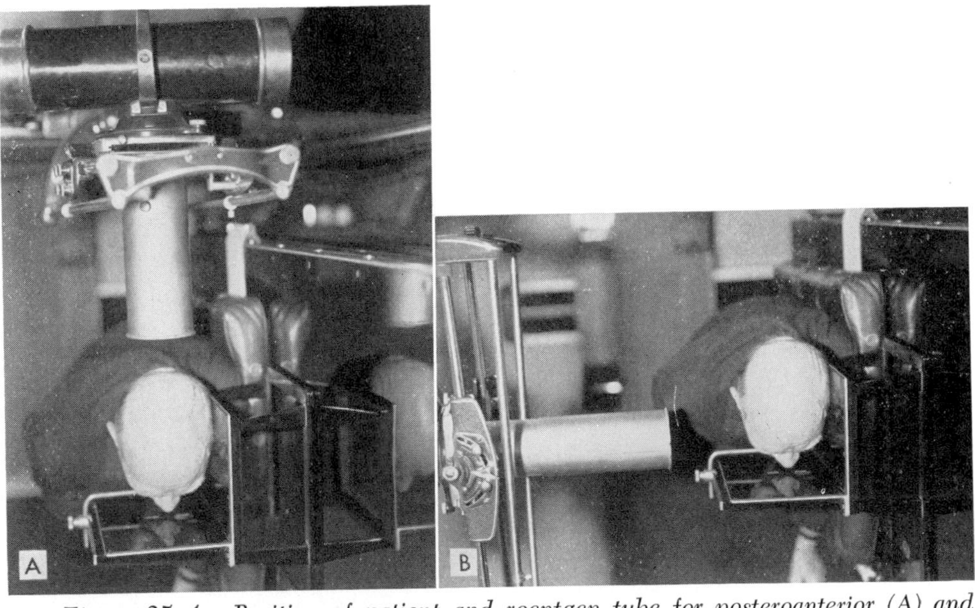

Figure 25–4. Position of patient and roentgen tube for posteroanterior (A) and lateral (B) films designed to localize an intraocular foreign body (see films in Figure 25–5).

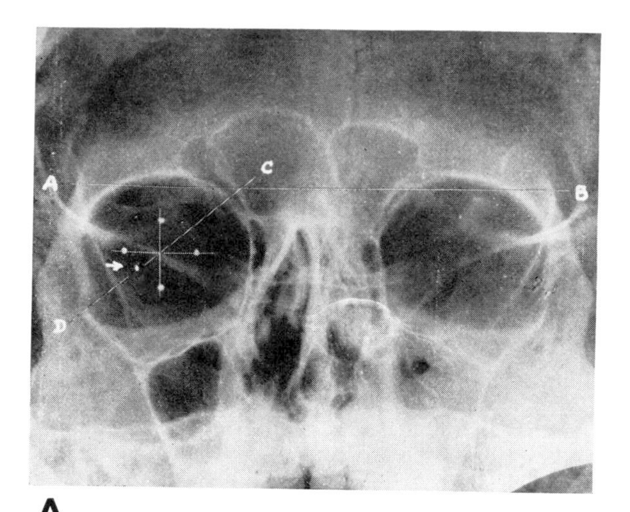

A

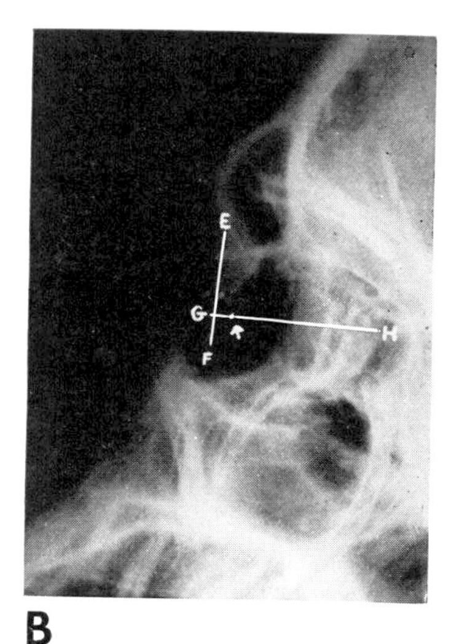

B

Three times natural size.

C Position of Body in Front View.

D Position of Body in Meridional Section.

Figure 25–5. Localization of an intraocular foreign body by use of a contact lens containing lead inserts, roentgen findings being transposed to appropriate charts for interpretation.

A. In the posteroanterior roentgenogram the line AB is drawn through the upper orbital rims. The diagonal line CD is drawn through the foreign body (arrow) and the center of the contact lens.

B. In the lateral roentgenogram the line EF is drawn anterior and tangential to the lens inserts, and locates the limbus. The line GH is drawn at right angles to EF, through the foreign body.

C. The angle between the lines AB and CD in the posteroanterior roentgenogram is transposed to the chart, C′D′. The distance of the foreign body from the lens center can now be measured directly, and corrections made for magnification.

D. The distance of the foreign body from EF in the lateral roentgenogram is measured directly, magnification is corrected, and it is plotted on the chart, on line G′H′. A second line I′J, representing the distance of the foreign body from the axis of the eyeball as previously determined, is then drawn perpendicular to the first.

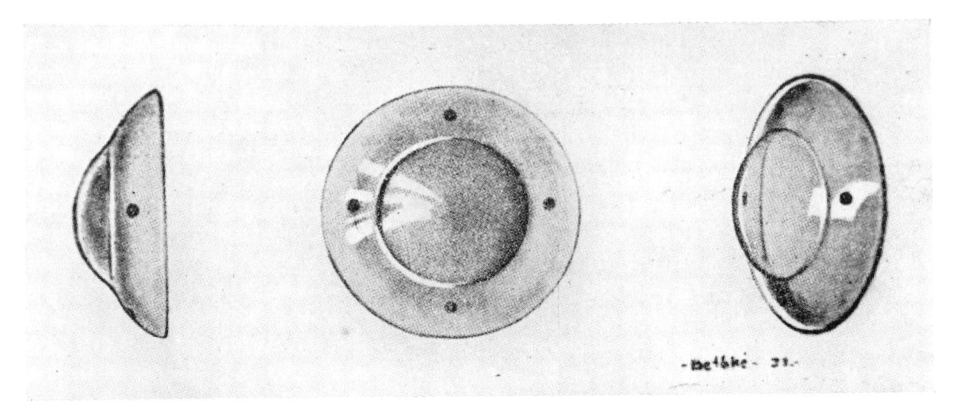

Figure 25–6. A contact lens containing four lead inserts for the localization of intraocular foreign bodies.

The injured eye is anesthetized with a few drops of 0.5 per cent tetracaine hydrochloride and this lens inserted by slipping it under the upper lid while the patient looks downward, and then lifting out the lower lid. An error in localization will occur if the lens does not fit the curves of the cornea and sclera, and dropping downward of a loose lens must be prevented by stabilization with Scotch tape, or it must be held in place while the films are taken.

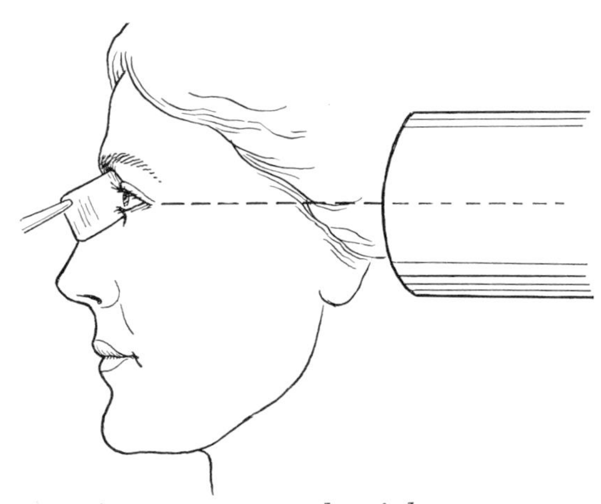

Figure 25–7. Bone-free roentgenography of the eye.

A dental film is held over and perpendicular to the inner canthus of the eye while the central beam of the x-ray is directed from the side to produce a shadow of the anterior segment of the eye, including the lids. This procedure is useful for identification and localization of small and questionably opaque foreign bodies, but is effective only in the anterior 8 to 12 mm. of the globe.

REMOVAL OF FOREIGN BODY FROM THE EYE

Whether a foreign body should be attracted from the posterior into the anterior chamber of the eye by a giant magnet and then removed through a corneal incision, or extracted by a small electromagnet through a scleral incision, has been a matter of some argument, which in the individual case is usually settled by the equipment available. In the absence of localizing roentgenograms, it is unlikely that a foreign body can be attracted by a small portable magnet, whereas a giant magnet may draw it into the anterior chamber with ease. As a rule, use of the giant magnet probably should be limited to the extraction of foreign bodies with smooth edges and not in excess of 3 mm. in diameter. Bodies smaller than 1 mm. may not be attracted to the giant magnet and are best localized accurately and approached directly through a scleral incision with a small portable magnet.

Direct removal of a foreign body is implemented by an incision through the sclera at the point of roentgenographic localization. The incision should be in a meridian of the globe, and about 1 mm. longer than the diameter of the object to be removed. The magnet tip is then placed in the incision and the current turned on intermittently until the foreign body appears on the magnet tip. Extraction of foreign bodies by the anterior route requires a giant magnet which is brought to within 1 mm. of the corneal surface with the patient in a sitting position. The foreign body, with its long axis remaining in the direction of the magnetic pull, is drawn through the vitreous to the posterior lens by opening and closing the circuit. It then passes around the equator of the lens and through the suspensory ligament, after which it is seen to move the iris forward. The current is then turned off, and the magnet tip is moved to the limbus opposite the point where the iris bulges. When the current is turned on, the foreign body is then drawn through the pupil and drops to the bottom of the anterior chamber when the magnet is removed. From this position it can be removed easily through a small corneal incision with the aid of a smaller magnet.

PROGNOSIS OF FOREIGN BODIES IN THE EYE

Immediate enucleation of the eye is required in about 50 per cent of cases where the foreign body penetrates and remains in the anterior chamber. Of the surviving eyes, the majority recover and retain useful vision of good quality, provided the foreign body has been successfully removed. Enucleation is necessary in almost 50 per cent of the cases in which the vitreous chamber has been penetrated. Of the remainder, 20 per cent of the patients in whom the foreign body has been successfully removed retain good vision. When the intraocular foreign body remains in place and becomes encapsulated, only about 10 per cent of patients retain visual function approximating normal.

SYMPATHETIC OPHTHALMIA

A decision must be made to preserve or to enucleate every seriously injured eye. The ultimate fate of the injured eye is not the only consideration. Sympathetic inflammation of the uninjured eye, caused by failure or delay of enucleation of the injured member, is a tragedy of catastrophic dimensions. Once such contralateral inflammation has become established, no benefit is to be derived from enucleation of the offending member. On the contrary, it should then be preserved, for when the inflammation finally subsides the vision sometimes proves to be better in the primarily involved eye than in the one inflamed secondarily. Intensive steroid therapy may depress the inflammatory reaction and prove of considerable benefit in such problems.

Extensive laceration of the globe with extrusion of lens and vitreous material into the wound warrants early enucleation. When a lacerated eye fails to show evidence of light perception, enucleation should be advised without more than a short delay. Laceration of the cornea and injury to the lens, with or without iris prolapse, and in the absence of vitreous injury, always is followed by a stormy convalescence and usually is complicated by chronic inflammation, secondary glaucoma, or both. At best, poor vision is to be expected. The progress of such an injury warrants a short period of observation, but the patient should be warned of the poor prognosis, the danger to his uninjured eye, and the likelihood that enucleation may be necessary at an early date.

The eye afflicted with intraocular suppuration following injury may be saved, but the visual result usually is poor. Even though sympathetic inflammation rarely develops subsequent to unilateral suppuration, it is probable that the majority of grossly infected eyes should be enucleated. Sympathetic inflammation has not been encountered when enucleation was done within a week following injury, but may occur following incomplete enucleation, especially if a small fragment of uvea is left in the orbit.

INDEX

Boldface folios indicate part titles

ABDOMEN, 495–539
distention of, compression fracture of vertebral body and, 579
injuries of, 504 (*see also* Thoraco-abdominal injuries)
characteristics of, 521
complications of, 530
diagnosis of, 504
errors in, objective vs. subjective, 511
examination in, 505
roentgen, 511, 512
history and, 505
tests in
laboratory, 514
special, 511
fractures and, 535
gunshot, 521
miscellaneous, 529
nonpenetrating
multiple injuries masking, 508
penetrating injuries vs., 509
observations in
inaccurate, 511
interpretation of, 511
pelvis fracture and, 536
penetrating
diagnosis of, 506
misleading signs in, 508
missile tracks and, 507
nonpenetrating injuries vs., 509
sequelae of, 530
skull fractures and, 536
spinal cord injuries and, 537
treatment of, 516
definitive, 517
drainage in, 520
urinary tract injuries and, 538
Abdomen (*continued*)
lower, injuries of, upper abdominal injuries vs., 501
silent, nonpenetrating abdominal injuries and, 510
splinting of, penetrating abdominal wounds and, 506
upper, injuries of, lower abdominal injuries vs., 501
Abdominal apoplexy, 530
Abscess
brain
post-traumatic, 709
skull fracture and, 668
of external ear, 691
Achilles tendon. *See* Tendo achillis
Acidosis, 18
correction of, 19
Acromioclavicular joint
derangement of, internal, 295
dislocations at
complete, 293
diagnosis of, differential, 295
treatment of, operative, 295
incomplete, 293
old unreduced, 295
injuries at, 292
subluxations at, painful persistent, 295
Acromion, fracture of, 237
ACTH, response to injury and, 15
Adrenal glands, complications involving, 96
Aerocoele, cranial, skull fractures and, 667
Age
anesthesia for reduction of fractures and, 41
bone repair and, 11

Age (*continued*)
burns and, 94
hip fractures and, 433
Airway, patent, importance of, 34
in head injuries, 686
in multiple injuries, 65
in prevention of shock, 25
"Alarm reaction," systemic response to injury and, 12
Albumin, blood, function of, 20
Alkalosis, 18
correction of, 19
Ambulance, speeding, patient welfare and, 37
Amputation
arterial injuries and, 98
of thumb, 130
traumatic, of finger, 129
Anemia
burns and, 93
hypoproteinemia and, 20
Anesthesia
for reduction of fractures, 40
for repair of injuries of hand, 119
local, in traumatic acute low-back pain, 624
surface, in traumatic acute low-back pain, 623
Anesthetist, responsibilities of, in prevention of shock, 25
Aneurysm, arterial, false, 100
Angiitis, obliterative, herniated intervertebral disc vs., 644
Aniridia, traumatic, 746
Ankle, 333–362 (*see also names of specific structures*)
anatomy of, 334
roentgen implications of, 335
architecture of, 333
ligaments of
injuries of, 336
rupture of, 342
shattered fractures of distal tibia involving, 361
sprain of, 336
severe, treatment of, 339
Annulus fibrosus, 563, 599, 639
Anoxia, tissue, shock and, 23
Anteroposterior ligament of ankle, rupture of, extensive, 344
Antibacterial agents, in trauma, 69–78
Antibacterial measures
in burns, 73
in open fractures, 63
Antibiotic(s), use of
general therapeutic, 76
prophylactic, 71
Anticoagulants
arterial repair and, 103
in conservative management of arterial injury, 105
Anxiety, emotional response to injury and, 30
Apprehension test, for subluxation of patella, 397
Arm (*see also names of specific structures*)
shoulder and, 233–296
Armamentarium, surgical
for arterial repair, 102
for open reduction, 56
Arteriovenous fistula
arterial injuries and, 100
carotid artery–cavernous sinus, skull fracture and, 669
Artery (Arteries)
injuries to, 98
complications of, 100
diagnosis of, 101
repair of
antibiotics and, 103
anticoagulants and, 103
infection and, 103
technique of, 104
timing of, 102
surgical, 101
treatment of, 101
conservative, 105
occlusion of, embolic, 106
Arthrodesis
in avascular necrosis of femoral head, 455
in nonunion of femoral neck fracture, 453
in nonunion of scaphoid fracture, 177
subtalar, primary, after compression fracture of calcaneus, 330
Arthroplasty
Smith-Peterson cup, in avascular necrosis of femoral head, 455
trochanteric, in nonunion of femoral neck fracture, 453

Arytenoid cartilage, injuries of, 710
Ascites, chylous, 530
Asepsis, open reduction and, 56
Asphyxiation (*see also* Airway, patent, *and* Tracheostomy)
  mandibular fractures and, 726
Astragalus. *See* Talus
Atlas. *See* Vertebra, cervical, first
Auditory apparatus
  injuries to, 691–703
  skull fractures extending into, 666
Auditory meatus, external, injuries of, 693
Avulsion, ring, of finger, 131
Axillary nerve, injuries of, 242
Axis. *See* Vertebra, cervical, second

BACTERIA, pathogenic, sensitivity of, to antibiotics, determination of, 70
Baker's cyst, 402
Ballance sign, in spontaneous rupture of spleen, 525
Battle's sign, in basal skull fracture, 657
Bennett's fracture, 135
  malunion of, 136
  reduction of, 136
Berlin's opacity, 748
Berman-Moorhead locator, for metallic foreign body
  in brain, 283
  in eye, 753
Biceps tendon
  distal, rupture of, 206
  long
    interposition of, in primary anterior dislocation of shoulder, 248
    rupture of, 285
    subluxation of, recurrent, 286
Birth palsy
  Erb-Duchenne, 240
  Klumpke-Déjerine, 241
  lower type, 241
  upper type, 240
Bite wounds, human, of hand, 126
Bladder
  injuries of, minor pelvic fractures and, 483
  rupture of, diagnosis of, 484
Blind nailing, of impacted valgus fractures of neck of femur, 437
Blood
  sequestration of, shock and, 22
  transfusion of
    in abdominal injuries, 516
    in treatment of shock, 27
Blood volume, restoration of, in treatment of shock, 26
Body fluids. *See* Fluids, body
Bone(s) (*see also names of specific bones*)
  cancellous, fracture of, 10
  cortical, fractures of, 10
  decalcification of, injury and, 4
  double, fracture of, 11
  features of, regional, 10
  repair of
    events in, 5
    fact(s) of, 7
    factors in
      local, 5
      regional, 9
      systemic, 11
    fallacies in, 11
    osteoblasts and, 6
    periosteal, 6
    pluripotentiality of mesenchyme in, 7
    theories of, 6
Brachial plexus, injuries of, 613
    pressure, 241
    traction, at birth, 239
Brackett operation, in nonunion of femoral neck fracture, 452
Bradford frame, in treatment of burns, 87
Brain
  abscess of
    post-traumatic, 709
    skull fracture and, 668
  anatomy of, 653
  arteries of, 654
  concussion of, 671
  contusion of, 672
  edema of, signs of, 687
  herniation of, 668
  injuries of, 671
  laceration of, hemorrhage and, 672
  sinuses of, 654
  skull and, 651–690
  veins of, 654

Bronchoscopy, chest injuries and, 547
Bronchus, rupture of, 555
Bryant's skin traction, femoral shaft fractures and, 415
Burn(s), 79–97
  absorption in, 83
  agents causing, 84
  antibacterial measures in, 73
  chemical, 96
  classification of, 82
  complications of, 94
    adrenal, 96
    cardiovascular, 95
    central nervous system, 96
    gastrointestinal, 95
    general, 95
    local, 94
    renal, 96
    respiratory, 95
  debilitation after, 84
  electrical, 96
  first-degree, 82
  full-thickness, 83
  general considerations in, 79
  grafting of, preparation for, 88
  infection in, 73
  injury in
    extent of, 79
    nature of, 79
    recognition of, 84
  location of, implications of, 81
  major
    prognosis in, 94
    treatment of, immediate, 89
  minor, treatment of, immediate, 89
  of hand, 126
    treatment of, 127
  partial-thickness, 83
  pathology of, 82
  radiation, 97
    of hand, 126
  second-degree, 82
  special mechanisms in, 84
  thermonuclear explosion, 97
  third-degree, 82
  transudation in, 83
  treatment of
    admission, 89
    "burn team" for, 91
    closed, 86
    immediate, 89
Burn(s) (*continued*)
  treatment of (*continued*)
    local, 85
      in certain areas, 87
    open, 86
    systemic, 91
      mistakes in, 93
Burn team, for treatment of burns, 91
Bursitis
  olecranon, 205
  prepatellar, 401
  radiohumeral, 204
  semimembranosus, 402
  subdeltoid, 286

CALCANEOCUBOID joint, derangement of, after compression fracture of calcaneus, 327
Calcaneus
  fractures of, 321
    classification of, 323
    compression
      disability after, 326
      late pain after, 326
      mobilization of, without reduction, 329
      pathology of, 324
      primary subtalar arthrodesis after, 330
      reduction of, immobilization and, 328
      treatment of, 329
    involving subtalar joint, 324
    not involving subtalar joint, 323
  thickened, after compression fracture, 327
  tip of, anterior superior, fracture of, 324
  tuberosity of, fracture of
      beak, 324
      horizontal, 324
      vertical, 323
Calcification, bone repair and, 7
Calcium
  bone repair and, 7
  dietary, bone repair and, 11
Calcium deposits, in tendons
    of foot, 304

Calcium deposits, in tendons (*continued*)
of hand, 128
of shoulder, 281
treatment of, indications for, 282
of wrist, 145
treatment of, 146
Capillary permeability
cell death and, 4
shock and, 22
Capitate bone
dislocations of, 168
fractures of, 168
Cardiac output, shock and, 23
Cardiac tamponade, crush injury of chest and, 555
Cardiovascular system, complications involving, burns and, 95
Carpal bones (*see also* Carpus *and names of specific bones*)
mechanism of, 140
Carpal canal, volar, 141
Carpus (*see also names of specific bones*)
dislocation of, marginal fracture of radius and, 168
mechanism of, 140
perilunate dislocation of other bones of, 162
old unreduced, without arthritis, 167
scaphoid fracture and, 166
"Carrying angle," of arm, 202
Cataract, traumatic, 746
Cauliflower ear, 692
Celiotomy, exploratory
diagnosis of abdominal injuries and, 504
multiple injuries and, 67
nonpenetrating abdominal injuries and, 509
penetrating abdominal wounds and, 506
suspected rupture of spleen and, 526
Cell(s), death of, injury and, 4
Cellulitis, clostridial, 75
Cephalhematoma, 660
Cerebral fungus, 668
Cerebrum
concussion of, 671
contusion of, 672
herniation of, 668
laceration of, hemorrhage and, 672
Cervical rib syndrome, 616
Chalcosis bulbi, 752
Charcot's joint, bone repair and, 12
Chest, 540–557
flail, 549
injuries of (*see also* Thoraco-abdominal injuries)
bronchoscopy in, 547
crush, 549
tracheostomy in, 551
internal, chest wall injury and, 542
open, 552
recognition of, 540
shock in, treatment of, 548
simple, of wall, 541
steering-wheel, 550
tracheal aspiration in, 546
tracheostomy in, 547
types of, 541
lower, severe injuries of, nonpenetrating abdominal injuries and, 510
wall of, injury of
intrathoracic injury and, 542
simple, 541
Chondroplasia, bone repair by, 7
Chordotomy, in avascular necrosis of femoral head, 456
Choroid, injuries of, 748
Chylothorax, 530
Chyluria, 530
Ciliary body, injuries of, 745
Circulation, regional, bone repair and, 9
Clavicle
fracture of, 289
complications of, 291
fixation of, 289
in infants, 291
reduction of, 289
treatment of, 289
outer end of, fracture of, 295
Coccygodynia, 494
Coccyx
anatomy of, 562
injuries of, 493
Cochlea, disorders of, post-traumatic, of central origin, 701
Collateral ligament(s)
cruciate ligaments and, of knee, rupture of, 389
fibular, 387

Collaterial ligament(s) (*continued*)
lateral
of ankle
sprain of
complications after, 339
inversion, 336
of knee, rupture of, 387
medial, of knee, 383
rupture of, 385
sprain of, 384
complications of, 385
tibial. *See* Collateral ligament, medial, of knee
Colles' fracture, 146
aftercare of, 150
complications of, 154
diagnosis of, 146
dilemma of, 153
immobilization for, duration of, 152
nonunion of, 156
old unreduced, 153
reduction of, 148
maintenance of, 149
reversed, treatment of, 152
shattered, treatment of, 151
stable, treatment of, 151
treatment of
definitive, 150
general principles of, 148
undisplaced, treatment of, 151
unstable, treatment of, 151
Colon, injuries of, 523
Coma, head injuries and, 655
Commotio retinae, 748
Concussion
cerebral, 671
corneal, 743
of iris, 745
Consciousness, state of, head injuries and, 656
Contact lens, with lead inserts, for roentgenographic localization of intraocular foreign body, 753
Convalescence, metabolism in, 12
"anabolic" phase, 14
"catabolic" phase, 12
final recovery phase, 14
Cornea
abrasions of, superficial, 743
concussion of, 743
foreign bodies in, embedded, 743
removal of, 744
Cornea (*continued*)
injuries of, 742
treatment of, 743
laceration of, 743
opacities of, 741
rupture of, 743
Corticosterone, response to injury and, 15
Cortisone, bone repair and, 12
Coxa plana, 420
diagnosis of, 420
differential, 421
pathology of, 420
treatment of, 422
Cranium, anatomy of, 653
Cruciate ligament(s)
anterior, of knee, 387
avulsion of tibial spine by, 388
"drawer test" of, 388
collateral ligaments and, of knee, rupture of, 389
combined, of knee, function of, 389
posterior, of knee, 389
Crush syndrome, shock and, 28
Crutch paralysis, 241
Cuboid bone, fracture of, 330
Cuneiform bones, fracture of, 330
Cyst
Baker's, 402
popliteal, 402

DEAFNESS. *See* Hearing, loss of
Debridement
of accidental wounds, 71
of open fracture wounds, 62
Dehydration, 17
electrolyte disturbances in, 17
hypertonic, 18
hypotonic, 17
rapid, 17
slow, 18
Deltoid muscle
nerve injuries and, 242
paralysis of, treatment of, 243
pseudoparalysis of, 243
Deoxycorticosterone, response to injury and, 15
Diaphragm, rupture of, 534
Diet, bone repair and, 11

Drugs, use of, in treatment of shock, 27
Drunkenness, accidental injuries and, 497
Duodenum, injuries of, 528
Dupuytren's contracture, of palmar fascia, 129
Dystrophy, vasomotor, reflex, 107

EAR
  external
    abscess of, 691
    injuries of, 691
  injuries of, 691–703
Elbow, 201–232
  anatomy of, 201
  dislocation of, 225
    aftercare of, 227
    anterior, humeral fracture and, 230
    reduction of, manipulative, 226
  epicondylitis of
    lateral, 204
    medial, 205
  epiphyses of, ossification of, 204
  fracture-dislocation of, 227
    anterior, 228
  injuries of, soft tissue, 204
  landmarks of, bony, 202
  sprain of
    fracture of distal humeral epiphyses vs., 212
    fracture of radial head vs., 221
  tennis, 204
Elbow joint, aspiration of, in fracture of head of radius, 221
Electrocardiography, in crush injury of chest, 555
Electroencephalography, head injuries and, 689
Electrolytes, body, response to injury and, 15
Electromyography, in injuries of roots of cervical nerves, 613
Embolectomy, in embolic arterial occlusion, 107
Embolism, arterial, 106
Enucleation, of eyeball, in sympathetic ophthalmia, 756
Epinephrine, response to injury and, 15
Epiphyseal injuries (*see also specific bones and anatomical regions*)
  importance of, 46
Escharotics, in local treatment of burns, 86
Esophagoscopy, rupture of esophagus and, 556
Esophagus
  injuries of, 556
  perforation of, spontaneous, 557
Ethmoid sinus, injury of, 706
Extensor carpi ulnaris tendon, subluxation of, Colles' fracture and, 156
Extensor pollicis longus tendon, rupture of, Colles' fracture and, 155
Extremity (Extremities)
  burns of, treatment of, local, 88
  injuries of
    thoraco-abdominal injuries vs., 502
    transportation after, 35
  lower, **297**
  upper, **111**
Eye, 740–757
  anatomy of, 740
  injuries of
    birth, 741
    sympathetic ophthalmia and, 756
Eyeball
  enucleation of, in sympathetic ophthalmia, 756
  foreign bodies in, 750
    diagnosis of, 752
    localization of, 752
    nature of material of, 751
    prognosis in, 756
    removal of, 755
Eyelids
  contusions of, 741
  injuries of, 741
  lacerations of, 742

FACE
  bones of, 726, 727
    fractures of, 726–739
  burns of, treatment of, local, 87
  injuries of, anatomical considerations in, 727

Facial nerve
  injury to
    in longitudinal fracture of petrous portion of temporal bone, 696
    in transverse fractures of the petrous portion of the temporal bone, 698, 700
Fascia
  palmar, 114
    Dupuytren's contracture of, 129
  plantar, inflammation of, after compression fracture of calcaneus, 327
Fat, body, injury and, 13, 14
Felon, 124
Femur
  condyle(s) of
    both, fracture of, 414
    single, fracture of, 413
  distal
    epiphysis of, injuries of, 414
    fracture of, 411
  fractures of
    dicondylar, 414
    dislocation of hip and, 470
    intertrochanteric
      complications of, 462
      type I, treatment of, 457
      type II, treatment of, 459
      type III, treatment of, 459
    mid-neck
      aftercare of, 441
      reduction of, open, 440
      treatment of, 439
    stiff knee after, 410
    subtrochanteric, treatment of, 461
    supracondylar, 411
    trochanteric, internal fixation of, 461
  head of
    avascular necrosis of, 454
      in posterior dislocation of the hip, 470
      treatment of, 455
    Axhausen's creeping substitution in, 432
    blood supply of, 431
    epiphysis of
      anatomy of, 419
      avulsion of, 429
      separations of, 419
      slipping of, 423
        diagnosis of, 424
          differential, 425

Femur (*continued*)
  head of (*continued*)
    epiphysis of (*continued*)
      slipping of (*continued*)
        pathology of, 423
        treatment of, 425
    resection of, in nonunion of femoral neck fracture, 453
  neck of, fractures of
      extracapsular, 456
        diagnosis of, 457
        treatment of, 457
      impacted valgus
        aftercare of, 439
        treatment of, 436
      intracapsular, 435
        complications after, 445
          associated with operative reduction, 445
          unassociated with operative reduction, 454
        loss of fixation after operative reduction of, 449
        nonunion of, after operative reduction, 450
        treatment of, 436
      vertical subcapital, treatment of, 443
  shaft of, fractures of, 415
      at birth, 415
      in adults, 416
        fixation of, 417
      in children, 415
  trochanter of
    greater, avulsion of, 429
    lesser, avulsion of, 430
Fibrinogen, function of, 20
Fibroplasia, injury and, 5
Fibrositis, chronic low-back pain and, 629
Fibula, 368
  shaft of, solitary fracture of, 370
  tibia and, fractures of
      internal fixation in, 377
      stable, 373
      unstable, 375
  use of, as bone graft, 369
Finger(s)
  amputation of, traumatic, 129
  avulsion of, ring, 131
  fracture of, 131
    of middle phalanx, 132
    of proximal phalanx, 133

Finger(s) (*continued*)
injuries of, 129
joints of
dislocation of, 134
fracture-dislocation of, 134
injuries of, 131
mallet, 132
trigger, Colles' fracture and, 155
Fingernail(s), 113
Fingertip, crushed, 129
Fistula
arteriovenous, arterial injuries and, 100
carotid artery–cavernous sinus, skull fracture and, 669
Fixation (*see also under* Fracture *and names of specific bones*)
internal
amount of, 54
basic principles of fracture treatment and, 54
contact compression and slotted plate for, 55
indications for, 56
materials for, 54
rigid, internal suture vs., 54
Flail chest, 549
Flat foot, spastic, compression fracture of calcaneus and, 326
Fluids, body
in treatment of burns, 91
replacement of, in treatment of burns, 92
response to injury and, 15
Foot, 299–332
anatomy of, 299
architecture of, 299
edema of, 301
prevention of, 302
flat, spastic, compression fracture of calcaneus and, 326
injuries of
immobilization and, 302
mobilization and, 303
problems common to, 301
soft tissue, 303
skeleton of, 299
sprain of, 307
tendons of, calcium deposits in, 304
treatment of, 305
tenosynovitis of, 305
Forearm, 179–200 (*see also names of specific structures*)
fractures of
comminuted, 200
multiple, 200
Foreign bodies
embedded
in cornea, 743
removal of, 744
in hand, 123
in sclera, 744
in paranasal sinuses, 709
inserted
complications of, 532
in gastrointestinal tract, 525
in genitourinary tract, 525
intraocular, 750
diagnosis of, 752
localization of, 752
nature of material of, 751
prognosis in, 756
removal of, 755
neck wounds from, 713
retained, in abdominal injuries, 519
dangers of, 531
Fracture(s) (*see also names of specific fractures and structures*)
abdominal injuries and, 535
aftercare of, 59
definition of, clinical, 6
deformity in, 42
correction of, 45
displacing forces in, 42
fixation of
external, 46
immobility and, 47
internal. *See* Fixation, internal
plaster of paris, 48 (*see also* Plaster of paris dressings)
traction for
continuous, 50
skeletal, 52
skin, 50
intra-articular, 11
open
aftercare of, 64
debridement in, 62
initial care of, 36
treatment of, 64
principles in, 62
treatment of wounds in, 62

Fractures(s) (*continued*)
reduction of, 38
anesthesia for, 40
delayed, 40
factors in, 39
manipulative, 43
technique of, 44
method for, choice of, 43
open, internal fixation and, 54
satisfactory
criteria of, 44
in adults, 44
in children, 45
timing of, 39
rehabilitation after, 61
repair of (*see also* Bone(s), repair of)
events in, local, 5
surgical emergency in, 39
treatment of
basic principles of, internal fixation and, 55
cardinal principles in, 32
goal of, 33
union of, clinical, criteria of, 60
Frontal sinus, injury of, 706
Fusion, spinal. *See* Vertebra(e), fusion of
Frozen shoulder, 287

GANGLION, of wrist, 128
Gangrene
arterial injuries and, 98
gas, 76
Gas gangrene, 76
Gas gangrene antitoxin, 76
open fractures and, 63
Gastrocnemius muscle, 390
Gastroepiploic vessels, rupture of, 530
Gastrointestinal tract
complications involving, burns and, 95
foreign bodies in, 525
injuries of, treatment of, 518
Gastroscopy, rupture of esophagus and, 556
Genitalia, burns of, treatment of, local, 87
Genitourinary tract
foreign bodies in, 525
injuries of, minor pelvic fractures and, 483

Glaucoma
concussion, 750
secondary, lens displacement and, 748
Glenohumeral ligaments, recurrent anterior dislocation of shoulder and, 255
Glenoid, recurrent anterior dislocation of shoulder and, 257
Glenoid meniscus, tear of, 286
Globulin, blood, function of, 20
"Golden period"
extension of, in accidental wounds, 72
for arterial repair, 102
open fractures and, 61
Graft
bone
in nonunion of scaphoid fracture, 177
use of fibula as, 369
skin
for burns, preparation for, 88
in scalp injuries, 659
vessel, arterial repair and, 104

HAMATE bone, injuries of, 170
Hamstring muscles, 391
Hand, 113–139
anatomy of, 113
attritional trauma of, 127
bite wounds of, human, 126
bones of, 117
burns of, 126
treatment of, 127
cold white, supracondylar fracture of humerus and, 209
degenerative conditions of, 127
foreign bodies in, embedded, 123
human bites of, 126
infections of, 124
injury of
debridement in, 120
extension of wound in, 121
inspection in, 120
penetrating, 124
repair of, 122
soft tissue, 117
tissue conservation in, 122
treatment of
immediate, 118
operative, 119

Hand (*continued*)
joints of, 117
lacerations of, 118
ligaments of, 117
nerves of, lacerated, repair of, 123
tendon(s) of, 114
blood supply of, 116
calcium deposits in, 128
divided, 119
location of, 121
pairing of, 122
repair of, 122
essentials in, 123
function of, 116
inflammation of, 127
tendon sheaths of, 114
infections of, 125
inflammation of, 127
Head (*see also* Brain, Scalp, *and* Skull)
anatomy of, 652
burns of, treatment of, local, 87
injuries of
examination of patient with, 655, 683
gunshot, 682
management of, 683
orders in, 686
pathology in, 655
sequelae of, 689
special senses and, **649**
Hearing, loss of
in blunt head injuries without fracture of temporal bone, 700
in longitudinal fracture of petrous portion of temporal bone, 697
Heart, injuries of, 555
Heart rate, shock and, 22
Hematemesis, nonpenetrating abdominal injuries and, 510
Hematoma(s)
after operative reduction of intracapsular femoral neck fracture, 448
in injuries of larynx and trachea, 710
of nasal septum, 705
of quadriceps muscle, 393
of scalp, 660
ossifying, of quadriceps muscle, 393
subdural
acute
brain injury and, 675
signs of, 687
treatment of, 675
Hematoma(s) (*continued*)
subdural (*continued*)
chronic, 677
treatment of, 677
subungual, 129
Hematotympanum, in longitudinal fractures of petrous portion of temporal bone, 696
Hematuria, nonpenetrating abdominal injuries and, 510
Hemopericardium, crush injury of chest and, 555
Hemorrhage
arterial injury and, 99
cerebral laceration and, 672
control of, in treatment of shock, 26
extradural
acute, brain injury and, signs of, 688
brain injury and, 673
treatment of, 674
in abdominal injuries, treatment of, 516
in laryngeal injuries, 712
initial care of, 34
intracerebral, massive, brain injury and, 681
intracranial, head injury and, 686
massive, multiple injuries and, 67
orbital, 741
retinal, 741, 748
retroperitoneal, spinal fracture and, 535
Hemothorax, 544
clotted, treatment of, 545
Heparin, arterial repair and, 103
Hip, 419–473 (*see also specific structures*)
dislocation of
anterior, 465, 471
central, 465, 473
fracture of femur and, 470
intrapelvic, 465, 473
obturator, 465, 471
posterior, 465
complications of, 470
diagnosis of, 466
pathology of, 466
treatment of, 469
sciatic. *See* Hip, dislocation of, posterior
traumatic, 465
types of, 465

Hip (*continued*)
  fractures of, 430
    atypical, 462
    classification of, 430
    due to metastases, 464
    in children, 462
    irradiation, 463
    shearing force and, 433
    treatment of, age and, 433
  sprain of, 430
Hippocratic method of reduction of primary anterior dislocation of shoulder, 247
Hormone, posterior pituitary, response to injury and, 15
Housemaid's knee, 401
Humerus
  distal
    epiphyses of
      fracture of, 212
        elbow sprain vs., 212
    fractures of, 206
      comminuted, 219
      in adult, 218
  epicondyle of
    lateral
      epiphysis of
        displacement of, 213
        fracture of, 213
      inflammation of, 204
    medial
      avulsion of, before ossification, 218
      epiphysis of
        fracture of, 215
          with intact elbow ligaments, 215
          with ruptured elbow ligaments, 216
      fracture of, elbow dislocation and, 227
      inflammation of, 205
  epiphysis of
    capitellar
      displacement of, 213
      fracture of, 213
        treatment of, 214
    trochlear, displacement of, 213
  fracture of
    dicondylar, 219
    elbow dislocation and, anterior, 230

Humerus (*continued*)
  fracture of (*continued*)
    intercondylar, 219
    supracondylar
      cold white hand and, 209
      dilemma of, 210
      displaced, 206
        anteriorly, 209
        fixation of, 209
        reduction of, 207
      greenstick, 206
      treatment of, 210
      types of, 206
      undisplaced, 206
    transcondylar, 219
  neck of, fractures of, in children, 277
  proximal
    epiphysis of, fractures of, 274
        growth disturbance after, 275
    fractures of, 265
      direct impact and, 265
      fixation of, 271
        mobilization after, 271
      indirect impact and, 266
      muscular violence and, 265
      reduction of
        contraindications to, 267
        indications for, 268
        manipulative, 268
          essentials of, 270
  shaft of
    distal, fractures of, 279
    fractures of, 277
      segmental, 279
    middle third, fractures of, 278
        complications of, 279
    proximal, fractures of, 277
  subluxation of, inferior, 273
  tuberosities of
    fracture of
      primary anterior dislocation of shoulder and, 251
      residual displacement in, 253
    greater, avulsion of, by spinati muscles, 266
    lesser, avulsion of, by subscapularis muscle, 265
Hydration, maintenance of, in treatment of burns, 93
Hygroma, subdural, 681
Hyoid bone, fractures of, 712
Hyperhydration, 20

Hypertension, intraocular, trauma and, 750
Hyphema, 745
Hypopotassemia, injury and, 15
Hypoproteinemia
  burns and, 93
  injury and, 20
  shock and, 23
Hypotension
  intraocular, trauma and, 750
  shock and, 23

IATROGENIC reactions, emotional response to injury and, 31
Ilium
  avulsion of, traumatic, 479
  spine of, anterior, avulsion of, 479
Infection(s)
  after operative reduction of intracapsular femoral neck fracture, 449
  arterial repair and, 103
  basal skull fractures and, 699
  clostridial, other than tetanus, 75
  in accidental wounds, prevention of, 69, 71
  in burns, 73
  in trauma, 69–78
  incidence of, in civilian surgery, 69
  middle palmar space, 126
  thenar space, 126
  wound, treatment of, 77
Inflammation, and repair, injury and, 3
Injury (Injuries) (*see also* Trauma, Wounds, *and under names of specific structures*)
  arterial, complications of, 100
  care of, initial, 33
  crushing, shock and, 28
  effect of, on tissue cells, 4
  examination after, 37
  history in, importance of, 37
  inflammation, repair and, 3
  initial care after, 33
  multiple
    examination in, 66
    nonpenetrating abdominal injuries and, 508

Injury (Injuries) (*continued*)
  multiple (*continued*)
    principles in, 65
    priorities in, 65
      therapeutic, 66, 496
    thoraco-abdominal injuries and, 497
  peripheral, thoraco-abdominal injuries vs., 502
  protein cesspool and, 3
  repair and, 3
  response to, 3–31
    emotional, 29
      iatrogenic reactions and, 31
      litigation and, 31
    factors in, endocrine, 14
    systemic, 12
  tetanus after, 74
  transportation after, 33, 34, 564, 608
  treatment of, preparation for, 37
  vascular, 98–109
Interosseous ligaments, of ankle, rupture of, 345
      treatment of, 346
Intervertebral disc(s), 639–647
  anatomy of, 639
  cervical
    displacement of, laterally, 603
    syndromes of, 599
      diagnosis of, aids in, 599
      operation for, 606
      treatment of, 606
  herniation of, 641
    diagnosis of, differential, 643
    examination in
      clinical, 644
      myelographic, 647
    mechanism of, 641
    myelography in, 647
    operation for
      choice of, 645
      indications for, 645
      technique of, 646
    studies in, laboratory, 647
  injuries of, 640
  protrusion of, sites of, in cervical region, 604
Intracranial pressure
  increased, head injuries and, 656
  multiple injuries and, 67
Intraocular tension, trauma and, 750
Iridodonesis, 747

Iris
concussion of, 745
injuries of, 745
laceration of, 746
Irrigation, of accidental wounds, 71
Ischemia, Volkmann's
in leg, 367
after treatment, 368
supracondylar fracture of humerus and, 210
Ischium, tuberosity of, avulsion of, by hamstring muscles, 478

JOINT(s) (*see also names of specific joints*)
Charcot's, bone repair and, 12
finger. *See under* Finger
of hand, 117
regional, bone repair and, 10

KEHR'S sign, in spontaneous rupture of spleen, 525
Kernig sign, positive, head injuries and, 657
Kidneys, complications involving, burns and, 96
Knee, 383–409 (*see also names of specific structures*)
dislocation of, 389
gliding mechanism of, 399
housemaid's, 401
injuries of, 383
quadriceps extensor mechanism, 391
injuries to, 393
stiff, after femoral fracture, 410
supports of
ligamentous, 383
muscular, 390
synovial cavities of
articular, 399
extra-articular, 400
thigh and, 383–409
Knee joint
aspiration of, 400
synovial cavity of, 399
Kocher's method of reduction of primary anterior dislocation of shoulder, 247
Kyphosis, 563

LABYRINTH, involvement of, in transverse fractures of petrous portion of temporal bone, 698
Labyrinthectomy, after transverse fracture of petrous portion of temporal bone, 700
Laparotomy. *See* Celiotomy
Laryngeal cartilages, fractures of, 710
Laryngoscopy, indirect, in laryngeal injuries, 711
Larynx
fractures of, complications of, 711
injuries of, 710–714
Lateral ligament, of ankle, rupture of, 342
extensive, 344
treatment of, 343
Leg, 363–382 (*see also names of specific structures*)
compartments of, 363
anterior, 364
lateral, 364
posterior, 365
soft parts of, 363
Volkmann's ischemic paralysis in, 367
after treatment, 368
Lens
displacement of, 747
injuries of, 746
Leukocytes, polymorphonuclear, injury and, 4
Litigation, emotional response to injury and, 31
Liver, injuries of, 527
Lordosis, 563
Low-back mechanism, 618–647
gravity and, 618
injuries to, other than intervertebral disc injuries
pain due to, 618–638 (*see also* Low-back pain)
Low-back pain
acute, traumatic, 619
aftercare of, 624
clinical picture in, 620
diagnosis of, 621
pathogenesis of, 619
phases of
primary, 619
secondary, 620
treatment of, 622
chronic, 625
etiology of, 625

Low-back pain (*continued*)
chronic (*continued*)
fibrositis and, 629
myositis and, 629
of postural origin, 625
exercises for, 628
muscle tests in, 625
treatment of, 627
osteoarthritis and, 630
osteoarthritis with nerve root compression and, 630
Lumbosacral plexus, malignant invasion of, herniated intervertebral disc vs., 644
Lunate bone
dislocation of, 160
diagnosis of, 161
treatment of, 162
dislocation of other carpal bones on, 162
old unreduced, without arthritis, 167
scaphoid fracture and, 166
excision of, after dislocation, 162
Lungs, function of, maintenance of, in multiple injuries, 65
Luxatio erecta, of shoulder, 261
Lymphatic vessels, injuries to, 108
Lymphedema, postoperative, 108

MALLEOLUS (Malleoli)
both, fractures of, 354
aftercare of, 356
immobilization for, extent of, 356
posterior tibial lip fracture and, 360
reduction of, open
contraindications to, 355
indications for, 355
fractures of, 347
pathology of, 348
lateral, impingement of calcaneus on, after compression fracture, 327
medial, fracture of, fibrous union after, 349
single, fracture of
stable, 350
unstable, 350
Mallet finger, 132
Mandible
angle of, fracture at, 716
body of, fracture of, 716
bilateral, 718
condyle of, fractures of, 724
displacement in, 717
treatment of, 724
edentulous, fractures of, displacement in, 718
fractures of, 715–726
aftercare of, 724
asphyxiation in, 726
complications of, 725
diagnosis of, 715
displacement in, 716
immobilization of, 719
arch bars for, 722
infection in, 725
intermaxillary wiring of, 720
eyelet, 721
multiple loop, 722
midline, 716
nonunion of, 725
reduction of, 719
open, 723
teeth in line of, 725
through body and opposite condyle, 717
treatment of, 719
neck of, fracture of, 717
Marjolin dislocation, of cervical vertebrae, 612
Mastoid process, avulsion of, fracture of petrous portion of temporal bone and, 699
Mastoidectomy, infection after basal skull fractures and, 700
Maxilla
alveolar process of, fracture of, 731
anterior, fracture of, comminuted, 735
fractures of, 730
horizontal, complete, 734
unilateral, 732
treatment of, 733
horizontal portion of, 732
tuberosity of, fracture of, 731
Maxillary sinus, injury of, 706
Maxillofacial injuries, 715–739 (*see also names of specific structures*)
Melena, nonpenetrating abdominal injuries and, 510

Meninges, 653
Meningitis
  head injuries and, 668
  post-traumatic, 709
  transverse fractures of petrous portion of temporal bone and, 699
Meniscectomy
  aftercare following, 407
  of torn meniscus of knee, 406
Meniscus (Menisci)
  glenoid, tear of, 286
  medial, of knee, tear of, diagnosis of, 404
  of knee, 402
    tear of
      mechanism of, 403
      pathology of, 404
      signs of, clinical, 405
      treatment of, indications for, 406
Metacarpal bones
  dislocation of, 134
  fractures of, 137
    Bennett's, 135
      malunion of, 136
      reduction of, 136
    types of, 138
Metacarpophalangeal joints, dislocation of, 134
Metatarsal bone(s)
  fifth, fracture of base of, 331
  fracture(s) of, 331
  fracture of neck of, 331
  march fracture of shaft of, 331
Midcarpal joint, 141
Missile track(s)
  irrigation of, in gunshot wounds of head, 683
  penetrating wounds of abdomen and, 507
Monteggia fracture, 193
  old unreduced, 197
  reverse, 197
Motorcycle injury, 479
Muscle(s) (*see also names of specific muscles*)
  regional, bone repair and, 9
  spasm of, reduction of, by continuous traction, 51
  tests of, in chronic low-back pain of postural origin, 625
Muscle spasm, reduction of, by continuous traction, 51
Muscle tests, in chronic low-back pain of postural origin, 625
Musculotendinous cuff, of shoulder
    injury of, primary anterior dislocation of shoulder and, 254
    interposition of, in primary anterior dislocation of shoulder, 249
    irregularity of, 287
    ruptures of, 283
      diagnosis of, 284
      treatment of
        conservative, 285
        operative, indications for, 285
Myelography
  in cervical intervertebral disc syndromes, 601, 605
  in herniation of intervertebral disc, 647
  in injuries of first and second cervical vertebrae, 612
  in injuries of roots of cervical nerves, 613
Myositis
  chronic low-back pain and, 629
  clostridial, 75
Myositis ossificans
  in radial head fracture with gross anterior displacement, 224
    prevention of, 225
  of quadriceps muscle, 393
Myringoplasty, for ruptured tympanic membrane, 694

NAVICULAR bone, fracture of, 330
Neck (*see also* Vertebra(e), cervical)
  burns of, treatment of, local, 87
  injury to, transportation after, 35
  wounds of, 712
Nerve(s) (*see also names of specific nerves*)
  cervical
    roots of
      avulsion of, 613
      involvement of, by protruding intervertebral discs, 604
  of hand, lacerated, repair of, 123
  of shoulder, injuries of, primary anterior dislocation of shoulder and, 252
  spinal, roots of, injury to, by herniated intervertebral disc, 641

Nervous system, central, complications involving, 96
Neurectomy, in avascular necrosis of femoral head, 456
Neuritis, herniated intervertebral disc vs., 644
Neurotrophic conditions, bone repair and, 12
Nitrogen, body, injury and, 13, 14
Norepinephrine, response to injury and, 15
Nose
  fractures of, 703
    comminuted, 705
    signs of, clinical, 704
    treatment of, 705
    without basal skull fracture, 729
  injuries to, 703–706
  skull fractures extending into, 665
  structure of, 729
Nucleus pulposus, 563, 599, 639
  herniation of, 633
Nutrient artery, significance of, in repair of fractured tibia, 371
Nystagmus, post-traumatic, 702

ODONTOID process, fracture of, 595, 611
Olecranon
  avulsion of
    with absent triceps function, 230
    with intact triceps function, 230
  fracture of, 230
    by direct impact, 232
    elbow dislocation and, anterior, 228
    indirect trauma and, 230
Ophthalmia, sympathetic, 756
Optic nerve, injuries of, 749
Orbicular ligament, pathology of, in fracture of shaft of ulna with dislocation of radial head, 193
Osgood-Schlatter disease, 398
Osteoarthritis
  chronic low-back pain and, 630
  with nerve root compression, chronic low-back pain and, 630
Osteochondritis dissecans, of talus, 319
Osteotomy
  for slipped femoral epiphysis, 427
  primary, for vertical subcapital femoral neck fracture, 443
    aftercare in, 445
Othematoma, 692
Otorrhea, cerebrospinal fluid
  head injuries and, 657
  skull fractures and, 667
Oxygen
  importance of, in multiple injuries, 65, 67
  supply of, multiple injuries and, 65
  transport of, multiple injuries and, 66
  use of
    in prevention of shock, 25
    in treatment of shock, 27

PAIN
  burns and, 84
  low-back. *See* Low-back pain
  reduction of, by continuous traction, 51
Palmar space, middle, infections of, 126
Palsy, birth. *See* Birth palsy
Pancreas, pseudocysts of, abdominal injury and, 532
Papilledema, head injuries and, 657
Paralysis
  birth. *See* Birth palsy
  crutch, 241
  Saturday night, 241
  Volkmann's ischemic
    in leg, 367
      after treatment, 368
    supracondylar fracture of humerus and, 210
Paranasal sinuses
  injuries of, 706–710
  skull fractures extending into, 665
Paronychia, 125
Patella
  dislocation of, 397
  fracture of
    avulsion
      with retraction, 396
      without retraction, 396
    comminuted, without retraction, 396
  subluxation of, 397

Patellar tendon
avulsion of, 395
rupture of, 395
Patellectomy, for comminuted patellar fracture without retraction, 396
Pellegrini-Stieda disease, sprain of medial collateral ligament of knee and, 385
Pelvis, 477–494
burst, 486
dislocation of, 486
aftercare in, 488
by hyperextension and abduction, 486
by hyperextension and adduction, 488
fracture of
abdominal injuries and, 536
avulsion, 478
stable, 482
fracture-dislocation of, 489
injuries of
combined, in children, 491
severe, nonpenetrating abdominal injuries and, 510
straddle, 484
unstable, 484
skeleton of, 477
telescoped, 488
Perianal area, burns of, treatment of, local, 87
Pericardium, injuries of, 555
Perichondritis, of articular cartilage, 691
Perineum, burns of, treatment of, local, 87
Periosteum, interposition of, in fractures of radius and ulna in children, 182
Peristalsis, absence of, penetrating abdominal wounds and, 506
Peritoneum, natural defenses of, 501
Peroneal nerve, 364
injury of, 365
Peroneal retinaculum, rupture of, 306
Phalanx (Phalanges). *See* Finger(s) *and* Toe(s)
"Pink plasma," significance of, in burned patients, 94
Plantaris tendon, rupture of, 367
Plasma, pink, significance of, in burned patients, 94
Plasma expanders, in treatment of burns, 92
Plaster of paris dressings
circular, 48
functions of, 47
padded, 48
splints, 49
types of, 48
unpadded, 48
Pneumocephalus
in longitudinal fractures of petrous portion of temporal bone, 697
paranasal sinus injuries and, 709
skull fractures and, 667
Pneumothorax, 542
tension, 543
Popliteal cyst, 402
Popliteus muscle, 390
Posture
effect of, on shock, 28
multiple injuries and, 66
Potassium, body
injury and, 13, 14, 15
replacement of, 17
Pressure dressings, for burned areas, 90
Prosthesis (Prostheses)
arterial repair and, 104
medullary, in nonunion of femoral neck fracture, 453
stem, in nonunion of femoral neck fracture, 453
Protein, body reserve of, 20
Protein cesspool, injury and, 3
Psychosis, after head injury, 689
Pubic ramus (rami), fracture of, 482
Pupil(s)
constriction of, head injuries and, 656
dilatation of, head injuries and, 656

QUADRICEPS extensor mechanism, of knee, 391
injuries to, 393
Quadriceps muscle
atrophy of, 392
rehabilitation of, 392
rupture of, incomplete, 393
Quadriceps tendon
avulsion of, 394
rupture of, 394
de Quervain's stenosing tenosynovitis, 127

Radial nerve, injury of, fracture of middle humeral shaft and, 279
Radiocarpal joint, 141
Radio-ulnar joint, distal, 144
subluxation at, 189
Radius
capitellum of, fracture of, elbow dislocation and, anterior, 230
epiphysis of, proximal, injuries to, 222
fracture of
Colles'. *See* Colles' fracture
marginal, dislocation of carpus and, 168
head of
dislocation of, fracture of shaft of ulna and. *See under* Ulna
fracture of, 221
aspiration of elbow joint in, 221
displaced, 222
elbow dislocation and, 227
anterior, 230
elbow sprain vs., 221
with gross anterior displacement, 224
with minimal displacement, 221
subluxation of, 200
shaft of
distal, fracture of, in adults, 188
fracture of, in adults, 188
proximal, fracture of, 189
ulna and
fracture of
in children, 179
immobilization in, 184
duration of, 185
optimal program of, 185
reduction of, 179
factors complicating, 181
treatment of, operative, 187
refracture of, in children, 186
shafts of, fracture of, in adults, 191
Rectum, injuries of, 523
Reduction
manipulative, technique of, 44
open
conditions necessary to, 56
internal fixation and, technique of, 58
timing of, 58
Rehabilitation
fracture treatment and, 61
litigation status and, 31
Relaxants, in traumatic acute low-back pain, 623
Respiratory tract
burns of, treatment of, 88
complications involving, burns and, 95
Rest, in traumatic acute low-back pain, 622
Resuscitation, response to, penetrating abdominal wounds and, 506
Retina
detachment of, 748
edema of, 748
injuries of, 748
Rhinorrhea, cerebrospinal fluid
blunt head injuries and, 708
head injuries and, 657
maxillary fractures and, 708
skull fractures and, 666
Rib(s)
cervical, symptoms due to, 616
fixation of, crush injury of chest and, 549
Rigidity, decerebrate, head injuries and, 657, 687
Roentgenography
aftercare of fractures and, 60
biplane, for locating intraocular foreign body, 753
bone-free, for locating intraocular foreign body, 753
Rule of Nines, for estimation of extent of burns, 80

Sacroiliac joint
instability of, permanent, 491
sprung, 483
Sacrum
anatomy of, 562
fracture of, 492
Saturday night paralysis, 241
Scalenus anticus syndrome, 615
Scalp
abrasions of, 658
anatomy of, 651
arteries of, 652
contusions of, 658
hematoma of, 660
injuries of, 658
infection in, 660

Scalp (*continued*)
lacerations of, 658
treatment of, 685
nerve supply of, 653
Scaphoid bone
cavitation of, after fracture, 174
dislocation of, 170
distal third of, fracture of, 172
fracture of, 170
diagnosis of, 171
immobilization in, duration of, 174
nonunion of
excision of fragments after, 176
intramedullary fixation in, 177
treatment of, 175
pathology of, 172
perilunate dislocation of other carpal bones and, 166
recent
immobilization in, 173
treatment of, 173
treatment during interval of indecision, 171
with perilunate dislocation of carpal bones, 166
proximal third of, fracture of, 172
waist of, fracture of, 172
Scapula
angle of
inferior, fracture of, 238
superior, injuries of, 239
avulsion of glenoid rim of, 237
body of, fractures of, 236
complications of, 237
coracoid process of, fractures of, 237
functions of, 236
grating, 239
injuries of, 236
neck of, fractures of, 237
Scapulectomy, effect of, 236
Scapulothoracic syndrome, 239
Sciatic nerve, injury of, in posterior dislocation of the hip, 470
Sclera
foreign bodies in, embedded, 744
injuries of, 744
rupture of, 744
Scoliosis, 563
Sensation, hand injuries and, 118
Senses, special, head and, **649**
Serratus muscle, nerve injuries and, 242
Sesamoid bones, of foot, fracture of, 332
Shock
arterial injury and, 102
burns and, 84, 91
cardiogenic, 21
chest injuries and, treatment of, 548
early deepening, nonpenetrating abdominal injuries and, 510
effects of, 22
etiology of, 22
factors in, toxic, 28
head injuries and, 655, 683
hematogenic, 21
in abdominal injuries, treatment of, 516
multiple injuries and, 66
neurogenic, 21
prophylaxis of, measures for, 24
signs of, clinical, 23
treatment of, 24
active, 26
preventive, 24
types of, 21
vasogenic, 21
Shoulder (*see also names of specific structures*)
abduction of, 234
adduction of, 234
anatomy of, 233
arm and, 233–296
derangement of, internal, 281
dislocation of, 243
anterior
old unreduced, 250
primary, 245
aftercare of, 254
diagnosis of, 246
reduction of, 246
complications following, 251
complications preventing, 248
recurrent, 255
aftercare of, 258
pathology of, 255
secondary, 257
treatment of, 258
posterior, 259
diagnosis of, 259
old unreduced, 261
primary, treatment of, 260
treatment of, 260
superior, 262
unusual, 261

Shoulder (*continued*)
fracture-dislocation of, 263
treatment of, 264
frozen, 287
cause of, 288
effects of, secondary, 287
management of, 288
pathology of, 288
treatment of, 288
movements of, 234
musculotendinous cuff of
injury of, primary anterior dislocation of shoulder and, 254
interposition of, in primary anterior dislocation of shoulder, 249
irregularity of, 287
ruptures of, 283
diagnosis of, 284
treatment of
conservative, 285
operative, indications for, 285
nerves of, injuries of, 239
primary anterior dislocation of shoulder and, 252
traction
at birth, 239
in adults, 241
in older children, 241
rotation of, internal, 234
snapping, 286
subluxation of, recurrent, 287
treatment of, 260
tendons of, calcium deposits in, 281
treatment of, indications for, 282
Siderosis bulbi, 752
Skier's sprain, 340
Skin
anatomy of, 81
grafting of
for burns, preparation for, 88
in scalp injuries, 659
of hand, 114
preparation of, for surgical repair, 120
physiology of, 81
Skull
brain and, 651–690
fractures of, 660
abdominal injuries and, 536
basal, mortality from, 699
Skull (*continued*)
fractures of (*continued*)
classification of, 660
comminuted, 664
complications of, 666
depressed, 661
compound, 664
extending into ear, 665
extending into nose and paranasal sinuses, 665
linear
compound, 664
simple, 661
ping-pong, 661
osteomyelitis of, head injury and, 669
Snapping shoulder, 286
Sodium, body, injury and, 13, 14
Speed, of ambulance, patient welfare and, 37
Spinal accessory nerve, injuries of, 242
Spinal cord
cervical
adnexa and, 598–617
anatomy of, 598
compression of, by intervertebral disc, 601
injuries of
abdominal injuries and, 537
caused by injury to vertebral column, 607
protection of, suspected fracture of cervical vertebrae and, 587
Spinal fusion. *See* Vertebra(e), fusion of
Spine. *See* Vertebral column
Spleen, rupture of, 525
Splenectomy, complications of, 526
Spondylolisthesis, 632
Spondylolysis, 632
Sprain
ankle, 336
severe, treatment of, 339
elbow
fracture of distal humeral epiphyses vs., 212
fracture of radial head vs., 221
of cervical vertebrae, 588
of foot, 307
of hip, 430
of medial collateral ligament of knee. 384
complications of, 385

Sprain (*continued*)
of wrist, 144
fracture of scaphoid bone vs., 170
skier's, 340
Stainless steel, internal fixation of fractures with, 54
Steering-wheel injury, of chest, 550
Sternoclavicular joint, dislocation at, 291
treatment of, 292
Subdeltoid bursa, thickened, 286
Subtalar joint
arthrodesis of, primary, after compression fracture of calcaneus, 330
derangement of, after compression fracture of calcaneus, 327
fractures of calcaneus involving, 324
Suggestion, emotional response to injury and, 30
Suicide, attempted, neck wounds and, 712
Surgeon, responsibilities of, in prevention of shock, 25
Surgery, civilian
infection in, 69
agents causing, 70
Sustentaculum tali, fracture of, 324
Suture, internal, rigid fixation vs., 54
Synovial cavity (cavities)
articular, of knee, 399
extra-articular, of knee, 400

TALONAVICULAR joint, dislocation at, 315
Talus
body of, fracture of, 317
displaced, 318
impacted, 318
dislocation of, 308
anterior, 309
lateral, 311
posterior, 309
total, 311
dislocation of other carpal bones on, 312
extrusion of, 312
fractures of, 315
injuries of, 307
neck of, fracture of, 315
osteochondritis dissecans of, 319
tubercle of, posterior, fracture of, 319
Tarsometatarsal joints, dislocation of, 330
Tarsus
dislocation of
at talonavicular joint, 313
subtalar, 312
T.A.T. *See* Tetanus antitoxin
Temperature, body
maintenance of, after injury, 37
rising, head injuries and, 656
Temporal bone
injuries of, 695
petrous portion of
avulsion of, 699
fractures of, 695
longitudinal, 696
transverse, 698
Tendo achillis
lengthening of, compression fracture of calcaneus and, 326
rupture of, 365
repair of, operative, 366
Tendon(s) (*see also names of specific tendons*)
interposition of, in fractures of radius and ulna in children, 181
of foot, calcium deposits in, 304
treatment of, 305
of hand, 114
blood supply of, 116
calcium deposits in, 128
divided, 119
location of, 121
pairing of, 122
repair of, 122
essentials in, 123
function of, 116
inflammation of, 127
of shoulder, calcium deposits in, 281
treatment of, indications for, 282
of wrist, calcium deposits in, 145
treatment of, 146
Tendon sheath(s)
of foot, inflammation of, 305
of hand, 114
infections of, 125
inflammation of, 127
Tendon sheath effusion, ganglion vs., 128
Tennis elbow, 204
Tenosynovitis
of foot, 305
of hand, 127

Tenosynovitis (*continued*)
 peroneal, after sprain of lateral collateral ligament, 339
 de Quervain's stenosing, 127
Teres minor muscle, nerve injuries and, 242
Tetanus, injury and, 74
Tetanus antitoxin
 burns and, 91
 injury and, 74
 open fractures and, 63
Tetanus toxoid
 burns and, 91
 open fractures and, 63
Thenar space, infections of, 126
Thermal trauma. *See* Burns
Thiersch grafts, in scalp injuries, 659
Thigh, 410–418 (*see also names of specific structures*)
Thoracic nerve, long, injuries of, 242
Thoraco-abdominal injuries, 495, 553
 characteristics of
  anatomical, 499
  clinical, 499
 civilian vs. military, 496
 contamination in, autogenous, 500
 extent of
  external evidence and, 499
  symptoms masking, 503
 localization of, symptoms masking, 503
 management of, 533
 military vs. civilian, 496
 mortality in, 534
 multiple, single agent producing, 500
 multiple injuries and, 497
 penetrating, posture and, 503
 peripheral injuries vs., 502
 physiology and, 499
 trauma sequence in, 500
 viscera and, vascular, 500
Thrombosis, mesenteric, 530
Thumb, amputation of, 130
Thyroid cartilage, injuries of, 710
Tibia
 anatomy of, 370
 condyle(s) of
  both, fracture of, 409
  fractures of, 407
  lateral, fracture of
   comminuted, 409
   uncomminuted, 408
Tibia (*continued*)
 distal, shattered fractures of, involving ankle joint, 361
 fibula and, fractures of
  internal fixation in, 377
  stable, 373
  unstable, 375
 fracture of, significance of nutrient artery in repair of, 371
 lip of
  anterior, fracture of, 361
  lateral, fracture of, 361
  posterior, fracture of, 357
   bimalleolar fracture and, 360
   requirements for correction of, paradoxical, 358
 shaft of, fractures of
  bone graft for, 380
   as primary procedure, 380
   in delayed union, 381
   in nonunion, 381
  compression by weight bearing in, 374
  solitary, 371
 spine of, avulsion of, by anterior cruciate ligament, 388
 tubercle of
  avulsion of, 398
  epiphysitis of, 398
 weight-bearing surface of, fractures of, 357
Tibial tendon, anterior, rupture of, 303
  treatment of, 304
Tibiofibular ligament, anterior, sprain of, external rotation, 340
"Tight calf"
 decompression of, by incision, 368
 penetrating wounds and, 367
Tissue fluid(s), pH of, injury and, 4
Tobacco, arterial injury and, 105
Toes, fractures of, 332
Tourniquet
 pneumatic, in repair of injuries of hand, 120
 use of, shock and, 28
Trachea, injuries of, 710–714
Tracheostomy
 chest injuries and, 547
  aftercare in, 547
  technique of, 548
 crush injury of chest and, 551
 head injuries and, 686

Tracheostomy (*continued*)
laryngeal injuries and, 712
mandibular fractures and, 726
multiple injuries and, 67
timing of, in multiple injuries, 65
tracheal injuries and, 710
Traction
continuous, 50
purposes of, 51
skeletal, 52
skin, 50
Transportation, of injured patient, 33, 34, 35, 564, 608
Trapezius muscle, nerve injuries and, 242
Trauma. *See also* Injury (Injuries)
antibacterial agents in, 69–78
attritional, of hand, 127
combined factors in, 502
force causing, effect of speed of, 501
general considerations in, **1**
infections in, 69–78
intraocular tension and, 750
thermal. *See* Burns
treatment of, general principles in, 32–68
Trendelenburg's sign, in nonunion of femoral neck fracture, 450
Triangular fibrocartilage, derangement of, Colles' fracture and, 154
Trigger finger, 128
Colles' fracture and, 155
Trunk, **475**
burns of, treatment of, local, 88
Tuber-joint angle, calcaneus fractures and, 322
Tumor
metastatic, extradural, herniated intervertebral disc vs., 643
primary, herniated intervertebral disc vs., 643
Tympanic membrane
injuries of, 693
perforation of, treatment of, 694

ULNA
coronoid of, fracture of, elbow dislocation and, 227
head of, subluxation of, Colles' fracture and, 155
olecranon of. *See* Olecranon
Ulna (*continued*)
radius and
fracture of, in children, 179
immobilization in, 184
duration of, 185
optimal program of, 185
reduction of, 179
factors complicating, 181
treatment of, operative, 187
refracture of, in children, 186
shafts of, fracture of, in adults, 191
shaft of, fracture of
dislocation of radial head and, 193
diagnosis of, 194
old unreduced, 197
treatment of, 196
in adults, 188, 190
styloid process of, fracture of, Colles' fracture and, 154
Ulnar nerve, injury to, in fracture of medial epicondyle epiphysis, 216
Unconsciousness, transportation during, 34
Uncus, herniation of, brain injury and, 674
Urethra, rupture of, straddle injury and, 485
Urinary tract
complications involving, burns and, 96
injuries of
abdominal injuries and, 538
minor pelvic fractures and, 483

VARIDASE, in clotted hemothorax, 545
Vasoconstriction, peripheral, shock and, 22
Vasodilatation, local, injury and, 4
Vasodilators, in conservative management of arterial injury, 106
Vasomotor dystrophy, reflex, 107
Veins, injuries to, 108
Vertebra(e) (*see also* Vertebral column)
cervical
anatomy of, 559
dislocations of, 588
bilateral, 589
Marjolin, 612
somersault, 612
unilateral, 589

Vertebra(e) (*continued*)
  cervical (*continued*)
    first and second
      anomalies of, congenital, 612
      dislocation at, 612
      fracture(s) of, 595
      fracture-dislocations of, 595
      injuries of
        special features of, 611
        supportive care after, 613
    injuries of, 587
      transportation after, 35
    second. *See* Vertebra(e), cervical, first and second
    sprains of, simple, 588
    subluxation of, 588
    third to seventh, fractures of, 591
  fracture(s) of
    compression, 571
      aftercare of, 580
      conditions predisposing to, 571
      disability after, 583
      etiology of, 571
      exercises after, 582
      prognosis in, 584
      reduction of
        maintenance of, 577
        methods of obtaining, 574
      sites of, 571
      treatment of, definitive, 573
      visceral complications of, 579
    hyperextension, 584
  fracture-dislocations of, 585
  fusion of
    aftercare in, 638
    indications for, 634
    technique of, 634
  laminae of, fractures of, 569
  lumbar
    anatomy of, 561
    defects of, 632
    slipping of, 632
  neural arch of, injuries of, 569
  pedicles of, fractures of, 570
  presacral, transitional, 632
  processes of
    articular, fractures of, 570
    spinous, fractures of, 568
        treatment of, 569
    transverse, fractures of, 565
        examination in, 566
        importance of, 567

Vertebra(e) (*continued*)
  processes of (*continued*)
    transverse, fractures of (*continued*)
        rehabilitation after, 568
        symptoms of, 566
        treatment of, 567
  thoracic, anatomy of, 561
Vertebral column, 558–598 (*see also* Vertebra(e))
  anatomy of, 558
  curves of, 563
  deviation of, 563
  fracture of, retroperitoneal hemorrhage and, 535
  injuries of
    assessment of patient's state in, 607
    associated injuries and, 565
    examination of, roentgen, 608
    transportation after, 34, 35, 564, 608
    treatment of, 609
  lumbosacral, unstable, 631
  movements of, 562
  support of, 563
Vertigo, post-traumatic, 702
Vessels, injuries to, 98–109
Vestibule
  disorders of, post-traumatic, of central origin, 701
  involvement of, in longitudinal fractures of petrous portion of temporal bone, 698
Vitallium, internal fixation of fractures with, 54
Vitreous body, injuries of, 749
Volkmann's ischemic paralysis
  in leg, 367
    after treatment, 368
  supracondylar fracture of humerus and, 210

WATER intoxication, 20
Wounds
  accidental, infection in
    agents causing, 71
    prevention of, 69, 71
  in open fractures, treatment of, 62
  initial care of, 36

Wrist, 140–178 (*see also names of specific structures*)
- architecture of, 140
- arthrodesis of, in nonunion of scaphoid fracture, 177
- dislocations at. *See names of specific bones*
- epiphyseal injuries at, 158
  - growth disturbance after, 159
  - sprain vs., 144
  - treatment of, 158
- fracture(s) at
  - Colles'. *See* Colles' fracture
  - involving capitate bone, 168
  - involving scaphoid bone, 170
- fracture-dislocation of, old unreduced, with arthritis, 167
- injuries of hamate bone, 170
- perilunate dislocation of carpal bones, 162
  - old unreduced, without arthritis, 167

Wrist (*continued*)
- perilunate dislocation of carpal bones (*continued*)
  - scaphoid fracture and, 166
- sprain of, 144
  - epiphyseal injuries vs., 144
  - fracture of scaphoid bone vs., 170
- tendons of, calcium deposits in, 145
  - treatment of, 146

ZYGOMA, fracture of, 735
- comminuted, 738
- diagnosis of, 736
- displaced, 738
- examination in, clinical, 736

Zygomatic arch, fracture of, 735, 737
- depressed, 737
- diagnosis of, 736
- examination in, clinical, 736